THE MANAGEMENT OF EATING DISORDERS AND OBESITY

SECOND EDITION

NUTRITION ◊ AND ◊ HEALTH

Adrianne Bendich, Series Editor

THE MANAGEMENT OF EATING DISORDERS AND OBESITY

SECOND EDITION

Edited by

DAVID J. GOLDSTEIN, MD, PhD

Department of Pharmacology and Toxicology, Indiana University School of Medicine and PRN Consulting, Indianapolis, IN

Foreword by

ALBERT J. STUNKARD, MD

Weight and Eating Disorders Program, Department of Psychiatry, University of Pennsylvania School of Medicine, Philadelphia, PA

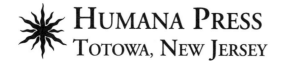

HUMANA PRESS
TOTOWA, NEW JERSEY

© 2005 Humana Press Inc.
999 Riverview Drive, Suite 208
Totowa, New Jersey 07512

www.humanapress.com

Due diligence has been taken by the publishers, editors, and authors of this book to assure the accuracy of the information published and to describe generally accepted practices. The contributors herein have carefully checked to ensure that the drug selections and dosages set forth in this text are accurate and in accord with the standards accepted at the time of publication. Notwithstanding, as new research, changes in government regulations, and knowledge from clinical experience relating to drug therapy and drug reactions constantly occurs, the reader is advised to check the product information provided by the manufacturer of each drug for any change in dosages or for additional warnings and contraindications. This is of utmost importance when the recommended drug herein is a new or infrequently used drug. It is the responsibility of the treating physician to determine dosages and treatment strategies for individual patients. Further it is the responsibility of the health care provider to ascertain the Food and Drug Administration status of each drug or device used in their clinical practice. The publisher, editors, and authors are not responsible for errors or omissions or for any consequences from the application of the information presented in this book and make no warranty, express or implied, with respect to the contents in this publication.

Cover design by Patricia F. Cleary
Production Editor: Robin B. Weisberg

For additional copies, pricing for bulk purchases, and/or information about other Humana titles, contact Humana at the above address or at any of the following numbers: Tel.: 973-256-1699; Fax: 973-256-8341; E-mail: humana@humanapr.com or visit our Website at www.humanapress.com

This publication is printed on acid-free paper. ∞
ANSI Z39.48-1984 (American National Standards Institute) Permanence of Paper for Printed Library Materials.

Printed in the United States of America. 10 9 8 7 6 5 4 3 2 1

eISBN 1-59259-865-X

Library of Congress Cataloging-in-Publication Data

The management of eating disorders and obesity / edited by David J. Goldstein.-- 2nd ed.
    p. ; cm. -- (Nutrition and health)
  Includes bibliographical references and index.
  ISBN 1-58829-341-6 (alk. paper)
  1. Eating disorders. 2. Obesity.
  [DNLM: 1. Bulimia--therapy. 2. Anorexia Nervosa--therapy. 3. Obesity--therapy. WM 175 M266 2005]
I. Goldstein, David J. (David Joel), 1947- II. Series: Nutrition and health (Totowa, N.J.)
  RC552.E18M364 2005
  616.85'2606--dc22

                                                                                2004009971

Series Editor's Introduction

The *Nutrition and Health Series* of books have had great success because each volume has the consistent overriding mission of providing health professionals with texts that are essential because each includes (1) a synthesis of the state of the science; (2) timely, in-depth reviews by the leading researchers in their respective fields; (3) extensive, up-to-date fully annotated reference lists; (4) a detailed index; (5) relevant tables and figures; (6) identification of paradigm shifts and the consequences; (7) virtually no overlap of information between chapters, but targeted, interchapter referrals; (8) suggestions of areas for future research; and (9) balanced, data-driven answers to patient/health professionals' questions that are based on the totality of evidence rather than the findings of any single study.

The series volumes are not the outcome of a symposium. Rather, each editor has the potential to examine a chosen area with a broad perspective, both in subject matter as well as in the choice of chapter authors. The editors, whose trainings are both research- and practice-oriented, have the opportunity to develop a primary objective for their book, define the scope and focus, and then invite the leading authorities to be part of their initiative. The authors are encouraged to provide an overview of the field, discuss their own research, and relate the research findings to potential human health consequences. Because each book is developed *de novo*, the chapters are coordinated so that the resulting volume imparts greater knowledge than the sum of the information contained in the individual chapters.

The Management of Eating Disorders and Obesity, Second Edition, edited by David J. Goldstein clearly exemplifies the goals of the *Nutrition and Health Series*. The first edition was widely acclaimed for its emphasis on data-driven clinical applications of the newest scientific discoveries in the areas of bulimia, anorexia, binge eating, and the complex, chronic disease of obesity. Dr. Goldstein, who is an internationally recognized leader in the fields of obesity and eating-disorder research, has enhanced the contents of the first edition even further with the addition of three timely, new chapters. The first two new chapters cover the internet and its value in the education and potential treatment of eating disorders in one chapter, and the use of the internet in education and treatment of obesity in a second chapter. The third critically important chapter reviews the role of hunger and satiety in obesity treatment. All of the original chapter authors, the most authoritative leaders in obesity and eating-disorder research, have updated the contents and have included recent references, figures, and graphs. Thus, Dr. Goldstein has developed a second edition that is destined to be the benchmark in the field because of its extensive, in-depth chapters covering the most important aspects of eating disorders and obesity, with emphases on human physiology, treatment, and disease prevention.

The book chapters are logically organized to provide the reader with a basic understanding of the clinical conditions of bulimia nervosa, anorexia nervosa, and obesity in the first chapter of each of the book's three major sections. Each section also contains chapters that address treatment options as well as prevention strategies. This logical sequence of chapters provides the latest information on the current standards of practice for clinicians, related health professionals including the dietitian, nurse, pharmacist, physical therapist, behaviorist, psychologist, and others involved in the team effort required for successful treatments. This comprehensive volume also has great value for academicians involved in the education of graduate students and postdoctoral fellows, medical students, and allied health professionals who plan to interact with patients with eating disorders including obesity.

Cutting-edge discussions of the roles of growth factors, hormones, cellular and nuclear receptors and their ligands, gene promoters, adipose tissue, and all of the cells directly involved in fat metabolism are included in well-organized chapters that put the molecular aspects into clinical perspective. Of great importance, the editor and authors have provided chapters that balance the most technical information with discussions of its importance for clients and patients as well as graduate and medical students, health professionals, and academicians.

Separate chapters in the three sections include specific, detailed information on the counseling of patients with bulimia and the pharmacological treatment of bulimia. There is a unique chapter that looks at the role of nutrition and dietary factors in the prevention of eating disorders. The anorexia section includes four chapters devoted to basic information, treatment strategies, detailed information on pharmacological therapies, and the new chapter on internet resources. The third section is the largest and contains three chapters on general aspects of obesity including the etiologies of obesity, medical consequences of obesity, as well as benefits of weight loss and a very practical chapter on binge eating in the obese.

Thirteen chapters are devoted to the treatment of obesity. These include an overview of current treatment options as well as a discussion of future treatments that are already in development. Critical to any weight-reduction program is exercise, and there is a comprehensive chapter on the role of physical activity, exercise, and nutrition in weight control. The importance of a team approach to the treatment of obesity as a chronic disease is extensively discussed in the chapter on lifestyle modification in the treatment of obesity. Specific treatment modalities are reviewed in separate chapters on very low-calorie diets, pharmacotherapies, combination therapies, the potential for genetic interventions, the new chapter on hunger and satiety, and surgical interventions that are discussed in detail, including drawings that depict the specific types of surgeries currently available. Each of these chapters presents an objective evaluation of the treatment and identifies the positives and negatives that have been seen during clinical studies, as well as cumulative data derived from clinical practice.

The final four chapters in the obesity treatment section examine the clinical experiences in a comprehensive weight-management program, the importance and value of a multidisciplinary team in the management of obesity, the potential for the internet to help in obesity treatment, and a most candid chapter on the barriers to obesity treatment. The final book chapter reviews the most medically relevant alternative to treatment–prevention of obesity—and examines the signs that could alert the health professional to the potential for the development of obesity, as well as outlines the steps to take to help prevent the overweight patient from moving to frank obesity.

There is a clear, data-driven message throughout the obesity section of the volume that obesity is a chronic disease. As with hypertension that can be controlled by drug therapy, so with obesity—therapy cannot stop once a particular weight-loss goal is reached. Like hypertension that reappears without chronic treatment, obesity can easily reappear if not treated as a chronic disease.

Detailed tables and figures assist the reader in comprehending the complexities of the disturbances in eating behaviors. Modulators of eating responses that are covered in this section include adrenergic receptors, cholecystokinin, γ-aminobutyric acid, histamine and serotonin receptors, insulin, leptin, neuropeptide Y, galanin, ghrelin, growth hormone, as well as substances that can be consumed in diet and/or supplements such as caffeine, ephedrine, aspirin and lithium, olestra, and yohimbine. Novel treatment options that are of great interest to clients and patients are included in several chapters that review more than 50 therapeutic agents. In-depth descriptions of behavioral modification programs, mental states, evaluation tools for documentation of patient eating habits, and many other valuable treatment aids are included in numerous chapters. Thus, *The Management of Eating Disorders and Obesity, Second Edition* is focused on answering questions commonly asked by clients and patients about why some diets do not work and why some "professional" sources advocate certain products that are available over the counter but may not "work." The overriding goal of this volume is to provide the health professional with the balanced documentation to assure the client/patient that eating disorders and obesity are complex states that transcend the simplistic view of just losing a few pounds.

Hallmarks of all chapters include bulleted key points at the beginning of each chapter as well as a detailed table of contents; complete definitions of terms with the abbreviations fully defined for the reader and consistent use of terms between chapters. There are numerous relevant tables, graphs, and figures as well as up-to-date references; all chapters include a conclusion section that provides the highlights of major findings. The Management of Eating Disorders and Obesity, Second Edition contains a highly annotated index and within chapters, readers are referred to relevant information in other chapters.

This important text provides practical, data-driven resources based on the totality of the evidence to help the reader understand the basics, treatments, and preventive strategies that are involved in bulimia, anorexia, and obesity. The overarching goal of the editor is to provide fully referenced information to health professionals so they may have a balanced perspective on the value of various treatment options that are available today as well as in the foreseeable future.

In conclusion, *The Management of Eating Disorders and Obesity, Second Edition*, edited by David J. Goldstein provides health professionals in many areas of research and practice with the most up-to-date, well-referenced and easy-to-understand volume on the importance of identifying and treating those already suffering from bulimia, anorexia, and/or obesity as well as providing strategies to prevent the development of these chronic, serious diseases. This volume will serve the reader as the most authoritative resource in the field to date and is a very welcome addition to the *Nutrition and Health Series*

Adrianne Bendich, PhD, FACN
Series Editor

Foreword

The 6 years since the publication of the first edition of *The Management of Eating Disorders and Obesity* has seen a sea change in our view of obesity. At the time of the first edition, obesity was still viewed as a fairly simple problem, with unfortunate, but not necessarily dire, consequences. Since that time, the importance of obesity has broken into our general awareness and into the medical literature in particular. The enormous increase in obesity, to the extent that two-thirds of Americans are overweight or obese, is now termed an "epidemic." This epidemic is destined to become even more severe as the huge increase in childhood obesity has its impact on obesity in later life. The serious health consequences of obesity are being increasingly recognized and Syndrome X has become a household word.

This situation in the treatment of obesity is a major reason for the consternation caused by the removal of fenfluramine from the market just as the first edition of this volume was published, because fenfluramine was the most effective pharmacological agent for the treatment of obesity yet employed and was a sound basis for medical treatment of the disorder. No other medication for obesity has yet taken its place.

In the face of the uncontrollable increase in obesity, the public is turning increasingly to popular fads. The explosion of interest in the Atkins Diet, and "low carbs" illustrates a near hysteria on the part of the general public. Forty million Americans are said to be currently following the not entirely benign Atkins Diet. In these frantic days, an important task of the practitioner is to forestall the more needless, and even harmful, results of the hysteria.

As befits an epidemic, public health efforts are being introduced in increasing measure to schools, communities, and in public communication, as through the internet. The focus of these methods is on the favorable changes in lifestyle that may help to prevent obesity from developing, control it when it develops, and, in some cases, reduce it. As outlined in *Food Fight* by Brownell and Horgen (1), the beginning of this effort is to think differently about foods, not as "good" or "bad," but in total calories of food intake. Next, public health and medical efforts should be combined to increase physical activity and to establish simple but sound eating habits that include smaller portion sizes. These activities had not been ones that, until now, the practitioner would have been able to pursue under the circumstances prevailing because they require services that had not been reimbursed. Awareness of the epidemic nature of obesity has led to the salutary consequence of the US Food and Drug Administration labeling obesity "a disease." This long-delayed action has important consequences. It makes it possible for the treatment of obesity to be reimbursed. For the first time, practitioners may be able to devote the time necessary for the successful treatment of obesity. Furthering at the individual level the efforts made at the public health level means that the practitioner can, for the first time, be able to advise patients on favorable lifestyle changes.

The eating disorders, in contrast to obesity, have been the subject of only modest change since the first edition of this volume. The greatest improvement has been in the management of bulimia nervosa. Intensive research has produced improvements in both the pharmacological and behavioral treatments of bulimia nervosa, and in their combination. The treatment of bulimia nervosa is still largely the province of specialists devoted to treatment of the disorder. But there is a critical role for the clinician in diagnosing it and referring patients for treatment. The earlier the treatment begins, the better its results, both in the short term and in the long term. Patients with bulimia nervosa should not be allowed to suffer without the effective help that is now available.

Binge-eating disorder has received increasing attention in recent years and it is now recognized as a widespread problem. A number of studies of pharmacological and psychological treatment have shown that these agents improve the symptoms of binge eating. This improvement, however, has not produced weight loss and the usefulness of this diagnosis has been questioned *(2)*.

The problem of anorexia nervosa is the most challenging among the eating disorders. Despite continuing research, little progress in treatment has been made. The most effective treatment for anorexia nervosa may well be Russell's *(3)* decades-old program of family therapy for young anorectics. As with bulimia nervosa, the practitioner can provide a valuable service in identifying patients with anorexia nervosa and carrying out the difficult task of getting them into treatment. The current status of the disorder is well described in the four chapters devoted to it.

Albert J. Stunkard, MD
Weight and Eating Disorders Program
Department of Psychiatry
University of Pennsylvania School of Medicine
Philadelphia, PA

REFERENCES

1. Brownell KD, Horgen K. Food Fight. Contemporary Books, Chicago, IL, 2004.
2. Stunkard AJ, Allison KC. Binge eating disorder: disorder or marker? Int J Eat Disord 2003;34:5107–5116.
3. Russell GFM, Szmukler GI, Dare C, Eisler I. An evaluation of family therapy in anorexia nervosa and bulimia nervosa. Arch Gen Psychiatry 1987;44:1047–1056.

Preface

The first edition of *The Management of Eating Disorders and Obesity* was published in 1999, just after the removal of fenfluramine and dexfenfluramine from the market because of the association of their use with development of valvular heart disease *(1)*. Dr. Albert J. Stunkard expressed the possibility that drug therapy would come to a "screeching halt" and that legal actions would cause prescribers to avoid obesity pharmacotherapies and cause pharmaceutical companies to discontinue development of future obesity therapies. Prescription of drugs for obesity treatment did decrease and the US Food and Drug Administration required additional evidence of safety prior to approval of new anti-obesity agents for marketing, but drug development did not stop. To the contrary, our improving understanding of the genetic basis of eating behaviors has expanded the number of molecular targets for obesity pharmacotherapies, and many novel molecular entities are being evaluated. Recently, the effects of ephedrine and similar compounds on blood pressure and the risk of stroke *(2,3)* have been more generally recognized, and ephedrine-containing products have been withdrawn from the market.

In 1999, I noted that eating disorders and obesity were common and their prevalence was increasing. Unfortunately, this trend has continued to the degree that obesity has been called an epidemic *(4)*. In 2004, the obesity-related mortality rate nearly overtook that of cigarette smoking. Underlying this increase in obesity is the abundance and variety of food, as well as the commercialization of the food industry, promoting more eating, larger portions, and high caloric density foods. Threats of litigation of "fast food" chains and social pressures may have encouraged these companies to add more healthful items to their menu and many have added low carbohydrate selections in an effort to capitalize on the recent trend for low carbohydrate diets. This is discussed in Chapter 19.

Obesity and associated diseases continue to cost society more than $100 billion in direct and indirect health costs annually. Treatment of eating disorders and obesity continue to be suboptimal. All tend to be best managed by experts and for obesity, maintenance of weight loss continues to be challenging, even in the best medically managed centers.

Associated with obesity is a societal stigma that leads in part to the emphasis on being thin and adds pressures toward attainment of lean body habitus, thus enhancing the development of the potentially life-threatening anorexia nervosa and bulimia nervosa. These eating disorders and obesity are disorders of ingestion—either too much or too little, too much control or too little, with purging behavior or without. All have significant health, social, and psychological consequences.

That is the bad news. So what is the good news? There is increasing awareness about eating disorders and their predispositions. Efforts are expanding on prevention, early identification, and intervention of eating disorders. Clinicians are developing treatment strategies incorporating newer technologies, including the internet, which might eventually reduce the cost while improving access to and effectiveness of therapy. Regarding obesity, there is greater focus on prevention, and strategies for prevention are being evaluated. Researchers are identifying the effects of maternal behaviors during pregnancy that "imprint" the fetus for increased postnatal weight gain and obesity-associated disease complications. As we learn about such effects, we may be able to recommend behaviors for pregnant women that would reduce the future risk for their infants. Increasing pressure for companies to improve the ingredients in their prepared foods has led many to respond in positive ways. School lunches have been placed under more scrutiny. Schools are attempting to educate students about nutrition and are attempting to encourage better eating and increased activity and exercise. More is understood about effective methods for maintenance of reduced weight and these methods are being incorporated into therapeutic programs. The molecular basis of obesity is being more effectively probed and many neuroendocrine mediators have been identified.

This second edition follows the structure of the first edition in that it consists of three major sections, one each for bulimia nervosa, anorexia nervosa, and obesity. Each section contains brief, practical, and timely reviews of the disorder or aspects of management. The reviews have been updated to incorporate recent findings and new chapters have been incorporated. The goal remains to provide assistance to practitioners who want to realize the maximal impact when caring for patients with eating disorders or obesity. Not only are present therapies described, but developing therapies are identified as well.

The unifying principle underlying the treatment of eating disorders and obesity is the establishment of healthful behaviors and the ideal of also attaining a healthy weight. So Drs. Romano and Blackburn and colleagues discuss the health consequences of bulimia nervosa (Chapter 1), anorexia nervosa (Chapter 5), and obesity (Chapter 10). Then Dr. Busk and colleagues discuss the health benefits of increased activity and exercise (Chapter 13). Increasing activity is important in alleviating the health consequences of obesity even without weight loss, as it has been identified as one of the behaviors that make weight maintenance more likely.

The treatment of the eating disorders can be challenging. Drs. Mitchell and Cook Myers discuss the nonpharmacological therapy of bulimia nervosa (Chapter 2) and Dr. Hsu discusses the strategy for treatment of anorexia nervosa (Chapter 6). Dr. Hudson and his colleagues and Dr. Kaye review the research on the pharmacotherapy of bulimia nervosa (Chapter 3) and anorexia nervosa (Chapter 7). They provide their experiences and strategies for treatment.

Ultimately, we should be trying to prevent the development of eating disorders and if they occur, we should attempt early treatment before the conditions become refractory to treatment. Once we have successfully treated the patient, we need to prevent relapse. Dr. Rock (Chapter 4) discusses the effects of nutrition on the development of eating disorders and how modification of nutrition can assist in preventing the development of, improving the treatment of, and preventing relapse of eating disorders.

Dr. Marcus (Chapter 11) provides an overview of binge-eating disorder. This is a more recently defined diagnosis that has had increasing research interest since the first edition. Dr. Marcus reviews much of the research related to treatment of binge-eating disorder and places this into perspective.

Dr. Foreyt and colleagues (Chapter 12) look at the present status of obesity and look forward to how today's needs may be met in the future. Part of the cause of obesity is the underlying genetics of the individual that becomes permissive for weight gain in an environment of excess *(5)*. As noted earlier, imprinting of the fetus and other environmental effects may also predispose individuals toward weight gain. These and other effects are discussed by Dr. Atkinson (Chapter 9).

Despite concerns about withdrawal from the market of obesity medications or greater regulatory restriction on obesity pharmacotherapy and despite possible increased stigmatization of obesity pharmacotherapy, two new obesity pharmacotherapies, orlistat and sibutramine, were approved for marketing in the United States, as is discussed by Dr. Bray (Chapter 16). New treatments continue to be explored and some of these have novel mechanisms that were not anticipated in 1999. Several of these may be approved for marketing during the next several years. Two that are anticipated in the near term are ciliary neurotrophic factor and rimonabant. In addition, some treatments are being used in combination with greater success than provided by individual agents, much as fenfluramine in combination with phentermine provided greater efficacy than did either agent individually *(4,6)*. Drs. Atkinson and Uwaifo report on use of combination therapy in Chapter 17. Combinations of drugs are used in other branches of medicine to improve control of disease or to lower blood pressure, cholesterol, control diabetes, and so on. It is reasonable to believe that use of medications with different mechanisms of action could produce better weight control. This greater efficacy led to the popularity of the fen-phen combination for weight reduction and other combinations are in use at present. Such combinations have not been adequately studied in large controlled trials, but we should expect such studies in the future.

The genetics of obesity has been further elucidated since the first edition and Dr. Fernandez (Chapter 18) provides an update on these findings and how they might relate to future therapeutics. He also attempts to address the genetic perspective on the role of environment and how to use genetic tools to better understand the interaction of nature and nurture.

Surgical solutions for obesity have, on average, resulted in greater and more sustained weight loss than other treatments. Recognition of this has led to increased interest and utilization of this alternative. Surgical therapy continues to generate media interest. The surgical procedures continue to be refined and developed to maximize weight loss and minimize adverse consequences. Dr. Shikora (Chapter 20) discusses these surgical techniques and management of the post-surgery patient.

Weight loss can be attained with very low calorie diets, discussed by Dr. Phinney (Chapter 15), and by calorie restricted diets with modification of lifestyle and eating behaviors, discussed by Drs. Fabricatore and Wadden (Chapter 14). Very low calorie diets require special monitoring to avoid problems. Dr. Phinney discusses this management. After initial weight loss, postreduction maintenance strategies are critical to prevent regain of weight. Dr. Fabricatore and Wadden discuss strategies for weight maintenance.

The low carbohydrate diet, commercialized by Dr. Atkins, and its variants, including the South Beach Diet, have become very popular. Recent research has provided scientific information from randomized clinical trials about the effects of a low carbohydrate diet. Michael Penn and I have summarized this information and provide it in the context of the role of hunger and satiety in the management of obesity (Chapter 19). We provide a hypothesis regarding the way the low carbohydrate diet may operate and note that we should expect that claims about diets and treatments should be tested scientifically.

A book on treatment would not be complete without covering the practical aspects of setting up and organizing the treatment practice. Drs. O'Neil and Rieder (Chapter 22) discuss the organization and use of a multidisciplinary program for treatment of obesity and Drs. Loper and Lutes (Chapter 21) discuss the practicalities of office practice and share their recent experience. Dr. Frank discusses the issues that prevent patients from achieving success in their effort to lose weight (Chapter 24). An enhanced understanding of these barriers to successful treatment will serve us well in our efforts to improve care of the obese patient.

The internet has provided access to information and treatment resources and potentially will provide a cost-effective adjunct to traditional therapy for patients with eating disorders and obesity. Internet resources are presented for eating disorders (Chapter 8) and obesity (Chapter 23). Although the use of the internet in therapy is very limited to date, we can expect the use of this medium to increase. It is hoped that providing this resource will benefit practitioners, particularly those in areas where consultant resources are limited. Although the Internal Revenue Service has just included the treatment of obesity as a tax deductible medical expense, it is still not covered by most health insurance policies and cost continues to be an issue. Indirect cost is also problematic in that intensive therapy is best and potentially entails missing work or obtaining child care. Use of the internet might alleviate some of this burden as well.

It is anticipated that incorporation of this information will enhance the effectiveness of practitioners in their management of patients with eating disorders and obesity.

I thank the Series Editor, Dr. Adrianne Bendich, Humana Press, and Paul Dolgert for their assistance in making this edition a reality. I also thank the chapter authors for their contributions.

David J. Goldstein, MD, PhD

REFERENCES

1. Connolly HM, Crary JL, McGoon MD, et al. Valvular heart disease associated with fenfluramine-phentermine. N Engl J Med 1997; 337:581–588.
2. Shekelle PG, Hardy ML, Morton SC, et al. Efficacy and safety of ephedra and ephedrine for weight loss and athletic performance. J Am Med Assoc 2003; 289: 1537–1545.
3. Bent S, Tiedt TN, Odden MC, Shlipak MG. The relative safety of ephedra compared with other herbal products. Ann Intern Med 2003; 138:468–471.
4. Weintraub M, Hasday JD, Mushlin AI, Lockwood D H. A double-blind clinical trial in weight control. Use of fenfluramine and phentermine alone and in combination. Arch Intern Med 1984; 144:1143–1148.
5. Kahn RC. The role of obesity in diabetes mellitus. Curr Opin Endocrinol Diabet 1996; 3:1–2.
6. Weintraub M. Long-term weight control study: conclusions. Clin Pharmacol Ther 1992; 51:642–646.

Contents

Contributors

RICHARD L. ATKINSON, MD • *Obtech Inc., Richmond, VA and Obesity Institute, MedStar Research Institute, Washington, DC*

GEORGE L. BLACKBURN, MD, PhD • *Center for the Study of Nutrition Medicine, Department of Surgery, Beth Israel Deaconess Medical Center, Harvard Medical School, Boston, MA*

GEORGE A. BRAY, MD • *Pennington Biomedical Research Center, Louisiana State University, Baton Rouge, LA*

MICHAEL F. BUSK, MD, MPH • *The National Institute for Fitness and Sport, Division of Pulmonary, Allergy, Critical Care and Occupational Medicine, and Department of Cellular and Integrative Physiology, Indiana University School of Medicine, Indianapolis, IN*

WILLIAM P. CARTER, MD • *Biological Psychiatry Laboratory, McLean Hospital and Department of Psychiatry, Harvard Medical School, Belmont, MA*

REED J. ENGEL, MD • *The National Institute for Fitness and Sport, Indianapolis, IN*

ANTHONY N. FABRICATORE, PhD • *Weight and Eating Disorders Program, Department of Psychiatry, University of Pennsylvania School of Medicine, Philadelphia, PA*

STACEY FARYNA, RD • *Division of Endocrinology and Metabolism, Indiana University Department of Medicine, Indianapolis, IN*

JOSÉ R. FERNÁNDEZ, PhD • *Division of Physiology and Metabolism, Department of Nutrition Sciences and Section in Statistical Genetics, Department of Biostatistics, University of Alabama at Birmingham, Birmingham, AL*

JOHN P. FOREYT, PhD • *Behavioral Medicine Research Center, Department of Medicine, Baylor College of Medicine, Houston, TX*

ARTHUR FRANK, MD • *The George Washington University Weight Management Program, Washington, DC*

DAVID J. GOLDSTEIN, MD, PhD • *Department of Pharmacology and Toxicology, Indiana University School of Medicine and PRN Consulting, Indianapolis, IN*

BARBARA C. HANSEN, PhD• *Obesity and Diabetes Research Center, Department of Physiology, University of Maryland School of Medicine, Baltimore, MD*

JODI HAZARD, MS • *The National Institute for Fitness and Sport, Indianapolis, IN*

JAMES I. HUDSON, MD, ScD • *Biological Psychiatry Laboratory, McLean Hospital and Department of Psychiatry, Harvard Medical School, Belmont, MA*

L. K. GEORGE HSU, MD, FRC PSYCH • *Department of Psychiatry, Tufts-New England Medical Center, Boston, MA*

WALTER H. KAYE, MD • *Anorexia and Bulimia Nervosa Research Module, Department of Psychiatry, University of Pittsburgh Medical Center, Western Psychiatric Institute and Clinic, Pittsburgh, PA*

JULIE J. KIM, MD • *Center for Minimally Invasive Obesity Surgery, Department of Surgery, Tufts-New England Medical Center, Boston, MA*

LALITA KHAODHIAR, MD • *Center for the Study of Nutrition Medicine, Department of Medicine and Surgery, Beth Israel Deaconess Medical Center, Harvard Medical School, Boston, MA*

MICHELE D. LEVINE, PhD • *Western Psychiatric Institute and Clinic, University of Pittsburgh Medical Center, Pittsburgh, PA*

JUDY LOPER, PhD, RD • *Central Ohio Nutrition Center, Inc., Columbus, OH*

RICHARD A. LUTES, MD • *Central Ohio Nutrition Center, Inc., Columbus, OH*

EDWARD T. MANNIX, PhD • *The National Institute for Fitness and Sport, Division of Pulmonary, Allergy, Critical Care and Occupational Medicine, and Department of Cellular and Integrative Physiology, Indiana University School of Medicine, Indianapolis, IN*

MARSHA D. MARCUS, PhD • *Western Psychiatric Institute and Clinic, University of Pittsburgh Medical Center, Pittsburgh, PA*

JAMES E. MITCHELL, MD • *Neuropsychiatric Research Institute, Department of Neuroscience, University of North Dakota School of Medicine and Health Sciences, Fargo, ND*

TRICIA COOK MYERS, PhD • *Neuropsychiatric Research Institute, Department of Neuroscience, University of North Dakota School of Medicine and Health Sciences, Fargo, ND*

PATRICK MAHLEN O'NEIL, PhD • *Weight Management Center, Department of Psychiatry and Behavioral Sciences, Medical University of South Carolina, Charleston, SC*

MICHAEL PENN, RPH • *Indiana University School of Medicine, Indianapolis, IN*

STEPHEN D. PHINNEY, MD, PhD • *University of California Davis School of Medicine, Sacramento, CA*

HARRISON G. POPE, JR., MD • *Biological Psychiatry Laboratory, McLean Hospital and Department of Psychiatry, Harvard Medical School, Belmont, MA*

WALKER S. C. POSTON II, PhD, MPH • *Department of Psychology, University of Missouri-Kansas City and Mid America Heart Institute, Kansas City, MO*

SHERRY RIEDER, PhD •*Weight Management Center, Department of Psychiatry and Behavioral Sciences, Medical University of South Carolina, Charleston, SC*

CHERYL L. ROCK, PhD, RD • *Department of Family and Preventive Medicine, University of California, San Diego, La Jolla, CA*

STEVEN J. ROMANO, MD • *Pfizer, Inc. and Department of Psychiatry, New York University School of Medicine, New York, NY*

SCOTT A. SHIKORA, MD, FACS • *Center for Minimally Invasive Obesity Surgery, Department of Surgery, Tufts-New England Medical Center, Boston, MA*

DAVID SMITH, MD • *Center for Minimally Invasive Obesity Surgery, Department of Surgery, Tufts-New England Medical Center, Boston, MA*

HELMUT O. STEINBERG, MD • *Division of Endocrinology and Metabolism, Department of Medicine, Indiana University School of Medicine, Indianapolis, IN*

ALBERT J. STUNKARD, MD • *Weight and Eating Disorders Program, Department of Psychiatry, University of Pennsylvania School of Medicine, Philadelphia, PA*

LISA TERRE, PhD • *Department of Psychology, University of Missouri-Kansas City, Kansas City, MO*

GABRIEL UWAIFO, MD • *Obesity Institute, Medstar Research Institute, Washington, DC*

THOMAS A. WADDEN, PhD • *Weight and Eating Disorders Program, Department of Psychiatry, University of Pennsylvania School of Medicine, Philadelphia, PA*

I Bulimia Nervosa

1 Bulimia Nervosa

Steven J. Romano

KEY POINTS

- Symptoms of binge eating and purging associated with bulimia nervosa are common, especially in teenage and young adult women, but males are also affected. Dancers, gymnasts, models, and wrestlers have high prevalence of bulimia nervosa.
- Diagnostic criteria have been established in the Diagnostic and Statistical Manual of Mental Disorders (DSM) by the American Psychiatric Association. Diagnosis can be difficult because patients may not complain of the condition or admit to the behaviors.
- Bulimia nervosa is commonly associated with psychiatric comorbidities such as depression and anxiety. Substance abuse is common.
- Medical complications can be life threatening.

1. INTRODUCTION

This chapter focuses on the psychiatric presentation, prevalence, and medical complications associated with bulimia nervosa and highlights comorbid psychopathology (Table 1). A more extensive discussion of etiological factors and treatment approaches can be found elsewhere in this text (*see* Chapters 2, 3, and 4).

Bulimia nervosa, like anorexia nervosa (*see* Chapter 5), represents a clinical syndrome with multiple factors that contribute to its etiology and affect clinical presentation. The term bulimia is from the Greek meaning "ox-hunger" and is an apt description of a primary feature of the disorder, binge eating. Interestingly, although Stunkard *(1)* described binge eating in obese patients decades ago, bulimia as part of a clinically distinct syndrome affecting normal-weight individuals and coupled with compensatory mechanisms to guard against weight gain, was not described in the medical literature until much later. At that time, Russell *(2)* put forth criteria for bulimia nervosa that included urges to engage in periods of overeating, attempts to avoid the "fattening" effect of food through vomiting or use of purgatives, and, similar to the central psychological feature of anorexia nervosa, the presence of a morbid fear of becoming fat. The latter feature underscored the anxiety and avoidance behavior that are an integral part of the syndrome. Bulimia nervosa was once postulated to be

From: *The Management of Eating Disorders and Obesity, Second Edition*
Edited by: D. J. Goldstein © Humana Press Inc., Totowa, NJ

Table 1
Chapter Overview

1. Introduction
2. Prevalence
3. Psychiatric Comorbidity
4. Clinical Description
5. Differential Diagnosis
6. Medical Complications
7. Conclusion

an affective subtype (a mood disorder), in part because of the preponderance of depressive features frequently accompanying the disorder's clinical presentation. The results of antidepressant treatment studies illustrating a specific response of bulimic symptoms strengthened that opinion. Nevertheless, newer information has led to an evolution in concept, and bulimia nervosa is now considered a primary eating disorder distinct from anorexia nervosa.

Since the initial description of bulimia nervosa, there has been an explosion of information, in both scientific and lay literature, regarding the apparent surge in bulimic-related behaviors. The recognition of the extent of eating-disorder behaviors in certain populations, such as college-aged women, and the description of a significant level of comorbid psychiatric symptomatology have led to advances in both the understanding of the biological underpinnings and efficacious approaches to treatment.

2. PREVALENCE

As the syndrome of bulimia nervosa was described in the medical literature only in the late 1970s and was not incorporated into the DSM until 1980, prevalence studies are few. Furthermore, the diagnostic criteria for bulimia nervosa have evolved to more specifically describe the symptoms of binge eating as part of a syndrome associated with purging and nonpurging compensatory behaviors and criteria for frequency and chronicity (illustrated in Table 2) (3). Thus, the early prevalence studies reflect the prevalence of specific behaviors, such as binge eating or, in a smaller number, vomiting. Those studies were generally in subpopulations, such as college-aged females. Thus, they do not accurately assess the prevalence of the syndrome of bulimia nervosa, as outlined in current diagnostic research criteria, in the general population.

Focusing on specific populations, a number of studies utilizing DSM-III criteria found the prevalence of bulimia to be approx 4 to 9% in high school- and college-aged students (4–7). Prevalence studies of binge eating in special populations described levels of disordered eating as high as, for example, 90% in ballet dancers (8). A study that focused on the assessment of vomiting in college students described a prevalence of 9.9% (9), and another study that examined attendees at a family-planning clinic found a prevalence of 2.9%.

Family studies in bulimia nervosa support a familial contribution. Increased rates of the eating disorders, including bulimia nervosa, were assessed by Strober (10) in a study comparing first- and second-degree relatives of anorexic patients with the relatives of a control group of non-anorexic, psychiatrically ill patients. More recent reports by

Table 2
Diagnostic and Statistical Manual of Mental Disorders Criteria for Bulimia Nervosa

---

A. Recurrent binge eating characterized by both
  1. Eating an amount of food that is definitely more than most people would eat
      i. During a similar time interval
      ii. Under similar circumstances
  2. Having a sense of lack of control over
      i. Amount of food eaten
      ii. Ability to stop eating
B. Recurrent inappropriate compensatory behaviors intended to prevent weight gain
  1. Self-induced vomiting
  2. Misuse of laxatives, diuretics, enemas, other medications
  3. Fasting
  4. Excessive exercise
C. Binge eating and compensatory behaviors occur at least twice a month for at least 3 mo.
D. Self-image is unduly influenced by body shape and weight
E. These behaviors do not occur exclusively during episodes of anorexia nervosa

---

Purging Type: During current episodes, the patient regularly engages in purging activities.
Nonpurging Type: During current episodes, the patient does not regularly engage in binge eating or purging, but uses other behaviors such as fasting or excessive exercise.

Lilenfeld et al. *(11)*, Strober et al. *(12)*, Stein et al. *(13)* further confirm that bulimia nervosa, as well as anorexia nervosa, is strongly familial. A number of studies indicated increased rates of affective disorders in the families of patients with anorexia nervosa and bulimia nervosa *(14–17)*. More studies need to be conducted to better elucidate familial patterns, clarify genetic variants, and to explore a potential link between bulimia and affective disorder. Regarding the latter, possible heritable biological vulnerability to a spectrum of psychopathology may exist to explain the observed increase in the incidence of affective disorder in families of bulimic patients. Functional dysregulation of serotonin, a potent neurohormone involved in both mood and appetitive behavior, may represent an etiological link and, along with potential disturbances in other neurotransmitter systems, is a focus of research interest.

Similar to anorexia nervosa, bulimia nervosa predominantly affects young women, although the age of onset tends to be later in adolescence. In contrast to anorexia nervosa, many patients with bulimia nervosa present in their 20s and 30s, often after having suffered with the disorder for a number of years. Although college-educated white females are most often described, clinical experience has appreciated a greater degree of heterogeneity than that generally regarded in anorexia nervosa, a situation that may reflect the relatively high incidence of dieting in populations at risk. Males appear to be affected more frequently by bulimia nervosa than by anorexia nervosa, representing perhaps as many as 10 to 15% of cases.

The prevalence and incidence data available on bulimia nervosa, although limited, provide a clue as to those populations most at risk for the development of clinically significant disturbances. In general, the single most important factor leading to an eating disorder is dieting, but significant sociocultural influences affect weight- and body-change behavior. Particular antecedents to dieting, such as equating beauty with thinness and viewing attractiveness as a prominent measure of success, both incorporated as values in Western society, represent such sociocultural influences and are more likely to affect young women. Dieting in this group is also peer-supported, leading to the persistence of periods of nutritional deprivation and subsequent development of disordered means of managing food intake in those unable to sustain restrictive dieting. Given the prevalence of dieting in this culture and the fact that dieting is considered the most potent stressor contributing to the development of an eating disorder in an otherwise vulnerable individual, the group at risk is expanding and represents a spectrum of personality types from a range of socioeconomic backgrounds. Of course, in those professions that are most likely to stress the aforementioned values, such as professional modeling, acting, and dance, a higher incidence of bulimia nervosa can be expected. In addition, professions that espouse body-change behavior in the service of improved performance, such as certain sports, would likely support the development of this disorder. Regarding the latter, wrestling is one of the few areas in which males are significantly influenced.

3. PSYCHIATRIC COMORBIDITY

Comorbid psychiatric symptomatology is frequently encountered in patients with bulimia nervosa. Affective symptoms are particularly common, as are features of anxiety and impulsivity. Some comorbid symptoms can be associated more directly with the primary eating disorder, whereas others may represent coexistent syndromes. The latter generally require thorough evaluation and subsequent management in order to enhance treatment response of the primary eating disorder.

The significance of depressive features presenting in a majority of patients with bulimia nervosa was evident in the earlier conceptualization of this syndrome as an affective subtype. This diagnostic construct was buttressed by the effectiveness of antidepressant treatment strategies (*see* Chapter 3). Currently, depressive features are most often viewed as secondary to the eating disturbance and often become less severe or abate with the treatment and resolution of the bulimic behaviors. The etiology of depressive symptoms in this setting may be, in part, physiological and linked to the negative effects and consequences of malnourishment and purging behaviors. In the case of some, for whom bulimia evolves into a strategy for reducing stress or moderating negative affective states such as anxiety or depression, depressive symptoms can emerge following control of bulimia. In other words, bulimia may be initially employed as a weight-reducing strategy but develop into a defense in the psychological sense, whereby removal of the behavior results in the emergence of negative affects previously held in check. This is more often the case in individuals manifesting significant comorbid character pathology. In others, affective symptoms may predate bulimia nervosa and represent a separate and primary psychiatric disorder.

Anxiety features are commonly associated with bulimia. Phobic avoidance of certain food items or meals is clearly an aspect of the primary eating disturbance, as is the anxiety associated with the ingestion of unwanted food or following a binge when the ability to purge is obstructed or delayed, as in the case of social interruption. Generalized anxiety, panic attacks, or obsessive–compulsive features may also be evident, with obsessive–compulsive features most often associated with eating or weight- and shape-related concerns. Certainly, the aforementioned anxiety symptoms can be evidence of other primary psychiatric disorders and should be thoroughly evaluated and pursued during an initial psychiatric evaluation.

Impulsivity is often observed in bulimic individuals and is a dimensional feature that seems to distinguish the personalities of patients with bulimia from those with restricting anorexia. Impulsivity in this regard may speak to the presence of a personality disorder as described in the fourth edition of the DSM. Especially apparent are traits associated with the dramatic cluster, which include borderline and histrionic personality disorders. Impulsivity may also be evidenced by certain concomitant behaviors, including substance abuse, sexual promiscuity, or shoplifting.

The rates of comorbid psychopathology have been assessed by a number of researchers and confirm many of the aforementioned clinical impressions. Lifetime rates of major depression in bulimia nervosa have been reported to be from 36 to 70% (18–20). The significance of concurrent depressive symptomatology at the time of presentation is well recognized and affects between one-third and one-half of the patients. The intensity of the depressive episode at presentation may influence the initial management of the individual with bulimia, which is addressed in more detail elsewhere in this text.

Supporting the clinical description of features associated with impulsivity and anxiety in many patients presenting with bulimia nervosa, the rates of personality disorders in both the dramatic cluster and the anxious cluster have been reported to be relatively high. In a more recent study, Braun et al. (21), employing the Structured Clinical Interview for DSM-Personality (SCID-P) diagnostic interview, established that one-third of the individuals in the bulimic subgroups met the criteria for a dramatic cluster personality disorder. One-third of those met the diagnosis for borderline personality disorder. In addition, one-third of the individuals in the bulimic subgroups met the criteria for a personality disorder in the anxious cluster, most often avoidant or obsessive–compulsive personality disorders. Interestingly, the rate of personality disorders from the anxious cluster was similar to the rate seen in the anorexic restrictor group. Previous studies assessing the rate of personality disorders in patients with bulimia nervosa revealed a wide range of findings. Specifically, the percentage of patients with at least one DSM-III-R personality disorder has been reported as 77% (22), 69% (23), 62% (24), 61% (25), 33% (26), and 28% (27).

The rate of substance abuse, including alcoholism, in patients with bulimia nervosa has been reported in a number of studies, and it varies from 18 to 33% (28–30). In all these studies, the rates in the bulimic groups were significantly greater than those for the control groups. More recently, Braun et al. (21) found that all bulimic subgroups had significantly higher rates of substance abuse in comparison with a subgroup of anorexic restrictors.

Given the breadth of psychopathology encountered in patients with bulimia nervosa discussed above, it may be helpful to consider an underlying biological disturbance or vulnerability that may contribute to the development of various behavioral outcomes. For example, the neurotransmitter serotonin has been implicated in several functional areas, including appetitive behavior, mood and affect modulation, and impulsivity, and serotonergic dysfunction has been proposed in the etiology of a spectrum of obsessive–compulsive syndromes. A disturbance in the functioning of serotonin neurotransmission or pathways could thus influence the modulation of normal behavior or the development of pathological symptomatology, leading to various clinical presentations. Further research will help elucidate the possible links that may underlie the comorbid presentation of bulimia and various other psychiatric conditions.

4. CLINICAL DESCRIPTION

The disorder of bulimia nervosa affects approx 2 to 3% of young women, although bulimic behaviors, as described earlier, may be encountered in many more. Such behaviors are generally precipitated by periods of restrictive dieting. Individuals with bulimia engage in regular episodes of binge eating, followed by compensatory behaviors that are an attempt to counteract the weight-gaining effect of ingested calories. Binge eating is characterized by the rapid consumption of large amounts of food over a distinct period of time, usually 1 to 2 hr. Binge eating is associated with the sense of losing control and is often followed by feelings of guilt or shame. Frequently, other dysphoric affective states, such as depression or anxiety, follow the binge eating and purging. Some patients report alleviation of dysphoria or even emotional numbing immediately following the episode, although this is short-lived. During a binge, an individual may consume a few thousand calories or more. Some individuals describe trigger foods, often a fattening sweet, such as chocolate, precipitating a binge, although the overall content of food consumed, by macro-analysis of nutritional content, varies. The bulimic individual almost exclusively binge eats in private, as the behavior of grossly overeating is humiliating. In this setting, embarrassment can lead to varying degrees of social avoidance and isolation.

Contributing further to avoidant behavior is the need to compensate for consumption, frequently in the form of purging. Most bulimic individuals induce vomiting during or after a binge, and some bulimic individuals use laxatives or diuretics alone. Recognizing the various compensatory behaviors encountered in this disorder, two subtypes are delineated: purging and nonpurging. Nonpurging compensatory behaviors include compulsive exercising and restrictive dieting or fasting between binges. In many individuals with bulimia nervosa, a variety of purging behaviors are utilized following binge eating in a desperate effort to avoid weight gain.

Another characteristic of bulimia nervosa is dissatisfaction with one's body shape or weight. For many, this may evolve into a significant degree of obsessional preoccupation. This is coupled with a self-evaluation that is overly influenced by these physical characteristics. Such overly critical self-evaluation can have a profound effect on self-esteem, as evidenced, in part, by the majority of patients presenting with comorbid depressive symptomatology. A notable degree of impulsivity is encountered in many individuals with bulimia nervosa, and associated behaviors reflecting this characterological dimension include, in some, substance abuse, sexual promiscuity, and stealing or shoplifting.

5. DIFFERENTIAL DIAGNOSIS

Few medical or psychiatric disorders present in such a manner as to confound the diagnosis of bulimia nervosa. Frequently, it is the finding of certain physical signs or symptoms in a young woman, who does not admit to binge-eating or purging behaviors, that leads the clinician on a search for some other primary medical diagnosis. Usually, the complaints are a direct result or consequence of self-induced vomiting and diuretic or laxative use. Signs and symptoms associated with gastritis, esophagitis, dehydration, or electrolyte disturbances lead to consultation with primary care physicians or to emergency room visits, postponing psychiatric consultation and evading more primary interventions.

Because significant affective symptoms frequently accompany the presentation of bulimia nervosa, and because bulimic individuals may initially be hesitant to admit to the extent of their eating-disorder behaviors, one needs to distinguish an eating disorder from a primary depressive disorder. Although antidepressants are effective treatment for both disorders, the treatment of bulimia generally requires a multimodal approach with more specific attention paid to particular eating-related behaviors and cognitions in order to achieve and sustain a marked improvement (*see* Chapter 2). Treatment of the associated depressive symptoms alone, without recognition of the underlying eating disorder, will lead to suboptimal management of both disturbances, with probable persistence of bulimia. One needs also to recognize or rule out personality disorders, because certain features associated with bulimia nervosa, such as impulsivity, may be seen as evidence of primary character pathology and limit further evaluation of disordered eating. Such patients may be initially referred for more dynamic psychotherapy, which may not address specific bulimic symptoms as appropriately as is generally required to effect a marked change. Importantly, one must distinguish bulimia from anorexia. If the patient is underweight and amenorrheic, and is binge eating and purging, she has anorexia nervosa, binge–purge subtype, rather than bulimia nervosa.

6. MEDICAL COMPLICATIONS

The majority of medical complications caused by bulimia nervosa are consequences of purging behaviors. Self-induced vomiting can lead to gastritis, esophagitis, periodontal disease, and dental caries, the latter caused by the corrosive effect of acidic stomach contents on the dental enamel. Gastric dilitation and gastric or esophageal rupture are rare medical emergencies that may lead to shock. Metabolic alkalosis with the development of clinically significant hypokalemia in patients who vomit is not unusual, and serum electrolytes will reveal typical indices. Electrocardiogram changes in this setting carry significant import, because arrhythmias can lead to cardiac arrest if hypokalemia and related disturbances are not effectively corrected. Use of diuretics can cause similar electrolyte disturbances. Metabolic acidosis can be encountered in those who use large numbers of stimulant-type laxatives. Dehydration, sometimes requiring intravenous hydration, can accompany each of the aforementioned purging behaviors. More often associated with bulimic behaviors are general physical complaints, such as fatigue and muscle aches. Although becoming less frequently encountered in clinical practice, long-term use of the emetic syrup of ipecac can lead to myopathies, including, most seriously, cardiomyopathy. The latter is not an infrequent cause of death in patients abusing this toxic substance.

7. CONCLUSION

Patients with bulimia nervosa or exhibiting the spectrum of eating-disorder behaviors associated with this syndrome have become increasingly common in clinical practice. This apparent increase in bulimic symptomatology has stimulated research interest that, in turn, has informed treatment strategies. Given the significant psychiatric and medical morbidity encountered in patients with bulimia nervosa, efforts should be made to improve recognition and ensure proper referral. The development of effective psychotherapies and adjunctive pharmacological treatments, in conjunction with the public's growing awareness, should encourage more individuals to present for management of their disorders. Further exploration into the biological underpinnings of bulimia, continued assessment of treatment outcome, and attempts to identify predictive patient characteristics should lead to more specific tailoring of therapy and enhancement of treatment response.

REFERENCES

1. Stunkard AJ. The current status of treatment of obesity in adults. In: Stunkard AJ, Stellar E, eds. Eating and Its Disorders. Raven, New York, NY, 1984, pp. 157–174.
2. Russell GFM. Metabolic, endocrine and psychiatric aspects of anorexia nervosa. Sci Basis Med Annu Rev 1969; 14:236–255.
3. American Psychiatric Association. Diagnostic and Statistical Manual of Mental Disorders, DSM-IV. American Psychiatric Association, Washington, DC, 1994, pp. 549–550.
4. Stangler RS, Printz AM. DSM-III: Psychiatric diagnosis in a university population. Am J Psychiatry 1980; 137:937–940.
5. Johnson CL. Bulimia: A descriptive survey of 316 cases. Int J Eat Disord 1982; 2:3–16.
6. Pyle RL, Mitchell JE, Eckert ED, Halvorson PA, Neuman PA, Goff GM. The incidence of bulimia in freshman college students. Int J Eat Disord 1983; 2:75–86.
7. Carter JA, Duncan PA. Binge eating and vomiting: A survey of a high school population. Psychol Schools 1984; 21:198–203.
8. Abraham SF, Mira M, Llewellyn-Jones D. Eating behaviors amongst young women. Med J Austr 1983; 2:225–228.
9. Halmi KA, Falk JR, Schwartz E. Binge-eating and vomiting: a survey of a college population. Psychol Med 1981; 11:697–706.
10. Strober M. A family study of anorexia nervosa. Paper presented at the International Conference on Anorexia Nervosa and Related Disorders. Swansea University College, Wales, UK, 1984.
11. Lilenfeld LR, Kaye WH, Greeno CG, et al. A controlled family study of anorexia nervosa and bulimia nervosa: psychiatric disorders in first-degree relatives and effects of proband comorbidity. Arch Gen Psychiatry. 1998; 55:603–610.
12. Strober M, Freeman R, Lampert C, Diamond J, Kaye W. Controlled family study of anorexia nervosa and bulimia nervosa: evidence of shared liability and transmission of partial syndromes. Am J Psychiatry. 2000; 157:393–401.
13. Stein D, Lilenfeld LR, Plotnicov K, et al. Familial aggregation of eating disorders: results from a controlled family study of bulimia nervosa. Int J Eat Disord. 1999; 26:211–215.
14. Winokur A, March V, Mendels J. Primary affective disorder in relatives of patients with anorexia nervosa. Am J Psychiatry 1980; 137:695–698.
15. Hudson PL, Pope HG, Jonas JM, Todd D. Family history study of anorexia nervosa and bulimia. Br J Psychiatry 1983; 142:133–138.
16. Gershon ES, Schreiber Jl, Hamovit JR, Dibble ED, Kaye W, Nurnberger JI, et al. Clinical findings in patients with anorexia nervosa and affective illness in their relatives. Am J Psychiatry 1984; 141: 1419–1422.
17. Rivinius TM, Biderman J, Hertzog DB, et al. Anorexia nervosa and affective disorders: a controlled family history study. Am J Psychiatry 1984; 141:1414–1418.
18. Piran, N, Kennedy S, Garfinkel PE, Owens M. Affective disturbance in eating disorders. J Nerv Ment Dis 1985; 173:395-400.
19. Walsh BT, Roose SP, Glassman AH, Gladis M, Sadik C. Bulimia and depression. Psychosom Med 1985; 47:123–131.
20. Laessle R, Kittl S, Fichter M, Wittchen HU, Pirke KM. Major affective disorder in anorexia nervosa and bulimia: a descriptive diagnostic study. Br J Psychiatry 1987; 151:785–789.
21. Braun DL, Sunday SR, Halmi KA. Psychiatric comorbidity in patients with eating disorders. Psychol Med 1994; 24:859–867.
22. Powers PS, Coovert DL, Brightwell BR, Stevens BA. Other psychiatric disorders among bulimic patients. Compr Psychiatry 1988; 29:503–508.

23. Wonderlich S, et al. DSM-III-R personality disorders in patients with eating disorders. Int J Eat Disord 1990; 9:607–616.
24. Gartner AF, Marcus RN, Halmi KA, Loranger AW. DSM-III-R personality disorders in patients with eating disorders. Am J Psychiatry 1989; 146:1585–1591.
25. Schmidt MB, Telch MJ. Prevalence of personality disorders among bulimics, non-bulimic binge eaters and normal controls. J Psychopath Behav Ess 1990; 12:170–185.
26. Ames-Frankel J, Devlin NJ, Walsh BT, et al. Personality disorder diagnoses in patients with bulimia nervosa: clinical correlates and changes with treatment. J Clin Psychiatry 1992; 53:90–96.
27. Herzog DB. Are anorexic and bulimic patients depressed. Am J Psych 1984; 141:1594–1597.
28. Hatsukami D, Eckert E, Mitchell JE, Pyle R. Affective disorder and substance abuse in women with bulimia. Psychol Med 1984; 14:701–704.
29. Mitchell J, Hatsukami D, Eckert E, Pyle R. Characteristics of 275 patients with bulimia. Am J Psychiatry 1985; 142:482–485.
30. Bulik C. Drug and alcohol abuse by bulimic women and their families. Am J Psychiatry 1987; 144: 1604–1606.

2 Counseling Patients With Bulimia Nervosa

Tricia Cook Myers and James E. Mitchell

KEY POINTS

- The first step of treatment is careful evaluation of physical, behavioral, and psychiatric status of the patient.
- The patient needs periodic monitoring of physical, behavioral, and psychiatric status as part of therapy.
- Counseling includes self-monitoring, prescription of regular and balanced meals, and behavioral and cognitive therapy.

1. INTRODUCTION

This chapter is designed to provide an introduction to the basic principles of counseling outpatients with bulimia nervosa who are being seen in a general medical setting. A summary of these principles and chapter outline is presented in Table 1. The purpose is not to make psychiatrists or counselors out of family physicians or other generalists, but rather to improve patient care and to briefly review some basic principles that can be useful in an office setting when working with these patients. Emphasis is placed on a few issues that may significantly increase the likelihood that cases of bulimia nervosa will be detected and that individuals with bulimia nervosa will become engaged in treatment and will take the first steps in the process of recovering from this disorder.

2. ASSESSMENT OF THE PATIENT

The first step for the physician is a thorough assessment of the patient. In the case of an individual with bulimia nervosa, this requires a detailed assessment of the various normal and abnormal eating and eating-related behaviors that may be present *(1)*. This assessment (*see also* Chapter 1) will lead the physician logically into treatment planning. Here, we discuss the issues that should be addressed in the assessment.

2.1. Weight

A careful weight history is essential. This includes an assessment of the patient's current height and weight (and calculations of the percent of ideal body weight), as well

From: *The Management of Eating Disorders and Obesity, Second Edition*
Edited by: D. J. Goldstein © Humana Press Inc., Totowa, NJ

Table 1
Chapter Overview

as high and low weight during adulthood, and, in particular, any history of being markedly overweight or underweight. Also, a family history of obesity is useful information in that there is a high heritability for adult body weight. As a corollary, it is very useful to evaluate how these patients feel at their current weight in general, and how they feel about specific body parts in particular. Many patients with eating disorders are very concerned about body weight, but others worry specifically about certain body parts, particularly their waist, hips, buttocks, and thighs. It is of note that these are the areas with which many young women in the general population are dissatisfied even if they are of normal weight.

2.2. Meal Pattern

It is useful to sketch out the meal pattern, including what the patient is eating and the frequency and timing of meals and snacks. Obtaining a specific dietary history is generally superior to a generalization about "usual" intake. Does the intake appear adequate? Most individuals with eating disorders markedly restrict food intake when not binge eating, and important goals of treatment are not only to suppress or eliminate binge eating, but also to increase the number of regular meals and snacks as a way of minimizing the dietary restriction that leads to binge eating.

2.3. Eating-Related Behaviors

There should be a very careful assessment of the presence of abnormal eating-related behaviors such as binge eating (2). This includes the age of onset, duration and frequency of the symptoms, and any periods of remission. Behaviors that should be assessed in addition to binge eating are as follow: self-induced vomiting, use of laxatives for weight control, use of diuretics or diet medication pills (number per day, type), and any use of serum of ipecac to stimulate vomiting (3). In obtaining this information, it is important to use a straightforward, nonjudgmental approach when questioning.

It is also important to elicit information about other behaviors that at times are associated with eating disorders, including excessive exercise, protracted fasting, chewing and spitting out food without swallowing it, ruminating food, and, in rare situations, the use of saunas or enemas for weight control.

2.4. Associated Psychiatric Problems

Many patients with eating disorders have other associated psychiatric problems (1,4). Most commonly, these include mood disturbances (usually depression), problems with anxiety, substance use disorders, including alcohol abuse, and personality disorders. The assessment should also evaluate the presence or absence of each of these associated problems, and appropriate diagnoses should be made when indicated. This again may impact significantly on treatment planning.

2.5. Current Symptoms

In obtaining information about current symptoms, the review of systems should focus on areas that are often problems for patients with eating disorders. In bulimia nervosa, these would include salivary gland hypertrophy, abdominal bloating and postprandial distress, symptoms of dehydration, constipation and diarrhea, edema, and any evidence of blood loss with vomitus or through laxative-induced diarrhea.

2.6. Screening

Generally, patients not only hesitate to initiate discussions about their bulimia nervosa, but they may also deny behaviors that might lead to diagnosis; there is evidence that fewer than 30% of general medical patients choose to discuss their eating disorder with their physician (5). Many patients with bulimia nervosa make every attempt to keep their disorders secret and because, unlike anorexia nervosa, there are often no overt signs of bulimia nervosa, many cases go undetected in primary care settings. Instead of discussing their eating behaviors, patients may complain of menstrual disturbances or generalized abdominal distress. As a consequence, physicians should routinely elicit information about dieting, patterns of eating, and body-image concerns, and may want to consider adding a two- to five-item screening tool to their review of systems when they routinely evaluate patients. Although there is no gold standard, validation is under way on several brief screening measures (6–8).

3. MEDICAL MONITORING

Fortunately, most patients with bulimia nervosa are medically stable, and the medical mortality from this disorder is very rare. However, there are certain issues that may be of concern and several laboratory parameters that often require monitoring (9).

3.1. Laboratory Evaluation

Serum electrolyte determination is usually the most important test for patients with bulimia nervosa. The classical pattern seen in bulimia nervosa patients is hypochloremic, and possibly hypokalemic, metabolic alkalosis. Evidence of severe alkalosis or hypokalemia is indicative of predisposition to organ failure. Fortunately, such severe abnormalities are rare. In attempting to correct a dehydration-associated alkalosis and hypokalemia, potassium supplementation should be accompanied by the strong advice to increase fluid intake because much of the potassium loss is attributable to the volume concentration. The presentation and physical examination can guide the choice of other laboratory tests. Any suggestion of pancreatitis or salivary gland changes should be evaluated with serum amylase, and lipase, and ipecac abuse should be evaluated with careful assessment of cardiovascular status *(3)*.

3.2. Dehydration

Laxative and diuretic abuse frequently results in profound dehydration acutely and reflex edema when they are discontinued. In managing abuse of these medications, the best approach is abrupt discontinuation of these drugs. In the case of laxative abuse, one sees reflex constipation after discontinuation; therefore, patients should be counseled to eat a high-fiber diet, avoid adding salt to their diet, and, if necessary, use a stool softener. Lactulose can be added if needed, but stimulant-type laxatives should be avoided if at all possible. Generally, fluid retention will remit within 7 to 10 d, and most patients will start having relatively regular bowel movements by then. Although some clinicians have advocated gradual reduction in the use of these drugs, this probably only prolongs the process and abrupt discontinuation should be encouraged.

4. SPECIFIC COUNSELING STRATEGIES

The following interventions should be considered: teaching the patient to begin self-monitoring *(10,11)*; the prescription of a pattern of regular, balanced meals *(12)*; and behavioral and cognitive-behavioral techniques for behavior control *(13–16)*. All of these can be inititiated by the physician; however, one-third of the cases probably will eventually require the involvement of a psychotherapist.

4.1. Self-Monitoring

Self-monitoring is very important for several reasons. Many patients with bulimia nervosa are not completely aware of the severity of their behavior. Thus, self-monitoring can be very useful to help patients begin to realistically appraise their current pattern. It also significantly improves eating behavior in bulimia nervosa. Patients are asked to record all food intake and any episodes of binge eating and vomiting with the times indicated. Patients can self-monitor using specific forms provided to facilitate this process or on a plain sheet of paper. It is important to have patients monitor not only the problem eating behaviors such as binge eating and vomiting, but also the healthier eating behaviors in hopes that these records can be used to point out both deficiencies and strengths in dietary intake *(13)*. It is important to remember, and to communicate to the patient, that dietary restriction during most of the day is a very important determinant of binge eating and that many patients will markedly decrease the frequency of their binge-eating and purging behavior if they develop a more regular pattern of intake. Self-monitoring forms can be very useful in shaping this improved pattern.

4.2. Prescription of Regular, Balanced Meals

The prescription of regular food intake, with at least minimal intake every 4 h, can be helpful for patients in terms of gaining control of their eating behavior (12). It is also important to remember that many patients seem to have lost a normal sense of hunger and satiety, and most try to restrict their intake early in the day knowing that they may binge eat later when returning home from work or school. Therefore, the physician, or the dietitian working in cooperation with the physician, should prescribe the regular intake of three meals and two to three small snacks, with enough calories to ensure that the patient will not be severely hungry at the end of the day, when binge eating is most likely to occur.

4.2.1. FLEXIBILITY

It is also important to try to encourage flexibility in the diet (12). Many patients with bulimia nervosa avoid certain "feared" foods. Often, these are foods that they perceive as high in fat content. Although it is important to encourage flexibility and variety from the beginning, often it is helpful to recommend that patients avoid feared foods early in treatment because these foods may precipitate binge eating. Thus, initially patients should eat only those foods that they are willing to eat without purging. Patients should later be encouraged to gradually reintroduce these foods into their diet.

4.2.2. SYMPATHETIC BUT FIRM APPROACH

It is important for the clinician to remember that both of these interventions-self-monitoring and nutritional counseling-are confrontational issues that patients with bulimia nervosa may strongly resist. Many bulimic patients will not self-monitor when initially asked to do so, and most will have a great deal of difficulty instituting a pattern of regular, balanced meals. A tolerant and sympathetic, yet firm, approach will often yield improved results. In particular, the physician must make sure that the records or homework assignments from the previous week are carefully reviewed with the patient. If the practitioner does not clearly place importance on the records, neither will the patient. Problems with self-monitoring and with the meal pattern should be pointed out, and specific suggestions should be offered.

4.3. Behavioral and Cognitive-Behavioral Counseling

The third intervention—the behavioral and cognitive-behavioral component—has been effective in controlled trials (1,4,10,13–15,17–22). Nevertheless, the typical practitioner will not have the time or expertise to embark on a full course of psychotherapy using these techniques. However, there are certain techniques that can be used if the opportunity arises while the practitioner sees the patient.

4.3.1. CONCENTRATE ON SUCCESS

Have patients concentrate on "what works." For example, if patients come in for an appointment and report that they have been able to go for several days without binge eating, it is important to focus on how this was accomplished. Were they busy doing other things? Were they able to eat regular meals and therefore were not as hungry? Were they feeling better about themselves for some other reason? If something works, it is a good idea to try to figure out what it was and to use it again.

4.3.2. TEACH NORMAL WEIGHT EXPECTATIONS

Most patients with bulimia nervosa are convinced that if they start eating regular, balanced meals, they will gain weight. With the exception of those patients who retain fluid during withdrawal from laxatives or diuretics, most patients with bulimia nervosa do not gain weight when they start eating regularly, although there are exceptions. It is best to encourage tolerance of minor weight gain or fluctuations but to stress that overall they should not gain a substantial amount of weight. Patients should be instructed to weigh themselves one morning each week in order to reassure themselves that the recommended dietary changes have not resulted in inordinate weight gain. Indeed, patients may be better able to control their weight, and their weight will be more stable over time, if they are able to control the binge-eating and vomiting behavior.

4.3.3. MAINTAIN AN ACTIVE LIFESTYLE

Put simply, it is important for patients to stay busy at the times when they are most prone to binge eating and vomiting, a strategy known as behavioral alternatives. Typically, patients engage in binge eating in the evening, when they are home alone. Therefore, if they engage in activities that are incompatible with binge eating and purging (e.g., call a friend, go to a public place), the behaviors will be much less likely to occur. Identifying high-risk periods and developing a repertoire of alternative behaviors at those times can prove quite useful.

4.3.4. IDENTIFY CUES

Many patients are able to identify specific cues in their environment that seem to be associated with binge-eating episodes. A frequent stimulus is hunger induced by a long period of dietary restriction. Another common trigger is boredom. Patients with bulimia nervosa tend to binge eat, and then vomit, during periods of time when nothing much else is going on. The behaviors often become institutionalized; individuals tend to engage in binge eating and vomiting at set times, such as right when they return home after work or school. Therefore, preplanning alternatives for high-risk times can be a very powerful deterrent to binge eating and vomiting.

4.3.5. HIGHLY STRUCTURED COUNSELING

Although all of these techniques can be quite useful, the literature suggests that the best counseling approach for patients with bulimia nervosa is a highly structured one. This includes individual or group therapy sessions conducted once or twice each week and involves a therapist specifically trained in cognitive-behavioral techniques *(23)*. Such therapy can result in dramatic reductions in the frequency of target behaviors and, in the majority of cases, will result in a complete remission of symptoms, as well as improvement in associated problems such as depression, self-esteem, and impaired interpersonal relationships.

4.4. Self-Help Manuals and Internet-Based Counseling

Recently, self-help manuals and Internet-based counseling (*see* Chapter 8) have been used to supplement treatment. Drug therapy has been combined with the use of a self-help manual provided to the patient, and use of a manual alone as the first choice in a stepped care approach to treatment has also been used. Internet-based counseling has also been used as an adjunct to office treatment. The results thus far obtained have been mixed, and further study is necessary before these strategies can be recommended.

5. MEDICATIONS AND REFERRAL FOR COUNSELING

Relative to initial treatment, however, the preferred sequence remains a matter of debate. Some advocate conservative management including the use of antidepressants; others favor an initial approach including psychotherapy with or without antidepressants *(21,23–29)*. The use of medications in treating bulimia nervosa is discussed in Chapter 3.

The practitioner should certainly consider referring patients to a professional counselor if cost is not an obstacle to obtaining these services and if therapists well trained in the techniques shown to work with these patients are available. Unfortunately, well-trained therapists are often unavailable, because many therapists are not formally trained in the specific forms of therapy shown to help these patients in controlled trials. Fortunately, medications that are helpful for many of these patients are widely available and decrease the need for referral.

The primary physician can encourage the patient to engage in self-monitoring, stress the importance of regular meal intake, and prescribe an antidepressant such as fluoxetine hydrochloride. Fluoxetine has been shown to help reduce binge-eating episodes in bulimia nervosa patients when prescribed at higher dosages (60 mg/d) *(21,25–26)*. Even at the higher dosage, most patients experience minimal or no side effects, and if any occur, such as nausea or insomnia, they are usually transitory. Therefore, the physician should be aggressive in escalating the dosage or might initiate treatment at 60 mg/d. Alternative selective seratonin reuptake inhibitors have not been studied systematically but are used clinically. However, if this regimen of physician encouragement, education, monitoring, and medication management is not found to be helpful, the patient may be referred to a professional counselor to facilitate recovery.

In the event that referral is necessary, communication between the general practitioner and counselor can be beneficial in several ways. This interplay can ensure that both professionals are receiving the same "message" from the patient regarding his or her progress in recovery. It also permits both professionals to provide the patient with a common approach. Additionally, this communication can keep counselors aware of any physical symptoms the patient may be experiencing and any changes in medication that may affect the patient's mental state.

However, it is important to remember that the advice and encouragement of the primary physician, who places a strong emphasis on improving the pattern of regular food intake and on self-monitoring of problematic and normal eating behavior, can go a long way in starting the patient in the process of recovery.

6. CONCLUSION

Treatment of bulimia nervosa begins with the initial evaluation. Because patients with bulimia nervosa often try to hide their eating behaviors, screening questions should be incorporated as a routine evaluation of patients. Eliciting specific eating behaviors during an initial evaluation will serve as an early guide to self-monitoring. Although many aspects of the disorder and its therapy can be generalized, each patient needs to be treated as an individual, with the patient's symptoms guiding both the laboratory evaluation and therapeutic recommendations. During therapy, the patient's behaviors should be periodically reevaluated. As treatment progresses, successful interventions and circumstances that produce setbacks to therapy need to be addressed in the treatment plan. Many patients will benefit from medication, although others will require referral to experts.

ACKNOWLEDGMENTS

This work was supported in part by the Neuropsychiatric Research Institute, a Center Grant on Eating Disorders Research from the McKnight Foundation, and a National Institutes of Health Obesity Center Grant.

REFERENCES

1. Lacey JH. Bulimia nervosa, binge-eating and psychogenic vomiting: a controlled treatment study and long-term outcome. Br Med J 1983; 286:1609–1613.
2. Mitchell JE, Hatsukami D, Eckert ED. Characteristics of 275 patients with bulimia. Am J Psychiatry 1985; 142:482–485.
3. Mitchell JE, Pomeroy C, Huber M. A clinician's guide to the eating disorders medicine cabinet. Int J Eat Disord 1988; 7:211–223.
4. Mitchell JE, Pyle RL, Pomeroy C, et al. Cognitive-behavioral group psychotherapy of bulimia nervosa: importance of logistical variables. Int J Eat Disord 1993; 14:277–287.
5. Fairburn CG, Cooper PJ. Self-induced vomiting and bulimia nervosa: an undetected problem. Br Med J 1982; 284:1153–1155.
6. Morgan JF, Reid F, Lacey JH. The SCOFF questionnaire: assessment of a new screening tool for eating disorders. Br Med J 1999; 4:1467–1468.
7. Freund KM, Boxx RD, Handleman EK, Smith AD. Secret patterns: validation of a screening tool to detect bulimia. J Women's Health Gend Based Med 1999; 8:1281–1284.
8. Anstine D, Grinenko D. Rapid screening for disordered eating in college-aged females in the primary care setting. J Adolesc Health 2000; 26:338–342.
9. Halmi KA. Medical aberrations in bulimia nervosa. In: Kaye WH, Gwirtsman HE, eds. A Comprehensive Approach to the Treatment of Normal Weight Bulimia. American Psychiatry Press, Washington, DC, 1985, pp. 37–46.
10. Agras WS, Rossiter EM, Arnow B, et al. Pharmacologic and cognitive-behavioral treatment for bulimia nervosa: a controlled comparison. Am J Psychiatry 1992; 149:82–87.
11. Connors ME, Johnson CL, Stuckey MK. Treatment of bulimia with brief psycho educational group therapy. Am J Psychiatry 1984; 141:1512–1516.
12. Boutacoff LI, Zollman MR, Mitchell JE. Healthy Eating: A Meal Planning System. Unpublished manual. University of Minnesota, Minneapolis, MN, 1984.
13. Fairburn CG, Kirk J, O'Connor M, Cooper PJ. A comparison of two psychological treatments for bulimia nervosa. Behav Res Ther 1986; 24:629–643.
14. Fairburn CG, Jones R, Peveler RC, et al. Three psychological treatments for bulimia nervosa: a comparative trial. Arch Gen Psychiatry 1991; 48:463–469.
15. Fairburn CG, Jones R, Peveler RC, Hope RA, O'Connor M. Psychotherapy and bulimia nervosa: the longer term effects of interpersonal psychotherapy, behavioral therapy, and cognitive behavior therapy for bulimia nervosa. Arch Gen Psychiatry 1993; 50:419–428.
16. Mitchell JE, Pyle RL, Hatsckami D. Bulimia Nervosa: Individual Treatment Manual. Unpublished manual. University of Minnesota, Minneapolis, MN, 1987.
17. Freeman CPL, Munro JKM. Drug and group treatments for bulimia/bulimia nervosa. J Psychosom Res 1988; 32:647–660.
18. Garner DM. Cognitive therapy for bulimia nervosa. Adolesc Psychiatry 1986; 13:358–390.
19. Kirkley BG, Schneider JA, Agras WS, Bachman JA. Comparison of two group treatments for bulimia. J Consult Clin Psychol 1985; 5:43–48.
20. Mitchell JE, Pyle RL, Eckert ED, Hatsukami D, Pomeroy C, Zimmerman R. A comparison study of antidepressants and structured intensive group psychotherapy in the treatment of bulimia nervosa. Arch Gen Psychiatry 1990; 47:149–157.

21. Mitchell JE, Raymond N, Specker S. A review of the controlled trials of pharmacotherapy in psycho-therapy in the treatment of bulimia nervosa. Int J Eat Disord 1993; 14:229–247.
22. Ordman AM, Kirschenbaum DS. Cognitive-behavioral therapy for bulimia: an initial outcome study. J Consult Clin Psychol 1985; 53:305–313.
23. Crosby RD, Mitchell JE, Raymond N, Specker S, Nugent S, Pyle R. Survival analysis of response to group psychotherapy in bulimia nervosa. Int J Eat Disord 1993; 13:359–368.
24. Abbott DW, Mitchell JE. Antidepressants vs. psychotherapy in the treatment of bulimia nervosa. Psychopharmacol Bull 1993; 29:115–119.
25. Fluoxetine Bulimia Nervosa Collaborative Study Group. Fluoxetine in the treatment of bulimia nervosa. Arch Gen Psychiatry 1992; 49:139–147.
26. Goldstein DJ, Wilson MG, Thompson VL, Potvin JH, Rampey Jr AH for the Fluoxetine Bulimia Nervosa Research Group. Long-term fluoxetine treatment of bulimia nervosa. Br J Psychiatry 1995; 166:660–666.
27. Herzog DB, Keller MB, Lavori PW. Outcome in anorexia nervosa and bulimia nervosa: a review of the literature. J Nerv Ment Dis 1988; 176:131–143.
28. Walsh T. Pharmacological treatment of bulimia. In: Halmi KA, ed. Psychobiology and Treatment of Anorexia Nervosa and Bulimia Nervosa. American Psychiatric Press, Washington, DC, 1992, pp. 329–431.
29. Walsh BT, Devlin MJ. The pharmacologic treatment of eating disorders. Psych Clin N Am 1992; 15: 149–160.

3 Pharmacological Therapy of Bulimia Nervosa

James I. Hudson, Harrison G. Pope, Jr., and William P. Carter

KEY POINTS

- Antidepressant medications have been shown to be effective in treating bulimia nervosa in placebo-controlled trials.
- Antidepressants should not be reserved only for bulimic patients who are depressed because antidepressants are equally effective in bulimic patients who are not depressed.
- Other medical treatments have been studied, but available data is sparse.
- Treatment with antidepressants does not preclude counseling or vice versa, but may be based on availabilty of counseling expertise.
- Some patients may require trials of different antidepressants to achieve efficacy.

1. INTRODUCTION

Pharmacological therapy is increasingly used in the management of patients with bulimia nervosa. Since the 1980s, many studies have reported beneficial effects of antidepressants and other agents for bulimia nervosa, and a large amount of clinical experience has also accumulated over this time period. In this chapter, we review the evidence for the efficacy of antidepressants and other medications, and provide guidelines for clinical practice based on this evidence and our experience (*see* Table 1).

2. EFFICACY OF ANTIDEPRESSANTS IN BULIMIA NERVOSA

2.1. Placebo-Controlled Studies of Marketed Antidepressants

We searched the literature for placebo-controlled trials of medications, marketed in the United States as "antidepressants," that have been studied in the treatment of bulimia nervosa and had adequate available documentation to permit analysis. We found 16 studies: 10 of tricyclic antidepressants *(1–10)*, 3 of selective serotonin reuptake inhibitors (SSRIs) *(11–13)*, 1 of monoamine oxidase inhibitors (MAOIs) *(14)*, and 2 of other

From: *The Management of Eating Disorders and Obesity, Second Edition*
Edited by: D. J. Goldstein © Humana Press Inc., Totowa, NJ

Table 1
Chapter Overview

antidepressant agents (trazodone *[15]*), bupropion *[16]*). All but one study *(13)* assessed acute treatment response in patients with active bulimia nervosa. The final study *(13)* assessed relapse prevention and involved treatment of patients with bulimia nervosa who had already responded to 8 wk of open-label treatment of bulimia. These studies are summarized in Table 2.

We excluded three studies of medications not marketed in the United States: one each of brofaromine *(17)*, isocarboxazid *(18)*, and mianserin *(19)*. The study of isocarboxazid found a significant benefit of drug vs placebo. The other two failed to find a significant difference between drug vs placebo but are difficult to interpret, in part because of very high placebo response rates. We also excluded one study *(20)* presented briefly in a letter to the editor (reporting an advantage of phenelzine and nomifensine vs placebo) and one study *(21)* that reported significant improvement of bulimic symptoms in patients with atypical depression.

The studies indicate that drugs from several different classes of antidepressants reduce the frequency of binges and the frequency of vomiting. Also, the great majority of studies have shown that antidepressants produce significant benefit on various measures of global improvement and of attitudes toward food and weight. In addition, the one study of relapse prevention *(13)* found that fluoxetine was associated with a significantly longer time to relapse of bulimia nervosa compared with placebo.

Furthermore, several studies have shown a significant improvement in the patients' depressive symptoms on medication vs placebo, although others have shown equivocal or no improvement on these indices. Interpretation of these results is limited by at least two considerations. First, only a minority of patients in these studies had current major depressive disorder, and many bulimic patients started treatment with little or no associated depressive symptomatology. Thus, when studies report that "depression" or "depressive symptoms" failed to improve, it cannot be determined whether this finding was caused by a failure of medication treatment to change these symptoms or whether it merely reflected a low baseline level of symptoms that could not be improved appreciably.

Table 2
Placebo-Controlled Studies of Antidepressants in Bulimia Nervosa [a]

Study (reference)	Drug (maximum dose)	Number of subjects [b]	Duration of trial [c]	Design [d]	Response to drug [e]
Tricyclics					
Mitchell and Groat, 1984 (1)	Amitriptyline 150 mg	32	8 wk	Parallel group	+
Hughes et al., 1986 (2)	Desipramine 200 mg	22	6 wk	Parallel group	++
Barlow et al., 1988 (3)	Desipramine 150 mg	47	6 wk	Crossover	++
Blouin et al., 1988 (4)	Desipramine 150 mg	10	6 wk	Crossover	++
McCann and Agras, 1990 (5)	Desipramine 300 mg	23	12 wk	Parallel group	++
Walsh et al., 1991 (6)	Desipramine 300 mg	68	6 wk	Parallel group	++
Pope et al., 1983 (7)	Imipramine 200 mg	19	6 wk	Parallel group	++
Agras et al., 1987 (8)	Imipramine 300 mg	20	16 wk	Parallel group	++
Mitchell et al, 1990 (9)	Imipramine 200 mg	74	12 wk	Parallel group	++
Alger et al., 1991 (10)	Imipramine 200 mg	15	8 wk	Parallel group	0
Selective serotonin reuptake inhibitors					
Fluoxetine Bulimia Collaborative Study Group, 1992 (11)	Fluoxetine 20/60 mg	387	8 wk	Parallel group	+/++
Goldstein et al., 1995 (12)	Fluoxetine 60 mg	398	16 wk	Parallel group	++
Romano et al., 2002 (13)	Fluoxetine 60 mg	150 [f]	52 wk [g]	Parallel group	++
Monoamine oxidase inhibitors					
Walsh et al., 1988 (14)	Phenelzine 90 mg	50	8 wk	Parallel group	++
Other antidepressants					
Horne et al., 1988 (15)	Bupropion 450 mg	81	8 wk	Parallel group	++
Pope et al., 1989 (16)	Trazodone	42	6 wk	Parallel group	++

[a] Restricted to medications marketed currently in the United States

[b] Number of subjects receiving drug or placebo who completed the trial or enough of the trial to be included in data analysis

[c] Period of time that subjects received active drug rather than total duration of the study

[d] All studies were randomized, placebo-controlled, double-blind trials; all but Romano et al. (13) were acute treatment of individuals with active bulimia nervosa; Romano et al. (13) was a relapse-prevention study of those who had responded to bulimia nervosa after 8 wk fluoxetine treatment

[e] For all studies except Romano et al. (13): ++, drug significantly superior to placebo in reducing frequency of binges and/or frequency of vomiting; +, some evidence that drug superior to placebo but not clearly significant; 0, little or no difference between drug and placebo. For Romano et al. (13): response of ++ indicates time to relapse was significantly longer for fluoxetine compared with placebo

[f] Subjects who were randomly assigned to fluoxetine or placebo after meeting response criteria after 8-wk treatment with fluoxetine

[g] Duration of randomized treatment following initial 8-wk treatment with fluoxetine.

Second, measures of "depressive symptoms" include many items in addition to depressed mood (such as sleep disturbance, appetite disturbance, and anxiety) that are not specific to depression, but occur in a wide range of conditions. Thus, when studies report that "depressive symptoms" improved, it is unclear what symptoms may have changed. In short, we can draw few definitive conclusions about the effects of antidepressants on depressive symptoms in patients with bulimia nervosa.

Because most of these studies were relatively small, it is difficult to assess whether there are any predictors of a favorable response to antidepressants among bulimic patients. One finding is quite clear, however: bulimic patients respond to antidepressant medications equally well regardless of whether they exhibit symptoms of depression. For example, one study (12,22) found that response to fluoxetine was independent of ratings on the Hamilton Rating Scale for Depression and independent of the presence or absence of current major depression or lifetime major depression. Also, two studies (2,15) specifically excluded bulimic patients with current major depressive disorder, but nevertheless found response rates comparable to those of studies that included depressed bulimic patients. Also, no study has found significantly different rates of improvement in nondepressed vs depressed patients.

Only 2 of the 16 studies, both using tricyclics (1,10), failed to find significant differences between drug and placebo on frequency of binges or frequency of vomiting episodes. However, these negative results may have been caused by methodologic limitations of the studies. In the first study (1), whereas the amitriptyline-treated group had a greater than 70% mean reduction in frequency of binges and vomiting, the placebo-treated group had a greater than 50% mean reduction, perhaps because "minimal behavioral therapy" was also employed. In the other study (10), only 7 patients were treated with imipramine; thus, the failure to find a significant drug–placebo difference in efficacy may have represented a type II error (failure to detect a significant difference when in fact one exists) because of the very small sample. On balance, then, the weight of the evidence strongly suggests that antidepressants are superior to placebo in the short-term treatment of bulimia nervosa.

For the most part, these studies have found antidepressants to be well tolerated and safe in the treatment of bulimia nervosa. The one important exception is that bupropion was associated with a high incidence of grand mal seizures (4 of 55 bupropion-treated patients) in the only controlled study using this drug in bulimia nervosa (15). Although it is impossible to assess the relative tolerance of bulimic patients to the various antidepressant medications, because studies have not compared medications directly to one another, it appears that the SSRI fluoxetine is the best-tolerated medication and that the MAOI phenelzine—despite excellent efficacy—is associated with more adverse effects than other agents.

After examining these studies, several methodologic limitations should be noted. First, most of the studies were of short duration, with a median of 8 wk, and all but five employed less than 3 mo of drug treatment. Thus, few address the potential long-term efficacy of these agents (see Subheading 2.2.). Second, many of the studies involved small sample sizes, with the majority reporting fewer than 15 patients per treatment group; only the three studies with fluoxetine enrolled more than 50 patients per group. It is noteworthy, however, that despite these small sample sizes, most of the studies nevertheless produced highly significant differences between drug and placebo, suggesting that antidepressants are associated with a large beneficial effect in bulimia nervosa. Third, two studies *(3,4)* used a crossover design, which has potential difficulties with maintenance of blinding and with carry-over effects. Fourth, although all studies used the frequency of eating binges or vomiting as the primary outcome measures, the studies varied considerably in their choice of secondary outcome measures, such as measures of global improvement, attitudes toward food and weight, and associated psychiatric symptoms.

A final consideration is that SSRIs have also been shown effective in placebo-controlled trials in the related condition, binge-eating disorder *(23–27)*, as discussed in Chapter 12.

2.2. Long-Term Antidepressant Studies

Only a few studies have examined the effect of antidepressant medications for more than 12 wk. Two of these were simple placebo-controlled trials *(8,12)*; one *(6)* was a complex design with placebo-controlled periods; one *(13)* was a relapse-prevention trial; two *(28–30)* were open-label tricyclic medication studies; and one *(18)* was an open-label follow-up of a placebo-controlled study of an MAOI.

In the two simple placebo-controlled trials, Agras and associates *(8)* found imipramine more effective than placebo, and Goldstein and colleagues *(12)* found fluoxetine more effective than placebo, both in 16-wk studies. Using a rather elaborate study design, Walsh and colleagues *(6)* randomized patients initially to either desipramine or placebo for 6 wk on a double-blind basis. At the end of 6 wk, they offered desipramine-responsive patients open maintenance treatment with desipramine for an additional 16 wk, and they offered placebo-treated nonresponders desipramine treatment for 6 wk. The placebo nonresponders who responded to desipramine were offered an additional 16 wk of open maintenance treatment with desipramine. Next, following this 24-wk total period of desipramine treatment, they randomized treatment responders to 26 wk of either desipramine or placebo. The investigators enrolled 80 subjects. Although they found good short-term response to desipramine, they gradually lost most subjects for a variety of reasons, such that only 21 patients entered and 11 completed the open maintenance period; and only 9 patients entered and 8 completed the final 24-wk period. Thus, this study documented high attrition using long-term desipramine therapy for bulimia nervosa.

In the relapse-prevention trial *(13)*, fluoxetine-treated subjects exhibited a significantly longer time to relapse than placebo-treated subjects. In addition, at endpoint, fluoxetine treatment was associated with significantly lower frequency of binges, frequency of vomiting, and global severity of illness compared with placebo.

Tricyclic medications were used nonblinded in two studies as one arm of treatment studies involving comparisons with psychotherapy alone or psychotherapy plus medications. One study *(28,29)* found that patients who received desipramine for 16 wk and then discontinued treatment were more likely to relapse by 32 wk and more likely to be doing poorly on 1-yr follow-up than patients who had received 24 wk of desipramine and then stopped. Another study *(30)* was designed to compare 20 wk of desipramine vs cognitive–behavioral therapy (CBT) vs combination treatment. However, this study was stopped prematurely because of a high drop-out rate, largely because of side effects in the group receiving desipramine treatment alone.

In the only long-term study using MAOIs, Kennedy and associates *(18)* reported that 1 yr after treatment in a placebo-controlled trial of isocarboxazid, 7 of 18 patients were doing well on isocarboxazid, and 11 patients had stopped the medication, mainly because of intolerable side effects.

Long-term studies of single agents are difficult to interpret because they do not reflect how medications are used in clinical practice, particularly in that there was no option of adding or switching drugs over the entire study interval. Extensive experience from clinical practice and data from several studies *(6,31–34)* have shown that most bulimic patients who fail to respond adequately to one antidepressant, or who tolerate it poorly, will achieve a beneficial response or better tolerance on another agent. Furthermore, in one of the single-agent studies *(28,29)*, medication was stopped after 16 or 24 wk and not reintroduced if symptoms reemerged. In clinical practice, one would usually stop medications only after at least 24 wk with an excellent response and would restart medication promptly if the patient had a relapse of symptoms. Thus, the single-agent studies almost certainly underestimate the efficacy of antidepressant treatment as it is actually practiced.

Our group reported two long-term open-label studies that followed patients using "doctor's choice" treatment. In these studies, patients who failed to respond to one agent were permitted to change to another. In the first *(32)*, we collected follow-up data for up to 2 yr on 20 bulimic patients who initially participated in a placebo-controlled study with imipramine *(7)*. At the time that the patients were last seen in follow-up, 10 (50%) of these subjects had experienced a complete remission of bulimic symptoms and 19 (95%) had experienced at least partial improvement. The only subject who did not exhibit improvement at last observation was a woman who had chosen to discontinue her antidepressant medication and who relapsed to her original level of bulimic symptoms. We also found that most subjects displayed a marked reduction in depressive symptoms, as well as bulimic symptoms, at follow-up. However, these encouraging findings were tempered by the observation that most subjects required one or more changes in antidepressant treatment over the course of the follow-up period, and only three subjects had successfully discontinued antidepressants at follow-up.

In the second long-term study *(33)*, we examined 36 bulimic patients who had participated in a placebo-controlled double-blind trial of trazodone. In this group, 26 patients had "pursued pharmacotherapy," meaning that they had been willing to try up to three different antidepressant medications if they had failed to respond. The remaining 10 subjects had not pursued pharmacotherapy to this degree. At follow-up, after 9 to 19 mo, 17 (65%) of those who had pursued pharmacotherapy had a remission of their bulimic symptoms, and 22 (88%) of this group had some improvement. By contrast, only 1 (10%) of the 10 patients who had failed to pursue pharmacotherapy exhibited a remission of bulimic symptoms, and 7 (70%) of these patients were unimproved or worse. These findings again suggest that considerable experimentation with antidepressants may be necessary to achieve an optimal result. Abandoning pharmacological treatment after only one or two trials may lead to inferior outcomes.

2.3. Open-Label Trials of Antidepressants

In addition to medications evaluated in placebo-controlled trials, several other antidepressants have been evaluated in open-label trials. They deserve mention either because they have proven to be useful treatment options in clinical practice or because they indicate possible future avenues for treatment.

Looking at tricyclics, we have consistently found nortriptyline effective in open-label trials *(31–33)*. Like desipramine, nortriptyline has two advantages relative to most other tricyclics: fewer anticholinergic effects and a well-established therapeutic range of plasma concentrations known to be effective in major depressive disorder. This range of plasma concentrations can be used as a confirmation of adequate dosage in the treatment of bulimia nervosa.

Although fluoxetine is the only member of the SSRI class whose efficacy has been established in placebo-controlled studies, case reports or small case series have reported beneficial effects for three other SSRIs currently marketed in the United States: fluvoxamine *(35,36)*, paroxetine *(37)*, and sertraline *(38)*.

Turning to MAOIs, we have reported tranylcypromine effective in open-label trials *(31–33)*. In clinical practice, we have found that tranylcypromine is often better tolerated than phenelzine.

As in the treatment of major depressive disorder, clinicians often employ *augmentation strategies*; in other words, they use a second medication to enhance the response of the first antidepressant. We have found that addition of lithium or triiodothyronine sometimes improves a partial response to antidepressants *(31–33)*.

Finally, considering newer types of antidepressants, we have found in our anecdotal experience that venlafaxine, a norepinephrine and serotonin reuptake inhibitor (NSRI), is often effective and well tolerated in bulimic patients. Milnacipran, another NSRI, was effective in an open-label case study *(39)*. Reboxetine, a noradrenaline reuptake inhibitor (NRI), was remarkably effective in treatment of bulimia nervosa in a small case study *(40)*. Also of note is one report *(41)* that the investigational 5-hydroxytrypamine (5-HT)-1_A agonist ipsapirone (which appears to have antidepressant properties *[42]*) is effective in bulimia nervosa. Thus, NSRIs, NRIs, and 5HT-1_A agonists represent promising possible new treatments for bulimia nervosa.

2.4. Theoretical Implications

Although it is beyond the scope of this chapter to discuss the theoretical implications of the above findings in detail, we should point out that there are logically two possible explanations for the efficacy of antidepressants in bulimia nervosa. One is that these drugs treat bulimia nervosa via the same chemical mechanism by which they treat depression; the alternative possibility is that these drugs possess two independent chemical mechanisms, one of which treats bulimia nervosa and the other of which treats depression. After inspecting the data, however, the second of these two possibilities would appear unlikely because we would have to postulate that each of the several different, chemically distinct families of antidepressants each possessed both an antidepressant mechanism and, by chance, an independent antibulimic mechanism. Although a single class of drugs might share two entirely independent chemical mechanisms, it would be most improbable that several unrelated classes would all share exactly the same two mechanisms. Therefore, the much more likely (and parsimonious) possibility is that antidepressants treat both bulimia nervosa and depression via a single chemical mechanism that operates at the same physiological "step" in the chain of "steps" required to produce each of the disorders. (For a more detailed discussion of this argument, we refer the reader to refs. *43* and *44*.)

2.5. Summary of Antidepressant Efficacy

The available data regarding antidepressant treatment of bulimia nervosa indicate that antidepressant agents from several chemical families are highly effective, at least in the short term, in the treatment of bulimia nervosa. These agents appear to not only reduce bulimic symptoms *per se*, but also to reduce associated symptoms of preoccupation with food and weight. The only antidepressant that appears contraindicated in bulimia nervosa is bupropion, because of the high risk of seizures in bulimic patients. Data regarding the long-term benefits of antidepressant treatment in bulimia nervosa are limited. Studies in which only a single antidepressant agent was administered have found high drop-out rates and frequent relapse. However, studies in which the physician was permitted to try a second or third antidepressant agent if the first one failed have produced much more promising results. Given that clinical practice allows the clinician to substitute a different agent if the first fails, these open-label studies probably reflect more accurately the prognosis of bulimia nervosa when treated with antidepressants under normal circumstances.

3. OTHER MEDICATIONS

Several types of medications other than antidepressants have been tried in bulimic patients. We summarize controlled trials of such medications marketed in the United States in Table 3. The table does not include 1- or 2-d studies because these trials are of largely theoretical interest in that they were not designed to provide information on the clinical utility of the compounds.

Most of these agents have not been shown unequivocally to be efficacious on the basis of the studies done, nor has any achieved widespread use in clinical practice. Nevertheless, several of these medications (such as valproate and carbamazepine) may have a role in the treatment of particular types of bulimic patients, especially those with concomitant bipolar disorder or cyclothymia. Others (such as topiramate and 5-HT$_3$ antagonists) may achieve more widespread use in the future.

3.1. Anticonvulsants

First, we consider four medications with anticonvulsant properties: carbamazepine, valproate, phenytoin, and topiramate. Two of these (carbamazepine and valproate) have mood-stabilizing properties useful in bipolar disorder. In a small placebo-controlled crossover study, Kaplan and colleagues *(45)* failed to find a beneficial effect of carbamazepine vs placebo in the overall analysis for treatment of bulimia nervosa. The weight gain associated with carbamazepine further decreases its utility in treating patients with bulimia nervosa.

Although it may not be useful routinely in the treatment of patients with bulimia nervosa, carbamazepine may have a role in the treatment of bulimic patients with cyclothymia or bipolar disorder. For example, Kaplan and associates *(45)* reported that a patient with bulimia nervosa and cyclothymia responded well to carbamazepine. Similarly, with regard to valproate, we *(46)* have reported a similar case of a woman with

Table 3
Placebo-Controlled Studies of Other Medications in Bulimia Nervosa[a]

Study (reference)	Drug (maximum dose)		Number of subjects [b]	Duration of trial [c]	Design [d]	Response to drug [e]
Kaplan et al., 1983 (45)	Carbamazepine[f]		6	6 wk	Crossover	0
Hsu et al., 1991 (62)	Lithium carbonate[g]		91	8 wk	Parallel group	0
Mitchell et al., 1989 (59)	Naltrexone	50 mg	16	3 wk	Crossover	0
Alger et al., 1991 (10)	Naltrexone	150 mg	15	8 wk	Parallel group	0
Faris et al., 2000 (63)	Ondansetron	24 mg	25	4 wk	Parallel group	++
Wermuth et al., 1977 (50)	Phenytoin[f]		19	6 wk	Crossover	+
Hoopes et al., 2003 (53)	Topiramate	400 mg	64	10 wk	Parallel group	++
Hedges et al., 2003 (54)						

[a] Restricted to medications marketed in the United States

[b] Number of subjects receiving drug or placebo who completed the trial or enough of the trial to be included in data analysis

[c] Period of time that subjects received active drug rather than total duration of the study

[d] All studies were randomized, placebo-controlled, double-blind trials

[e] ++, drug significantly superior to placebo in reducing frequency of binges and/or frequency of vomiting; +, some evidence that drug superior to placebo, but not clearly significant; 0, little or no difference between drug and placebo

[f] Dose not specified, but plasma levels adjusted to therapeutic range for use in epilepsy

[g] Dose varied between 600–1200 mg, with median level of 0.62 mEq/L

bulimia nervosa and bipolar disorder who responded to valproate. Given the high comorbidity between bulimia nervosa and bipolar disorder (47), this combination of disorders is encountered frequently. In our anecdotal experience, bulimic symptoms in patients with concomitant bipolar disorder or cyclothymia appear to respond well when these patients are treated in the standard manner for bipolar disorder. Specifically, bulimic patients with hypomanic or manic symptoms often respond to mood stabilizers alone; and bulimic patients with past, but without current, hypomania or mania, often respond to mood stabilizers, either alone or in combination with cautiously administered antidepressants.

There is some evidence from an open-label trial (48,49) and a placebo-controlled trial (50) that phenytoin may be useful in bulimia nervosa (see further discussion elsewhere [51, 52]). However, the results of the placebo-controlled trial indicated a very modest effect, and phenytoin has not enjoyed widespread acceptance in contemporary clinical practice (52).

In a promising study (53,54), topiramate was significantly more effective than placebo in reducing the frequency of days during which subjects experienced episodes of binge eating and purging, as well as in improving other aspects of the disorder. An open-label case series (55) also reported beneficial effects of topiramate in five patients with bulimia nervosa and comorbid mood or anxiety disorders. Also of relevance is that topiramate was effective in a placebo-controlled trial in the related condition, binge-eating disorder (56).

3.2. Opiate Antagonists

On the basis of encouraging open studies (57,58), Mitchell and colleagues (59) and Alger and associates (10) conducted placebo-controlled trials of naltrexone in bulimia nervosa. Mitchell and colleagues (60) also conducted a 2-d trial of intravenous naloxone, a related opiate antagonist. These trials failed to show a beneficial effect of opiate antagonists. However, the studies are difficult to interpret because the 50 mg dose of naltrexone used in the study of Mitchell and colleagues was less than others have used for successful treatment in open-label trials (57,58), and the study by Alger and associates had only seven patients on medication.

3.3. Lithium

On the basis of an encouraging open trial (61), Hsu and associates (62) conducted a placebo-controlled study of lithium carbonate in 91 bulimic patients. Although this study found little overall advantage of lithium vs placebo, interpretation of the results is hampered by a large placebo response rate (perhaps augmented by the use of concomitant minimal behavior therapy) and by plasma levels of lithium that are lower (mean level of 0.62 mEq/L in this trial) than those used in the treatment of bipolar disorder (0.8–1.2 mEq/L). Thus, it is unclear whether lithium might be effective in bulimia nervosa. As mentioned above, we have sometimes added small doses of lithium to augment the effects of antidepressant medications. However, because of the propensity for weight gain on lithium and the many more attractive alternative medication treatments for bulimia nervosa, use of lithium alone would appear to have little place currently in the treatment of most bulimic patients.

3.4. 5-HT₃ Antagonists

One open-label trial *(63)* of 5 patients and one placebo-controlled trial *(64)* of 28 patients reported efficacy of the $5-HT_3$ receptor antagonist ondansetron in bulimia nervosa. The authors speculate that the effect of ondansetron on bulimic symptoms and behaviors was mediated by afferent vagal effects. However, there are also many other candidates for ondansetron's mechanism of action, including effects on serotoninergic neurotransmission. Currently, ondansetron is marketed in the United States as an antiemetic. Its expense for continued treatment, as well as only modest evidence for efficacy, have limited its use in clinical practice.

4. STUDIES OF ANTIDEPRESSANTS AND BEHAVIORAL THERAPY

Five studies *(9,28,36,65,66)* have compared the outcome of bulimic patients receiving antidepressants with that of patients receiving CBT or the combination of antidepressant and CBT. Mitchell and colleagues *(9)* randomly assigned 171 bulimic patients to one of four treatments for 12 wk: imipramine 200 mg; placebo; intensive group CBT plus imipramine; and CBT plus placebo. The investigators found significant benefits for all three active treatments vs placebo. In comparisons among the active treatments, CBT and CBT plus imipramine were both significantly superior to imipramine alone in improvement of bulimic symptoms. Agras and associates *(28)* randomly assigned 73 bulimic patients to one of three treatments: desipramine up to 350 mg/d; individual CBT; and desipramine up to 350 mg plus CBT. The total treatment period was 24 wk; after 16 wk, half of the desipramine-treated subjects were randomly discontinued from medication for the final 8 wk. Subjects were evaluated at 16, 24, and 32 wk after initiation of treatment. The authors found that CBT and CBT plus desipramine were superior to desipramine alone at 16 wk and that the 32-wk outcome of CBT plus desipramine given for 24 wk was superior to that of the group that had received desipramine alone for 16 wk. Subsequently, subjects were reevaluated at 1 yr. Subjects who had received desipramine treatment for 16 wk had a significantly inferior outcome compared to those in the other three groups. In the intervening 28 wk after the completion of the active study period, only 4 of the subjects (1 in each treatment group) had received antidepressant treatment.

Fichter and associates *(65)* treated 40 bulimic patients for 5 wk with either intensive inpatient CBT or fluoxetine 60 mg plus intensive inpatient individual CBT. They found no significant difference in outcome between the two groups, but they did find that both groups had improved significantly compared with baseline. Next, Leitenberg and colleagues *(36)* enrolled 21 bulimic patients in a 20-wk study to compare the effects of three treatments: desipramine, individual CBT, and desipramine plus individual CBT. They stopped this study prematurely because of a high number of dropouts in the desipramine-alone group, largely caused by side effects from medication.

Finally, in the most ambitious and methodologically rigorous study thus far, Walsh and colleagues *(66)* treated 120 bulimic women for 16 wk in a randomized trial with five treatment arms: (1) CBT alone plus placebo, (2) supportive psychotherapy plus placebo, (3) CBT plus medication, (4) supportive psychotherapy plus medication, and (5) medication alone. The medication treatment was a two-stage intervention, in which a second antidepressant (fluoxetine 60 mg/d) was employed if the first (desipramine up to 300 mg/d) was either ineffective or poorly tolerated. The results showed significant improvement of symptoms for CBT vs supportive psychotherapy and for medication in combination with psychological treatment vs psychological treatment alone. Furthermore, CBT plus medication was significantly superior to medication alone, but supportive psychotherapy plus medication was not superior to medication alone. Finally, there was no difference in efficacy between CBT plus placebo and medication alone.

The results of these studies of antidepressants vs behavioral therapy must be interpreted with regard to a number of methodological limitations. First, except in the study by Walsh and associates (66), there is no control psychological treatment. Thus, in most of the studies, it is not possible to judge what portion of the improvement in behavioral therapy represented an actual therapy-specific effect, and what portion represented a nonspecific "placebo" effect from extensive human contact.

Second, drug therapy in these studies does not mirror actual clinical practice. By allowing treatment with only a single agent (or in the case of the study by Walsh and colleagues [66], two agents), it seems likely that the studies may have underestimated the efficacy of antidepressants as they are used in the field, as we have discussed above in our consideration of long-term studies using single antidepressant agents. Indeed, the best results of medication in comparison with psychotherapy were obtained in the only study to allow use of two medications (66). Furthermore, one of the studies of medication vs CBT specifically showed that the response rate to antidepressants was much improved when a second antidepressant trial was allowed after the conclusion of the 12-wk comparison study (34).

Third, in one (21) of the studies, antidepressant treatment was simply stopped after a fixed period of time, regardless of whether it appeared clinically appropriate to do so. Although it might be argued that such a strategy is "fair," in that CBT, by comparison, is typically given for a time-limited period, such a technique is incompatible with ordinary clinical practice in antidepressant treatment.

Fourth, when comparing any psychological therapy to a drug therapy, it is difficult to estimate the magnitude of the "responsibility effect." Specifically, if patients fail to respond to a drug, they usually assume that the drug has failed, through no fault of their own. But if they fail to respond to a psychological therapy such as CBT, they may feel some responsibility for their own failure. Thus, the responsibility effect may cause patients in psychological therapy to overestimate their degree of improvement, both in their own minds and when reporting to investigators, in order to minimize any sense of failure. Because psychological therapies are usually administered nonblinded, by investigators with positive expectations, the responsibility effect may be further magnified. It is difficult to judge the degree to which this effect may bias findings in favor of psychological therapies vs drug therapies in bulimic patients.

In summary, it appears reasonable to conclude that CBT and antidepressants both represent effective treatments for bulimia nervosa. However, as a result of the methodologic limitations described above, little can be concluded regarding the relative efficacy of the two techniques. Future comparison studies should be designed to mimic medication treatment as given optimally in clinical practice and to control for the responsibility effect, if possible, by using placebo psychological therapies, administered by individuals who communicate comparable enthusiasm for the benefit of their treatment. Without these refinements, head-to-head comparisons of psychological and pharmacological therapies may be misleading

Table 4
Treatment Guidelines for Bulimia Nervosa

1. Select cognitive–behavioral therapy or pharmacological therapy.
2. If cognitive–behavioral therapy is chosen, strongly consider pharmacological therapy if response to cognitive behavioral therapy is inadequate.
3. If pharmacological therapy is chosen, begin with SSRI.
4. If partial response and maximum dose limited by side effects, consider a second SSRI
5. If no response, try venlafaxine or a tricyclic (generally desipramine or nortriptyline); monitor tricyclic concentrations if response inadequate.
6. If still no response, try topiramate or MAOI.
7. With response, continue therapy for at least 6 mo.
8. If relapse occurs, restart medication promptly and continue for at least 6 mo prior to attempting discontinuation.

5. PRACTICAL CONSIDERATIONS: TREATMENT GUIDELINES

In this section, we offer guidelines for the pharmacological management of bulimic patients based on the scientific literature, our clinical experience, and discussion with other experienced clinicians. These guidelines, summarized in Table 4, are admittedly somewhat subjective. The clinician should feel free to modify his or her approach based on the circumstances of individual patients and his or her own clinical experience.

The first practical question to be addressed by the clinician is whether to begin with drug treatment or some other therapy in a bulimic patient who presents for treatment for the first time (*see* Chapter 2). Given the ambiguity of the evidence for the relative efficacy of CBT vs antidepressants, as discussed above, there is no clear "best treatment" for bulimia nervosa at this time. Therefore, some clinicians may prefer to begin with a trial of CBT in bulimic patients, reserving pharmacological therapy for those who fail to respond or who improve in some aspects of their eating disorder, but nevertheless continue to display significant residual bulimic or depressive symptoms. Alternatively, many clinicians may prefer to begin with pharmacological treatment, especially if expert CBT is not readily available. In any event, both of these two modalities should be actively considered in any new bulimic patient.

There may be special cases in which antidepressants are particularly indicated, such as bulimic patients with severe depressive symptoms or suicidal ideation. However, it is important to note that *antidepressants should not be reserved only for bulimic patients who are depressed, because antidepressants are equally effective in bulimic patients without depression.*

If drug treatment is selected, one passing question to be addressed is whether to choose an antidepressant or some other agent from the list of nonantidepressant drugs that have been tried in bulimia. Here, the decision seems clear: aside from special cases (such as patients with concomitant bulimia nervosa and bipolar disorder), antidepressants are the treatment of choice.

Once the decision is made to choose an antidepressant, which drug should be chosen? Although, as we have shown in this review, there is no clear evidence that one family of antidepressants is more efficacious than another, the data suggest that drugs of the SSRI class may have fewer side effects than those in other families of antidepressants. Therefore, we generally start with a trial of an SSRI, usually citalopram or fluoxetine.

We do not have an established algorithm for the choice of drugs for subsequent trials, and the three of us differ somewhat in our preferred approach. Generally speaking, our approach to pharmacological therapy of bulimic patients is virtually identical to our approach for depressed patients. Hence, if a patient fails to respond to an SSRI, we switch to a different class of medication. However, if the patient has had a partial response but cannot increase the dose because of adverse effects, we will often try a second SSRI (indeed, we have found that some patients respond to a second SSRI even when they completely fail to respond to the first).

Our choice for a second, non-SSRI agent is usually venlafaxine, and then tricyclics. For tricyclics, we prefer desipramine or nortriptyline because they have less anticholinergic effect than the other tricyclics and because the dose can be optimized by achieving plasma concentrations comparable to those established as efficacious in major depressive disorder. Thus, desipramine concentrations of at least 160 ng/mL or nortriptyline concentrations of 50–140 ng/mL appear optimal. Even though there are no published reports of its efficacy in bulimia nervosa, we often use venlafaxine as a second choice for three reasons: it is chemically distinct from SSRIs in that it has noradrenergic effects in addition to serotonergic effects, we have found anecdotally that SSRI nonresponders often respond to venlafaxine, and it has fewer adverse effects than tricyclics.

We usually reserve MAOIs for a third or subsequent trial, and we have had better experience with tranylcypromine than phenelzine, particularly because tranylcypromine seems less likely to induce weight gain. We note that MAOIs should not be used in conjunction with SSRIs and that the clinician should allow a generous wash-out period between trials of SSRIs and MAOIs (at least 2 wk in either direction, except when going from fluoxetine to an MAOI, in which case we recommend 5 wk in view of the long half-life of fluoxetine). When selecting alternatives for a third trial, we also consider using topiramate.

We have had good results at times with trazodone but usually do not use this agent for a first or second trial. Finally, we recommend considering augmentation strategies for tricyclics and SSRIs, using lithium 600 mg or triiodothyronine 25–50 µg daily.

Having chosen a medication, we need to consider the dose and the duration of treatment. We recommend using doses of medication that are equal or slightly greater than doses used in the treatment of major depressive disorder. For example, fluoxetine 20 mg is often an effective dose for major depressive disorder. However, this dose was not markedly superior to placebo treatment in a large trial (11), whereas 60 mg was unequivocally superior to placebo. For tricyclics, as mentioned above, we suggest using doses that achieve plasma concentrations established as the therapeutic range for major depressive disorder. We have had success clinically with this approach, and one study of desipramine (2) found that nonresponding bulimic patients whose level was less than the therapeutic level for depression improved when their dose was raised into the therapeutic range.

Turning to duration of treatment and guidelines for discontinuation, we recommend an approach identical to that used in the treatment of major depressive disorder. We first conduct serial trials of antidepressants as outlined above in an attempt to achieve either a remission or marked improvement of bulimic symptoms. Once this level of response has been achieved, we treat for 6–12 mo before considering discontinuation of medication. We discontinue medication at a time when the patient can tolerate the possibility of relapse and then monitor the patient carefully. If relapse occurs, we restart medication promptly and treat for another 6–12 mo before attempting discontinuation again.

Overall, although our approach to antidepressant therapy in bulimic patients is very similar to the one we use in depressed patients, there are three differences of note. First, we tend to use somewhat higher doses, as discussed above. Second, we are more sensitive to the issue of possible weight gain as a side effect. As mentioned above, this consideration is one of our reasons for preferring tranylcypromine over phenelzine for MAOI therapy. Finally, because of their association with weight gain in patients with mood disorders, we are somewhat less likely to use tricyclics and lithium, even though they have not been associated with weight gain in reported studies of bulimic patients. Third, because of the risk of seizures, we do not use bupropion.

REFERENCES

1. Mitchell JE, Groat R. A placebo-controlled, double-blind trial of amitriptyline in bulimia. J Clin Psychopharmacol 1984; 4:186–193.
2. Hughes PL, Wells LA, Cunningham CJ, Ilstrup DM. Treating bulimia with desipramine: a double-blind, placebo-controlled study. Arch Gen Psychiatry 1986; 43:182–186.
3. Barlow J, Blouin J, Blouin A, Perez E. Treatment of bulimia with desipramine: a double-blind crossover study. Can J Psychiatry 1988; 33:129–133.
4. Blouin AG, Blouin JH, Perez EL, Bushnik T, Zuro C, Mulder E. Treatment of bulimia with fenfluramine and desipramine. J Clin Psychopharmacol 1988; 8:261–269.
5. McCann UD, Agras WS. Successful treatment of nonpurging bulimia nervosa with desipramine: a double-blind, placebo-controlled study. Am J Psychiatry 1990; 147:1509–1513.
6. Walsh BT, Hadigan CM, Devlin MJ, Gladis M, Roose SP. Long-term outcome of antidepressant treatment for bulimia nervosa. Am J Psychiatry 1991; 148:1206–1212.
7. Pope HG Jr, Hudson JI, Jonas JM, Yurgelun-Todd D. Bulimia treated with imipramine: a placebo-controlled, double-blind study. Am J Psychiatry 1983; 140:554–558.
8. Agras WS, Dorian B, Kirkley BG, Arnow B, Bachman J. Imipramine in the treatment of bulimia: a double-blind controlled study. Int J Eating Disorders 1987; 6:29–38.
9. Mitchell JE, Pyle RL, Eckert ED, Hatsukami D, Pomeroy C, Zimmerman R. A comparison study of antidepressants and structured intensive group psychotherapy in the treatment of bulimia nervosa. Arch Gen Psychiatry 1990; 47:149–157.
10. Alger SA, Schwalberg MD, Bigaouette JM, Michalek AV, Howard LJ. Effect of a tricyclic antidepressant and opiate antagonist on binge-eating behavior in normal-weight bulimic and obese, binge-eating subjects. Am J Clin Nutr 1991; 53:865–871.
11. Fluoxetine Bulimia Collaborative Study Group. Fluoxetine in the treatment of bulimia nervosa: a multicenter placebo-controlled, double-blind trial. Arch Gen Psychiatry 1992; 49:139–147.
12. Goldstein DJ, Wilson MG, Thompson VL, Potvin JH, Rampey AH Jr., for the Fluoxetine Bulimia Nervosa Research Group. Long-term fluoxetine treatment of bulimia nervosa. Br J Psychiatry 1995; 166:660–666.
13. Romano SJ, Halmi KA, Sarkar NP, Koke SC, Lee JS. A placebo-controlled study of fluoxetine in continued treatment of bulimia nervosa after successful acute fluoxetine treatment. Am J Psychiatry 2002; 159:96–102.
14. Walsh BT, Gladis M, Roose SP, Steward JW, Stetner F, Glassman AH. Phenelzine vs placebo in 50 patients with bulimia. Arch Gen Psychiatry 1988; 45:471–475.
15. Horne RL, Ferguson JM, Pope HG Jr, et al. Treatment of bulimia with bupropion: a controlled multicenter trial. J Clin Psychiatry 1988; 49:262–266.
16. Pope HG Jr, Keck PE Jr, McElroy SL, Hudson, JI. A placebo-controlled study of trazodone in bulimia nervosa. J Clin Psychopharmacol 1989; 9:254–259.

17. Kennedy SH, Goldbloom DS, Ralevski E, Davis C, D'Souza JD, Lofchy J. Is there a role for selective monoamine oxidase inhibitor therapy in bulimia nervosa? a placebo-controlled trial of brofaromine. J Clin Psychopharmacol 1993; 13:415–422.

18. Kennedy SH, Piran N, Warsh JJ, et al. A trial of isocarboxazid in the treatment of bulimia nervosa. J Clin Psychopharmacol 1988; 8:391–396.

19. Sabine EJ, Yonace A, Farrington AJ, Barratt KH, Wakeling A. Bulimia nervosa: a placebo controlled double-blind therapeutic trial of mianserin. Br J Clin Pharmac 1983; 15:195S–202S.

20. Price WA, Babai MR. Antidepressant drug therapy for bulimia: current status revisited. J Clin Psychiatry 1987; 48:385.

21. Rothschild R, Quitkin MH, Quitkin FM, et al. A double-blind placebo-controlled comparison of phenelzine and imipramine in the treatment of bulimia in atypical depressives. Int J Eating Disorders 1994; 15:1–9.

22. Goldstein DJ, Wilson MG, Ascroft RC, Al-Banna M. Effectiveness of fluoxetine therapy in bulimia nervosa regardless of comorbid depression. Int J Eat Disord 1999; 25:19–27.

23. Hudson JI, McElroy SL, Raymond NC, et al. Fluvoxamine in the treatment of binge-eating disorder: a multi-center placebo controlled, double-blind trial. Am J Psychiatry 1998; 155:1756–1762.

24. McElroy SL, Casuto LS, Nelson EB, et al. Placebo-controlled trial of sertraline in the treatment of binge-eating disorder. Am J Psychiatry 2000; 15:1004–1006.

25. Arnold LM, McElroy SL, Hudson JI, Welge JA, Bennett AJ, Keck PE Jr. A placebo-controlled randomized trial of fluoxetine in the treatment of binge-eating disorder. J Clin Psychiatry 2002; 63: 1028–1033.

26. McElroy SL, Hudson JI, Mlhotra S, Welge, JA, Nelson EB, Keck PE Jr. Citalopram in the treatment of binge-eating disorder: a placebo-controlled trial. J Clin Psychiatry 2003; 64:807–813.

27. Carter WP, Hudson JI, Lalonde JK, Pindyck L, McElroy SL, Pope HG Jr. Pharmacologic treatment of binge-eating disorder. Int J Eating Disord 2003; 34:514–588.

28. Agras WS, Rossiter EM, Arnow B, et al. Pharmacologic and cognitive–behavioral treatment for bulimia nervosa: a controlled comparison. Am J Psychiatry 1992; 149:82–87.

29. Agras WS, Rossiter EM, Arnow B, et al. One-year follow-up of psychosocial and pharmacologic treatments for bulimia nervosa. J Clin Psychiatry 1994; 55:179–183.

30. Leitenberg H, Rosen JC, Wolf J, Vara LS, Detzer MJ, Srebnik D. Comparison of cognitive–behavior therapy and desipramine in the treatment of bulimia nervosa. Behav Res Ther 1994; 32:37–45.

31. Pope HG Jr, Hudson JI, Jonas JM. Antidepressant treatment of bulimia: preliminary experience and practical recommendations. J Clin Psychopharmacol 1983; 3:274–281.

32. Pope HG Jr., Hudson JI, Jonas JM, Yurgelun-Todd, D. Antidepressant treatment of bulimia: a two-year follow-up study. J Clin Psychopharmacol 1985; 5:320–327.

33. Pope HG Jr, McElroy SL, Keck PE Jr, Hudson JI. Long-term pharmacotherapy of bulimia nervosa. J Clin Psychopharmacol 1989; 9:385–386.

34. Mitchell JE, Pyle RL, Eckert ED, Hatsukami D, Pomeroy C, Zimmerman R. Response to alternative anti-depressants in imipramine nonresponders with bulimia nervosa. J Clin Psychopharmacol 1989; 9:291–293.

35. Spigset O, Pleym H. Case report of successful treatment of bulimia nervosa with fluvoxamine. Pharmacopsychiatry 199; 24:180.

36. Ayuso-Gutierrez JL, Palazón M, Ayuso-Mateos JL. Open trial of fluvoxamine in the treatment of bulimia nervosa. Int J Eating Disorders 1994; 15:245–249.

37. Prats M, Diez-Quevedo C, Avila C, et al. Paroxetine treatment for bulimia nervosa and binge eating disorder. Abstract 308. Abstracts of the Sixth International Conference on Eating Disorders, New York, NY, April 1994.

38. Roberts JM, Lydiard RB. Sertraline in the treatment of bulimia nervosa. Am J Psychiatry 1993; 150:1753.

39. El-Giamal N, de Zwaan M, Bailer U, Strnad A, Schussler P, Kasper S. Milnacipran in the treatment of bulimia nervosa: a report of 16 cases. Eur Neuropsychopharmacol 2003; 13:73–79.

40. El Giamal N, de Zwaan M, Bailer U, et al. Reboxetine in the treatment of bulimia nervosa: a report of seven cases. Int Clin Pschopharmacol 2000; 15:351–356.

41. Geretsegger C, Greimel KV, Roed IS, Hesselink JMK. Ipsapirone in the treatment of bulimia nervosa: an open pilot study. Int J Eating Disorders 1995; 17:359–363.

42. Heller AH, Beneke M, Kuemmel B, et al. Ipsapirone: evidence for efficacy in depression. Psycho-pharmacol Bull 1990; 26:219–222.

43. Hudson JI, Pope HG Jr. Affective spectrum disorder: does antidepressant response identify a family of disorders with a common pathophysiology? Am J Psychiatry 1990; 147:552–564.

44. Hudson JI, Mangwth B, Pope HG Jr, et al. Family study of affective spectrum disorder. Arch Gen Psychiatry 2003; 60:170–177.

45. Kaplan AS, Garfinkel PE, Darby PL, Garner DM. Carbamazepine in the treatment of bulimia. Am J Psychiatry 1983; 140:1225–1226.

46. Herridge PL, Pope HG Jr. Treatment of bulimia and rapid-cycling bipolar disorder with sodium valproate. J Clin Psychopharmacol 1985; 5:229–230.

47. Hudson JI, Pope HG Jr, Yurgelun-Todd D, Jonas JM, Frankenburg FR. A controlled study of lifetime prevalence of affective and other psychiatric disorders in bulimic outpatients. Am J Psychiatry 1987; 144:1283–1287.

48. Green RS, Rau JH. Treatment of compulsive eating disturbances with anticonvulsant medication. Am J Psychiatry 1974; 131:428–31.

49. Rau JH, Green RS. Compulsive eating: a neuropsychologic approach to certain eating disorders. Compr Psychiatry 1975; 16:223–231.

50. Wermuth BM, Davis KL, Hollister LE, Stunkard AJ. Phenytoin treatment of the binge-eating syndrome. Am J Psychiatry 1977; 134:1249–1253.

51. Hudson JI, Pope HG Jr. The role of anticonvulsants in the treatment of bulimia. In: McElroy SL, Pope HG Jr, eds. Use of Anticonvulsants in Psychiatry. Oxford Health Care, Clifton, NJ, 1988, pp. 141–154.

52. Pope HG Jr, Hudson JI. New Hope for Binge Eaters: Advances in the Understanding and Treatment of Bulimia. Harper and Row, New York, NY, 1984.

53. Hoopes S, Reimherr F, Hedges D, et al. 1: Topiramate in the treatment of bulimia nervosa: a randomized, double-blind, placebo-controlled trial. J Clin Psychiatry 2003; 64:1335–1341.

54. Hedges D, Reimherr F, Hoopes S, et al. 2: Treatment with topiramate is associated with improvements in psychiatric measures of bulimia nervosa: a randomized, double-blind, placebo-controlled trial. J Clin Psychiatry 2003; 64:1449–1454.

55. Barbee JG. Topiramate in the treatment of severe bulimia nervosa with comorbid mood disorders: a case series. Int J Eat Disord 2003; 33:468–472.

56. McElroy SL, Arnold LM, Shapira NA, et al. Topiramate in the treatment of binge-eating disorder associated with obesity. Am J Psychiatry 2003; 60:255–261.

57. Jonas JM, Gold MS. Naltrexone reverses bulimic symtoms. Lancet 1986; 1:807.

58. Jonas JM, Gold MS. Treatment of bulimia with the opiate antagonist naltrexone: preliminary data and theoretical implications. In: Hudson JI, Pope HG Jr, eds. Psychobiology of Bulimia. American Psychiatric Press, Washington, DC, 1987, pp. 115–127.

59. Mitchell JE, Christenson G, Jennings J, et al. A placebo-controlled, double-blind crossover study of naltrexone hydrochloride in outpatients with normal weight bulimia. J Clin Psychopharmacol 1989; 9: 94–97.

60. Mitchell JE, Laine DE, Morley JE, Levine AS. Naloxone but not CCK-8 may attentuate binge-eating behavior in patients with the bulimia syndrome. Biol Psychiatry 1986; 21:1399–1406.

61. Hsu LKG. Treatment of bulimia with lithium. Am J Psychiatry 1984;141:1266–1262.

62. Hsu LKG, Clement L, Santhouse R, Ju ESY. Treatment of bulimia nervosa with lithium carbonate: a controlled study. J Nerv Ment Dis. 1991;179:351–355.

63. Hartman BK, Faris PL, Kim SW, et al. Treatment of bulimia nervosa with ondansetron. Arch Gen Psychiatry 1997; 54:969–970.

64. Faris PL, Kim SW, Meller WH, et al. Effect of decreasing afferent vagal activity with ondansetron on symptoms of bulimia nervosa: a randomized, double-blind trial. Lancet 2000; 355:792–797.

65. Fichter MM, Leibl K, Rief W, Brunner E, Schmidt-Auberger S, Engel RR. Fluoxetine versus placebo: a double-blind study with bulimia inpatients undergoing intensive psychotherapy. Pharmacopsychiatry 1991; 24:1–7.

66. Walsh BT, Wilson GT, Loeb KL, et al. Medication and psychotherapy in the treatment of bulimia nervosa. Am J Psychiatry 1997; 154:523–531.

4 Prevention of Eating Disorders

A Nutritional Perspective

Cheryl L. Rock

KEY POINTS

- Patients with eating disorders have a biological predisposition, but certain dietary intakes associated with dieting and subclinical eating disturbances may precipitate or exacerbate underlying biochemical disturbances.
- Impaired nutritional status can perpetuate eating disorders and make them intractable to treatment. Improving nutritional status can help prevent relapse.
- Nutritional intervention should be part of the therapy of eating disorders.
- Prevention entails intervention on sociocultural pressures, self-esteem, and excessive dieting.
- Although a universal approach to intervention is important, early identification of high-risk individuals is an important aspect of prevention and can be most cost and resource efficient.

1. INTRODUCTION: NUTRITION AND EATING DISORDERS

The clinical eating disorders are only the most extreme form of pathological eating attitudes and behaviors. Many people engage in pathological weight-control behaviors without meeting the current diagnostic criteria for anorexia or bulimia nervosa and may be regarded as having subclinical eating disorders. As described by Fairburn and Beglin (1), a broad spectrum of eating disorders appears to exist in the general population as a continuum of dieting behavior and weight concerns, especially among women. The current prevalence of the clinical eating disorders in the general population has been estimated to be 0.5–1% for anorexia nervosa, 2% for bulimia nervosa, and 2% for binge-eating disorder (BED [2]). However, at least 30% of women of reproductive age have been shown to be practicing some pathological weight-control activities, with 15% regularly engaging in bulimic behaviors, including both binge eating and purging (3,4).

Among adolescents, the prevalence rates for pathological weight-control activities are even higher. In a US nationally representative sample of 6728 adolescents in grades 5 to 12, 45% of the girls and 20% of the boys reported that they had been on a diet, and disordered eating (binge–purge cycling) was reported by 13% of the girls and 7% of the

From: *The Management of Eating Disorders and Obesity, Second Edition*
Edited by: D. J. Goldstein © Humana Press Inc., Totowa, NJ

Table 1
Chapter Overview

boys *(5)*. More than half of females and nearly one-third of males in a large ($N = 81,247$) statewide population-based sample of 9th and 12th graders reported disordered eating and weight-control behaviors (fasting or skipping meals, use of diet pills, vomiting, use of laxatives or smoking cigarettes, and binge eating) *(6)*. Frequent dieting and binge eating occur more often among overweight or obese adolescents *(7)*, and the pattern of dieting with subsequent loss of control and overeating has been suggested to increase risk for weight gain and obesity. Longitudinal studies of adolescents support this theory because frequent dieters have been observed to be more likely to become obese *(8,9)*. Given the current epidemic of obesity in the United States *(10,11)*, the relationship between dieting behavior and increased risk for subsequent obesity has important public health and clinical implications.

In the patient with bulimia nervosa (*see* Chapter 1), dieting appears to play a key etiologic role. The onset of bulimia nervosa typically follows a period of dieting to lose weight *(12)*, and a causative link between dietary restraint and bulimia is strengthened by similar observations of obese patients who binge eat and of normal subjects following a period of food deprivation *(13,14)*. The abnormal eating patterns that develop with repeated episodes of dieting and binge eating serve to perpetuate the disorder. The physiological consequences of these abnormal eating patterns contribute to its often intractable nature.

In the pathogenesis of anorexia nervosa (*see* Chapter 5), nutritional factors are among both precipitating and perpetuating factors *(15)*. Dieting or other purposeful changes in food choices triggers the onset of the disorder, and the physiological and psychological consequences of starvation serve as perpetuating factors that can impede progress toward recovery. Nutritional rehabilitation is the first goal of treatment *(16)*, although other components of therapy are necessary to prevent relapse.

The link between nutritional patterns, unhealthful eating attitudes, and risk for eating disorders suggests that dieting behavior and food cognitions may be a critical area of focus for preventive efforts *(17,18)*, especially when targeted toward vulnerable individuals and high-risk populations. Effective prevention or early intervention should address nutritional issues because of the role of these factors in the development of the clinical eating disorders. Across the spectrum of eating pathology in the general population, efforts to promote healthy eating attitudes and behaviors may reduce risk for consequent psychological and other health problems.

This chapter reviews the issues related to the influences of dietary patterns and nutritional status on eating disorders, the risk factors associated with the development of eating disorders, and suggestions for prevention and early intervention for eating disorders (Table 1). Abnormal nutritional status and dietary patterns are the central features of eating disorders. The objectives of this chapter are to provide the scientific background supporting this relationship, the likely characteristics of at-risk individuals, and potential interventions.

2. DIETING, DIETARY RESTRAINT, AND DISORDERED EATING PATTERNS

2.1. Dieting

In the United States, concern with body weight and dieting is so common that it may be considered normative behavior. In a nationally representative sample of US adults, 44% of women and nearly 29% of men were trying to lose or maintain weight by eating less and/or increasing physical activity *(19)*. In addition, overweight and obesity occur in a high proportion of both adolescent and adult respondents. However, the dieters identified in population survey studies may not necessarily be obese. In fact, a substantial proportion of those who are dieting (particularly adolescents and young women) are not overweight *(5,20)*. Individuals who try to either lose or maintain weight restrict their dietary intake most commonly by chronic or intermittent dieting rather than by exercise or other approaches to promote weight control.

Despite the high prevalence of dieting, this behavior does not necessarily achieve successful long-term weight loss. In fact, dietary restraint may even reduce the likelihood of successful weight loss. Most long-term dieters do not lose substantial amounts of weight *(19)*. Instead, the result of dieting behavior is chronic, purposeful restriction of food intake, irrespective of changes in body weight. The associated eating pattern and related attitudes toward food are not equivalent to, or synonymous with, the concept of weight cycling. Weight cycling is defined as weight loss (often substantial) and regain; and although there is some overlap, the nutritional issues and possible consequences of weight cycling may be quite different from those associated with dieting behavior, food rules, and episodic restriction that does not necessarily produce significant weight fluctuations.

2.2. Dietary Restraint

As reviewed by Polivy *(21)*, evidence from numerous investigations conducted over the past few decades indicates that dietary restriction, the basic element of dieting, appears to play an important etiologic role in the development of disordered eating patterns. In the classic starvation studies by Keys et al. *(14)*, previously normal eaters were observed to become increasingly focused on food when dietary intake was restricted and to binge eat when they were permitted access to food following dietary restriction. Among the etiologic factors in bulimia nervosa, dieting appears to be a crucial precondition for development of this eating disorder. Food deprivation associated with dieting and dietary restraint sets the stage for the development of binge eating and purging behaviors, which are typically followed by more strict dieting, in a cycle that becomes self-perpetuating *(22,23)*. Binge eating among the obese *(see* Chapter 12), now recognized as occurring in a substantial proportion of that patient population *(13)*, occurs more often among those patients attempting to adhere to the most limited diets or those who are prescribed more severe dietary restrictions *(24,25)*. Approximately half of patients with anorexia nervosa also have binge-eating behaviors *(15)*, while still maintaining a low body weight. Notably, anorexia nervosa patients in this subgroup are likely to have a longer duration of illness than those who do not have this behavior, which suggests causality that may be attributed in part to the chronicity of the dietary restriction in these patients *(26)*.

Although dieting behavior appears to be an important etiologic factor in the development of eating pathology in the majority of cases, results from some recent studies of patients with bulimia nervosa and BED suggest that a subset of individuals in these groups may begin binge eating prior to dieting. In a study in which the temporal relationship between dieting and binge eating was examined in 221 women with bulimia nervosa, 20 of the women reported binge eating prior to the onset of dieting *(27)*. Similarly, a proportion of obese individuals who binge eat or have BED do not report a history of dieting prior to binge-eating onset *(28)*. An important methodological issue is that criteria used to identify dietary restriction, when examining the temporal pattern or identifying a subgroup, can vary substantially. Dieting has been defined very differently across studies *(29)*, often based on subject report of a weight loss of 10 or 20 lb as being indicative of dietary restriction. However, such weight loss is not the typical result of the episodic but chronic dieting behavior exhibited by most women who are attempting to control or lose weight.

2.3. Consequences of Restrained Eating

The best-supported explanation for a mechanism by which dietary restriction may cause disordered eating patterns is based on the concept of restrained eating. The food cognitions and eating behaviors of individuals who are purposefully limiting their intake (i.e., restrained eaters) differ from those who are not dieting or restricting food intake, when observed under experimental conditions *(21)*. Restrained eaters in feeding studies typically eat more food following a preload when they believe that they have already deviated from a diet by eating something "fattening." This behavior occurs regardless of the actual amount of energy consumed in the preload and is in marked contrast to a presumed spontaneous regulation of intake to meet energy needs, which would be evident if the individual ate less following a more energy-dense preload. Believing that one has already "blown" a strict diet, a restrained eater eats more than would be eaten otherwise, resulting in a dietary pattern that alternates between undereating and overeating.

In addition to promoting episodes of binge eating, chronic dieting also causes cognitive changes characteristic of eating disorders, such as difficulty concentrating on a task and resistance to psychotherapeutic counseling (15,16). In fact, many affective and cognitive abnormalities characteristic of eating disorders, especially in low-weight anorexia nervosa, may directly result from chronically inadequate intake of energy and essential nutrients (30). Nutritional rehabilitation is now considered an essential, initial component of treatment of anorexia nervosa that enables other etiologic aspects of the disorder to be addressed, permitting sustained weight recovery (16). Therapeutic counseling strategies simply cannot be effective when the patient is cognitively impaired and is focused on food as a result of semistarvation. Dietary restriction also contributes to depression (14), which may be state related in patients with disordered eating patterns. In many instances, the affective changes associated with eating disorders may be caused by the abnormal nutritional status and erratic eating patterns rather than being present as a distinct comorbid condition (15). Following recovery from bulimia nervosa, patients identify regular meal patterns that permit adequate dietary intake and avoidance of excessive food restrictions as being among the most helpful strategies to stop binge eating (31).

Women who engage in pathological dieting behavior without meeting the full diagnostic criteria for an eating disorder have nutritional characteristics similar to those characteristics observed in patients with clinical eating disorders. Eating pathology in these women is typified by a chronic or intermittent restriction of energy intake, driven primarily by the avoidance of foods perceived as energy dense or "fattening" (32,33). Early studies suggested that patients with eating disorders primarily avoided dietary carbohydrate, but it is now apparent that avoidance of dietary fat, coupled with binges that consist of highly palatable and typically high-fat foods, is the pattern of eating behavior that typifies the eating pattern of clinical, as well as subclinical, anorexia and bulimia nervosa (33–35).

3. IDENTIFYING THE PATIENT AT RISK

3.1. Risk Factors

Much of the current knowledge of possible risk factors for eating disorders has been gained from studies of clinical populations. Perceptions of risk factors or correlates with illness may be somewhat limited or distorted by the nature of the subgroup that has been studied, because many individuals with eating disorders do not seek treatment. Epidemiological studies have mainly examined prevalence, rather than specific risk factors. These studies have focused on Caucasian females aged 14–40 yr, in whom eating disorders have been believed to be more common (6). However, although clinical eating disorders have been historically identified more often in non-Hispanic white females than in other subgroups of the population, current data suggest that eating disorders occur in a more diverse population, including males and individuals from lower socioeconomic groups and from minority populations (36,37). Higher prevalence rates among specific groups, such as athletes and patients with diabetes mellitus, support the concept that increased risk occurs with conditions that impart great importance to dietary restraint and weight concerns.

Table 2
Various Factors Associated With Increased Risk for Eating Disorders

• Female gender	• Dieting and other weight-control behaviors
• Family dysfunction	• Low self-esteem
• Body dissatisfaction	• Family history (i.e., genetic factors)
• Profession or pursuit that stresses maintaining a certain body weight (i.e., dance, modeling, acting, athletics)	• Diseases for which management involves emphasis on diet and diet regulation (i.e., diabetes mellitus, cystic fibrosis)

Table 2 lists various risk factors associated with eating disorders. Sociocultural norms set the stage and genetic factors probably affect susceptibility, but personal characteristics and behavioral factors also contribute variably to individual risk. Personal characteristics include both psychological and behavioral factors. Psychological risk factors include low self-esteem, high levels of body dissatisfaction, high concern for appearance, and lower scores on measures of emotional well-being *(6,15,18)*. As a behavioral factor, dieting has been found to be specifically linked to risk for eating disorders in community-based studies. In a longitudinal study of London schoolgirls (of whom 31% were dieting), about one-fifth of the dieters progressed to an eating disorder during a 12-mo period of observation. The results correspond to an eightfold increase in the risk for meeting diagnostic criteria for an eating disorder in dieters vs nondieters *(38)*. Among the dieters, those individuals subsequently diagnosed with an eating disorder had an increase in self-reported depressive symptoms compared with the dieters who did not develop an eating disorder. Depression was the only factor that discriminated between outcomes. Patton *(38)* proposed that key influences, including societal pressures to attain low body weight, operate to initiate dieting, rather than, specifically, the eating disorder. The individual who develops an eating disorder as a consequence of dieting may have focused excessively on body shape and weight, resulting in diminished self-esteem or other psychological vulnerabilities.

In a 3-yr prospective analysis of sixth- and seventh-grade girls, Killen et al. *(39)* examined the relationship between the onset of eating-disorder symptoms and baseline measures on a variety of indices, including pubertal development, body mass index, and questionnaires that addressed concerns with weight, dieting, and psychological characteristics assessed by the Eating Disorder Inventory (EDI). Measured weight concerns, based on the results of a questionnaire consisting of items ranking the degree of fear of weight gain, worry about weight, diet history, and perceived fatness, were found to be significantly associated with risk for onset of symptoms, although this measure also correlated with both Restraint and relevant EDI subscales.

3.2. Degree of Food Restriction

The degree of food restriction, which can be evaluated by dietary assessment, may also be an early indicator of increased risk. Comparison of food records from 18-yr-old women in a nonclinical population, representative of a continuum of eating attitudes and behaviors, revealed that reduced energy intake was the most notable dietary characteristic associated with greater eating pathology *(32,33)*.

3.2.1. NORMAL ENERGY REQUIREMENTS

Much has been learned about energy requirements and energy expenditure over the last few years because of improved measurement technologies, such as the doubly labeled water method. Normal levels of energy intake that are currently recommended are at least 1600 kcal/d for very sedentary women and some older adults; at least 2200 kcal/d for teenage girls, active women, and sedentary men; and at least 2800 kcal/d for teenage boys, many active men, and very active women *(40)*. In the clinical setting, individual energy requirements can be estimated with the Harris-Benedict equation *(41)*, which is:

Women: $BEE = 655 + 9.6 (W) + 1.8 (H) - 4.7 (A)$

Men: $BEE = 66 + 13.7 (W) + 5 (H) - 6.8 (A)$

where BEE = Basal energy expenditure (kcal/d), W = weight (kg), H = height (cm), and A = age (yr). To estimate the average total daily energy expenditure, multiply $BEE \times 1.3$. To convert to kJ/d, multiply by 4.184.

In estimating the energy requirement, figures derived from this formula may overestimate the needs of sedentary women, underestimate the basal needs of athletic women, and may also underestimate energy requirements for older men (>65 yr of age) *(42,43)*. The energy cost of exercise also has a potentially large effect on total daily energy expenditure by further increasing the daily requirement. When comparing these figures to reported estimates of energy intake, it is important to recognize that substantial underreporting of energy intake has been verified with modern objective measures of energy expenditure *(44)*. The degree of underreporting of energy intake is higher in overweight or obese (vs normal weight) individuals, women (vs men), and individuals representing minority groups (vs non-Hispanic whites).

3.2.2. MACRONUTRIENTS

Current dietary recommendations for the distribution of energy among the macronutrients (e.g., carbohydrate, protein, fat) in adolescent and adult diets are that carbohydrate should contribute 45–65%, protein should contribute 10–35%, and fat should contribute 20–35% of energy, in a dietary pattern that is composed of a variety of foods, such as grain products, vegetables, fruits, low-fat dairy products, and sources of high-quality protein *(44)*. Dieters at risk of developing eating disorders typically modify their energy intakes and food choices to a more extreme degree than is advised for healthy weight control (e.g., a deficit of 500–1000 kcal/d relative to energy expenditure). Individuals at risk for eating disorders also often adopt various idiosyncratic eating behaviors, such as consuming large amounts of diet soft drinks and caffeinated beverages in an effort to control hunger despite semistarvation.

3.2.3. ADOLESCENTS

Clearly, not all those who purposely restrict dietary intake will develop an eating disorder. As noted in Subheading 3.1., other personal, socioenviornmental, and genetic factors will influence whether a dieting adolescent or adult will develop an eating disorder. Distinguishing dieting behavior that is not developing into an eating disorder from the intensive or extreme dieting that represents increased risk is particularly challenging in the adolescent patient. Some impulsive eating behaviors, including occasional binges or conspicuous overeating, are often a normal component of this phase of psychological and physical development. As an example, although vegetarian food patterns are common among patients with eating disorders *(45)*, experimenting with alternative diets such as vegetarianism is common among adolescents and should not necessarily be considered abnormal.

3.3. Role of Patient's Attitudes Toward Dieting, Body Weight, and Food Selection

The patient's attitude toward dieting, body weight, and food choices is an important element that links dieting behavior with risk for eating disorders *(12,15)*. Intense concern with diet as it relates to the dieter's gaining weight or becoming fat is the predominant attitude in the individual at increased risk. The desire for thinness is the primary determinant for food choices, which can be revealed with a thorough and empathetic interview. In contrast, the dieter with lower risk of developing an eating disorder will exhibit occasional "slips" or deviations from the diet without great psychological distress. Eating in secret, as well as being unsatisfied with eating patterns, suggests the presence of bulimia nervosa *(46)*. Excessive concern with body image, because it has become a measure of self-worth and a major determinant of mood, is a clear indicator of increased risk for eating disorders in the dieter.

4. NUTRITION IN PREVENTION AND EARLY INTERVENTION

The primary factors that set the stage for development of eating disorders, such as sociocultural pressures, self-esteem, and excessive dieting, are appropriate targets for prevention efforts. Obviously, some of these factors are more amenable to change than others. Recognition of risk factors and early identification of a developing problem are feasible activities for those providing primary and preventive medical care. A general guideline is to discourage strict dieting and instead to emphasize the benefits of increased physical activity and healthful food choices as more effective approaches to weight control in the long term, even if the patient is overweight. As described above, patients at high risk for eating disorders have a singular and intense focus on diet and food choices that is mainly directed toward calories, rather than nutrient composition or health benefits. Working with a registered dietitian, patients at risk can learn to approach foods with a more normal attitude, recognizing the many aspects of foods that relate to overall health and enjoyment. For adolescents and school-age children, preventive efforts also need to target the parents, who may express unwarranted concerns or attitudes toward a child's body weight or eating patterns and create an environment that unintentionally encourages the development of eating disorders *(18,47)*.

4.1. Anorexia Nervosa

For the underweight patient with subclinical or clinically diagnosable anorexia nervosa, weight restoration is the most critical component of treatment *(16)*. However, weight restoration alone does not indicate recovery, and forcing weight gain without psychological support and counseling is ill-advised.

Restoration of body weight in the underweight patient is usually best approached with the goal of a slow, yet steady, rate of weight gain *(16,48,49)*. Depending on the patient's initial level of energy intake, progressive increases at a rate of 200–250 kcal/wk (837–

Table 3
Basic Principles and Goals of Nutritional Intervention in Anorexia Nervosa

1. Increased energy intake to promote weight restoration, applying a weekly, stepwise increase to achieve the goal weight gain (i.e., 0.5–1.0 kg/wk).

2. Specific meal plan and dietary guidelines to promote normalization of intake, including some limitations on the number of foods that patients may refuse to eat and accommo-dating patient preferences that permit nutritional adequacy and weight gain.

3. A new approach to food choices, based on nutrient contributions and other qualities, rather than energy content.

4. Formerly forbidden foods introduced with reassurance and sensitivity to a fear of uncon-trollable eating and weight gain.

5. Adequate dietary calcium to permit improved bone mineralization as weight is restored and hormonal abnormalities are corrected.

6. Low-dose daily multiple vitamin with minerals especially if patients are chronically ill.

7. Avoidance of strategies to reduce energy intake and manage hunger (such as overuse of caffeine-containing beverages, chewing gum) or promote energy expenditure (such as excessive exercise).

1046 kJ/wk) usually result in a goal weight gain of 0.5–1.0 kg/wk. During the process of restoring normal body weight, accumulation of extracellular water may occur and is clinically evident as edema. Most patients with anorexia nervosa have significant osteopenia. The decrease in bone mineral density occurs soon after amenorrhea devel-ops (50,51). Peak bone mass is a major determinant of the risk for osteoporosis, and the majority of bone mineralization occurs in girls during the second decade, so emphasis on weight restoration is critical in adolescent anorexia nervosa. Current evidence sug-gests that improvement in bone mineralization in these patients is associated with weight restoration and the resolution of hormonal abnormalities, and that the problem will not be corrected by calcium supplementation or hormone therapy alone (52,53). Dietary calcium plays a permissive role in osteoporosis: an adequate amount must be provided by the diet if positive balance is to occur with correction of the hormonal abnormalities. Basic principles and goals of nutrition intervention in anorexia nervosa are listed in Table 3.

The nutritional counseling process in the early intervention and treatment of anorexia nervosa consists of establishing and monitoring dietary and behavioral goals in a stepwise manner, with the application of counseling strategies to help the patient expand his or her diet. Typically, the patient is terrified of weight gain and may be struggling with hunger and urges to binge eat, yet the food choices allowed (by the patient) are too limited to enable sufficient energy intake. Thus, individualized guidance and a meal plan that provides a framework for meals and food choices can be very helpful. Specific strategies for effective nutrition intervention and counseling techniques have been described (48,49). Cognitive restructuring, which involves challenging deeply held beliefs and thought patterns with more accurate and healthy perceptions and interpretations, also includes nutrition education and the provision of factual information regarding dieting, nutrition, and the relationship between starvation and physical symptoms. Nutrition counseling begins with assessment and the development of short- and long-term goals, as rapport and a trusting relationship develop, and extends over some time, with counseling sessions scheduled at a frequency that is individualized for the patient and his or her needs.

As a component of the intervention, nutrition education for anorexia nervosa patients usually incorporates some type of food-group system as a theoretical basis for the food plan that is developed. The goal is to teach a new approach to food choices, emphasizing nutrient density (the contribution of essential nutrients such as protein, vitamins, and minerals) or other health-promoting qualities, rather than to prescribe another rigid diet. Working with a food plan in the outpatient or private practice setting, patients can be guided toward increased quality and quantity of the diet (48,49). Formerly forbidden foods are gradually introduced, using strategies such as including foods that have positive attributes or planning the meal environment so that the fear of overeating can be managed.

4.2. Bulimia Nervosa

For the patient with bulimia nervosa, meal planning, encouraging a pattern of regular eating, and discouraging dieting are all part of early intervention, in addition to teaching about body-weight regulation, adverse effects of dieting, and physical consequences of bulimic behavior (54). The primary goal of nutritional management is to normalize the patient's eating pattern, which is typically very chaotic and characterized by an overall pattern of food rules, restrictions, or dieting, regularly interspersed with episodes of binge eating and purging. Although many patients with bulimia nervosa desire weight loss (whether or not they are truly overweight), it is important to communicate that the primary goal of intervention is to normalize eating patterns and discontinue purging behavior.

Cognitive–behavioral therapy (CBT), which is well established as an effective treatment of bulimia nervosa, includes dietary guidance and nutrition education as core components of the therapy (16,54) (see Chapter 2). The primary nutritional aspects of CBT include education about the effects of dieting on the physical and psychological problems, meal planning, encouraging a pattern of regular eating, and discouraging dieting. Didactic nutrition education includes teaching about body-weight regulation, energy balance, psychological and physiological effects of starvation, misconceptions about dieting and weight control, and physical consequences of bulimic behavior. Patients are encouraged to eat three planned meals (plus two to three planned snacks) each day, with a minimum of 1500 kcal/d to prevent hunger, because hunger has been shown to greatly increase susceptibility to binge eating. Helping the patient expand her diet to begin to include forbidden foods (initially, under controlled circumstances) is usually necessary and helpful. Severe and self-imposed dietary restraint regarding specific food types and choices also promotes perpetuation of the binge-eating pattern. Other strategies that are helpful include keeping food records, weighing no more than once per week, and stimulus control (i.e., not shopping while hungry). Nutritional counseling includes developing a food plan and individualized guidance with specific dietary goals that are established and monitored as the diet is expanded and a regular eating pattern is established. Additional counseling strategies have been previously summarized (48,49).

Table 4
Basic Principles and Goals of Nutritional Intervention in Bulimia Nervosa

1. Regular pattern of nutritionally balanced, planned meals and snacks.
2. Adequate energy intake in the meal plan, with the goal of weight maintenance.
3. Adequate dietary fat and fiber intake, with the goal of promoting meal satiety.
4. Avoidance of dieting behavior, excessive exercise, and associated strategies (such as overuse of caffeine-containing beverages).
5. Inclusion of formerly forbidden foods in the diet, with the goal of minimizing food avoidances, using behavioral strategies.
6. Dietary record keeping and review to assess progress and plan strategies.
7. Weighing at scheduled intervals only.

Many patients with bulimia nervosa benefit from detailed assistance with meal planning, reassurance with estimating portion sizes, and reinforcement in modifying abnormal thoughts and beliefs about food and weight. Strategies to maximize meal satiety may be helpful for the patient with bulimia nervosa (or even the anorexia nervosa patient of the bulimic subtype) *(48,49)*, as long as the importance of weight restoration in the low-weight patient and adequate total energy intake are recognized and addressed. Well-balanced meals with adequate amounts of fat and fiber, eaten while sitting down, are examples of these strategies. Patients who are being weaned off laxatives need adequate dietary fiber (from grains rather than from excessive amounts of raw vegetables and fruits) to encourage normal gastrointestinal function. Fluid retention and dramatic weight fluctuations should be anticipated following a reduction in vomiting and laxative and diuretic abuse. Secondary hyperaldosteronism and reflex peripheral edema are the result of volume depletion and dehydration *(55)*, but this problem resolves with sustained discontinuation of purging behavior. Working with individual food attributions and beliefs is used as the basis for expanding the diet to include formerly forbidden foods and to minimize food restrictions. As another example of specific strategies, food that is preportioned and labeled with energy and nutrient content can provide some reassurance to patients who are expanding their allowed food choices. Adding foods to formerly restricted meals can be approached in a stepwise manner, beginning with one meal and then moving on to the next. Table 4 lists basic principles and goals of nutrition intervention in bulimia nervosa.

4.3. Eating Disorder Not Otherwise Specified

Eating disorder not otherwise specified (EDNOS) is a large and heterogeneous diagnostic category that is applicable for individuals who have clinically significant eating disorders but who fail to meet all of the diagnostic criteria for the main eating disorders, anorexia nervosa or bulimia nervosa. Eating-disorder patients with the EDNOS diagnosis are similar to those patients with anorexia nervosa or bulimia nervosa, but represent a subclinical condition. For example, some women menstruate at a very low body weight, possibly because of a biological adaptation to the low weight, although they are otherwise comparable to the patient who meets the full diagnostic criteria for anorexia nervosa (which includes amenorrhea for at least three consecutive menstrual cycles). Another example is an obese individual who has lost a substantial amount of weight from extreme and unhealthy eating patterns and cognitive distortions related to food and weight, but whose current weight is in the normal range.

Because this is a heterogeneous group, the nutritional management of a patient with a diagnosis of EDNOS is determined by the specific eating behaviors and attitudes and clinical problems that are present. In general, the same issues, principles and treatment strategies relevant to the other eating disorders are applicable to these patients.

4.4. Binge-Eating Disorder

BED (*see* Chapter 11) is included in the category of EDNOS at this time, until sufficient evidence accumulates to support the specific diagnostic criteria for this disorder. Patients with BED do not use purging behaviors on a regular basis, yet they binge eat regularly, so they are typically obese. Patients with BED are usually identified when they seek treatment for their obesity, rather than presenting for treatment of an eating disorder. In fact, more than 20% of individuals seeking weight-loss treatment from university or commercial programs report binge-eating problems and related psychological distress (56). The characteristics and behaviors of patients with BED have been compared with those of non-binge-eating obese patients in several studies, and a consistent finding is that patients with BED are typically more obese than non-binge-eating obese patients (57). Another consistent finding is that patients with BED, compared to non-binge-eating obese patients, have an increased frequency of psychiatric symptoms and diagnoses (mainly major depression), independent of degree of obesity (58). Also, a pattern of dieting behavior preceding binge eating is not characteristic of patients with BED, in contrast with the temporal sequence that occurs in the majority of patients with bulimia nervosa. Approximately 50% of patients with BED report that they started binge eating before they started dieting or trying to lose weight (59,60). Concern that dietary restriction increases the susceptibility to binge eating may not be as relevant in the treatment of BED, in contrast with anorexia and bulimia nervosa.

Patients with BED typically have a generalized and consistent lack of control over their eating patterns and food choices, even when they are not binge eating. In the adaptation of CBT to the treatment of BED, the goal is reduced frequency of binge eating and also a pattern of overall moderation of food intake. A framework or meal plan for regular meals may be useful for many patients. The goal is to promote a healthy overall pattern of eating and exercise, and achieving that goal is accomplished by planning and by identifying and modifying maladaptive thoughts and beliefs that lead to overeating and binge eating. Similar to the management of a patient with bulimia nervosa, nutritional guidance emphasizes three planned meals and two to three planned snacks each day, no more than a 3-h interval between meals or snacks, a varied and balanced diet, and food servings that are of average portion size.

The vast majority of these patients are obese, and efforts that are focused solely on eliminating binge eating have not been shown to result in weight loss in the majority of patients with BED (60–64). Also, studies suggest that guidance toward energy restriction through the application of behavioral weight-control strategies does not appear to exacerbate binge eating in these patients (61). However, the long-term effects on weight management that may be achieved in these patients by behavioral intervention programs that incorporate energy restriction are unknown.

4.5. General Interventions

Attitudes about health, body weight, and self-esteem can also be addressed with individual patients at risk as part of a prevention and early intervention effort. For example, many patients need encouragement to accept themselves as they are. At critical points and in susceptible individuals, attitudes about nutrition expressed by health professionals, and even public health messages about diet and weight, can reinforce dieting and weight concerns and can contribute to the development of eating disorders. Even usual patient care activities such as the measurement of body weight and casual discussion during the examination can reinforce, or possibly even counter, the societal pressures that encourage inappropriate dieting. If not thoughtfully considered, these messages can promote an unhealthy focus on body weight and diet composition. Sensitivity to these issues should be reflected in the formulation of dietary or nutritional guidelines and communications, particularly when addressing women and age groups at high risk.

4.6. Organized Efforts to Prevent Eating Disorders

Given the utility of preventing a chronic condition that can be challenging to treat, the development of interventions to prevent eating disorders is an area of great interest. As recently reviewed (18,65,66), developing and testing an organized effort to prevent eating disorders involves some unique barriers and challenges. Because dieting behavior and eating disturbances have been identified as important factors associated with increased risk, several intervention programs have specifically focused on dieting behavior (18,67). Other major targets have included improving self-esteem and self-efficacy, and improving media-related knowledge, attitudes, and behavior. Eating disorder prevention programs can be generally grouped as either universal approaches, such as those provided in schools or for other populations that include both high- and low-risk participants, or targeted interventions that are aimed toward high-risk individuals or groups.

One of the major challenges in designing interventions is that the development of an eating disorder in any given individual is known to be a heterogeneous process, with numerous determinants and etiological factors contributing to risk (66). The sociocultural environment, personal psychological characteristics, developmental events, family environment, and various behavioral patterns all contribute in various degrees to the development of the disorder. Unfortunately, prevention interventions have some constraints, targeting only a limited number of the various domains and risk factors. Responses to any particular intervention are likely to reflect the applicability of the area of focus to the members of the heterogeneous group who are the target of the efforts. Also, the programs described in the current scientific literature are usually quite limited in depth, especially those tested in classroom settings. The time frame of the intervention and the follow-up is typically quite limited, and long-term outcomes are not available. As recently summarized (66), the majority of these studies have not described a positive behavioral effect, although increased knowledge or attitudinal effects have been observed in several studies.

4.6.1. UNIVERSAL APPROACHES

The majority of prevention programs that have been reported to date have been universal approaches, most often in a school and involving a curriculum as the intervention.

For example, Killen et al. *(68)* investigated the effect of a prevention curriculum designed to modify eating attitudes and pathological weight control behaviors in sixth- and seventh-grade girls enrolled in four US middle schools. The goals of the curriculum were to teach the harmful effects of unhealthful weight control practices, provide information on alternative and healthier approaches (involving diet and exercise), and teach coping skills for resisting adverse sociocultural influences that promote excessive dieting and thinness. Although energy restriction was discouraged, some aspects of diet modification were encouraged as a healthier approach (as an aspect of disease prevention), such as choosing higher fiber, lower fat foods. Although a significant increase in knowledge was observed in those who received the curriculum, there were no significant differences between treatment and control groups for any measure of eating attitudes and unhealthful weight-control practices *(68)*.

In a study involving female university students, Huon *(69)* evaluated the effect of peer-group discussions that focused on dieting and body image. Half of the groups were instructed to focus on barriers that impede change in these areas (i.e., media promotion of the thin image, poor self-esteem), whereas the remainder focused on strategies to facilitate change. Facilitating strategies included participating in physical activities that are enjoyed, identifying and pursuing broader life goals, learning to value individuality, increasing self-confidence, and developing skills to resist social pressures. Participants in the discussion groups that focused on helpful strategies to facilitate change exhibited more changes toward developing a positive body image and giving up dieting. In all cases, however, the discrepancy between actual and ideal weights remained unchanged.

In another school-based approach targeting girls aged 11–12 yr, a 5-wk eating disorders prevention program was compared to a control intervention focusing on increasing vegetable and fruit intake *(70)*. Both of the interventions promoted a decrease in dietary restraint at 6 mo follow-up, and a marginally significant improvement in self-esteem was observed in the eating disorders prevention arm.

A recently reported primary prevention study in a group of 500 seventh grade girls utilized a universal approach that involved an 8- to 15-wk curriculum that emphasized the recognition of sociocultural influences, improved body image, and media message interpretation *(71)*. Compared to a control group, the intervention group subjects reported a significant improvement in measures of knowledge and body image at 6-mo follow-up. However, eating-related behaviors, such as skipping meals and dieting, were unaffected by program participation.

As an example of a universal approach applied in a community (rather than school) setting, Neumark-Sztainer et al. *(72)* tested an eating disorders prevention intervention in 226 Girl Scouts. This study focused on improving body acceptance and interpretation of media messages about body image. At 3-mo follow-up, the program was found to have a significant positive effect on media-related attitudes and behaviors, including internalization of sociocultural ideas. However, significant changes were not noted for dieting behaviors in response to the intervention.

4.6.2. Targeting High-Risk Groups

Targeting the intervention toward individuals at high risk has been suggested to be a more efficacious approach, and a few such programs have been tested and reported.

In a randomized controlled study, adolescent girls with body-image concerns ($N = 148$) were assigned to a healthy weight-control intervention, dissonance-based intervention, or wait-list group and were followed for 6 mo *(73)*. The dissonance-based intervention involves a series of verbal, written, and behavioral exercises encouraging participants to critique the thin-body ideal, aiming for a reduction in thin-ideal internalization. Participants in both interventions reported decreased thin-ideal internalization, negative affect, and bulimic symptoms at follow-up. However, no effects on body dissatisfaction or dieting were observed, and effects diminished over time. Using a variety of communication modalities, other targeted prevention programs are being developed and tested. For example, Zabinski et al. *(74)* developed an Internet-based eating disorders prevention program that is currently under study, targeting high-risk female university students.

4.6.3. INTEGRATED PROGRAMS

A current view is that it may be feasible, and also desirable, to integrate the prevention of eating disorders and obesity *(75)*, particularly in the interventions aimed toward adult women and adolescents. With the concurrent high prevalence of both obesity and pathological weight-control practices that may lead to eating disorders, especially in these subgroups, integrated prevention programs that promote healthy eating attitudes and behaviors may be an appropriate approach. Irving and Neumark-Sztainer *(75)* note that such a program could conceptually and practically include behavioral targets, such as reducing unhealthy weight control practices (e.g., binge eating, excessive restraint) and promoting healthy eating and physical activity practices (e.g., regular meal patterns, reduced intake of energy-dense foods, increased physical activity). Another area of focus that is relevant to both eating disorders and obesity is media literacy, which involves becoming a critical, active consumer of media messages. Media messages promote attitudes and behaviors that contribute to risk for both eating disorders and obesity, and restructuring attitudinal and behavioral responses to these messages may help to reduce the risk for these weight-related problems.

5. CONCLUSION

Nutritional intervention in patients with eating disorders, or in those at increased risk for eating disorders, presents some distinct challenges. Altered nutritional status and disordered eating patterns contribute to the protracted course experienced by some patients and the development of irreversible sequelae, such as bone loss. Current evidence suggests that preventive efforts addressing the crucial nutritional issues are likely to face some barriers, such as the multifaceted etiologic factors that contribute to the development of the disease, and some of these influencing factors may not be amenable to change. However, the link between dieting, food restriction, and risk for eating disorders is well established, and the importance of addressing these issues in the patient at risk cannot be overstated, given the severity of the adverse medical and psychological consequences that may result. Both eating disorders and obesity are weight-related problems that are linked by behavioral and attitudinal factors that must be addressed, and linking these targets in an effort to promote healthy weight management is a feasible and promising new area of discussion and research.

REFERENCES

1. Fairburn CG, Beglin SJ. Studies of the epidemiology of bulimia nervosa. Am J Psychiatry 1990; 147: 401–408.
2. Schweiger U, Fichter M. Eating disorders: clinical presentation, classification and aetiological models. Baillieres Clin Psych 1997; 3:199–216.
3. Drewnowski A, Yee DK, Kurth CL, Krahn DD. Eating pathology and DSM-III-R bulimia nervosa: a continuum of behavior. Am J Psychiatry 1994; 151:1217–1219.
4 Krahn DD, Demitrack MA, Kurth C, Drewnowski A, Jordan KA, Reame NE. Dieting and menstrual irregularity. J Women's Health 1992; 1:289–291.
5. Newmark-Sztainer D, Hannon PJ. Weight-related behaviors among adolescent girls and boys. Arch Pediatr Adolesc Med 2000; 154:569–577.
6. Croll J, Neumark-Sztainer D, Story M, Ireland M. Prevalence and risk and protective factors related to disordered eating behaviors among adolescents: relationship to gender and ethnicity. J Adolesc Health 2002; 31:166–175.
7. Ackard DM, Neumark-Sztainer D, Story M, Perry C. Overeating among adolescents: prevalence and associations with weight-related characteristics and psychological health. Pediatrics 2003; 111:67–74.
8. French SA, Perry CL, Leon GR, Fulkerson JA. Changes in psychological variables and health behaviors by dieting status over a three-year period in a cohort of adolescent females. J Adolesc Health 1995; 16: 438–447.
9. Stice E, Cameron RP, Killen JD, Hayward C, Taylor CB. Naturalistic weight-reduction efforts prospectively predict growth in relative weight and onset of obesity among female adolescents. J Consult Clin Psychol 1999; 67:967–974.
10. Mokdad AH, Ford ES, Bowman BA, et al. Prevalence of obesity, diabetes, and obesity-related health risk factors, 2001. JAMA 2003; 289:76–79.
11. Ogden CL, Flegal KM, Carroll MD, Johnson CL. Prevalence and trends in overweight among US children and adolescents, 1999–2000. JAMA 2002; 288:1728–1732.
12. Kirkley BG. Bulimia: clinical characteristics, development, and etiology. J Am Diet Assoc 1986; 86: 486–472.
13. Marcus MD. Binge eating in obesity. In: Fairburn CG, Wilson GT, eds. Binge Eating. Guilford Press, New York, NY, 1993, pp. 77–96.
14. Keys A, Brozek J, Henschel A, Mickelson O, Taylor HL. The Biology of Human Starvation. University of Minnesota Press, Minneapolis, MN, 1950.
15. Garner DM. Pathogenesis of anorexia nervosa. Lancet 1993; 341:1631–1635.
16. American Psychiatric Association. Practice guidelines for eating disorders. Am J Psychiatry 2000; 157(Suppl):1–39.
17. Austin SB. Population-based prevention of eating disorders: an application of the Rose Prevention Model. Prev Med 2001; 32:268–283.
18. Rosen DS, Neumark-Sztainer D. Review of options for primary prevention of eating disturbances among adolescents. J Adolesc Health 1998; 23:354–363.
19. Serdula MK, Williamson DF, Anda RF, Levy A, Heaton A, Byers T. Weight control practices in adults: results of a multistate telephone survey. Am J Public Health 1994; 84:1821–1824.
20. Paeratakul S, York-Crow EE, Williamson DA, Ryan DH, Bray GA. Americans on diet: results from the 1994–1996 Continuing Survey of Food Intakes by Individuals. J Am Diet Assoc 2002; 102:1247–1251.
21. Polivy J. Psychological consequences of food restriction. J Am Diet Assoc 1996; 96:589–592.
22. Walsh BT. Binge eating in bulimia nervosa. In: Fairburn CG, Wilson GT, eds. Binge Eating. Guilford Press, New York, NY, 1993, pp. 37–49.
23. Polivy J, Herman CP. Etiology of binge eating: psychological mechanisms. In: Fairburn CG, Wilson GT, eds. Binge Eating. Guilford Press, New York, NY, 1993, pp. 173–205.
24. Garner DM, Wooley SC. Confronting the failure of behavioral and dietary treatments for obesity. Clin Psychology Rev 1991; 11:729–780.
25. Loro AD, Orleans CS. Binge eating in obesity. Addictive Behav 1981; 6:155–166.
26. Garner DM. Binge eating in anorexia nervosa. In: Fairburn CG, Wilson GT, eds. Binge Eating. Guilford Press, New York, NY, 1993, pp. 50–76.

27. Mussell MP, Mitchell JE, Fenna CJ, Crosby RD, Miller JP, Hoberman HM. A comparison of onset of binge eating versus dieting in the development of bulimia nervosa. Int J Eating Dis 1997; 21:353–360.
28. Spurrell EB, Wilfley DE, Tanofsky MB, Brownell KB. Age of onset for binge eating: are there different pathways to binge eating? Int J Eating Dis 1997; 21:55–65.
29. Mussell MP, Mitchell JE, de Zwann M, Crosby RD, Seim HC, Crow SJ. Clinical characteristics associated with binge eating in obese females: a descriptive study. Int J Obesity 1996; 20:324–331.
30. Rock CL, Vasantharajan S. Vitamin status of eating disorder patients: relationship to clinical indices and effect of treatment. Int J Eating Dis 1995; 18:257–262.
31. Gannon MA, Mitchell JE. Subjective evaluation of treatment methods by patients treated for bulimia. J Am Diet Assoc 1986; 86:520–521.
32. Rock CL, Demitrack MA, Drewnowski A. Eating pathology, fat avoidance and serum estradiol concentrations in young women. Int J Eating Dis 1996; 20:427–431.
33. Rock CL, Gorenflo DM, Drewnowski A, Demitrack MA. Nutritional characteristics, eating pathology and hormonal status in young women. Am J Clin Nutr 1996; 64:566–571.
34. Hetherington MM, Altemus M, Nelson ML, Bernat AS, Gold PW. Eating behavior in bulimia nervosa. Am J Clin Nutr 1994; 60:864–873.
35. Drewnowski A, Pierce B, Halmi KA. Fat aversion in eating disorders. Appetite 1988; 10:19–31.
36. Gard MCE, Freeman CP. Dismantling of a myth: review of eating disorders and socioeconomic status. Int J Eating Dis 1996; 20:1–12.
37. Wilfley DE, Schreiber GB, Pike KM, Striegel-Moore RH, Wright DJ, Rodin J. Eating disturbance and body image: comparison of a community sample of adult black and white women. Int J Eating Dis 1996; 20:377–387.
38. Patton GC. Eating disorders: antecedents, evolution and course. Ann Med 1992; 24:281–285.
39. Killen JD, Taylor CB, Hayward C, et al. Pursuit of thinness and onset of eating disorder symptoms in a community sample of adolescent girls: a three-year prospective analysis. Int J Eating Dis 1994; 16: 227–238.
40. US Department of Health and Human Services. US Department of Agriculture. Nutrition and Your Health: Dietary Guidelines for Americans, 5th Ed. Home and Garden Bulletin No. 232. US Government Printing Office, Washington, DC, 2000.
41. Harris JA, Benedict FG. A Biometric Study of Basal Metabolism in Man. The Carnegie Institute, Washington, DC, 1919.
42. Owen OE, Kavle E, Owen RS, et al. A reappraisal of caloric requirements in healthy women. Am J Clin Nutr 1986; 44:1–19.
43. Owen OE, Holup FL, D'Alessio DA, et al. A reappraisal of the caloric requirements of men. Am J Clin Nutr 1987; 46:875–885.
44. Panel on Macronutrients, Panel on the Definition of Dietary Fiber, Subcommittee on Upper Reference Levels of Nutrients, Subcommittee on Interpretation and Uses of Dietary References Intakes, and the Standing Committee on the Scientific Evaluation of Dietary Reference Intakes, Institute of Medicine. Dietary Reference Intakes for Energy, Carbohydrate, Fiber, Fat, Fatty Acids, Cholesterol, Protein, and Amino Acids. National Academies Press, Washington, DC, 2002.
45. Rock CL, Curran-Celentano J. Nutritional disorder of anorexia nervosa. Int J Eating Dis 1994; 15: 187–203.
46. Freund KM, Graham SM, Lesky LG, Moskowitz MA. Detection of bulimia in a primary care setting. J Gen Intern Med 1993; 8:236–242.
47. Lifshitz F, Moses N. Nutritional dwarfing: growth, dieting, and fear of obesity. J Am Coll Nutr 1988; 7:367–376.
48. Rock CL. Nutritional management of anorexia and bulimia nervosa. Balliere's Clin Psychiatry 1997; 3:259–273.
49. Rock CL, Yager J. Nutrition and eating disorders: a primer for clinicians. Int J Eating Dis 1987; 6: 267–280.
50. Bachrach LK, Katzman DK, Litt IF, Guido D, Marcus R. Recovery from osteopenia in adolescent girls with anorexia nervosa. J Clin Endocrinol Metab 1991; 72:602–606.
51. Hergenroeder AC. Bone mineralization, hypothalamic amenorrhea, and sex steroid therapy in female adolescents and young adults. J Ped 1995; 126:683–689.

52. Ward A, Brown N, Treasure J. Persistent osteopenia after recovery from anorexia nervosa. Int J Eating Dis 1997; 22:71–75.
53. Klibanski A, Biller BMK, Schoenfeld DA, Herzog DB, Saxe VC. The effects of estrogen administration on trabecular bone loss in young women with anorexia nervosa. J Clin Endocrinol Metab 1995; 89: 898–904.
54. Fairburn CG, Marcus MD, Wilson GT. Cognitive-behavioral therapy for binge eating and bulimia nervosa: a comprehensive treatment manual. In: Fairburn CG, Wilson GT, eds. Binge Eating. Guilford Press, New York, NY, 1993, pp. 361–404.
55. Mitchell JE, Specker SM, DeZwaan M. Comorbidity and medical complications of bulimia nervosa. J Clin Psychiatry 1991; 52(Suppl):13–20.
56. Devllin JM. Assessment and treatment of binge-eating disorder. Psych Clin North Am 1996; 19:761–772.
57. Telch CF, Agras WS, Rossiter EM. Binge eating increases with increasing adiposity. Int J Eating Dis 1988; 7:115–119.
58. Marcus MD, Wing RR, Ewing L, Kern E, Gooding W, McDermott M. Psychiatric disorders among obese binge eaters. Int J Eating Dis 1996; 19:45–52.
59. Wilson GT, Nonas CA, Rosenblum GD. Assessment of binge-eating in obese patients. Int J Eating Dis 1993; 13:25–33.
60. Mussell MP, Mitchell JE, Weller CL, Raymond NC, Crow SF, Crosby RD. Onset of binge eating, dieting, obesity, and mood disorders among subjects seeking treatment for binge eating disorder. Int J Eating Dis 1995; 17:395–410.
61. Marcus MD, Wing RR, Fairburn CG. Cognitive treatment of binge eating versus behavioral weight control in the treatment of binge eating disorder. Ann Behav Med 1995; 17:S090.
62. Wilfley DE, Agras WS, Telch CF, et al. Group cognitive–behavioral therapy and group interpresonal therapy for the nonpurging bulimic individual: a controlled comparison. J Consult Clin Psychol 1993; 61:296–305.
63. Carter JC, Fairburn CG. Cognitive–behavioral self-help for binge eating disorder: a controlled effectiveness study. J Consult Clin Psychol 1998; 66:616–623.
64. Tech CF, Agras WS, Rossiter EM, Wilfley D, Kenardy J. Group cognitive–behavioral treatment for the nonpurging bulimic: an initial evaluation. J Consult Clin Psych 1990; 58:629–635.
65. Pratt BM, Woolfenden SR. Interventions for preventing eating disorders in children and adolescents (Cochrane Review). In: The Cochrane Library, Issue 2. Update Software, Oxford, UK, 2003.
66. Pearson J, Goldklang D, Striegel-Moore RH. Prevention of eating disorders: challenges and opportunities. Int J Eating Dis 2002; 31:233–239.
67. Paxton SJ, Wertheim EH, Pilawski A, Durkin S, Holt T. Evaluations of dieting prevention messages by adolescent girls. Prev Med 2002; 35:474–491.
68. Killen JD, Taylor BC, Hammer LD, et al. An attempt to modify unhealthful eating attitudes and weight regulation practices of young adolescent girls. Int J Eating Dis 1993; 13:369–384.
69. Huon GF. Towards the prevention of dieting-induced disorders: modifying negative food- and body-related attitudes. Int J Eating Dis 1994; 16:395–399.
70. Baranowski MJ, Hetherington MM. Testing the efficacy of an eating disorder prevention program. Int J Eating Dis 2001; 29:119–124.
71. Steiner-Adair C, Sjostrom L, Franko DL, et al. Primary prevention of risk factors for eating disorders in adolescent girls: learning from practice. Int J Eating Dis 2002; 32:401–411.
72. Neumark-Sztainer D, Sherwood NE, Coller T, Hannan PJ. Primary prevention of disordered eating among preadolescent girls: feasibility and short-term effect of a community-based intervention. J Am Diet Assoc 2000; 100:1466–1473.
73. Stice E, Trost A, Chase A. Healthy weight control and dissonance-based eating disorder prevention programs: results from a controlled trial. Int J Eating Dis 2003; 33:10–21.
74. Zabinski MF, Wilfley DE, Pung MA, Winzelberg AJ, Eldredge K, Taylor CB. An interactive Internet-based intervention for women at risk of eating disorders: a pilot study. Int J Eating Dis 2001; 30:129–137.
75. Irving LM, Neumark-Sztainer D. Integrating the prevention of eating disorders and obesity: feasible or futile? Prev Med 2002; 34:299–309.

II ANOREXIA NERVOSA

5   Anorexia Nervosa

Steven J. Romano

KEY POINTS

- Anorexia nervosa occurs primarily in teenage and young adult women, but males are also affected. The affected individuals are generally members of middle and upper socioeconomic strata.
- Diagnostic criteria have been established in the Diagnostic and Statistical Manual of Mental Disorders (DSM) by the American Psychiatric Association. Patients often deny having the behaviors and may hide them.
- Anorexia nervosa is commonly associated with psychiatric comorbidities, such as depression and anxiety. Many have obsessional ideation and compulsive, eating-related behaviors.
- Medical complications can be life threatening.

1. INTRODUCTION

This chapter reviews the clinical syndrome of anorexia nervosa, including prevalence, psychiatric comorbidity, differential diagnosis, and associated medical complications (Table 1).

Anorexia nervosa is a disorder best conceptualized as a clinical syndrome because a single, specific etiology is lacking. Although recent sociocultural pressures have perhaps contributed to an increased prevalence, and at least to a much greater and often sensationalized focus in the media, the disorder is not new. Descriptions of anorexia in the medical literature were evident as early as the 17th century. These were antedated by colorful descriptions of the ritual of self-starvation, a striking feature of the currently conceptualized syndrome, in the stories of medieval Christian saints. Perhaps the earliest medical report of anorexia nervosa was that of Richard Morton, whose detailed descriptions of a "nervous consumption" appeared in his textbook *Phythisiologia, seu Exercitationes de Phthisi* (later translated into English and subtitled *A Treatise of Consumptions*) in 1689 *(1)*. Morton's attention focused substantially on the physical manifestations of the disorder, and he noted with curiosity the absence of fever or other signs of known disease. In 1860, Louis-Victor Marce described a "hypochondriacal delirium," underscoring a significant psychiatric contribution to the condition *(2)*. Continued focus on the psychological aspects of anorexia was apparent in Charles Laseque's article "L'

From: *The Management of Eating Disorders and Obesity, Second Edition*
Edited by: D. J. Goldstein © Humana Press Inc., Totowa, NJ

Table 1
Chapter Overview

anorexie hysterique" in 1873 and was complemented by the description of the physical consequences of starvation by William W. Gull *(3,4)*. It was not until the second half of this century, however, and after more classic psychoanalytic formulations (such as refusal to eat interpreted as the fear of oral impregnation) failed to effect treatment course that a fundamental shift in our understanding of anorexia nervosa occurred. This was catalyzed by the writings and insights of Hilda Bruch, who psychotherapeutically explored the emotional machinations of her patients *(5)*. Her elaboration of a number of central psychological features revolutionized our view and advanced our nosological categorization of anorexia nervosa specifically and the eating disorders in general. Bruch highlighted features of anorexia nervosa that helped to distinguish the syndrome from other psychiatric or physical disorders that may have certain elements, such as weight loss, in common. She underscored a body-image disturbance, seen to variable degrees and sometimes to near-delusional proportion, as well as cognitive distortions and inaccuracies that influence the anorexic's interpretation of somatic stimuli. The latter, she purported, was associated with the anorexic's denial of the need to eat and of the complications of starvation. Bruch highlighted the patient's sense of personal ineffectiveness, a feature common to many suffering from this disorder. As is apparent, many of the aforementioned features of anorexia nervosa illustrated by Bruch persist as key elements in our current psychiatric research criteria.

2. PREVALENCE

Anorexia nervosa occurs mainly in females, with approx 5% of patients being male *(6–8)*. Although onset of anorexia nervosa beyond the late 20s or early 30s is recognized, the majority of patients present to the physician during adolescence or college age.

Certain groups appear to be at particular risk for developing clinically significant disordered eating and thus have the potential for such behavior to evolve into anorexia nervosa. Most have experienced a period of nutritional restriction that may be either willful or situationally imposed. Regarding the former, voluntary dieting in an attempt to achieve a more attractive appearance, a prevalent behavior in Western culture and particularly among young females who are more vulnerable to societal pressures and media images, is probably the most frequent antecedent. Restrictive dieting accompanying attempts at improving performance lend greater risk to those in such professions as ballet and gymnastics or, in the case of males, those engaged in sports such as wrestling. In this setting, weight-reducing and body-changing behaviors may be supported and, in fact, encouraged by authority figures, such as coaches and parents. Interestingly, in males who engage in eating-disorder behaviors to enhance performance, the behavior generally remits following the disengagement from the activity. This may, in part, be owing to the lack of peer support for weight manipulation that is not in the service of performance augmentation. Regarding severe nutritional restriction that is situationally imposed, the possibility of establishing disordered eating patterns has been described in some patients following surgery or a period of significant medical illness. Keys best illustrated the induction of eating-disorder behavior and other psychological morbidity through sustained nutritional restriction in a study conducted on a group of healthy males (9). In that study, disordered eating behavior more typical of patients with primary anorexia was expressed in a significant proportion of males and was accompanied by frequent depressive symptoms, highlighting the noxious effects of severe caloric restriction.

2.1. Racial Background

Earlier reviews and general clinical experience reflect a predominance of cases occurring in Caucasians and those in the middle to upper socioeconomic strata. The author's experience directing a busy outpatient clinic in a large metropolitan center is that there appears to be a growing number of patients in non-white populations. This is especially true of those minorities who have assimilated to the dominant culture and who are from families in higher socioeconomic classes. Prevalence data need to be derived from minority populations, such as African-Americans and Hispanics, to support this clinical impression.

2.2. Population Surveys

A number of studies have attempted to quantify the prevalence and incidence of anorexia nervosa. In a survey of school girls in London ages 12–18, the overall prevalence was 1 severe case in approx 200 girls with 1 case per 100 girls in the age range of 16 to 18 yr (10). The findings of a few studies reflect the clinical impression that anorexia nervosa may be increasing in prevalence over the past few decades. Theander, examining the incidence of anorexia in a region of Sweden from 1930 to 1960, described an incidence of 0.24 per 100,000 population per year but underscored a rather sharp rise during the prior decade (1951–1960) (11). In Monroe County, New York, the incidence of 0.35 per 100,000 population between the years 1960 and 1969 increased to 0.64 per 100,000 in the years 1970–1976 (12). A Swiss study that reviewed case histories of anorexia and sampled three decades illustrated a significant rise in incidence: 0.38 per 100,000 for the years 1956–1958, 0.55 per 100,000 for the years 1963–1965, and 1.12 per 100,000 for the years 1973–1975. Again, these studies together appear to substantiate a trend of increasing incidence and prevalence suggested by clinical experience.

2.3. Family Studies

A number of family studies demonstrate a familial contribution to the development of anorexia nervosa. In a study by Holland et al., concordance rates were 9 out of 16 for monozygotic twins and 1 out of 14 for dizygotic pairs *(13)*. An earlier study by Theander presented a calculated 6.6% risk for a female sibling of an anorexic proband *(11)*. These findings are striking given the relatively rare occurrence of the disorder in the general population. In a comparison of families of anorexic probands with families of nonanorexic, psychiatrically disordered probands, increased rates of the eating disorders (including anorexia nervosa and bulimia nervosa) was reported by Strober in the first- and second-degree relatives of those subjects *(14)*. More recent studies by Lilenfeld et al. *(15)*, Stein et al. *(16)*, Fairburn et al. *(17)*, and Strober et al. *(18)* further confirm that anorexia, as well as bulimia, is strongly familial. Halmi, in an interesting study that compared 57 mothers of anorexics with mothers of age- and gender-matched controls, found a significantly higher rate of obsessive–compulsive disorder (OCD) in the mothers of anorexics *(19)*. This finding resonates with the noted obsessional preoccupations and ritualistic behaviors that are characteristic of many anorexic patients. Interestingly, the role of serotonin in disturbances of appetitive behavior, as well as its putative link to obsessive–compulsive syndromes, perhaps suggests a spectrum of disorders character- ized by serotonergic dysfunction. Significant comorbid affective psychopathology, as well as a noted elevation of the prevalence of affective disorders in families of anorexic probands, adds further support to this hypothesis.

3. PSYCHIATRIC COMORBIDITY

Comorbid psychiatric symptomatology is not uncommon in patients presenting with anorexia nervosa. Such symptoms must be distinguished from other coexisting syn- dromes that often require separate and specific intervention adjunctive to management of the eating disorder. A wide array of psychiatric features may be observed, including anxiety, depressed affect and mood, obsessive–compulsive symptoms, and features of personality disorders. Many of these "features" may be conceptualized as dimensions of the primary eating disturbance, rather than true comorbid syndromes, and some may be worsened or modified by the physiological consequences of starvation, malnourishment, and purging behaviors.

3.1. Mood and Anxiety Disorders

Anxiety is prominent and is often expressed in terms of phobic avoidance, for instance, of certain foods, types of clothing, or situations involving meals. The majority of anorexics present with some degree of affective disturbance, most often sadness, although they frequently deny a depressed mood. This denial of a depressed mood may reflect the anorexic's general level of denial, especially in the early phases of evaluation and treat- ment. It is not unusual to observe a constricted, even bland affective display, perhaps most frequently encountered in the more emaciated patient and possibly reflecting a compro- mised physical condition. Certainly, a percentage of these patients present with signifi- cant depressive symptomatology, and some meet criteria for major depression. The latter group clearly has treatment implications, particularly when associated with thoughts of suicide or a significant past history of severe depressive episodes.

Obsessive–compulsive symptoms are often closely linked to primary eating-disorder pathology. Many of the preoccupations or obsessional ideas expressed by the anorexic patient are directly associated with diet, body shape, and weight. Similarly, most compulsive, even ritualistic behaviors pertain to the preparation and ingestion of meals, dieting, weighing, and exercise. Still, a significant number of anorexics may present with obsessions or compulsive behaviors distinct from eating- or weight-related concerns, with a noticeable minority meeting the criteria for OCD.

Some studies have examined more formally the incidence of comorbid psychiatric disorders in patients with anorexia nervosa. In more recent studies, Toner et al. cited a 40% lifetime history of depression in a 5- to 14-yr follow-up involving 47 individuals, which compared with a 12% rate in controls (20). A lifetime history of 68% was established by Halmi et al. (19) in a 10-yr follow-up of 62 anorexics. This compared with a rate of 21% in the control population. An earlier survey by Gershon found the diagnosis of major depression in 13 (54%) of the anorexic patients studied. The aforementioned studies are referenced to emphasize the frequent association of clinically significant affective disturbance in patients with anorexia nervosa.

Both Toner et al. (20) and Halmi et al. (19) assessed the prevalence of anxiety disorders in their studies, including OCD, generalized anxiety disorder, and phobias. The lifetime prevalence of anxiety disorders in these two studies was remarkably similar: 65% in the Halmi study and 60% in the Toner study, with the most commonly encountered disorders being social phobia and OCD. Regarding social phobia, Halmi found a lifetime prevalence of 34%. In the same study, the lifetime prevalence of OCD was 26%. Additionally, Thiel et al. (21) found that 37% of 93 patients who met DSM-III-R criteria for anorexia nervosa or bulimia nervosa also met the criteria for OCD and suggested that the prevalence may be correlated with the severity of the eating disorder. The latter would imply that in severe cases of anorexia, OCD should be addressed early in the evaluation process because the treatment plan and outcome may be influenced by this concomitant condition.

3.2. Personality Disorders

Certain personality characteristics may also be evident, especially those associated with the anxious cluster of personality disorders described in the DSM. These include avoidant traits, perfectionism, and other obsessional characteristics and dependent features. Anorexics of the bulimic subtype may exhibit traits associated with the dramatic cluster of personality disorders, including impulsive behavior and borderline features.

The assessment of comorbid personality disorders in patients with anorexia nervosa has varied widely and reflects, to some degree, the methods and instruments used and the fact that the presence of significant axis I psychopathology can influence the presentation of "personality" features. Recently, a few published studies employed DSM-III-R criteria and utilized more structured interview techniques for assessment of personality disorders. Gartner et al. (22) noted a 33% incidence of personality disorders in restricting anorexics compared with 80% in the study by Wonderlich et al. (23), 23% in the study by Herzog et al. (24), and, most recently, 23% in a study by Braun et al. (25). All of these rates pertained to restrictor-type anorexics. In the Braun et al. study, all personality disorders diagnosed in anorexic restrictors were from the anxious cluster of personality

Table 2
Diagnostic and Statistical Manual of Mental
Disorders Diagnostic Criteria for Anorexia Nervosa

1. Refusal to maintain body weight at or above a minimal normal for height and age.
    a. Weight loss leading to less than 85% of expected body weight.
    b. Lack of weight gain with growth leading to less than 85% of expected weight.
2. Intense fear of weight gain or becoming fat, despite being underweight.
3. Disturbed weight and shape perception.
    a. Undue influence of body weight or shape on self-evaluation.
    b. Denial of seriousness of current low body weight.
4. In postmenarcheal females, absence of at least three consecutive menstrual cycles without hormone administration.
5. a. Restrictive type: During current episodes, the patient does not regularly engage in binge eating or purging.
    b. Binge-eating/Purging type: During current episodes, the patient regularly engages in binge eating or purging.

disorders. Interestingly, 38% of the bulimic-subtype anorexics met criteria for a person-ality disorder in the dramatic cluster, which was similar to the incidence of these person-ality disorders in the normal-weight bulimics studied.

3.3. Psychosis

Psychoticism is rare in anorexics, although, historically, the syndrome was once specu-lated to be a *forme fruste* of schizophrenia. Of note, the degree of body-image distortion in some anorexics may appear to be of delusional proportion, but, again, the disturbance is circumscribed to areas central to the primary eating disorder.

4. DESCRIPTION OF THE DISORDER

The diagnostic criteria for anorexia nervosa are summarized in Table 2. This includes descriptions of the two subtypes: restricting type and binge-eating/purging type.

The most striking behavior in individuals with anorexia nervosa is the persistent and willful restriction of intake that can lead to death in 5–7% of patients within 10 yr of the onset of their disorder. Another distinguishing psychological feature is the irrational fear of becoming fat, frequently in concert with a grossly distorted view of one's self as overweight. This persists even in the presence of severe emaciation and in the face of life-threatening medical sequelae. The patient often exhibits a phobic response to food, particularly fatty and other calorically dense items. Anorexics develop an obsessive preoccupation with food, eating, dieting, weight, and body shape, and they frequently exhibit ritualistic behaviors involving choosing, preparing, and ingesting meals. An example of ritualistic behavior is cutting food into very small pieces or chewing each bite a specific number of times.

Early in the course of the illness, a patient begins to restrict many food items, as is typical of most dieters. As the disorder progresses, though, the anorexic's menu becomes grossly constricted and she develops greater rigidity. Minor variation in meal content can produce tremendous anxiety. Unlike the average dieter, the anorexic continues her pursuit of thinness to an extreme and becomes dependent on the daily registration of weight loss. This fuels even more restrictive dieting. Extreme dieting is often complicated by other weight-reducing behaviors. Exercise is frequently compulsive and hyperactivity in underweight patients is a curious but often encountered concomitant. Weakness, muscle aches, sleep disturbances, and gastrointestinal complaints, including constipation and postprandial bloating, are common physical findings. Amenorrhea, reflecting endocrine dysfunction, is present in females, and lack of sexual interest is frequently observed in both males and females.

Some anorexics engage in bulimic behaviors, including binge eating and purging. Often, purging behavior, such as self-induced vomiting or the misuse of laxatives and diuretics, is seen in the absence of binge eating. The coupling of purging with self-starvation compounds the medical consequences of the disorder. Furthermore, as a manifestation of their denial, anorexics generally minimize their symptoms and the negative consequences of their disorder and are thus rarely motivated for treatment. Unfortunately, denial, as well as the aforementioned characteristics of the illness, is intensified with weight loss, frustrating attempts at engaging the patient in a meaningful therapeutic process. Family and friends become increasingly anxious, even angry, as their loved one regresses and their efforts are thwarted by mounting opposition. Superficial compliance, as is sometimes seen, belies a profound resistance.

Psychosocial dysfunction is common in patients with anorexia. Although educational accomplishments are often seen in adolescent patients, social relations become increasingly constricted, and sexual interest is generally diminished or absent.

Those familiar with patients suffering from anorexia nervosa or who have attempted to treat them will immediately admit to the tenacity of their patients' distorted beliefs. Through the efforts of those dedicated to the study and management of anorexia nervosa, earlier recognition of potentially dangerous eating behaviors and improved treatment strategies should help both the clinician's task and the sufferer's outcome.

5. DIFFERENTIAL DIAGNOSIS

The classical features of anorexia nervosa—that is, the intense fear of becoming fat coupled with the relentless pursuit of thinness—is generally absent in medical and psychiatric conditions that might confound the diagnosis. The term anorexia, which itself refers to absence of appetite, is a misnomer in the case of the syndrome of anorexia nervosa. True anorexia, such as that which might be seen in many medical conditions or diseases, would be accompanied by telltale signs or symptoms of those illnesses (e.g., as in gastrointestinal disease or many cancers).

Lack of appetite or decreased intake, with or without subsequent weight loss, is encountered in a number of psychiatric disorders, such as depression, hysterical conversion and other psychosomatic disorders, schizophrenia, and certain delusional disorders. Each of these is associated with a cluster of other substantiating symptomatology. Examples include persistent mood disturbance and associated depressive ideation in major depression, fear of choking in a patient with globus hystericus, or fear of poisoning, predicated on false belief or delusional ideation, in patients with paranoid delusions. Some patients with OCD may exhibit what appear to be bizarre behaviors around food, eating, or meal preparation, but, on further exploration, their behavior is in response to obsessional ideation (e.g., the fear of contamination). Such patients, in contrast to those with anorexia nervosa, generally admit their discomfort with the need to perform such compelling and often excessive or senseless acts. In summary, although comorbid psychopathology may be encountered in patients with anorexia nervosa, including symptoms of depression or OCD, the hallmark of anorexia nervosa (i.e., the morbid fear of becoming fat and the relentless pursuit of thinness) is absent in the aforementioned psychiatric syndromes. In none of these syndromes does the goal of weight loss drive the behavior.

6. MEDICAL COMPLICATIONS

The majority of the medical consequences, including physiological and metabolic changes, that are observed in anorexia nervosa, are present in starvation states or are a direct result of purging behaviors. With nutritional rehabilitation and the discontinuation of purging behaviors, these aberrations can be expected to resolve.

6.1. Hematological and Electrolyte Abnormalities

Common abnormalities in hematopoiesis include leukopenia with a relative leukocytosis. With nutritional rehabilitation, the depressed white cell count returns to normal and does not require further medical workup. Metabolic alkalosis with associated hypokalemia, hypochloremia, and elevated serum bicarbonate is frequently seen in patients who induce vomiting. A metabolic acidosis may be encountered in some patients who abuse large quantities of stimulant-type laxatives. Volume depletion associated with dehydration in those who fast or purge can increase aldosterone, leading to potassium excretion from the kidneys, which results in hypokalemia. In addition, this indirect renal loss of potassium can compound direct loss through self-induced vomiting. The aforementioned electrolyte disturbances are often associated with the physical symptoms of lethargy and weakness.

Emaciation and electrolyte disturbances can be associated with other significant abnormalities, especially in those patients who purge. An electrocardiogram may show flattening or inversion of T-waves, ST-segment depression, and a prolonged QT interval. Severe hypokalemia can lead to serious arrhythmias and the risk of cardiac arrest. The risk of heart failure is associated with the injudicious rapid refeeding of emaciated anorexics and must be avoided during the period of weight restoration.

6.2. Chemistry Abnormalities

Laboratory tests reflecting liver function may reveal elevation of serum enzymes, most likely indicating some degree of fatty degeneration. This may be observed in the state of emaciation as well as during the period of refeeding. In younger patients, serum cholesterol levels may be elevated. Carotinemia, which normalizes with weight restoration, is often seen in malnourished anorexics. Parotid gland enlargement and an associated elevation in amylase are often seen in anorexic patients who binge and self-induce vomiting.

6.3. Gastrointestinal Complications

Delay in gastric emptying because of extended caloric restriction may cause a sense of postprandial discomfort and early satiety. Both are frequently observed and contribute to the persistence of restricting behavior in anorexia nervosa. Constipation caused by fluid and caloric restriction is common and frequently requires management strategies. In patients who self-induce vomiting, gastritis and esophageal erosions are possible complications. Acute gastric dilatation and esophageal rupture are rare medical emergencies and can lead to shock and death in patients who binge.

6.4. Long-Term Complications

In those patients whose illness persists for several years or longer, the risk of osteoporosis evolves. The degree to which bone density can be reversed with sustained nutritional rehabilitation is unclear. Chronic gynecological abnormalities, such as amenorrhea, can lead to difficulty in conceiving. This author has treated several cases of anorexics who have been prescribed fertility agents to compensate for difficulty in conceiving, the latter clearly linked to the compromised medical condition associated with the primary eating disorder. This situation can lead to complicated pregnancies and premature births. In such cases, it is imperative that infertility specialists ensure that presentation difficulties are not linked to anorexia nervosa in an underweight patient with a history of amenorrhea or irregular menses. Other long-term complications include skeletal-muscular injuries, such as sprains and fractures, resulting from compulsive physical exertion in a compromised patient, and the persistence of a generally compromised medical state.

7. CONCLUSION

Anorexia nervosa is a severe psychiatric disorder of unclear etiology associated with significant morbidity and mortality. Over the past few decades, greater research focus and the attempts by many to delineate effective treatment strategies has led to earlier recognition, as well as the flourishing of treatment centers to address the spectrum of eating-disorder psychopathology. An apparently increasing incidence of anorexia nervosa over the past several decades has been described in a few prevalence studies. Unfortunately, Western society's continued emphasis on the achievement of a slim profile along with the desire to complement thinness with muscular fitness as a key feature of female attractiveness ominously predicts a greater pressure to diet and exercise excessively. This pressure to diet and exercise leads to a heightened possibility of developing clinically significant eating disorders in vulnerable individuals. With the recognition of the chronicity of some features of anorexia nervosa, particularly disordered attitudes regarding body shape and food, there is a need in the mental health field to vigorously research the biological underpinnings of anorexia, establish more effective psychotherapeutic interventions and pharmacological therapies, and, perhaps most importantly, outline preventive strategies aimed at populations at risk.

REFERENCES

1. Morton R. Phythisiologia seu Exercitationes de Phthisi. S Smith, London, UK, 1689.
2. Marce L-V. On a form of hypochondriacal delirium occurring consecutive to dyspepsia, and characterized by refusal of food. J Psychol Med Mental Pathol 1860; 13:264–266.
3. Lasegue C. De l'anorexie hysterique. Arch Gen Med 1873; 1:385–403.
4. Gull W. Anorexia nervosa. Lancet 1888; 1:516–517.
5. Bruch H. Eating Disorders: Obesity, Anorexia Nervosa and the Person Within. Basic Books, New York, NY, 1973.

6. Decourt N. A study of adolescent males with anorexia nervosa. Rev Neuropsychiatr Infant 1964; 12: 499–512.
7. Dally PJ. Anorexia Nervosa. Grune and Stratton, New York, NY, 1969.
8. Halmi KA. Anorexia nervosa: demographic and clinical features in 94 cases. Psychosom Med 1974; 36: 18–22.
9. Keys A, et al. The Biology of Human Starvation, Vols. 1 and 2. The University of Minnesota Press, Minneapolis, MN, 1950, pp. 68–81, 819–921.
10. Crisp AH, Palmer RL Kalucy RS. How common is anorexia nervosa? Br J Psychiatry 1976; 128:549–554.
11. Theander S. Anorexia nervosa. Acta Psychiatr Scand 1970; 214:1–300.
12. Jones DJ, Fox MM, Babigian HM, Hutton HE. Epidemiology of anorexia nervosa in Monroe County, NY: 1960–1976. Psychos Med 1980; 42:551–567.
13. Holland AJ, Hall A., Murray R, Russell GFM, Crisp AH. Anorexia nervosa: a study of 34 twin pairs and one set of triplets. Br J Psychiatry 1984; 145:414–419.
14. Strober M. A family study of anorexia nervosa. Paper presentation. International Conference on Anorexia Nervosa and Related Disorders. Swansea University College, Wales, UK, 1984.
15. Lilenfeld LR, Kaye WH, Greeno CG, et al. A controlled family study of anorexia nervosa and bulimia nervosa: psychiatric disorders in first-degree relatives and effects of proband comorbidity. Arch Gen Psychiatry. 1998; 55:603–610
16. Stein D, Lilenfeld LR, Plotnicov K, et al. Familial aggregation of eating disorders: results from a controlled family study of bulimia nervosa. Int J Eat Disord. 1999; 26:211–215.
17. Fairburn CG, Cowen PJ, Harrison PJ. Twin studies and the etiology of eating disorders. Int J Eat Disord. 1999; 26:349–358.
18. Strober M, Freeman R, Lampert C, Diamond J, Kaye W. Controlled family study of anorexia nervosa and bulimia nervosa: evidence of shared liability and transmission of partial syndromes. Am J Psychiatry. 2000; 157:393–401.
19. Halmi KA, Eckert E, Marchi PA, Sampugnaro V, Apple R, Cohen J. Comorbidity of psychiatric diagnoses is anorexia nervosa. Arch Gen Psychiatry 1991; 48:712–718.
20. Toner BB, Garfinkel PE, Garner DM. Affective and anxiety disorders in the long term follow-up of anorexia nervosa. Int J Psychiatry Med 1988; 18:357–364.
21. Thiel A, Broocks A, Ohlmeier M, Jacoby G, Schussler G. Obsessive–compulsive disorder among patients with anorexia nervosa and bulimia nervosa. Am J Psychiatry 1995; 152:72–75.
22. Gartner AF, Marcus RN, Halmi K, Lonanger AW. DSM-III-R personality disorders in patients with eating disorders. Am J Psychiatry 1989; 146:1585–1591.
23. Wonderlich SA, Swift WJ, Slotnick HB, et al. DSM-III-R personality disorders and eating disorder subtypes. Int J Eat Disord 1990; 9:607–616.
24. Herzog DB, Keller MB, Lavori PW, Kenny GM, Sacks NR. The prevalence of personality disorders in 210 women with eating disorders. J Clin Psychiatry 1992; 53:147–152.
25. Braun DL, Sunday SR, Halmi K. Psychiatric comorbidity in patients with eating disorders. Psychol Med 1994; 24:859–867.

6 Treatment of Anorexia Nervosa

L. K. George Hsu

KEY POINTS

- It is challenging to engage the patient in therapy.
- The family needs to be engaged in therapy.
- Goals of therapy are weight restoration, normalization of attitudes, normalization of eating pattern, correction of physical complications, and weight maintenance.
- Inpatient therapy is likely to be required initially.
- Treatment is time consuming. It requires patience and persistence. The expertise of the therapist is an important component of therapy.
- The potential for relapse needs to be considered as part of therapy.

1. INTRODUCTION

Anorexia nervosa, although it continues to be a relatively rare disorder (1), has one of the highest mortality rates among psychiatric disorders (2,3).

Despite intense research, the pathogenesis of anorexia nervosa remains elusive. Various genetic studies (4–9) have yet to identify candidate genes for anorexia nervosa, and the role of various neurotransmitters and peptides in the pathogenesis of anorexia nervosa remains unclear (10,11). However the increase of the incidence of anorexia nervosa (1,12), particularly in non-Western cultures (13–16), suggests that cultural factors are likely to be involved.

Various suggestions for specific targets of treatment for anorexia nervosa (17–20) have yet to be formally tested and studied. Furthermore, very few controlled treatment studies have been conducted since the publication of the first edition of *The Management of Eating Disorders and Obesity*. Treatment of anorexia nervosa, therefore, continues to be largely empirical and should focus on the major areas of impairment. Treatment of an anorectic patient can sometimes be an exasperating experience for the clinician because of the patient's tendency to deny illness, to defy treatment recommendations, to sabotage treatment plans, and sometimes to be openly hostile towards her care givers. Despite these impediments, the learning experience gained through the treatment process can be very rewarding. A step-by-step approach to the management of a patient with anorexia nervosa is described in this chapter (Table 1).

From: *The Management of Eating Disorders and Obesity, Second Edition*
Edited by: D. J. Goldstein © Humana Press Inc., Totowa, NJ

2. MAKING A DIAGNOSIS

The fourth edition of the Diagnostic and Statistical Manual of Mental Disorders (DSM-IV) *(21)* provides a set of criteria for the diagnosis of anorexia nervosa (*see* Chapter 5). Clinicians are sometimes confused by the lack of clear distribution between the two subtypes of anorexia nervosa, restrictive and bulimic, and among anorexia nervosa and bulimia nervosa, and binge-eating disorder (*see* Chapter 12). The clinical features are summarized in Table 2. In addition, although controversial, the criteria may be too rigid regarding the presence of ammenorhea and weight phobia.

Another potential source of diagnostic confusion is the presence of menstrual cycles even in some very emaciated, usually chronic, anorectic women. For this reason, several investigators have questioned whether amenorrhea should be a necessary criterion for the diagnosis of anorexia nervosa *(22)*. Therefore, it seems reasonable that if a patient fulfills all other DSM-IV criteria for anorexia nervosa except for the presence of amenorrhea, a diagnosis of anorexia nervosa should still be given, and the patient treated accordingly.

A third potential source of confusion is the clinical status of partial syndromes and the subtyping of anorexia nervosa. There is some evidence that partial anorexia nervosa and full anorexia nervosa may be very similar in terms of clinical features and outcome *(23)*. As well, separation of anorexia nervosa into the restrictive subtype (ANR) and bulimic subtype (ANBP) may not be very meaningful because crossover from ANR to ANBP is common in follow up studies *(24,25)*. Clinicians should therefore treat partial syndrome anorexia nervosa and subtypes of anorexia nervosa with equal vigor.

Finally, recent reports, mostly from East Asia *(26)*, suggest that the characteristic "weight phobia" may not always be present in anorexia nervosa patients who otherwise fulfill all criteria. Overall, this absence of weight phobia is probably encountered in less

Table 2
Comparison of Anorexia Nervosa, Bulimia Nervosa, and Binge-Eating Disorder

	Anorexia nervosa		Bulimia nervosa	Binge-eating disorder
	Restrictive	Bulimic		
Weight	Very low	Low	Usually normal	Usually overweight
Eating pattern	Marked restriction	Marked restriction with occasional lapses	Cycles of fasting, binging, and vomiting	Repeated binge episodes
Binge eating	None	Occasional	Frequent	Frequent
Vomiting/purging	None or occasional	Occasional to frequent	Frequent	None or occasional
Fear of fat	Marked	Marked	Marked	None or moderate
Menstrual abnormality	Amenorrhea usually	Amenorrhea usually	Irregular or none	Usually none

than 10% of cases in this country. Furthermore, some patients who initially denied weight phobia or otherwise do not meet full criteria may later become full syndrome cases. When making a diagnosis of anorexia nervosa when weight phobia is absent, the clinician must be careful to rule out physical causes of weight loss. Patients who lack a physical cause for weight loss should be considered to have anorexia nervosa because some patients might be helped at an earlier stage in their illness. Therefore, patients who do not meet full criteria should always be offered treatment.

Because anorexia nervosa is much more common in females than in males, the female pronoun is used in the following discussion. Nevertheless, males also can have anorexia nervosa, and most of the discussion generalizes to males.

3. ENGAGING THE PATIENT AND FAMILY

Usually the anorexia nervosa patient is not concerned about her illness, and sometimes even the family may not be aware of the serious consequences of the illness. Some recent attempts (27) have been made to assess the patient's readiness to change based on a transtheoretical model of change (28). Briefly, according to this model originally designed for smoking cessation, patients may be classified into five stages according to their readiness to change. The five stages are precontemplation, contemplation, preparation, action, and maintenance. Most patients with anorexia nervosa, when first seen by a physician, are probably in the precontemplation or contemplation stage (29). Some investigators have suggested matching treatment to stage of change (27), but this strategy requires more study.

To increase the patient's awareness of her own illness and its serious consequences, it is probably best to take a nonconfrontive psychoeducational approach. Sharing information about anorexia nervosa in a matter-of-fact way such as its prevalence ("you are not the only person with this problem"), clinical features, intermediate and long-term outcome ("eventually the consequences of self-starvation may catch up with you"), treatment goals and approaches ("how you can feel better about yourself without starving yourself") may increase the patient's motivation to change. In younger patients, it is imperative to speak to the parents (after getting the patient's permission) about these same issues.

Sometimes the patient and the family may find it helpful to contact other patients and families through local self-help organizations (see Chapter 8). Books such as *The Golden Cage (30)*, *Fat Is a Feminist Issue (31)*, or *Fasting Girls (32)* may also be helpful.

4. EVALUATING THE PATIENT

At the initial evaluation, the patient's height and weight should be measured. A history of weight and menstrual function changes before and after onset of illness, along with a history of the eating pattern (meals eaten, items of food eaten, binge eating, vomiting, laxative abuse, diet pills or diuretic abuse, and cigarette, alcohol, and substance use) and exercise and activity pattern, should be obtained from the patient. Sleep patterns, social and interpersonal relations, and work or school performance should also be assessed. If possible, a family member or friend can serve as an independent informant to help refine this history. This is especially important when denial accompanies the patient's illness. Such informants are also useful in treatment planning.

Anorexia nervosa is often associated with other psychiatric disturbances. Depression, anxiety, and alcohol and substance abuse are common. Compulsive rituals, if present, are usually centered around concerns about weight, eating, or food preparation, although checking, cleaning, and other rituals sometimes occur. Obsessive thoughts are almost always focused on eating and weight. About 5% of anorexia nervosa patients have a schizophreniform psychosis. Although anorexia nervosa patients who developed psychotic features often retain their weight phobia, the psychosis should be treated independently. Many patients who are in remission from schizophrenia and are taking maintenance medications express concerns about their weight but they rarely develop full-blown anorexia nervosa.

Abnormal physical and laboratory findings are very common in anorexia nervosa. Most of them occur as a result of starvation and malnutrition and normalize when the patient's weight and nutritional status improves *(33)*. Because of acute starvation and emaciation, certain abnormalities, such as electrolyte disturbances and infection, may be life-threatening and should be immediately corrected. Electrolytes and electrocardiogram should be routinely assessed until normalized. Full blood count and tuberculin test (tuberculosis was a major cause of death in anorexia nervosa before 1960) should also be done. Serum amylase is raised in those who are vomiting and may be helpful in monitoring this behavior during treatment. Decreased bone density occurs probably because of reduced calcium intake, decreased estrogen secretion, and increased cortisol levels *(34,35)*. Other tests should be ordered if clinically indicated.

5. SETTING TREATMENT GOALS

Because the treatment needs of individual patients may differ and the needs of specific patients may change over the course of what is usually a long illness, flexibility and sensitivity on the part of the physician are essential, and treatment goals should always be clearly formulated and revised as needed.

5.1. Weight Restoration

With an emaciated patient, the primary goal of treatment is weight restoration *(36,37)*, and the clinician should not ignore the starvation while attempting to understand the underlying causes. Keyes and associates *(38)* clearly established the effects of starvation, and many of the symptoms of anorexia nervosa occur directly as a result of the self-imposed starvation. Improvement in the patient's nutritional status not only is therefore lifesaving, but it may also improve her morbid mental attitudes *(39)*. The latter may seem paradoxical, but many clinicians have clearly documented an improvement in the fat phobia in conjunction with weight gain *(33,40)*.

5.2. Normalization of Attitudes

In the context of restoring the patient's nutritional status, a second important treatment goal is to change her relentless pursuit of thinness, her lack of confidence, and her misguided striving for specialness and individuality. Weight restoration can rarely be achieved successfully without some concomitant change in the patient's distorted attitudes *(39)*.

5.3. Normalization of Eating Pattern

A third treatment goal is the improvement of the patient's eating pattern. Increasing the normal range of foods eaten along with the amount eaten helps to diminish the rigid and often painful restrictions that the patient with anorexia nervosa sets for herself. Very often, an anorectic patient will prefer to eat by herself, attaching a sense of shame and guilt to eating in the presence of others. This reduces the socialization of the patient because eating with others is an important social interaction. Finally, for the bulimic anorectic, cessation of the starve–binge–purge cycle is a major treatment goal.

5.4. Correction of Physical Complications

A fourth major goal is the treatment of physical complications (such as hypokalemia, dehydration, or osteoporosis). A fifth major goal is the treatment of concurrent psychiatric symptoms such as depression, anxiety, or obsessive–compulsive symptoms.

5.5. Weight Maintenance

After weight restoration, the major goal of continuation treatment is the maintenance of a healthful weight. As we discuss later, this is often the most difficult task to achieve.

As already mentioned, treatment goals may need to be individualized. In a chronic anorexia nervosa patient who has many failed hospitalizations and treatment efforts, treatment goals may need to be modified *(41)*. In these chronic patients, attempts to fully restore weight may precipitate depression or even suicide, and great clinical acumen is needed to help these patients live with their illness.

Despite the fact that male anorexia nervosa patients often struggle with different psychosocial issues than their female counterparts *(42)*, the treatment goals for these patients are similar to those of female anorexia nervosa patients.

6. DETERMINING THE TREATMENT SETTING

In-patient treatment may be lifesaving for an emaciated patient *(43)*. It may also foster an otherwise fragile treatment alliance so that meaningful psychotherapy can be initiated. In addition, complications can be effectively diagnosed and managed in an inpatient setting. However, although the short-term benefits of inpatient treatment are indisputable, the long-term goals are still doubtful *(25)*. Most clinicians will recommend in-patient treatment for a patient who weighs less than 75% of average weight, has severe metabolic disturbances, is feeling suicidal, or has failed to improve after a period of outpatient or partial program treatment *(21)*.

Traditionally, inpatient treatment is continued until the patient has reached a reasonably healthy body weight *(39,40)*. In the current climate of managed care, inpatient treatment is used for the stabilization of a patient's medical condition. The day hospital or partial program is now increasingly utilized to implement weight and nutritional restoration as well as psychotherapy. Common sense would suggest that weight restoration and improvement in eating behavior may be more difficult to achieve in a day hospital or outpatient setting, because close monitoring and staff support are not possible except for a part of the day. Nevertheless, no treatment data exist to favor one approach over the other. Crisp et al. *(44)* compared traditional outpatient treatment, outpatient therapy, and no treatment. In this report, both treatments were similar to each other and superior to no treatment. However, randomization to the treatment conditions was most probably compromised, and the patients may not have been matched in terms of severity of illness.

Once weight has been restored and other physical abnormalities are corrected, there is little controversy over the treatment setting for such therapy because it probably makes little difference whether psychotherapy is conducted in an inpatient or outpatient setting. The treatment goal is to improve the patient's dysfunctional body and self-attitudes.

7. RESTORING WEIGHT AND IMPROVING EATING HABITS

The fact that weight restoration is successful in a specialized eating-disorder in-patient program for more than 85% of patients is attested to by different authors working in different programs (39,40,43,45,46). It would appear that these inpatient programs have a number of common characteristics:

1. Weight and nutritional restoration occur in conjunction with psychotherapy.
2. Weight gain is gradual and not precipitous.
3. Staff support is utilized to encourage the patient to eat meals.
4. The patient's self-defeating behaviors such as purging or fighting with the family over meals are contained and controlled in the program.

These findings suggest that a competent and experienced team of clinicians, consisting of a psychiatrist, an individual therapist, nursing staff, and registered dietitian, who implement a rational and reasonable program consistently, will be successful in the majority of patients. It also suggests that specialized approaches, such as behavior therapy, tube feeding, hyperalimentation, and pharmacotherapy, are usually not needed in achieving weight and nutritional restoration. However, as we discuss later, short-term success, although probably life saving, unfortunately does not guarantee long-term recovery.

The discussion of a "target" weight is one of the important initial tasks of weight restoration. This should be done in the context of a discussion of the importance of a healthy body weight including a healthy bone mass. Currently, most clinicians probably use body mass index of 18.5 kg/m^2 as the minimal healthy weight for a patient over the age of 16 yr. Although achievement of this minimal weight may not be always be possible during inpatient treatment, the patient and the family should accept this as an ultimate goal of treatment.

An emaciated patient should be gradually refed, beginning with 800–1000 cal/d and increasing by 300 cal every 2 or 3 d. Rapid refeeding may lead to massive edema or acute gastric dilation, and may increase resistance on the part of the patient.

As mentioned, it is important during the early stages of treatment that a staff member sit with the patient during mealtimes to gently encourage her to eat and to calm her fears about eating. It is preferable that the staff member sit with the patient for at least 30 min after eating, to help her understand and accept the fullness after a meal and to ensure that purging does not occur.

A patient given an apparently adequate number of calories (e.g., 2500 cal) who is not gaining weight is either self-inducing vomiting or disposing of food surreptitiously. Additionally, many patients may continue to exercise excessively while in the hospital, even repetitively jumping in a closet. An experienced treatment team will usually be able to prevent this from happening. It is the experience of many clinicians that there are three periods during the weight-gain process that are the most difficult: the initial 5 lb or so, the time when she reaches about 80% to 85% of target weight, and when she approaches target weight. Patients often will stop gaining weight or even lose weight at each of these milestones. Support and encouragement together with close monitoring and psychotherapy will usually get the patient through these difficult times. Patience on the part of the clinician is essential.

8. CHANGING DYSFUNCTIONAL ATTITUDES

Data are slowly emerging that some forms of individual psychotherapy may be effective in anorexia nervosa *(47–49)*, although more research is needed to identify the particular elements of psychotherapy that may be most effective *(50)*.

Many authors have written about the psychotherapy of anorexia nervosa patients. The following authors may be particularly helpful to those who want to get acquainted with the literature: Bruch *(51)*, Beckman *(52)*, Garner and Bemis *(53)*, Goodsitt *(54)*, Levenkron *(55)*, and Reinhart *(56)*. Although they wrote from different theoretical perspectives, their writings demonstrate a number of striking similarities in terms of treatment goals and therapeutic techniques. They believe that the therapist should be active and should function in the therapeutic encounter as a parent, teacher, guide, and coach. The therapist should explain, evoke, exhort, teach, prescribe for, soothe, and calm the patient. A major therapeutic element in the treatment of the anorexia nervosa patient is, therefore, the personality of the therapist.

There are a number of goals in therapy. The first is to help the patient to get in touch with her inner feelings and experiences, to identify and to verbalize them. Many anorectics have difficulty doing this, and success in this area is usually the first step toward recovery.

Another goal is to identify dysfunctional thought patterns, usually expressed as fear of fat and guilt regarding eating food. Many different dysfunctional thoughts enter into the struggle over whether to eat or not: magnification ("this will put a ton of weight on me"), distorted thinking ("eating this is bad, not eating is good"), overgeneralization ("if I start to gain an ounce of weight, it will not stop until I become 300 lbs"), or personalization ("if I eat this, nobody will like me"). Many patients actually do not want to lose more weight. They do so only because they feel that only by continuing to lose weight can they guarantee that they will not become fat.

Such dysfunctional thoughts extend into other areas of life and seriously impair interpersonal relationships. Because of the lack of data, it is unclear whether anorexia nervosa patients demonstrate more dysfunctional thinking than, say, a depressed patient of similar age, gender, and socioeconomic background. However, because these dysfunctional thoughts clearly impair their recovery, common sense suggests that a therapist should work hard to change them.

Several dysfunctional thinking patterns are commonly encountered. "Mind-reading" is particularly common: "he doesn't talk to me, and I know he doesn't like me," or "he doesn't talk to me because he thinks I'm fat." "Should" and "should not" are also common: "he should have known I am upset." A process of cognitive restructuring *(57)* is usually emphasized to gently challenge the patient's assumptions and to guide her in thinking more rationally. Questions such as, "Is it really true that you will gain 10 lbs by eating this food?, "What is the evidence for thinking that he thinks you are fat?", "What is the worst that can happen to you if he doesn't like you?", are usually used to provoke the patient to reconsider her conclusions.

Another goal is to help the patient to solve problems so that she can to decide what action to take when she feels conflicted and indecisive. For instance, a patient may debate endlessly with herself whether to eat lunch. With further exploration, the therapist may find that the patient is using food restriction to confront day-to-day problems, whether it is conflict with her mother or inability to do schoolwork. Starving herself makes her "feel better," it is something she is "good at." Helping her to develop an alternative set of problem-solving skills, and to think through the pros and cons of each approach, including that of self-starvation, is a crucial therapeutic task.

Although it may be simplistic to say that anorexia nervosa patients fear growing up, it is true that they are often struggling with some developmental issues: issues relating to individuation, identity formation, acceptance of one's self, and relationship with peers of both the same and opposite gender. Adolescence certainly has a different impact on males and females, and many authors have stated that young women may be particularly vulnerable to developing anorexia nervosa because of their relationship orientation (i.e., the importance they place on interpersonal relationships) and their tendency to focus on the body (58). The therapeutic task is, therefore, aimed at helping the patient to balance her self-acceptance with what she perceives of others' acceptance of her. In this connection, Brumberg's discussion (32) on the historical and contemporary cultural influences on women's perception on food, self, and weight may be particularly illuminating. Many patients may benefit from putting their eating disorder in a wider cultural perspective.

9. WORKING WITH THE FAMILY

Family therapy is one of very few treatments that has been demonstrated to be effective in younger (under age of 18 yr) patients with a shorter duration (under 2 yr) of illness (59,60). Although its effectiveness may be less apparent 5 yr later (49), any treatment that shortens the duration of this devastating illness is welcome. Therefore, the therapist must make every attempt to engage the family. This is not to suggest that the family is somehow causing the patient to develop anorexia nervosa; in fact, the therapist must not blame the family for the illness. Living with a person who seems to be starving herself to death generates many fears and anxieties, and it is understandable that family members feel overprotective, angry, and frustrated. They may sometimes use apparently overnurturing and rigid means to try to respond to this difficult situation.

Nevertheless, most family members are willing to learn more effective means to help the patient and to cope with her illness. The very least the therapist can do is to listen to the family to understand their perspective. The therapist can also educate the family regarding the treatment and outcome of the illness. In this process the therapist can discuss with the family members their questions and concerns.

One of the most common questions families ask is how they can get the patient to eat more. The best way to respond is to ask what they have been doing so far. This may lead to a discussion of whether each parent has responded differently to the illness and to differences in their opinions of how the anorectic behaviors should be handled. Without having to take sides, the therapist may point out how different responses may be appropriate in different situations. It may, at that time, be possible for the therapist to encourage the parents to work out a plan of action that both of them feel comfortable adopting and applying consistently until the next family session.

The initial family sessions should, therefore, always focus on helping the family to manage the patient's eating behavior. The family should meet with the dietitian to work out a meal plan appropriate for weight gain or weight maintenance, and details of food preparation (who does the cooking and the way the food is prepared), mealtimes, and who eats together (given the fact that family members' schedules are often different) should be discussed in detail.

After the patient's weight is stable and she is eating satisfactory, family sessions can focus on more general issues such as individuation, boundaries, alliances, and communication. The overall plan is to move the family communication and interaction away from food and weight to more direct and open sharing of feelings and thoughts and more constructive problem solving and conflict resolution.

10. PHARMACOTHERAPY AND THE TREATMENT OF CONCURRENT DISTURBANCES

Pharmacotherapy in anorexia nervosa has had a long history (see Chapter 7). One of the earliest publications endorsing the use of medication was that by Dally and Sargant (46), who proposed using chlorpromazine for allaying fear and resistance during refeeding. Since then, quite a few medication studies have been published, including a few that are randomized controlled trials (61).

It would appear that pharmacotherapy in anorexia nervosa is usually instituted for one or more of the following reasons:

1. Depressed, sad mood is common in anorexia nervosa, and some have suggested that anorexia nervosa may be a variant of a major depressive disorder (62).
2. Obsessionality and perfectionism are quite prevalent in anorexia nervosa, particularly the restrictive subtype (63).
3. The overvalued idea of pursuit of thinness or fear of fat may, at least in theory, occur on a continuum with a delusional thought (64).
4. Neurotransmitter and imaging studies suggest that multiple neuronal system disturbances may occur in anorexia nervosa (17).
5. Multiple concurrent physical disorders occur in anorexia nervosa, and most are related directly to the malnutrition. Among these physical disorders, low bone density has recently been the subject of targeted treatment (32,33).

Several recent studies have involved the use of olanzapine (64,65), haloperidol (66), sertraline (67), fluoxetine, chlorpromazine, and amisulpride (68). All have been shown to be of some benefit but conclusive evidence is lacking. Until more definitive data appear, physicians may use clinical acumen and judgment to use medications for targeted symptoms while watching out diligently for side effects.

11. PREVENTING RELAPSE

As already mentioned, relapse prevention is the most difficult task in the treatment of anorexia nervosa. It is often helpful to set a minimal weight that the patient must maintain during follow-up. If their weight falls below this minimal level, admission to a medical or psychiatric unit for stabilization is implemented. Many patients will maintain their weight above this level if only to avoid inpatient admission, and, in time, some will grow out of their weight phobia.

Many follow-up studies have found anorexia nervosa to be a chronic disorder *(3)*. The 1-yr relapse rate after weight restoration in an inpatient setting may be as high as 50–60% *(69,70)*.

Unfortunately, there are very few treatment studies designed to prevent relapse. The value of family therapy for younger, nonchronic patients has already been mentioned *(59)*. Preliminary data from pilot studies found cognitive therapy *(60)* and fluoxetine *(71)* to yield encouraging data.

12. OUTCOME

The 4- to 10-yr outcome of anorexia nervosa has been extensively studied *(3,25)*. In summary, about 50% recover in terms of weight and menstrual function, 5% die, and the remainder are in various stages of recovery. For those who recover, the duration of illness after initiation of treatment is about 5 yr. Prognostic indications for poor outcome include longer duration of illness, lower body weight during illness, vomiting, poor premorbid personality, poor family functioning, and repeated failed hospitalizations. Thus, early identification of patients with anorexia nervosa may be important for improving the likelihood of successful treatment.

Several studies have focused on the 20-yr outcome of the disorder *(72–74)*. Although the data are somewhat conflicting, it would appear that most patients either recover or die from the illness by the time they reach about 40 to 45 yr of age. The two most common causes of death in anorexia nervosa are complications of malnutrition/emaciation and suicide *(25,75,76)*. Deaths from effects of malnutrition and emaciation are more likely during the first 10 yr of illness, and there is some evidence to suggest that rigorous treatment during the acute phase of the illness might have decreased the early mortality rate. The suicide rate apparently increases as the duration of illness lengthens, and careful monitoring and treatment of concurrent depression may be able to prevent suicide in this group of chronic patients. Nevertheless, the long-term efficacy of our current treatment for anorexia nervosa remains unknown.

Finally, it must be remembered that because anorexia nervosa has a usual onset of illness at about age 16 to 19, a 20-yr follow-up would have tracked these patients only to their late 30s or early 40s. Therefore, studies of even longer duration of follow-up may be necessary to demonstrate the full course and duration of illness.

13. CONCLUSION

Treatment of anorexia nervosa is time consuming. It requires skill, persistence, and patience. From time to time, there have been claims of major breakthroughs in the treatment of anorexia nervosa, but invariably these claims have proven to be empty because their efficacy could not be supported by rigorous follow-up data. Little progress has been made in the treatment of anorexia nervosa since the last review, and controlled treatment studies for both the acute phase and relapse prevention are urgently needed.

REFERENCES

1. Lucas AR, Crowson CS, O'Fallon WM, Melton LJ. The ups and downs of anorexia nervosa Int J Eat Disor 1999; 26:397–405.
2. Keel PK, Dorer DJ, Eddy KT, Franko D, Charatan D, Herzog D. Predictors of mortality in eating disorders. Arch Gen Psychiatry 2003; 60:179–183.

3. Steinhausen HC. The outcome of anorexia nervosa in the 20th century. Am J Psychiatry 2002; 159: 1284–1293.

4. Eastwood H, Brown KM, Markoviz D, Pieri L. Variation in the ESRI and ESR2 genes and genetic susceptibility to AN. Mol Psychiatry 2002; 7:86–89.

5. Frisch A, Laufer N, Daniziger Y, et al. Association of AN with the high activity allele of COMT gene. Mol Psychiatry 2001; 6:243–245.

6. Gorwood P, Ades J, Bellodi L, et al for the EC Framework Factors in Healthy Eating Consortium. The 5-HT(2A)-1438G/A polymorphism in AN. Mol Psychiatry 2002; 7:90–94.

7. Kipman A, Bruins-Slot L, Boni C, et al. The 5HT(2A) gene promoter polymorphism as a modifying rather than a vulnerability factor in AN. Eur Psychiatry 2002; 17:227–229.

8. Koronyo-Hamaoui M, Danziger Y, Frisch A, et al. Association between AN and the hskCa3 gene. Mol Psychiatry 2002; 7:82–85.

9. Urwin RE, Bennetts B, Wilchen B, et al. AN (restrictive subtype) is associated with a polymorphism in the novel norepinephrine transporter gene promoter polymorphic region. Mol Psychiatry 2002; 7: 652–657.

10. Frank GK, Kaye WH, Weltzin TE, et al. Altered response to meta-chlorophenylpiperazine in AN. Int J Eat Disord 2001; 30:57–68.

11. Otto B, Cuntz U, Fruehauf E, et al. Weight gain decreases elevated plasma ghrelin concentrations of patients with AN. Eur J Endocrinol 2001; 145:669–673.

12. Moller-Madsen S, Nystrup J. Incidence of anorexia nervosa in Denmark. Acta Psychiatr Scand 1992; 86:197–200.

13. Lai K. AN in Chinese adolescents. J Adolesc 2000; 23:561–568.

14. Perera H, Wickramasinghe V, Wanigasinghe K, Perera G. AN in early adolescence in Sri Lanka. Ann Trop Pediatr 2002; 22:173–177.

15. Ung EK. Eating disorders in Singapore. Ann Acad Med Singapore 2003; 32:19–24.

16. White VO, Gardner JM. Presence of AN and BN in Jamaica. West Indian Med J 2002; 51:32–34.

17. Barbarich NC, Kaye WH, Jimmerson D. Neurotransmitter and imaging studies in AN. Curr Drug Target CNS Neurol Disorders 2003; 2:61–72.

18. Gutierrez E, Vazquez R. Heart in the treatment of patients with AN. Eur Weight Disord 2001, 6:49–52.

19. Hadley SJ, Walsh BT. Gastrointestinal disturbances in AN and BN. Curr Drug Target CNS Neurol Disord 2002; 2:1–9.

20. Wheatland R. Alternative treatment considerations in AN. Med Hypotheses 2002; 59:710–715.

21. American Psychiatric Association. Diagnostic and Statistical Manual of Mental Disorders, 4th Ed. American Psychiatric Association, Washington, DC, 1994.

22. Garfinkel PE, Lin E, Georing P, et al. Should amenorrhoea be necessary for the diagnosis of anorexia nervosa? Bri J Psychiatry 1996; 168:500–506.

23. Crow SJ, Agras WS, Halmi K, Mitchell J, Kraemer KC. Full syndromal versus subthreshold AN, BN and BED. Int J Eat Disord 2002; 32:309–318.

24. Eddy KT, Keel PK, Dorer DJ, Delinsky SS, Franko DL, Herzog DB. Longitudinal comparison of AN subtypes. Int J Eat Disord 2002; 31:191–201.

25. Hsu LKG. The outcome of anorexia nervosa: a reappraisal. Psychol Med 1988; 18: 807–812.

26. Hsu LKG, Lee S. Is weight phobia always necessary for a diagnosis of anorexia nervosa? Am J Psychiatry 1993; 150:1466–1471.

27. Touyz S, Thornton C, Rieger E. The incorporation of the Stage of Change Model in the day hospital treatment of patients with AN. Eur Child Adol Psychiatry 2003; 12(Suppl 1):165–171.

28. Prochaska JO, DiClemente CC. Stages and processes of self change in smoking. J Consult Clin Psychol 1983; 155:390–395.

29. Rieger E, Touyz S, Benmont PJ. The AN Stages of Change Questionnaire. Int J Eat Disord 2002; 32:24–38.

30. Bruch H. The Golden Cage. Open Books, London, UK, 1978.

31. Orbach S. Accepting the symptom: a feminist psychoanalytic treatment of anorexia nervosa. In Garner DM, Garfinkel PE, eds. Handbook of Psychotherapy for Anorexia Nervosa and Bulimia. Guilford, New York, NY, 1985; pp. 83–106.

32. Brumberg JJ. Fasting Girls. Harvard University Press, Cambridge, MA, 1988.

33. Hsu LKG. Eating Disorders. Guilford, New York, NY, 1990.
34. Gordon CM, Grace E, Emans SJ, et al. Effects of oral dehydroepiandrosterone on bone density in young women with AN. J Clin Endocrinol Metab 2002; 87:4935–4941.
35. Grinspoon S, Thomas L, Miller K, Herzog D, Klibanski A. Effects of recombinant human 1GF-I and oral contraceptive administration on bone density in AN. J Clin Endocrinol Metab 2002; 87:2883–2891.
36. American Dietetic Association. Position of the American Dietetic Association on nutrition intervention in AN. J Am Diet Assoc 2001; 101:810–819.
37. American Psychiatric Association. Practice guidelines for eating disorders. Am J Psychiatry1993; 150:212–228.
38. Keyes A, Brozek J, Henschel A, Michelson O, Taylor HL. The Biology of Human Starvation, Vol. 1. University of Minnesota Press, Minneapolis, MN, 1950, p. 828.
39. Morgan HG, Russell GFM. Value of family background and clinical features as predictors of long-term outcome in anorexia nervosa: four year follow-up study of 41 patients. Psychol Med 1975; 5:355–371.
40. Garfinkel PE, Garner DM. Anorexia nervosa: a multidimensional perspective. Basic Books, New York, NY, 1982.
41. Crisp AH. Anorexia Nervosa: Let Me Be. Plenum, London, UK, 1980.
42. Andersen AE. Males with Eating Disorders. Brunner/Mazel, New York, NY, 1990.
43. Powers PS, Powers HP. Inpatient treatment of anorexia nervosa. Psychosomatics 1984; 25:512–527.
44. Crisp AH, Norton K, Gowers S, . A controlled study of the effect of therapies aimed at adolescent and family psychopathology in anorexia nervosa. Br J Psychiatry 1991; 159:325–333.
45. Crisp AH, Hsu LKG, Harding B, Hartshorn J. Clinical features of anorexia nervosa. J Psychosom Res 1980; 24:179–191.
46. Dally PJ. Anorexia Nervosa. Grune Stratton, New York, NY, 1969.
47. Dare C, Eisler I, Russell G, Treasure J, Dodge L. Psychological therapies for adults with AN. Br J Psychiatry 2001; 178:216–221.
48. Robin AL, Siegel PT, Moye AW, Gilroy M, Dennis AB, Sikand A. A controlled comparison of family versus individual therapy for adolescents with AN. Am J Acad Child Adolesc Psychiatry, 1999; 38: 1482–1489.
49. Eisler I, Dare C, Russell G. Family and individual therapy in AN. Arch Gen Psychiatry 1997; 54: 1025–1030.
50. Kaplan AS. Psychological treatments for AN. Can J Psychiatry 2002; 47:235–242.
51. Bruch H. Eating Disorders: Obesity, Anorexia Nervosa, and the Person Within. Basic Books, New York, NY, 1973.
52. Griffin ME, Frazier SH, Robinson DB, Johnson AM. The internist's role in the successful treatment of anorexia nervosa. Proc Staff Meet Mayo Clin 1957; 32:171–182.
53. Garner DM, Bemis KM. Cognitive therapy for anorexia nervosa. In: Garner DM , Garfinkel PE ,eds. Handbook of Psychotherapy for Anorexia Nervosa and Bulimia. Guilford, New York, NY, 1985, pp. 107–146.
54. Goodsitt A. Self-psychology and the treatment of anorexia nervosa. In: Garner DM , Garfinkel PE, eds. Handbook of Psychotherapy for Anorexia Nervosa and Bulimia. Guilford, New York, NY, 1985, pp. 55–82.
55. Levenkron S. The Best Little Girl in the World. Contemporary Books, Chicago, IL, 1983.
56. Reinhart JB, Kenna MD, Succop RA. Anorexia nervosa in children: outpatient management. J Am Acad Child Psychiatry 1972; 11:114–131.
57. Burns DD. Feeling Good. Signet/New American Library, New York, NY, 1981.
58. Striegel-Moore RH. A feminist perspective on the etiology of eating disorders. In: Brownell KD , Fairburn CG , eds. Eating Disorders and Obesity. Guilford, New York, NY, 1955, pp. 224–229. .
59. LeGrange D. Family therapy for adolescent AN. J Clin Psychol 1999; 55:727–739.
60. Lock J. Treating adolescents with eating disorders in the family context. Child Adolesc Psychiatr Clin North Am 2002; 11:331–42.
61. Zhu AJ, Walsh BT. Pharmacologic treatment of eating disorders. Can J Psychiatry 2002; 47:227–234.
62. Pope HG, Jr. Hudson JI. Is bulimia nervosa a heterogeneous disorder? Lessons from the history of medicine. Int J Eat Disord 1988; 7:155–166.
63. Halmi KA, Sunday SR, Strober M, et al. Perfectionism in AN. Am J Psychiatry 2000; 157:1799–1805.

64. Mehler C, Wewetzer C, Schulze U, Warnke A, Theisen F, Dittmann R. Olanzapine in children and adolescents with chronic AN. Eur Child Adolesc Psychiatry 2001; 10:151–157.
65. Powers PS, Santana CA, Bannon YS. Olanzapine in the treatment of AN. Int J Eat Disord 2002; 32:146–154.
66. Cassano GB, Miniati M, Pini S. Six month open trial of haloperidol as an adjunctive treatment for AN. Int J Eat Disord 2003; 33:172–177.
67. Santonastaso P, Friederici S, Favaro A. Sertraline in the treatment of restricting AN. J Child Adolesc Psychopharmacol 2001; 11:143–150.
68. Ruggiero GM, Laini V, Mauri MC, et al. A single blind comparison of amisulpride, fluoxetine and clomipramine in the treatment of restricting AN. Prog Neuropsych Pharmacol Biol Psychiatry 2001; 25:1049–1059.
69. Russell GFM, Szmukler GI, Dare C, Eisler I. An evaluation of family therapy in anorexia nervosa and bulimia nervosa. Arch Gen Psychiatry 1987; 44:1047–1056.
70. Hsu LKG, Crisp AH, Harding B. Outcome of anorexia nervosa. Lancet 1979; 1:62–65.
71. Kaye WH, Nagata T, Weltzin TE, et al. Double blind placebo controlled administrates of fluoxetine in restrictive type AN. Biolog Psychiatry 2001; 49:644–652.
72. Ratnasuriya RH, Eisler I, Szmukler GI, Russell GFM. Anorexia nervosa: outcome and prognostic factors after 20 years. Brit J Psychiatry 1991; 158:947.
73. Crisp AH, Callender JS, Hallek C, Hsu LKG. Long term mortality in AN. Brit J Psychiatry 1992; 161:104–107.
74. Theander S. Outcome and prognosis in anorexia nervosa and bulimia: some results of previous investigations, compared with those of a Swedish long-term study. J Psych Res 1985; 19:493–508.
75. Sullivan PF. Mortality in AN. Am J Psychiatry 1995; 152:1073–1074.
76. Nielsen S, Moller-Madsen S, Isager T, Jorgensen J, Pagsberg K, Theander S. Standardized mortality in eating disorders. J Psychosom Res 1998; 44:413–434.

7
Pharmacological Therapy for Anorexia Nervosa

Walter H. Kaye

KEY POINTS

- The initial treatment of patients with anorexia nervosa usually is as hospital inpatients. As a consequence, most studies of medications for anorexia nervosa are generally initiated in inpatients.
- Although many different medications have been studied for effects on anorexia nervosa, few have been evaluated in double-blind, placebo-controlled trials.
- The endpoint of most pharmacotherapy studies has been weight gain. Other endpoints, such as obsessional thinking and mood, should also be evaluated.
- The best studied medication is fluoxetine, and it should be the first therapy used. It appears to be of benefit in preventing relapse after hospital discharge.

1. INTRODUCTION

People with anorexia nervosa have abnormal eating behaviors with associated cognitive misconceptions concerning body image and disturbances of mood as well as alterations of a wide variety of hormonal and metabolic systems (*see* Chapter 5 for further description of anorexia nervosa). Currently, many investigators conceptualize these disorders as being caused by a combination of cultural-social, psychological, and biological factors *(1,2)*. In general, the response of patients with anorexia nervosa to psychotherapeutic or pharmacological treatments has been limited. The purpose of this chapter is to review the evidence for the efficacy of available drug treatments for anorexia nervosa and guidelines for pharmacological therapy (Table 1).

2. RELATIVE VALUE OF CLINICAL TRIALS

Most medication trials have been done in anorexics who were inpatients in an attempt to find an agent that might accelerate restoration of weight. Some studies also determined whether the medication influenced mood or anorectic attitudes. A wide variety of psychoactive medications have been administered to people with anorexia nervosa in open,

From: *The Management of Eating Disorders and Obesity, Second Edition*
Edited by: D. J. Goldstein © Humana Press Inc., Totowa, NJ

Table 1
Chapter Overview

1. Introduction
2. Relative Value of Clinical Trials
   2.1 Design Issues
   2.2. Study Questions
3. Overview of Medication Trials
   3.1. Neuroleptics
   3.2. Appetite Stimulants
   3.3. Prokinetic Agents, Stimulation of Gastric Emptying
   3.4. Antidepressants
   3.5. Serotonin-Specific Medications
   3.6. Atypicals
4. Guidelines for Clinical Treatment
5. Conclusion

uncontrolled trials. Most have been open trials of medications, and the medications have been reported to be beneficial in the treatment of anorexia nervosa. Unfortunately, few studies of medication evaluated in rigorous double-blind, placebo-controlled trials have been reported in patients with anorexia nervosa. In the reported double-blind trials, in contrast to the positive claims from open trials, results have been, for the most part, more modest. Double-blind studies report limited success in treatment of specific problems, such as slow rate of weight gain during refeeding, disturbed attitudes toward food and body image, depressed mood, or gastrointestinal discomfort. Although double-blind placebo-controlled trials are more rigorous and, generally, easier to interpret, some valuable information can be gleaned from uncontrolled trials. Open trials have suggested possible efficacy of L-dopa *(3)*, phenoxybenzamine *(4)*, diphenylhydantoin *(5,6)*, stimulants *(7)*, and naloxone *(8)*. None of these observations has been studied appropriately under double-blind, controlled conditions. Nevertheless, although these medications have not been rigorously studied, they should not be dismissed. Ignoring such studies opens the possibility of overlooking useful therapeutic agents. Rather, we should encourage subsequent controlled trials. In the meantime, the clinician must rely on the psychopharmacological principles of balancing risks and benefits. If the patient has had multiple treatment failures or is severely incapacitated by dysphoric mood or obsessional thoughts, the use of novel treatment strategies should be considered.

2.1. Design Issues

Few double-blind, placebo-controlled pharmacological studies have been done in patients with anorexia nervosa. One problem with determining the efficacy of pharmacotherapy in anorexia nervosa is that often medications have been given in association with other therapies. For example, drug trials during inpatient weight restoration are confounded by the effects of refeeding, structure of the inpatient unit, and other factors. Moreover, there is a ceiling on the rate of inpatient weight gain because of limitations on the amount of food that anorexics can eat. Thus, it may be unclear whether it was the medication or the therapy that resulted in improvement. Furthermore, the criterion for improvement has often been weight gain, not a normalization of thinking and a reduction in fears of being fat. It is important to emphasize that getting anorexics to gain weight can be accomplished in structured settings without medication. However, what is more difficult is getting anorexic patients to maintain weight in the long term when they are not in a structured treatment setting. The majority of medication trials have been short term and usually associated with a weight-gaining program assessing the effect of medication on the rate of weight gain. Few follow-up studies have evaluated whether any medications produce permanent beneficial effects.

2.2. Study Questions

We think that there are probably more important questions to now assess in pharmacologic treatments. First, could a medication help underweight anorexics gain weight in an outpatient setting? Second, could medication help anorexics maintain weight as outpatients? When assessing the effect of medication on weight, it is important that the trial be long enough to determine whether significant changes in weight occur. This length of time might be at least 4 mo. In trials, a placebo-control group is essential because some anorexics will improve with minimal interventions. If medications are given in association with other therapies, these therapies should be similar for groups on placebo and active medication. Groups of subjects given placebo and active medications should be randomly allocated to treatment, or even stratified to balance factors known to affect outcome. These confounding factors include age of onset, duration of illness or age at study, restrictor-type vs bulimic/purging-type anorexia, and gender. Importantly, it should be determined whether active medication affects symptoms and function. That is, is there a reduction in "core" anorexia nervosa symptoms, obsessionality, depression, and anxiety? Finally, because few anorexics rapidly and spontaneously improve, the use of a washout period is probably not necessary.

3. OVERVIEW OF MEDICATION TRIALS

The first generation of treatment studies focused mainly on attempts to increase the rate of weight gain of emaciated patients in a hospital setting. This strategy is of limited usefulness, since inpatient treatment, consisting of nursing care, behavior modification, and supportive psychotherapy, succeeds in restoring the weight of over 85% of emaciated anorectics (9). Thus, it may be difficult to prove that an active medication or psychotherapies are effective in such a setting.

Relapse within 1 yr after successful inpatient weight restoration is very common (10). For example, the Maudsley study (11) reported that only 23% of the patients had a good outcome at 1 yr after discharge despite intensive outpatient individual or family therapy. Thus, it can be argued that if a treatment method is effective, it should demonstrate that it could maintain a healthy body weight and prevent relapse in patients after discharge from the hospital. In fact recent studies have suggested that specialized psychotherapies (12,13), or selective serotonin reuptake inhibitor (SSRI) medication (14) may improve outcome.

As defined by the revised third edition of the Diagnostic and Statistical Manual of Mental Disorders (DSM-III-R), anorexia nervosa is characterized by certain core symptoms such as "refusal to maintain body weight, an intense fear of gaining weight or becoming fat, and feeling fat." These body-image distortions and the fear of being fat tend to be persistent, recurrent, intrusive, and continuous ruminations. Moreover, many anorexics have "perfectionistic" thinking in that they feel that they think, do, and say things exactly correctly and better than other people. Many anorexics incessantly exercise and have odd, ritualized eating behaviors. Studies using medication and psychological treatments have not tended to report whether these treatments reduce these core symptoms.

Finally, although not a focus of this chapter, recent controlled trials have demonstrated benefits of family therapy, insight-oriented therapy, and supportive psychotherapy *(11,13,15,16)*. Family therapy techniques appear to be particularly helpful in younger patients with anorexia nervosa. Follow-up studies suggest that these interventions may also help prevent relapse in patients who achieve weight restoration. Recent studies have begun more systematic evaluation of the potential benefits of manualized cognitive behavioral and family therapies for this disorder *(17–19)*.

3.1. Neuroleptics

Two neuroleptics, pimozide *(20)* and sulpiride *(21),* have been investigated in anorexia using controlled treatment trials. Both drugs had limited success in accelerating weight gain or altering anorectic attitudes for some patients for part of the study, but overall drug effect was marginal. These studies do not support the use of pimozide or sulpiride in the routine treatment of anorexia nervosa. Whether other "traditional" neuroleptics are useful remains unknown.

3.2. Appetite Stimulants

Two drugs, tetrahydrocannabinol (THC) and clonidine, were tested because of anecdotal reports of appetite stimulation. THC was not useful and, in fact, may have been detrimental because it increased dysphoria in some patients *(22)*. Clonidine was also found to have no therapeutic effect on increasing weight restoration as compared to placebo *(23)* even with doses that effected hemodynamic parameters.

3.3. Prokinetic Agents, Stimulation of Gastric Emptying

When underweight, patients with anorexia nervosa have delayed gastric emptying *(24)*. In general, gastric emptying improves with refeeding. Still, delayed gastric emptying could perpetuate the disorder in some patients by limiting the quantity of food that may be comfortably eaten. Also, delayed gastric emptying could influence the learning of abnormal associations to the presence of food in the stomach, which may persist even when the pathophysiology has been reversed.

Studies of prokinetic drugs in anorexia nervosa have been limited to parenteral preparations or to experiments with small uncontrolled groups of patients *(25–28)*. Szmukler *(29)* administered cisapride to underweight hospitalized anorexics who were in a weight-gaining program. Subjects got either 10 mg of cisapride three times a day or placebo in a double-blind, placebo-controlled design. It was found that gastric emptying improved significantly, but equally, in both subjects who received cisapride or placebo. Subjective measures of distress during meals and measures of hunger improved more in the group on cisapride. Both groups gained similar amounts of weight. The authors suggest that cisapride could be an adjunct to the management of patients who have marked distress associated with meals and who have evidence of delayed gastric emptying.

3.4. Antidepressants

There has been controversy as to whether anorexia nervosa and major depressive disorders share a common diathesis. However, critical examination of clinical phenomenology, family history, antidepressant response, biological correlates, course and outcome, and epidemiology yield limited support for this hypothesis *(30–32)*. This focus has tended to obscure investigations of other psychiatric symptoms commonly observed in this illness. At least three lines of evidence suggest that anorexia nervosa may be related to obsessive–compulsive disorder (OCD) and/or anxiety disorders. First, anorexics have a high prevalence of obsessive–compulsive symptoms or disorders *(30,33–35)*, as well as other anxiety disorders *(36)*. For example, Strober *(33)* described the anorexic personality as being markedly obsessional in character makeup, introverted, self-denying, prone to self-abasement with limited spontaneity, overly formalistic, and stereotyped in thinking despite being industrious. He noted that these characteristics persisted after short-term weight restoration. Second, adult women with OCD have an increased incidence of prior anorexia nervosa *(37)*. Third, anorexics have disturbances of serotonergic *(38)* activity that persist after long-term weight recovery. A disturbance of this neurotransmitter system has been implicated in OCD *(39)*.

Because of the high incidence of mood disturbances in anorexics, several antidepressants have been studied in controlled treatment trials. These include amitriptyline *(40–42)*, and lithium *(43)*. None of these medications appears to significantly improve mood compared with the effects of placebos. Some partial effects were noted for weight gain, improved attitude, and weight maintenance following discharge, but benefits were relatively minor. Thus, the benefit of using antidepressants in anorectics remains unknown but worthy of further study. Although antidepressants do not appear to be indicated as a routine part of weight-restoration programs, they should be tried when an affective disorder is present.

3.5. Serotonin-Specific Medications

Several lines of evidence support the possibility that serotonin-specific medication might be useful in the treatment of anorexia nervosa. First, for more than 50 yr *(44)*, investigators have raised the possibility that anorexia nervosa shares similarities with OCD. Only serotonin-specific medication has been found to be useful in treating OCD. Moreover, serotonin reuptake blockers have been reported to be useful in the treatment of body-dysmorphic disorder *(45)*, which are symptoms that seem to share some overlap with anorexia nervosa and OCD. Second, we have found *(38)* that women recovered from anorexia nervosa had *increased* cerebrospinal fluid (CSF) concentrations of 5-hydroxy indole acetic acid (5-HIAA), the major serotonin metabolite, compared to control women. Additionally, women who were recovered from anorexia nervosa continued to have modest, but significant, increases in negative mood, obsessionality, perfectionism, and core eating-disorder symptoms *(46)*. Studies in humans and animals suggest that serotonin activity is related to behavioral inhibition. Considerable numbers of studies show that reduced CSF 5-HIAA concentration correlates with impulsive aggressive behaviors. Recent studies from our group show persistent alterations of serotonin 2A receptors after recovery from anorexia nervosa *(47,48)*, which may be a compensatory downregulation as a result of increased synaptic serotonin. Together, these data raise the possibility that increased serotonin activity could be associated with inhibition of and an obsessive need with exactness and perfectionism. These data also suggest that the efficacy of serotonergic medications could also be related to a reduction of obsessional and perfectionistic behaviors, and improvement in mood. The evidence supporting the role of abnormal serotonin activity suggests that serotonin contributes to the pathogenesis of eating disorders.

Studies using serotonin-specific medication support the serotonergic hypothesis. Crisp et al. *(49)* found that clomipramine was associated with increased appetite, hunger, and caloric consumption when administered to anorexics during the early stages of refeeding and weight restoration. Initial reports on cyproheptadine, a drug that is thought to act on the serotonergic and histaminergic system *(50)*, indicated that it might have beneficial effects on weight gain, mood, and attitude in some patients *(51,52)*. Reanalysis of this cyproheptadine data in comparison to trials of amitriptyline or placebo found cyprohep-tadine to significantly improve weight gain in restrictor anorectics, whereas amitriptyline was more effective in those anorectics with bulimic behavior *(53)*.

Gwirtsman and colleagues *(54)* reported that an open trial of fluoxetine, a highly specific SSRI, helped six chronic, refractory anorexic patients gain weight, reduce depression, and decrease obsessive thoughts about food and ritualistic preoccupations. In a preliminary open trial *(55)*, fluoxetine was administered to 31 anorexic patients. This study was designed to determine whether fluoxetine could improve outcome in anorexia nervosa by helping patients maintain a healthy and normal weight in an out-patient setting after weight restoration. Thus, most were treated after inpatient hospital-ization and weight restoration. At the time of follow-up (11 ± 6 mo on fluoxetine), 29 of the 31 patients had maintained their weight at or above 85% average body weight (ABW) (97 ± 13% ABW for the group) outside of a hospital setting. Restrictor-type anorexics responded significantly better than bulimic- and/or purging-type anorexics. These open trials raised the possibility that fluoxetine might help patients with anorexia nervosa gain and/or maintain a healthy body weight.

Recently, our group reported a double-blind, placebo-controlled trial of fluoxetine in 35 patients with restrictor-type anorexia nervosa *(14)*. Subjects were started on fluoxetine after they achieved weight restoration (approx 90% of ideal body weight) during a hos-pitalization. Anorexics were randomly assigned to fluoxetine ($n = 16$) or placebo ($n = 19$) after inpatient weight restoration and then were followed as outpatients for 1 yr. After 1 yr of outpatient follow-up, 10 of 16 (63%) subjects had a good outcome on fluoxetine, whereas only 3 of 19 (16%) had a good outcome on placebo ($p = 0.006$). Aside from improved outcome, fluoxetine administration was associated with a significant reduction in obsessions and compulsions and a trend toward a reduction in depression. These data suggest that fluoxetine may help some patients with anorexia nervosa maintain a healthy body weight as outpatients.

It is important to note that SSRIs may have little effect on reducing symptoms and preventing hospitalization in malnourished, underweight anorexics *(56,57)*. Women with anorexia nervosa, when malnourished and underweight, have reduced plasma tryp-tophan availability *(58)* and reduced CSF 5-HIAA *(59)*, the major metabolite of seroto-nin in the brain. Additionally, low estrogen values during the malnourished state may reduce serotonin activity by effects on gene expression for serotonin receptors *(60)* or the serotonin transporter *(61)*. SSRIs are dependent on neuronal release of serotonin for their action. If malnourished anorexics have compromised release of serotonin from presynaptic neuronal storage sites and reduced synaptic serotonin concentrations, then a clinically meaningful response to an SSRI might not occur (62). The possibility that fluoxetine is effective for anorexics only after weight restoration is supported by the fact that a change of serotonin activity is associated with weight gain. For example, CSF 5-HIAA levels are low in underweight anorexics, normal in short-term weight-restored anorexics, and elevated in long-term weight-restored anorexics (63). If CSF 5-HIAA levels accurately reflect central nervous system serotonin activity, then these data imply that a substantial increase in serotonin activity occurs after weight gain.

The use of serotonin-specific medications in the treatment of anorexia nervosa is promising, but many questions remain. First, only one double-blind, placebo-controlled study has been completed in a relatively small number of restrictor-type anorexics. Several studies in progress by several groups, in a larger group of patients, seek to replicate and extend these findings. Second, it is not known whether fluoxetine has similar efficacy in underweight and weight-restored anorexics. Third, more data are needed to determine whether there are differential effects between restrictor-type and bulimic- and/or purging-type anorexics. Fourth, it needs to be determined which symptoms respond to serotonin-specific medications: core anorexic symptoms, depression, anxiety, obsessionality, or eating behavior. For example, binge–purge-type anoretics might do better when dosed in the morning to enhance potential for absorption because purging often occurs later in the day.

3.6. Atypicals

There have been a number of uncontrolled studies (64–69) that have raised the possibility that olanzapine may useful in anorexia nervosa because it reduces anxiety and improves mood, and perhaps reduces core eating disorder symptoms. Additionally, there is a possibility that olanzapine may aid in normalization of body weight in anoretics. Although studies of serotonin and dopamine abnormalities in anorexia nervosa support a rationale for why drugs such as olanzapine may be useful, it is important to note that there are no controlled trials proving that this is an effective treatment. The actual number of individuals treated in all of these trials is small, so little is known about dose or side effects. Some individuals do not like or tolerate the sedative effects of olanzapine or have difficulties with the possible effects related to weight gain. Although it is important to consider new treatments, the results of such open trials must be viewed with caution.

4. GUIDELINES FOR CLINICAL TREATMENT

Anorexia nervosa is a relatively rare disorder with a high relapse rate. We strongly support use of the recent American Psychiatric Association (APA) guidelines for eating disorders (70), which describe comprehensive treatment of anorexia nervosa. Table 2 summarizes guidelines for clinical treatment.

The first line of treatment for underweight anorexics should be refeeding and weight restoration. As noted above, although this is difficult, most anorexics will gain weight in a structured eating-disorders treatment program without the use of medication. Weight gain alone tends to reduce exaggerated obsessionality and dysphoric mood in many anorexics patients (71). There is limited evidence that fluoxetine, and possibly other SSRI medications, help prevent relapse after weight restoration. Only recently has it been shown that fluoxetine, given in a double-blind, placebo-controlled manner, may provide

Table 2
Guidelines for Clinical Treatment

- Begin refeeding and weight restoration
- Institute pharmacologic therapy
- Continue therapy for at least 3 mo
- Resumption of menstruation
- Normalization of caloric needs
- Remediation of physical complications
- Remission of pathological eating and body-image distortions
- Reevaluate need for continuing pharmacologic therapy

substantial long-term benefits in terms of helping patients maintain weight after discharge from the hospital.

It is important to emphasize that some physiological and cognitive alterations persist for months after achieving goal weight. These include increased energy needs, menstrual disturbances, several neurotransmitter disturbances, urges to engage in disordered eating patterns, and body-image distortions. Thus, treatment should continue for at least 3 to 6 mo after achieving goal weight, preferably until there is resumption of menstrual periods, normalization of caloric needs, remediation of any physical complications, and sufficient remission of pathological eating and body-image distortions so that daily activities are not disturbed.

The dose of serotonin-specific medication that may be useful for the treatment of anorexia nervosa remains to be determined. The dose should be titrated, balancing side effects and therapeutic effects. It has been our experience that when anorexics have a successful response to fluoxetine, it is often accompanied by a reduction in motor activity and an improvement in sleep. Thus, it is often useful to administer these drugs late in the day.

It is very difficult to get many restrictor-type anorexics to take medication. Some patients had repeated bouts of weight loss until they were persuaded to try medication. Some anorexics had increased dysphoria during the first week of fluoxetine administration, a phenomenon noted with clomipramine treatment of OCD (72). These symptoms were transient and usually disappeared by d 10 of treatment. Thus, we forewarned and supported anorexics during this early period of anxiety to prevent discontinuation of medication. Finally, although these preliminary results are encouraging, it should be emphasized that only a few patients had a dramatic response with a large reduction in symptoms. For most patients, symptoms were reduced, but continued to be present.

5. CONCLUSION

Few clinical trials have evaluated the efficacy of medications in patients with anorexia nervosa, and even fewer studies have been placebo controlled. As a consequence, several medications are used to help patients regain weight without sufficient clinical evidence of their efficacy. Maintenance of weight and reduction of core symptoms of anorexia nervosa is of greater concern, but clinical evidence of drug efficacy for these effects is negligible.

At present the APA guidelines should be used to guide treatment of anorexia nervosa. The first medication to consider, given that it has evidence of efficacy in placebo-controlled trials, is fluoxetine. If fluoxetine treatment is unsuccessful, other pharmacotherapies can be tried, despite lack of evidence for their efficacy.

Rigorously designed trials of pharmacotherapies in anorexia need to be performed to develop additional treatments for this serious condition.

REFERENCES

1. Garner DM, Garfinkel PE. The eating attitudes test: an index of the symptoms of anorexia nervosa. Psychol Med 1979; 9:273–279.
2. Ploog D. The Psychobiology of Anorexia Nervosa. Springer-Verlag, Berlin, Germany and New York, NY, 1984.
3. Johanson AJ, Knorr NJ. L-Dopa as treatment for anorexia nervosa. In: Vigersky RA, ed. Anorexia Nervosa. Raven Press, New York, NY, 1977, pp. 363–372
4. Redmond DE, Swann A, Heninger GR. Phenoxybenzamine in anorexia nervosa. Lancet 1976; 2:397.
5. Green RS, Rau JH. Treatment of compulsive eating disturbances with anticonvulsant medication. Am J Psych 1974; 131:428–432.
6. Green RS, Rau JH. The use of diphenylhydantoin in compulsive eating disorders: Future studies in anorexia nervosa. In: Vigersky RA, ed. Anorexia Nervosa. Raven Press, New York, NY, 1977, pp. 377–385.
7. Wulliemier JF, Rossel F, Sinclair K. La therapie comportementale de l'anorexia. J Psychosom Res 1975; 19:267–272.
8. Moore R, Mills IH, Forster A. Naloxone in the treatment of anorexia nervosa: effect on weight gain and lipolysis. J R Soc Med 1981; 74:129–131.
9. Halmi KA, ed. Anorexia Nervosa. Williams and Wilkins, Baltimore, MD, 1980
10. Hsu LKG. The treatment of anorexia nervosa. Am J Psychiatry 1986; 143:573–581.
11. Russell GF, Szmukler GI, Dare C, Eisler I. An evaluation of family therapy in anorexia nervosa and bulimia nervosa. Arch Gen Psychiatry 1987; 44:1047–1056.
12. Gowers S, Norton K, Halek C, Crisp AH. Outcome of outpatient psychotherapy in a random allocation treatment study of anroexia nervosa. Int J Eat Disord 1994; 15:165–177.
13. Treasure J, Todd G, Brolly M, Tiller J, Nehmed A, Denman F. A pilot study of a randomised trial of cognitive analytical therapy vs educational behavioral therapy for adult anorexia nervosa. Behav Res Ther 1995; 33:363–367.
14. Kaye WH, Nagata T, Weltzin TE, et al. Deep D. Double-blind placebo-controlled administration of fluoxetine in restricting- and restricting–purging–type anorexia nervosa. Biol Psychiatry 2001; 49:644–652.
15. Dare C, Eisler I, Russell G, Treasure J, Dodge L. Psychological therapies for adults with anorexia nervosa: randomised controlled trial of out-patient treatments. Br J Psychiatry 2001; 178:216–221.
16. Eisler I, Dare C, Russell GF, Szmukler G, Le Grange D, Dodge E. Family and individual therapy in anorexia nervosa: a 5-year follow-up. Arch Gen Psychiatry 1997; 54:1025–1030.
17. Fairburn CG, Shafran R, Cooper Z. A cognitive behavioral theory of anorexia nervosa. Behav Res Ther 1999; 37:1–13.
18. Kleinfield EI, Wagner S, Halmi KA. Cognitive–behavioral treatment of anorexia nervosa. Psychiatr Clin North Am 1996; 19:715–737.
19. Lock J, Le Grange D. Can family-based treatment of anorexia nervosa be manualized? J Psychother Pract Res 2001; 10:253–261.
20. Vandereycken W, Pierloot R. Pimozide combined with behavior therapy in the short-term treatment of anorexia nervosa: a double-blind placebo-controlled cross-over study. Acta Psychiatr Scand 1982; 66:445–450.
21. Vandereycken W. Neuroleptics in the short-term treatment of anorexia nervosa: a double-blind placebo-controlled study with sulpiride. Br J Psychiatry 1984; 144:288–292.
22. Gross H, Ebert MH, Faden VB, et al. A double-blind trial of δ 9-tetrahydrocannabinol in primary anorexia nervosa. J Clin Psychopharmacol 1983; 3:165–171.

23. Casper RC, Schlemmer RFJ, Javaid JI. A placebo-controlled crossover study of oral clonidine in acute anorexia nervosa. Psychiatry Res 1987; 20:249–260.
24. Szmukler GI, Young GP, Lichtenstein M, Andrews JT. A serial study of gastric emptying in anorexia nervosa and bulimia. Aust N Z J Med 1990; 20:220–225.
25. Domstad PA, Shih WJ, Humphries L, DeLand FH, Digenis GA. Radionuclide gastric emptying studies in patients with anorexia nervosa. J Nucl Med 1987; 28:816–819.
26. Russell DM, Freedman ML, Feiglin DH, Jeejeebhjoy KN, Swinson RP, Garfinkel PE . Delayed gastric emptying and improvement with domperidone in a patient with anorexia nervosa. Am J Psych 1983; 140:1235–1236.
27. Saleh JW, Lebwohl P. Metoclopramide-induced gastric emptying in patients with anorexia nervosa. Am J Gastroenterol 1980; 74:127–132.
28. Stacher G, Bergmann H, Wiesnagrotzki S, et al. Intravenous cisapride accelerates delayed gastric emptying and increases antral contraction amplitude in patients with primary anorexia nervosa. Gastro-enterology 1987; 92:1000–1006.
29. Szmukler GI, Young GP, Miller G, Lichtenstein M, Binns DS. A controlled trial of cisapride in anorexia nervosa. Int J Eat Disord 1995; 17:347–357.
30. Strober M, Katz JL. Depression in the eating disorders: A review and analysis of descriptive, family, and biological findings. In: Garner DM, Garfinkel PE, eds. Diagnostic Issues in Anorexia Nervosa and Bulimia Nervosa. Brunner/Mazel, New York, NY, 1988, pp. 80–111.
31. Rothenberg A. Differential diagnosis of anorexia nervosa and depressive illness: a review of 11 studies. Compr Psychiatry 1988; 29:427–432.
32. Swift WJ, Andrews D, Barklage NE. The relationship between affective disorder and eating disorders: a review of the literature. Am J Psych 1986; 143:290–299.
33. Strober M. Personality and symptomatological features in young, nonchronic anorexia nervosa patients. J Psychosom Res 1980; 24:353–359.
34. Hudson JI, Pope HG Jr, Jonas JM, Yurgelun-Todd D. Phenomenologic relationship of eating disorders to major affective disorder. Psychiatry Res 1983; 9:345–354.
35. Solyom L, Freeman RJ, Miles JE. A comparative psychometric study of anorexia nervosa and obsessive neurosis. Can J Psychiatry 1982; 27:282–286.
36. Toner BB, Garfinkel PE, Garner DM. Long-term follow-up of anorexia nervosa. Psychosom Med 1986; 48:520–529.
37. Kasvikis YG, Tsakiris F, Marks IM. Past history of anorexia nervosa in women with obsessive compul-sive disorder. Int J Eat Disord 1986; 5:1069–1075.
38. Kaye WH, Gwirtsman HE, George DT, Ebert MH. Altered serotonin activity in anorexia nervosa after long-term weight restoration: does elevated cerebrospinal fluid 5-hydroxyindoleacetic acid level corre-late with rigid and obsessive behavior? Arch Gen Psychiatry 1991; 48:556–562.
39. Zohar J, Insel TR. Obsessive–compulsive disorder: psychobiological approaches to diagnosis, treat-ment, and pathophysiology. Biol Psychiatry 1987; 22:667–687.
40. Moore R. Amitriptyline therapy in anorexia nervosa. Am J Psych 1977; 13:1303–1304.
41. Needlemen HL, Waber D. The use of amitriptyline in anorexia nervosa. In: Vigersky RA, ed. Anorexia Nervosa. Raven Press, New York, NY, 1977, pp. 357–362.
42. Bieberman J, Herzog DB, Rivinus et al. Amitriptyline in the treatment of anorexia nervosa: a double-blind placebo-controlled study. J Clin Psychopharmacol 1985; 5:10–16.
43. Gross HA, Ebert MH, Faden VB, Goldberg SC, Nee LE, Kaye WH. A double-blind controlled trial of lithium carbonate primary anorexia nervosa. J Clin Psychopharmacol 1981; 1:376–81.
44. Kaye WH, Weltzin T, Hsu LKG. Anorexia nervosa. In: Hollander E, ed. Obsessive–Compulsive Related Disorders. American Psychiatric Press, Washington, DC, 1993, pp. 49–70.
45. Hollander E, Liebowitz MR, Winchel R. Treatment of Body-Dysmorphic Disorder With Serotonin Reuptake Blockers. American Psychiatric Press, Washington, DC, 1989, pp. 768–770.
46. Srinivasagam NM, Kaye WH, Plotnicov KH, Greeno C, Weltzin TE, Rao R. Persistent perfectionism, symmetry, and exactness after long-term recovery from anorexia nervosa. Am J Psychiatry 1995; 152: 1630–1634.
47. Frank G, Kaye WH, Meltzer CC, et al. Reduced 5-HT 2A receptor binding after recovery from anorexia nervosa. Biological Psychiatry 2002; 52:896–906.

48. Bailer UF, Price JC, Meltzer CC, et al. Altered 5-HT$_{2A}$ receptor activity after recovery from bulimia-type anorexia nervosa. Neuropsychopharmacology 2004; 29:1143–1155

49. Crisp AH, Lacey JH, Crutchfield M. Clomipramine and "drive" in people with anorexia nervosa: an inpatient study. Br J Psychiatry 1987; 150:355–358.

50. Stone CA, Wenger HC, Ludden CT. Antiserotonin–antihistamine properties of cyproheptadine. J Pharm Experi Ther 1961; 131:73–81.

51. Goldberg SC, Halmi KA, Eckert ED, Casper RC, Davis JM. Cyproheptadine in anorexia nervosa. Br J Psychiatry 1979; 134:67–70.

52. Halmi KA, Eckert E, Falk JR. Cyproheptadine for anorexia nervosa. Lancet 1982; 1:1357–1358.

53. Halmi KA, Eckert E, LaDu TJ, Cohen J. Anorexia nervosa: treatment efficacy of cyproheptadine and amitriptyline. Arch Gen Psychiatry 1986; 43:177–181.

54. Gwirtsman HE, Guze BH, Yager J, Gainsley B. Fluoxetine treatment of anorexia nervosa: an open clinical trial. J Clin Psychiatry 1990; 51:378–382.

55. Kaye WH, Weltzin TE, Hsu LK, Bulik CM. An open trial of fluoxetine in patients with anorexia nervosa. J Clin Psychiatry 1991; 52:464–471.

56. Ferguson CP, La Via MC, Crossan PJ, Kaye WH. Are serotonin selective reuptake inhibitors effective in underweight anorexia nervosa? Int J Eat Disord 1999; 25:11–17.

57. Attia E, Haiman C, Walsh BT, Flater SR. Does fluoxetine augment the inpatient treatment of anorexia nervosa? Am J Psychiatry 1998; 155:548–51.

58. Schweiger U, Warnhoff M, Pahl J, Pirke KM. Effects of carbohydrate and protein meals on plasma large neutral amino acids, glucose, and insulin plasma levels of anorectic patients. Metabolism 1986; 35: 938–943.

59. Kaye WH, Gwirtsman HE, George DT, Jimerson DC, Ebert MH. CSF 5-HIAA concentrations in anorexia nervosa: reduced values in underweight subjects normalize after weight gain. Biol Psychiatry 1988; 23:102–105.

60. Fink G, Sumner BE. Oestrogen and mental state. Nature 1996; 383:306.

61. McQueen JK, Wilson H, Dow RC, Fink GJ. Oestradiol-17 β increases serotonin transporter (SERT) binding sites and SERT mRNA expression in discrete regions of female rat brain. J Physiol (Lond) 1996; 495.

62. Tollefson GD. Selective serotonin reuptake inhibitors. In: Schatzberg AF, Memeroff CB, eds. Textbook of Psychopharmacology. American Psychiatric Press, Washington, DC, 1995.

63. Kaye WH, Ebert MH, Raleigh M, Lake R. Abnormalities in CNS monoamine metabolism in anorexia nervosa. Arch Gen Psychiatry 1984; 41:350–355.

64. Barbarich N, McConaha C, Gaskill J, et al. An open trial of olanzapine in anorexia nervosa. In press.

65. Hansen L. Olanzapine in the treatment of anorexia nervosa. Br J Psychiatry 1999; 175:592.

66. Jensen VS, Mejlhede A. Anorexia nervosa: treatment with olanzapine. Br J Psychiatry 2000; 177:87.

67. La Via MC, Gray N, Kaye WH. Case reports of olanzapine treatment of anorexia nervosa. Int J Eat Disord 2000; 27:363–366.

68. Malina A, Gaskill J, McConaha C, et al. Olanzapine treatment of anorexia nervosa: a retrospective study. Int J Eat Disord 2003; 33:234–237.

69. Powers PS, Santana CA, Bannon YS. Olanzapine in the treatment of anorexia nervosa: an open label trial. Int J Eat Disord 2002; 32:146–154.

70. American Psychiatric Association. Practice guideline for eating disorders: I. disease definition, epidemiology, and natural history. Am J Psychiatry 1993; 150:212–228.

71. Pollice C, Kaye WH, Greeno CG, Weltzin TE. Relationship of depression, anxiety, and obsessionality to state of illness in anorexia nervosa. Int J Eat Disord 1997; 21:367–376.

72. Zohar J, Insel TR, Zohar-Kadouch RC, Hill JL, Murphy DL. Serotonergic responsivity in obsessive–compulsive disorder: effects of chronic clomipramine treatment. Arch Gen Psychiatry 1988; 45:167–172.

8 The Internet and Eating Disorders

David J. Goldstein

KEY POINTS

- Because therapeutic expertise is not generally available and finances for medical care are constrained, use of the Internet in medical therapy will expand to meet those needs.
- Numerous sites are available for dissemination of educational material for patients, families, and health care professionals.
- Various organizations are attempting to develop and evaluate therapeutics on the Internet.

1. INTRODUCTION

The cost of medical care continues to be an issue for governmental organizations and companies. As a consequence, there are efforts to reduce costs. The "medicalization" of the eating disorders with the use of pharmaceuticals to displace costs of more intensive counseling is one trend toward reduction of health care expense. The development of Internet resources to substitute for personalized counseling is another.

Online resources can be beneficial additions for health care professionals and patients. For professionals, they can be a source of information and can be used as supplements for patients to augment the benefits provided during office visits. This can be of benefit in both the integrated eating-disorders clinic and the smaller practice that has a limited support system.

Patients should be informed of these resources and guided to avoid strictly commercial and fad sites. This chapter summarizes available online information sources, the patient perspective, and support groups. Table 1 outlines the chapter.

2. THE INTERNET AS A SOURCE OF INFORMATION

If one enters "eating disorders" into an Internet search engine, one will obtain approx 1.5 million hits. Thus, although there is a substantial amount of information available on the Internet, accessing this information via search engines is not efficient *(1)* and the priority of hits does not reflect a factual or noncommercial priority. Additionally, although much of the available medical information tends to be good, it is generally at an academic reading level that is beyond most patients *(1)*.

From: *The Management of Eating Disorders and Obesity, Second Edition*
Edited by: D. J. Goldstein © Humana Press Inc., Totowa, NJ

Table 1
Outline of Chapter

1. Introduction
2. The Internet As a Source of Information
2.1. Disease Information: Eating Disorders
2.2. Nutrition and Exercise Information
2.3. Patient Perspectives
2.4. Self-Help Groups
3. The Internet As a Source for Counseling
3.1. Online Counseling Sites
3.2. E-mail As an Adjunct
4. Conclusion

As a consequence, several reputable sites that are noncommercial or that separate commercial content from information sharing are provided here. Many of these include a description of the information or services that they provide. This list is not exhaustive and it is acknowledged that organizations and Internet addresses may change. Some of the listed organizations provide handouts for patients and some may provide information that might assist a practitioner caring for patients with eating disorders or help in identifying referral services.

2.1. Disease Information: Eating Disorders

The Academy for Eating Disorders (AED) (www.aedweb.org) is a professional organization whose goal is to promote research in the eating disorders in an effort to improve the treatment, education, and prevention of eating disorders. The AED publishes the *International Journal of Eating Disorders*. Their address is 6728 Old McLean Village Drive, McLean, VA 22101; Phone: 703-556-9222; Fax: 703-556-8729; aed@degnon.org.

The American Academy of Family Physicians (www.familydoctor.org) provides handouts for patient use. The handout for anorexia nervosa is found at familydoctor.org/handouts/063.html. A handout designed for teens can be found at familydoctor.org/handouts/277.html.

The Anorexia File, Center for Current Research (www.lifestages.com/health/anorexia.html) provides information on recent research on treatments for anorexia nervosa.

The Center for Change, Incorporated (centerforchange.com) is a facility for treatment, but their website provides information about eating disorders including a list of and links to recent publications. Their address is 1790 North State Street, Orem, UT 84057; Phone: 801-224-8255; Toll Free: 888-224-8250; Fax: 801-224-8301.

The Center for the Study of Anorexia and Associated Disorders (www.health.gov/NHIC/NHICScripts/Entry.cfm?HRCode=HR2111) provides treatment for eating disorder patients and their families. The center offers specialized training for professionals who treat people with eating disorders and seeks to educate the community about the growing incidence of eating disorders. The center provides information and outreach services. The address is 1841 Broadway, 4th Floor, New York, NY 10023; Phone: 212-333-3444; Fax: 212-333-5444.

The Eating Disorders Coalition for Research, Policy & Action (www.EatingDisorders Coalition.org) is an advocacy group for people with eating disorders, their families, and professionals who work with them to promote federal support for improved access to care. Their address is 611 Pennsylvania Avenue SE, Suite 423, Washington, DC 20003-4303; Phone: 202-543-9570.

Eating Disorder Recovery Online, Arizona Center for Eating Disorder Recovery (www.ederecovery.com) provides information, a chat room, online assessments, and both group and individualized counseling for pay. The chat room adress is www.edrecovery.com/chatroom/index.html.

The Eating Disorder Referral and Information Center (www.EDreferral.com/) is an international eating-disorder referral organization dedicated to the prevention and treatment of eating disorders. The center provides information and treatment resources for all forms of eating disorders.

The Harvard Eating Disorders Center (www.hedc.org) conducts research and provides information. The center's address is 15 Parkman Street, Boston, MA 02114; Phone: 617-236-7766; Fax: 617-236-2068.

The International Association of Eating Disorders Professionals (IAEDP) (www.iaedp.com) offers nationwide education, training, certification, and a semiannual conference for practitioners who treat people with eating disorders. The IAEDP address is 427 center Pointe Circle, Suite 1819, Altamonte Springs, FL 32706; Phone: 309-346-3341; 800-800-8126; Fax: 309-346-2874.

The National Association of Anorexia Nervosa and Associated Disorders (ANAD) (www.anad.org) is dedicated to alleviating the problems of eating disorders, especially anorexia nervosa and bulimia. ANAD provides educational and self-help for both patient and parents. The address is P.O. Box 271, Highland Park, Illinois 60035; Phone: 312-831-3438; Fax: 847-433-4632; Advocacy: anadadvocacy@aol.com; Information: anad20@aol.com.

The goal of the National Eating Disorders Association (NEDA) (www.NationalEating Disorders.org), the largest consumer advocacy organization in the United States, is the elimination of eating disorders and body dissatisfaction by employing far-reaching and comprehensive strategies to prevent young people from developing eating disorders. The NEDA also seeks to ensure that those who suffer from eating disorders receive access to the information, care, and support. The NEDA provides information about eating disorders and body-image concerns and referrals for centers, physicians, counselors, therapists, and so on. The NEDA also has an online store that provides educational and training materials. The address is 603 Stewart St, Suite 803, Seattle, WA 98101; Phone: 206-382-3587 (office); 800-931-2237 (information and referral helpline); Fax: 206-829-8501; info@nationaleatingdisorders.org.

The Pennsylvania Educational Network for Eating Disorders (PENED) (http://trfn.clpgh.org/pened/) provides education, support, and referral information on the causes, treatment, and prevention of eating disorders and related issues. PENED's address is 7805 McKnight Road, Pittsburgh, PA 15237; Phone 412-366-9966; Fax: 412-487-6850.

2.2. Nutrition and Exercise Information

The American Dietetic Association (www.eatright.org), a professional society for dietitians, promotes the science of dietetics and nutrition, and public and professional education in these areas. ADA activities and services include continuing education programs, nutritional research, scholarships, consumer publications, educational publications for professionals, public awareness campaigns, and promulgation of educational standards. The address is 216 West Jackson Boulevard, Suite 800, Chicago, IL 60606-6995; Phone: 800-366-1655 (nutrition hotline), 312-899-0040, 900-CALL-AN-RD; media@eatright.org.

The Food and Nutrition Information Center, US Department of Agriculture (www.nal. usda.gov/fnic/) provides information on food, human nutrition, and food safety to consumers and professionals. The address is National Agricultural Library, 10301 Baltimore Avenue, Room 105, Beltsville, MD 20705-2351; Phone: 301-504-5719; Fax: 301-504-6409.

The site at www.webhealthcentre.com provides health calculators for determination of body mass index (BMI) and energy utilization. The BMI calculator permits the determination of BMI and interpretation related to level of appropriateness of weight (i.e. underweight, normal, normal, overweight, obese, morbid obesity). It also provides the lower and upper range of normal for that individual assuming normal range of musculature. The energy calculator permits the determination of the minimal (basal) and ambulatory caloric utilization for an individual of a given gender, age, height, and weight.

My.webmd.com provides information on food and nutrition, sports and fitness, and health e-tools. Food and nutrition contains articles on diet, exercise, nutrition, including interviews with experts and bulletin boards that permit individuals to ask for advice from these experts. This site also includes some recipes. Sports and fitness contains calculators for target heart rate and calories expended with different exercise regimes. Health e-tools has a diet and exercise log including a dessert wizard that permits one to calculate the amount of exercise required to offset the calories of a specific dessert, target heart rate calculator, and calorie calculator. Although typically used for weight loss, this can also be utilized for weight maintenance or weight gain.

The President's Council on Physical Fitness and Sports (www.fitness.gov) promotes, encourages, and motivates the development of physical fitness and sport participation for Americans of all ages through its work with partners in government and the private sector. It provides recognition and incentive programs for individuals and organizations and materials on fitness and physical activity. The address is 200 Independence Avenue, SW, Room 738-H, Washington, DC 20201; Phone: 202-690-9000; Fax: 202-690-5211.

2.3. Patient Perspective

There are multiple Internet sites that provide stories by patients about their conditions. A couple of these are The Close to You Family Resource Network, which has an eating disorders site that lists stories of patients at closetoyou.org/eatingdisorders/byyou/posts.htm and Healthyplace.com, which provides stylized stories at www.healthyplace.com/communities/eating_disorders/site/eating_disorders.htm.

2.4. Self-Help Groups

Although many patients value self-help interactions, these need to be approached with caution given the potential for dissemination of inaccurate and potentially dangerous information.

The Eating Disorder Recovery Online, Arizona Center for Eating Disorder Recovery provides an online chat room (www.edrecovery.com/chatroom/index.html).

The Center for Counseling and Health Resources Inc. (www.caringonline.com) provides information and online support.

The Center for Eating Disorders of St. Joseph Medical Center (www.eating-disorders.com/) provides an eating disorders discussion forum and offers the ability to ask questions of experts.

Eating Disorders Anonymous (EDA) (www.EatingDisordersAnonymous.org) provides information about local support group meetings. EDA's address is 18233 M. 16th Way, Phoenix, AZ 85022.

New Realities Eating Disorders Recovery Centre has a good self-assessment questionnaire, as well as useful information.

Psychforums.com (www.psychforums.com/forums/index.php) provides a discussion group for patients with anorexia nervosa and bulimia nervosa.

Something fishy (www.something-fishy.org/online/chatcenter.php) provides a discussion groups for eating disorders.

It is valuable to know whether patients are utilizing these and what they are learning so that interventions can be modified to accrue benefits and avoid detriments from these interactions.

3. THE INTERNET AS A SOURCE FOR COUNSELING

No publications are available on the use or success of these programs. Until such information is available, they should be used with caution and considered an adjunct to face-to-face counseling.

One study evaluated an Internet health education program designed to improve body satisfaction and reduce weight and shape concerns (2). This study evaluated the change in body-image perception and drive for thinness in 60 women randomized to the Internet or a control program. At the conclusion of the program, the women trained in using the Internet program had significantly greater improvements in both body image and drive for thinness. This finding provides some support that the Internet might be of benefit as an adjunct to counseling.

3.1. Online Counseling Sites

The Eating Disorder Recovery Online, Arizona Center for Eating Disorder Recovery (www.EDrecovery.com) provides for pay online assessments, both group and individualized counseling. Eating Disorder Recovery Online, Arizona Center for Eating Disorder Recovery, Tucson, Arizona; Phone: 888-520-1700, 520-323-3734; Chat room: http://www.edrecovery.com/chatroom/index.html Nutrition Consulting.Com provides consulting for eating disorders (anorexia, bulimia, and binge eating) and weight issues via telephone and e-mail or in person in the metropolitan New York area.

3.2. E-Mail as an Adjunct

One study has been published on the use of e-mail as an adjunct to counseling in anorexia nervosa *(3)*. Patients were to have obligatory contacts by e-mail between visits. The patients were to report on their eating behaviors. Although this was not a controlled study, the patients considered use of e-mail to be helpful and all patients showed improvement. The authors hypothesized that the e-mail contacts were beneficial because they increased therapeutic contact, permitted "talking on demand," and increased the frequency of confronting eating behaviors, enhancing honesty and integrity. They also noted that relatively little time was required by the counselors.

4. CONCLUSION

The number of sites and the volume of information related to eating disorders is extraordinary. Nevertheless, little information is available on the usefulness of the Internet for providing information or for counseling. An educated professional can identify information for the patient and can utilize this to supplement patient care. It may be that the Internet can be used to supplement office counseling to improve patient outcomes. However, the ways that the Internet can be used to enhance treatment requires study.

ACKNOWLEDGMENTS

The author thanks Dr. James E. Mitchell, Fargo, ND, for his suggestions and the National Eating Disorders Association.

REFERENCES

1. Berland GK, Elliott MN, Morales LS, et al. Health information on the Internet: accessibility, quality, and readability in English and Spanish. JAMA 2001; 285:2612–2621.
2. Winzelberg AJ, Eppstein D, Eldredge KI, et al. Effectiveness of an Internet-based program for reducing risk factors for eating disorders. J Consult Clin Psychol 2000; 68:346–350.
3. Yager J. E-mail as a therapeutic adjunct in the outpatient treatment of anorexia nervosa: Illustrative case material and discussion of the issues. Int J Eat Disord 2001;41:536–544.

III OBESITY

9 Etiologies of Obesity

Richard L. Atkinson

KEY POINTS

- Obesity is an exceedingly complex group of diseases and probably should be characterized as a syndrome.
- Simply overeating does not result in long-term obesity.
- More than 350 genes or gene markers have been identified that are associated with obesity and may contribute to the etiology of obesity in animals and humans.
- The etiologies that contribute to obesity that physicians can influence include dietary and exercise patterns, endocrine and metabolic diseases, and drugs.
- More research is needed to uncover the causes of obesity and to develop therapies.

1. INTRODUCTION AND OVERVIEW

This chapter examines some of the evidence to date for the various etiologies of obesity. Table 1 provides an outline of the chapter and the major factors thought to contribute to the etiology of obesity.

The common feature of all obese people is an excess accumulation of adipose tissue. However, obesity is not a single disease. More than 300 different genes and gene markers have been identified that are associated with obesity (*see* Chapter 18 for a discussion on recent research on the genetics of obesity), and there are numerous environmental factors that appear to be necessary for the expression of obesity *(1–2)* (*see* Table 2). A prevailing current hypothesis is that, in most people, obesity is the interaction of the environment and a genetic predisposition to accumulate excess adipose tissue. Usually, both the genetic factor(s) and the environmental factors must be present for obesity to occur. This hypothesis is undoubtedly true for the vast majority of obese people. The previous belief of many lay people and health professionals that obesity is simply the result of a lack of willpower and an inability to discipline eating habits is no longer defensible (*see* Chapter 24 for a summary of lay and professional attitudes about obesity) despite its continued popularity. It is likely that few or no cases of obesity are simply the result of overeating, rather than a more complex interaction of environmental and genetic factors. The classic studies of Sims et al. *(3)* provide evidence that simply

From: *The Management of Eating Disorders and Obesity, Second Edition*
Edited by: D. J. Goldstein © Humana Press Inc., Totowa, NJ

Table 1
Chapter Overview

overeating does not result in long-term obesity. In these studies, forced overfeeding of young lean males resulted in weight gain averaging only about 21% over baseline, despite dramatic increases in energy intake for months. Furthermore, this overfeeding did not result in long-term obesity *(3)*.

The hypothesis that obesity is almost always a product of a genetic predisposition interacting with the environment has been challenged by recent evidence that animals infected with certain viruses develop obesity *(4–6)*. Preliminary data suggest that one or more of these viruses may contribute to obesity in humans, but additional research must be done. As is shown here, we are only in our infancy of understanding of the etiologies of obesity.

2. GENETIC FACTORS CONTRIBUTING TO OBESITY

2.1. Single-Gene Defects

Single-gene defects as models of obesity in animals have been known for many years, and more recently have been described in humans *(1)*. The two most prominent single-gene defects that cause obesity in animals and/or humans include *ob/ob* and *db/db*, the genes coding for leptin and leptin receptor, respectively. Others include the *agouti, tubby*, and *proopiomelanocortin* genes *(1)*. Coleman's *(7–9)* early descriptions of two mouse models, the obese *(ob/ob)* and the obese and diabetic *(db/db)*, stimulated a series of research studies that culminated with the identification of the gene defects responsible for each of these disorders. The *ob* gene, first described by Zhang et al. *(10)*, codes for leptin.

Table 2
Potential Explanations Advanced for the Epidemic of Obesity

1. Reduced activity
   a. Greater affluence, more cars, less heavy labor
   b. Cable TV, increased channels
   c. Computers in workplace and home
   d. Computer games, handheld and desktop
   e. Fears of violence or kidnapping of children
   f. Organized sports for children, reduced outside playing time
2. Changes in food intake
   a. Increasing affluence among population, food more affordable
   b. Easier access to food in environment
   c. Expansion of fast food sources and availability
   d. Change in character of food (high fat, refined carbohydrates)
   e. Larger portion sizes
3. Two-income families, less attention to meal preparation
4. Worldwide epidemic of obesity-producing virus

Leptin is made in adipose tissue and is postulated to signal the brain regarding insufficiency of food intake and decreasing levels of adipose tissue stores in the body. Leptin deficiency is an autosomal recessive trait that produces massive obesity in ob/ob mice and in a small number of humans reported with this defect *(10–15)*. Coleman *(7,8)* showed that ob/ob mice must be food restricted to half of the energy intake of their lean siblings to achieve a comparable body weight, and even then, their body fat is greater.

When injected with leptin, both ob/ob mice and humans lose weight down toward the levels of their unaffected siblings *(11–13,16)*. The altered gene in the db/db mouse codes for the leptin receptor, and apparently results in a defective or absent receptor site. Defects in the comparable gene in rats produce the Zucker obese rat model. Neither db/db mice nor Zucker rats lose weight when injected with leptin.

Only a tiny fraction of obese people have a single-gene disorder as the etiology of their obesity. Such individuals tend to gain weight continually until they die of some complication of obesity. Recent studies have identified a very small number of humans with leptin deficiency, and a somewhat larger number with leptin receptor defects *(14–18)*. It has been disappointing to learn that obese people have high levels of leptin, and appear to be resistant to its action in reducing body fat *(19)*.

There are several other rare obesity syndromes owing to genetic or familial causes as reviewed by Chagnon et al. *(1)* and Bray et al. *(20)*. For example, the Prader-Willi syndrome (obesity, mental retardation, short stature, small hands and feet) probably represents a mutation in affected individuals *(20)*. Of the 24 genes specifically identified with human obesity *(1,21)*, most contribute only very modestly to the obesity in a given individual. Bouchard et al. *(21)* maintain a constantly updated website on the human obesity genome at http://obesitygene.pbrc.edu.

2.2. Polygenic Obesity

In the majority of both animals and humans, the genetic contribution to obesity is not a single-gene defect, but is the result of a combination of genetic factors (Chapter 18 summarizes recent advances in the genetics of human obesity with emphasis on leptin and the leptin receptor). As noted earlier, Bouchard, Chagnon and colleagues *(1)* identified more than 300 genes or gene markers that are involved in the etiology of obesity, and 24 chromosomes have genes or gene markers that definitely contribute to obesity *(21)*. Some genes promote obesity and some appear to be protective. The implications of this number of genes being involved in obesity are that there may be dozens to thousands of different types of obesity.

2.3. Clinical Studies

Twin studies provide the most impressive clinical evidence that genetic factors play an important role in the etiology of obesity in humans *(22–25)*. Stunkard et al. *(23)* studied identical and nonidentical twins who were reared together and others who were reared apart. They found a high correlation of body weight among identical twins, even if they were reared apart, and concluded that as much as 70% of the variance of obesity could be attributed to genetic factors. Allison et al. *(24)* confirmed these results in a separate set of 53 twin pairs from multiple countries. They concluded that the heritability of body mass index was between 0.50 and 0.70 *(24)*. Bouchard et al. *(25)* did very careful studies in twins who were isolated in the Canadian wilderness with no access to foods other than those provided by the investigators. Identical twins were overfed for a period of 100 d and the gains in body weight and adipose tissue were evaluated. There was a closer association of both body weight and intra-abdominal adipose tissue (visceral fat) within twin pairs compared to among twin pairs. Recent studies suggest that the heritability of obesity in twins may differ among the sexes *(22)*.

Bogardus et al. *(26)* evaluated potential mechanisms by which genetic factors may contribute to obesity. Studies of resting metabolic rate show that the variation within families is less than the variation among families. This study suggests that energy metabolism is involved in regulating the body weight, and may contribute to the etiology of obesity. Potential candidate genes that could affect energy metabolism are the genes for the various uncoupling proteins. Uncoupling protein-1 (UCP-1) in brown fat plays a major role in energy metabolism in rodents, but there appears to be little brown fat in adult humans. Fleury et al. *(27)* first described the links between uncoupling protein-2 (UCP-2) and obesity and hyperinsulinemia. However, many studies have not been able to associate genetic differences in UCP with the prevalence of obesity *(1,25,28)*. Even when associated, the contribution of UCP mutations to obesity is very small, about 1–3% of the variance.

3. ENVIRONMENTAL FACTORS CONTRIBUTING TO OBESITY

3.1. Environmental Programming of Genetic Expression

Although the gene pool of an individual is fixed at conception, environmental factors may determine how these genes are expressed. There is intense interest on the role of environmental factors during intrauterine life and early infancy in the production of disease later in life.

3.1.1. Intrauterine Factors

The German blockade of the Netherlands during World War II resulted in many pregnant women undergoing starvation during some or most of their pregnancies. People born during the "Dutch famine" have been followed by their government for many years and in 1976, Ravelli et al. *(29)* reported that there was an increased prevalence of obesity in this population. If mothers were starved during the first 6 mo of pregnancy, the progeny were obese and had the "metabolic syndrome" in later life. If starved in the last 3 mo, progeny tended to be thinner than normals.

Epidemiological studies demonstrate that babies with a low birth weight and particularly babies who are born small for gestational age have a higher prevalence of obesity in adulthood *(30)*. The causes for small-for-dates babies are not clear, but abnormalities of the placenta may play a role. Low birth weight may be the result of a number of environmental factors including maternal undernutrition and smoking. Conversely, babies with high birth weights, and particularly those whose mothers had gestational diabetes, are at increased risk for obesity *(30–32)*.

Animal studies have confirmed that nutritional and hormonal manipulations during intrauterine life lead to obesity and metabolic syndrome in adulthood. Female rats exposed to an intrauterine environment of gestational diabetes produced by giving the drug streptozotocin to their mothers during pregnancy, develop gestational diabetes when they grow up and become pregnant *(33)*. This effect may go out to three generations.

Rhesus monkeys whose mothers were injected with androgen during pregnancy develop obesity, insulin resistance, and a syndrome similar to polycystic ovary syndrome when they become adults *(34,35)*.

3.1.2. Environmental Factors in Early Development

Overfeeding shortly after birth may lead to obesity and diabetes later in life in both humans and animals *(36,37)*. Underfeeding shortly after birth has been postulated to result in obesity later in life in humans, but studies are inconclusive *(36)*.

It is apparent that numerous environmental factors have the ability to alter gene expression. This effect may not be confined to fetal or early life. The phenomenon of sudden weight gain in adult humans and animals in response to environmental stressors that leads to obesity that then persists has been noted by many clinicians. For example, rats fed a high-fat diet for a brief period will become obese, but lose the weight if returned to a chow diet. If the high-fat diet is given for an extended time, permanent obesity ensues. Similar mechanisms may be operating in humans.

3.2. Familial and Ethnic Factors

Environmental factors of a familial nature including ethnic food preferences, eating patterns, dietary composition differences (e.g., high-fat diets), and activity levels, play a role in the etiology of obesity. Studies of energy expenditure in individuals and families show that differences are greater between families vs within families *(26)*. This may be the result of genetic factors affecting energy metabolism, but could also be owing to learned patterns of activity. Different ethnic groups demonstrate marked differences in the character and amounts of foods eaten. Factors that may influence total calorie intake include the frequency and timing of eating and the use of spices, oils and fats, and preferred food sources (e.g., rice, wheat).

3.3. Diet Composition and Eating Patterns

In considering factors that may have played a role in the epidemic of obesity, increases in food intake are high on the list (Table 2). People in the United States and across the

Table 3
Mechanisms of Obesity on High-Fat Diets

1. Increased food intake
   a. Increased energy content of fat for same volume or weight
   b. Greater palatability of high-fat foods
   c. Generally lower chewing and swallowing time for high-fat foods
   d. Lower degree of satiety from high-fat foods
2. Greater efficiency of storage with excess intake
3. Differences among individuals in oxidation of dietary fatty acids

world are becoming more affluent and able to afford more food and more commercially prepared foods, which tend to have a higher energy density. Ease of access to food has increased with more restaurants, especially fastfood restaurants that have quite inexpensive, high-fat, high-calorie foods as their staples. Portion sizes have increased since the 1980s. With more leisure-time activity, especially watching TV, food intake increases.

Excessive calorie intake above daily energy requirements is necessary for the development of obesity, but it is incorrect to assume that simple overeating is responsible for all obesity. As noted in Chapter 19, there is evidence that the quality of the foods ingested also is important in producing obesity. In animal studies, diets high in fat produce a greater degree of obesity than those high in carbohydrate (CHO). There are several reasons that increased dietary fat produces obesity (Table 3). Fat contains more than twice as many calories per gram as protein or CHO. Eating the same volume of food results in much greater energy intake on a high-fat diet than on a low-fat diet. Also, high-fat foods are more palatable than low-fat foods. Fat adds a desirable "mouth feel" to foods that animals and humans prefer. Fatty foods are usually low in dietary fiber, are softer, and require less time to chew and swallow than other types of foods. This is particularly true of high-fat desserts. Because there is less processing time for high-fat foods, it is easier to eat larger amounts. Finally, there is evidence that high-fat foods do not produce satiety as well as do high-CHO foods (38). Experiments in which subjects were fed a high- or low-fat preload before a meal showed that total energy intake was greater with the high-fat preload. The subjects did not perceive the increased energy of the preload, ate a comparably sized meal, and thus obtained a greater total energy intake. Tremblay et al. (39) noted that the combination of a high-fat appetizer and simultaneous consumption of alcohol results in a significantly higher total energy intake as compared to an equicaloric low-fat, no-alcohol appetizer.

The predisposition to gain fat on a high-fat diet is partially genetically determined. West et al. (40) studied nine strains of inbred mice. Within each strain, half of the mice were fed a high-fat diet, the other half was fed a low-fat diet, and the differences in weight gain and fat gain were determined. There were marked differences in weight and fat gain, supporting the Flatt hypothesis, although differences in food intake contributed to the fat gain. Rissanen et al. (41) reported on human twins who differed in body weight and had different preferences for dietary fat. The fatter twin preferred and ate more fat than the leaner twin. This suggests that although genetic factors are important, environmental factors play a major role in the preference for dietary fat and its contribution to obesity.

Ravussin and Smith *(42)* postulated that some humans, upon gaining weight, lose the ability to make new fat cells to store the excess fat in adipose tissue, so they begin to deposit fat in muscle, liver, and other tissues. This produces insulin resistance and contributes to the metabolic syndrome and to diabetes. More studies are needed to prove this theory.

Fat is stored more efficiently than CHO or protein when the diet contains more energy than is necessary for weight maintenance *(43–46)*. The cost of storing excess fat as a percentage of ingested energy is significantly less than the cost of making fat from CHO or protein. The capacity of different people or animals to oxidize fat in the diet to match fat intake varies from individual to individual. Many animals or humans are able to increase fat oxidation to match fat intake only after some degree of fat storage. Flatt *(44,45)* has postulated that on changing from a low- to a high-fat diet, individuals who lack the ability to match fat oxidation to fat intake will gain weight. The rationale for this hypothesis is that there are only two fates for ingested fat: oxidation or storage. Humans have a very limited capacity to convert any of the energy in fat to either protein or CHO *(44,45)*. Therefore, if the percentage of fat in the diet increases, fat oxidation must immediately increase to prevent storage of the additional fat calories.

The ability to oxidize fat apparently is influenced by genetic factors. Boozer et al. *(47)* demonstrated that not all calories are equal when they fed four groups of rats a similar number of kcal, but different percentages of fat. The rats on the high-fat diet (48% of kilocalories as fat) gained almost 50% more body fat over a 6-wk period than rats on an equicaloric low-fat diet (12% of kilocalories as fat). Similar observations have been made in humans. Danforth noted that comparable weight gain with overfeeding required many fewer kilocalories on a high-fat diet than on a low-fat diet *(48)*. Lissner et al. *(49)* kept calories constant, but switched from a high-fat to a low-fat diet, and noted weight loss. Prewitt et al. *(50)* also switched from a high-fat to a low-fat diet and found that the subjects could not maintain body weight, despite increasing the daily energy intake of low-fat foods.

The studies above suggest that the level at which body weight is regulated is determined in part by the percentage of fat calories in the diet. Not all investigators agree. The arguments pro and con are summarized in two editorials by Bray and Popkin vs Willett, respectively *(51,52)*.

3.4. Amount of Physical Activity

The amount of daily physical activity clearly contributes to the maintenance of body weight (*see* Chapter 13 on the role of exercise). Obese people are less active than lean people. Prentice and Jebb *(53)* observed that obesity is more common in lower vs upper socioeconomic groups, and that the factor that correlated best with the degree of obesity was activity. Degree of obesity was negatively correlated with daily physical activity.

Explanations for the epidemic of obesity focus on changes in activity since the 1980s in the United States (Table 2). With increasing affluence and mechanization, there are more cars, labor-saving devices, and less need for heavy labor. Greater penetration in homes of televisions, computers, and computer games increases sedentary time, especially for children. Fear of violence, secondary to drug dealing, and fear of kidnapping influence parents to keep children in the house or to limit outside exercise to organized sports. Long car travel to little league games, soccer practice, and so forth mean less actual time playing outside for children.

It is important to recognize that greater activity levels do not necessarily require greater amounts of formal exercise. Although all exercise is activity, the activities of daily living make an important contribution to total daily energy expenditure. Zurlo et al. *(54)* studied subjects in their indirect calorimeter facility and found that spontaneous activity, or "fidgeting," was correlated with body weight and adiposity. The difference in energy expenditure from "fidgeting" amounted to as much as 600 kcal/d, an amount that could account for a sizable difference in body weight. These findings were confirmed by Levine et al. *(55)*. It is not clear whether deliberately attempting to increase fidgeting will assist in weight loss or maintenance, but encouragement by physicians for patients to try as much as possible to minimize inactivity may be helpful. Epstein et al. *(56)* found that this strategy was useful in treating childhood obesity. Children were limited to a fixed amount of time in sedentary activities, and left to their own devices during nonsedentary times. Another group was assigned specifically to exercise. The decreased sedentary-behavior group had a decrease in overweight of 20 vs 13% for the exercise group, and at 1 yr, the differences were 19 vs 9%. Gortmaker et al. *(57)* and Robinson et al. *(58)* evaluated the role of TV viewing on obesity in children. TV clearly contributes to obesity in children, and reducing time watching TV was effective in preventing obesity.

3.5. Drugs

It is not well recognized, but numerous drugs may produce an increase in food intake or body weight. Glucocorticoids produce fat gain, particularly truncal adiposity, in a high percentage of users. Insulin and oral hypoglycemics (sulfonylureas and thiazolidinediones) promote weight and adipose tissue gain in diabetics. Phenothiazines, atypical antipsychotic agents, and some antidepressants, such as tricyclics and selective serotonin reuptake inhibitors, may produce weight gain. Cyproheptadine and valproic acid also have been implicated in the etiology of obesity in some patients. Finally, β-adrenergic antagonists such as propranolol are postulated to reduce sympathetic nervous system activity and lead to weight gain or difficulty in losing weight.

3.6. Stress

3.6.1. Emotional Stress

Several types of stress may contribute to obesity; perhaps the most studied of which is emotional stress. Depression is associated with weight gain in about 10 to 20% of cases. Weight gain is particularly common in seasonal depression (seasonal affective disorder [SAD]), which occurs in the winter months predominantly in northern latitudes. Some studies have suggested that SAD and its associated weight gain may be treated by exposure to artificial sunlight. On an anecdotal basis, many patients report that the onset of obesity occurred with some major emotionally stressful event in their lives. However, it is difficult to identify a suitable control group for such events. Multiple studies have shown that surgery, such as tonsillectomy, is associated with an increased incidence of obesity compared to unoperated controls in the period after surgery *(59,60)*.

3.6.2. Central Nervous System Damage

Injury to selected areas of the central nervous system (CNS) from accidents or neoplasms is known to cause obesity in a small number of patients *(61)*. Probably the most common type of injury is head trauma from automobile accidents. Pituitary or hypothalamic tumors are the most common types of neoplasms associated with the onset of obesity *(61)*.

3.6.3. SURGICAL PROCEDURES

Surgical procedures in the CNS may produce trauma to critical areas and produce obesity *(61)*. However, there are many anecdotal cases of obesity following surgery on other parts of the body, as noted for obesity after tonsillectomy. It is unclear whether damage to the CNS occurs during surgery in these cases, or if there is some other factor that alters CNS biochemistry. Animal studies show that lesions of the ventromedial hypothalamus, for example, leads to massive obesity, which is then defended by the body's normal mechanisms against starvation *(62)*.

3.6.4. INFECTIOUS DISEASES

An ominous potential etiology of obesity is that of infectious disease. Bray *(61)* reported a small number of patients who developed obesity after tuberculosis or other infections of the CNS that produced anatomical damage. Such bacterial infections causing obesity are rare and the CNS mechanisms easily understood. What is more disquieting is the possibility that viral infections may cause obesity. There are seven known animal models of virus-induced obesity. Lyons et al. *(63)* described massive obesity that occurred in mice after infection with canine distemper virus, a virus that is similar to human measles virus. Carter et al. *(64)* described obesity and stunting in chickens resulting from a rous-associated virus. Several strains of scrapie agent produce obesity, apparently by damaging the brain *(65)*. Borna virus produces widespread abnormalities including lympho-monocytic inflammation of the hypothalamus, hyperplasia of pancreatic islets, elevated serum glucose and triglycerides levels, stunting, and an increased body fat *(66)*. Dhurandhar et al. *(67)* described an unusual type of obesity in chickens in India owing to an avian adenovirus. This adenovirus caused the deposition of increased visceral fat, but paradoxical reductions in serum cholesterol and triglycerides. In a small study, about 20% of obese humans selected randomly from an obesity treatment program in Bombay, India, had antibodies that reacted with this chicken adenovirus *(68)*. The patients with antibodies weighed significantly more and had significantly lower serum cholesterol and triglycerides. Dhurandhar and Atkinson demonstrated that infection with a human adenovirus, Ad-36, produced increased adipose tissue and paradoxically lower serum cholesterol and triglycerides in chickens, mice, and nonhuman primates *(5,6)*. Obese humans who have antibodies to Ad-36 have lower serum cholesterol and triglycerides than do antibody negative individuals *(69)*. More research is urgently needed to determine whether obesity in humans may be due to viral infections.

4. ENDOCRINE AND METABOLIC DISEASES AS AN ETIOLOGY OF OBESITY

Endocrine disease is a commonly sought etiology of obesity, but is rarely found (Chapter 21 includes discussions of the evaluation of obese patients in obesity treatment programs). Thyroid disease is most often blamed for causing obesity, particularly in adolescents. However, hypothyroidism very rarely produces significant weight gain and treatment of thyroid deficiency rarely results in much weight loss. In the experience of the author, the presence of hypothyroidism makes it difficult for patients to lose weight while participating in an obesity treatment program, but with thyroid hormone replacement, weight loss in response to diet, exercise, and behavior modification including diet and exercise, with or without drug therapy, proceeds as predicted. An unusual cause of obesity reported by anecdote is hyperthyroidism. The author has taken care of four patients who reported the onset of weight gain simultaneously with the onset of symptoms suggestive of hyperthyroidism, and who were documented with elevated thyroid hormone levels and depressed thyroid-stimulating hormone (TSH) levels. Because thyroid disease is commonly found in obese patients, it is wise to check the serum thyroxine (T4) and TSH before starting a weight-reduction program.

Cushing's syndrome resulting from treatment with exogenous glucocorticoids is the most common form of endocrine obesity. Weight gain with glucocorticoid treatment may be large, in the range of 25 to 50 kg in extreme cases. Weight gain of these levels in spontaneously appearing Cushing's disease (pituitary tumor) or Cushing's syndrome owing to an adrenal adenoma certainly may be seen, but these diseases are exceedingly rare. Insulinomas are another rare cause of endocrine obesity. They promote deposition of adipose tissue and overeating due to periods of hypoglycemia.

Pseudohypoparathyroidism, hypothalamic disease, and hypogonadism are very rare causes of obesity. Although the average physician is not likely to ever see such patients in the primary care of medicine, endocrine diseases should be kept in mind because they are associated with treatable conditions that may markedly improve quality of life for these unfortunate people.

5. ABNORMAL REGULATION OF BODY WEIGHT OR BODY FAT

Keesey *(62,70)* advanced the hypothesis that individuals have a "body weight set point" that represents a body weight or an adipose tissue mass that is defended from change. Not all authors agree with this concept *(44,45,71)*. Flatt *(44,45)* suggested that the apparent "regulation" of body weight is the result of a confluence of factors that eventually lead to a stable body weight. If the equilibrium is disturbed, there are compensatory changes and a "settling" of the body weight or body fat at a new level. In the final analysis, the argument may be about semantics, but it is quite clear that the body weights of animals and humans do fluctuate in a fairly narrow range, and that single perturbations such as reduction of daily energy intake promote biochemical changes in the body that limit the reduction in weight and adipose tissue mass *(62,70)*. Conversely, overfeeding results in compensatory changes that limit weight gain. These biochemical changes, particularly in the case of underfeeding, are perfectly understandable survival traits that undoubtedly have been incorporated into the gene pool of all living creatures to deal with the periodic shortages of food or even famines that plagued the world for most of the time that life has been on Earth. Because surpluses of food have been rare throughout history, it would not be surprising that the mechanisms to deal with overfeeding are not as powerful as those dealing with underfeeding. These biochemical responses cause little inconvenience or health problems for the normal-weight individual who wishes to lose weight for cosmetic purposes. However, for the significantly obese person who needs to lose weight for health purposes, these "protective" mechanisms are frustrating indeed.

The discovery of leptin and its effects on body fat stores has given credence to the concept of regulation of fat stores in the body *(7–19)*. Leptin signals the brain regarding the amount of fat that is stored in the body, and abnormal genes for leptin or leptin receptors are associated with massive obesity in humans and animals. Treatment with leptin reduces body fat content of genetically obese mice, normal mice, and mice made obese by feeding a high-fat diet *(11–13)*. However, serum leptin levels are strongly correlated with adipose tissue mass *(19)*, suggesting that leptin "resistance" occurs. These data illustrate that leptin is not part of a simple negative feedback regulatory loop.

It appears that lowering the fat content of the diet from 35% of kilocalories, which is the typical American diet, to about 20% or less, which is the diet of primitive cultures, may lower the level at which body weight is defended. Likewise, exercise or increased activity may lower the defended body weight. These have been incorporated into behavioral treatments of obesity, but with a poor success rate. Obesity drugs and obesity surgery, particularly jejuno-ileal bypass surgery and gastric bypass surgery, are more passive methods of lowering the level at which body weight is regulated *(72,73)*. Other chapters (*see* Chapter 20) in this book discuss the success of treatment of obesity with these methods. More research is needed to determine if there is active regulation of body weight as postulated in the "body weight set point" theory, or if weight regulation is simply an interaction of a variety of factors that influence food intake, activity levels, and metabolic rate.

6. CONCLUSION

Obesity is an exceedingly complex group of diseases and probably should be characterized as a syndrome. With research in the area only just begun, more than 350 genes or gene markers have been identified that are associated with obesity and may contribute to the etiology of obesity in animals and humans. This suggests that there may be thousands of different types of obesity. The presence of a genetic tendency to obesity does not mean that obesity is inevitable, since environmental factors are critical for the expression of the genetic potential. Physicians should be aware of the factors that contribute to obesity that can be manipulated, such as dietary and exercise patterns, endocrine and metabolic diseases, and drugs. Research into obesity and its etiologies has been sparse, but the accelerating pace of research into obesity promises to provide new answers and point the way to new treatments for obesity.

REFERENCES

1. Chagnon YC, Rankinen T, Snyder EE, Weisnagel SJ, Perusse L, Bouchard C. The human obesity gene map: the 2002 update. Obes Res 2003; 11:313–367.
2. Friedman JM. A war on obesity, not the obese. Science 2003; 299:856–858.
3. Sims EA, Danforth E Jr, Horton ES, Bray GA, Glennon JA, Salans LB. Endocrine and metabolic effects of experimental obesity in man. Recent Prog Horm Res 1973; 29:457–496
4. Dhurandhar NV. Infectobesity: obesity of infectious origin. J Nutr 2001; 131:2794S–2797S.
5. Dhurandhar NV, Israel BA, Kolesar JM, Mayhew GF, Cook ME, Atkinson RL. Increased adiposity in animals due to a human virus. Int J Obes Relat Metab Disord 2000; 24:989–996.
6. Dhurandhar NV, Whigham LD, Abbott DH, et al. Human adenovirus Ad-36 promotes weight gain in male rhesus and marmoset monkeys. J Nutr 2002; 132:3155–3160.
7. Coleman DL. Obese and diabetes: two mutant genes causing diabetes-obesity in mice. Diabetologia 1979; 14:141–148.
8. Coleman DL. Genetics of obesity in rodents. In: Bray GA, ed. Recent Advances in Obesity Research: II. Newman Publishing, London, UK, 1978, pp. 142–152.
9. Coleman DL. Effects of parabiosis of obese with diabetes and normal mice. Diabetologia 1973; 9: 294–298.

10. Zhang Y, Proenca R, Maffei M, Barone M, Leopold L, Friedman RM. Positional cloning of the mouse obese gene and its human homologue. Nature 1994; 372:425–431.
11. Pelleymounter MA, Cullen MJ, Baker MB, et al. Effects of the obese gene product on body weight regulation in ob/ob mice. Science 1995; 269:540–543.
12. Halaas JL, Gajiwala KS, Maffei M, et al. Weight-reducing effects of the plasma protein encoded by the obese gene. Science 1995; 269:543–546.
13. Campfield LA, Smith FJ, Guisez Y, Devos R, Burn P. Recombinant mouse OB protein: evidence for a peripheral signal linking adiposity and central neural networks. Science 1995; 269: 546–549.
14. Montague CT, Farooqi IS, Whitehead JP, et al. Congenital leptin deficiency is associated with severe early-onset obesity in humans. Nature 1997; 387:903–908.
15. Strobel A, Issad T, Camoin L, Ozata M, Strosberg AD. A leptin missense mutation associated with hypogonadism and morbid obesity. Nature Genet 1998; 18:213–215
16. Farooqi IS, Matarese G, Lord GM, et al. Beneficial effects of leptin on obesity, T cell hyporesponsiveness, and neuroendocrine/metabolic dysfunction of human congenital leptin deficiency. J Clin Invest 2002; 110:1093–1103.
17. Clement K, Vaisse C, Lahlou N, et al. A mutation in the human leptin receptor gene causes obesity and pituitary dysfunction. Nature 1998; 392:398–401.
18. Clement K, Vega N, Laville M, et al. Adipose tissue gene expression in patients with a loss of function mutation in the leptin receptor. Int J Obes Relat Metab Disord 2002; 26:1533–1538.
19. Considine RV, Sinha MK, Heiman ML, et al. Serum immunoreactive-leptin concentrations in normal-weight and obese humans. N Engl J Med 1996; 334:292–295.
20. Bray GA, WT Dahms, RS Swerdloff, RH Fiser, RL Atkinson, RE Carrel. The Prader-Willi syndrome: a study of 40 patients and a review of the literature. Medicine 1983; 62:59–80.
21. Bouchard C, Snyder EE. Obesity Gene Map. Website: (http://obesitygene.pbrc.edu).
22. Schousboe K, Willemsen G, Kyvik KO, et al. Sex differences in heritability of BMI: a comparative study of results from twin studies in eight countries. Twin Res 2003 ;6: 409–421.
23. Stunkard A, Sorensen TIA, Hanis C, et al. An adoption study of human obesity. N Engl J Med 1986; 314:193–198.
24. Allison DB, Kaprio J, Korkeila M, Koskenvuo M, Neale MC, Hayakawa K. The heritability of body mass index among an international sample of monozygotic twins reared apart. Int J Obes Relat Metab Disord 1996; 20:501–506.
25. Bouchard C, Tremblay A, Despres JP, et al. The response to long-term overfeeding in identical twins. N Engl J Med 1990;24;322:1477–1482.
26. Bogardus C, Lillioja S, Ravussin E, et al. Familial dependence of the resting metabolic rate. N Eng J Med 1986; 315:96–100.
27. Fleury C, Neverova M, Collins S, et al. Uncoupling protein-2: a novel gene linked to obesity and hyperinsulinemia. Nature Genetics 1997; 15:269–272.
28. Dalgaard LT, Pedersen O. Uncoupling proteins: functional characteristics and role in the pathogenesis of obesity and Type II diabetes. Diabetologia 2001; 44:946–965.
29. Ravelli GP, Stein ZA, Susser MW. Obesity in young men after famine exposure in utero and early infancy. New England Journal of Medicine 1976; 295: 349–353.
30. Rogers I; EURO-BLCS Study Group. The influence of birthweight and intrauterine environment on adiposity and fat distribution in later life. Int J Obes Relat Metab Disord 2003; 27:755–777.
31. Catalano PM, Kirwan JP, Haugel-de Mouzon S, King J. Gestational diabetes and insulin resistance: role in short- and long-term implications for mother and fetus. J Nutr 2003; 133: 1674S–1683S.
32. Gillman MW, Rifas-Shiman S, Berkey CS, Field AE, Colditz GA. Maternal gestational diabetes, birth weight, and adolescent obesity. Pediatrics 2003; 111:e221–226.
33. Oh W, Gelardi NL, Cha CJ. The cross-generation effect of neonatal macrosomia in rat pups of streptozotocin-induced diabetes. Pediatr Res 1991; 29:606–610.
34. Dumesic DA, Abbott DH, Eisner JR, Goy RW. Prenatal exposure of female rhesus monkeys to testosterone propionate increases serum luteinizing hormone levels in adulthood. Fertil Steril 1997; 67:155–163.
35. Eisner JR, Dumesic DA, Kemnitz JW, Colman RJ, Abbott DH. Increased adiposity in female rhesus monkeys exposed to androgen excess during early gestation. Obes Res 2003; 11:279–286.
36. Martorell R, Stein AD, Schroeder DG. Early nutrition and later adiposity. J Nutr 2001; 131:874S–880S.

37. Plagemann A, Heidrich I, Gotz F, Rohde W, Dorner G. Obesity and enhanced diabetes and cardiovascular risk in adult rats due to early postnatal overfeeding. Exp Clin Endocrinol 1992; 99:154–158.
38. Rolls BJ, Kim-Harris S, Fischman MW, Foltin RW, Moran TH, Stoner SA. Satiety after preloads with different amounts of fat and carbohydrate: implications for obesity. Am J Clin Nutr. 1994; 60:476–487.
39. Tremblay A, St-Pierre S. The hyperphagic effect of a high-fat diet and alcohol intake persists after control for energy density. Am J Clin Nutr 1996; 63:479–482.
40. West DB, Boozer CN, Moody DL, Atkinson RL. Dietary obesity in nine inbred mouse strains. Am J Physiol 1992; 262:R1025–R1032.
41. Rissanen A, Hakala P, Lissner L, Mattlar CE, Koskenvuo M, Ronnemaa T. Acquired preference especially for dietary fat and obesity: a study of weight-discordant monozygotic twin pairs. Int J Obes Relat Metab Disord 2002; 26:973–977.
42. Ravussin E, Smith SR. Increased fat intake, impaired fat oxidation, and failure of fat cell proliferation result in ectopic fat storage, insulin resistance, and type 2 diabetes mellitus. Ann N Y Acad Sci 2002; 967:363–378.
43. Jequier E. Thermogenesis induced by nutrient administration in man. Infusionsther Klin Ernahr 1984; 11:184–188.
44. Flatt JP. Effect of carbohydrate and fat intake on postprandial substrate oxidation and storage. Top Clin Nutr 1987; 2:15–27
45. Flatt JP, Ravussin E, Acheson KJ, Jequier E. Effects of dietary fat on postprandial substrate oxidation and on carbohydrate and fat balances. J Clin Invest 1985; 76:1019–1024.
46. Horton TJ, Drougas H, Brachey A, Reed GW, Peters JC, Hill JO. Fat and carbohydrate overfeeding in humans: different effects on energy storage. Am J Clin Nutr 1995; 62:19–29.
47. Boozer CN, Schoenbach G, Atkinson RL. Dietary fat and adiposity: a dose–response relationship in adult rats fed isocalorically. Am J Physiol 1995; 268:E546–550.
48. Danforth E, Jr. Diet and obesity. Am J Clin Nutr 1985; 41:1132–1145.
49. Lissner L, Levitsky DA, Strupp BJ et al. Dietary fat and the regulation of energy intake in human subjects. Am J Clin Nutr 1987;46:886–892.
50. Prewitt TE, Schmeisser D, Brown PE, et al. Changes in body weight, body composition, and energy intake in women fed high- and low-fat diets. Am J Clin Nutr 1991, 54:304–310.
51. Bray GA, Popkin BM. Dietary fat affects obesity rate. Am J Clin Nutr 1999;70:572–573.
52. Willett WC. Dietary fat and obesity: an unconvincing relation. Am J Clin Nutr 1998; 68:1149–1150.
53. Prentice AM, Jebb SA. Obesity in Britain: gluttony or sloth? BMJ 1995; 311:437–439.
54. Zurlo F, Ferraro RT, Fontvieille AM, Rising R, Bogardus C, Ravussin E. Spontaneous physical activity and obesity: cross-sectional and longitudinal studies in Pima Indians. Am J Physiol 1992; 263: E296–E300.
55. Levine JA, Schleusner SJ, Jensen MD. Energy expenditure of nonexercise activity. Am J Clin Nutr 2000; 72:1451–1454.
56. Epstein LH, Valoski AM, Vara LS, et al. Effects of decreasing sedentary behavior and increasing activity on weight change in obese children. Health Psychol 1995; 14:109–115.
57. Gortmaker SL, Must A, Sobol AM, Peterson K, Colditz GA, Dietz WH. Television viewing as a cause of increasing obesity among children in the United States, 1986–1990. Arch Pediatr Adolesc Med 1996; 150:356–362.
58. Robinson TN. Television viewing and childhood obesity. Pediatr Clin North Am 2001; 48:1017–1025.
59. Barr GS, Osborne J. Weight gain in children following tonsillectomy. J Laryngol Otol 1988; 102:595–597.
60. Camilleri AE, MacKenzie K, Gatehouse S. The effect of recurrent tonsillitis and tonsillectomy on growth in childhood. Clin Otolaryngol 1995; 20:153–157.
61. Bray GA. Syndromes of hypothalamic obesity in man. Ped Annals 1984; 13:525–536.
62. Keesey RE; Powley TL. The regulation of body weight. Ann Rev Psychol 1986; 37: 109–133.
63. Lyons MJ, Faust IM, Hemmes RB, Buskirk DR, Hirsch J, Zabriskie JB. A virally induced obesity syndrome in mice. Science 1982; 216:82–85.
64. Carter JK, Ow CL, Smith RE. Rous-Associated virus type 7 induces a syndrome in chickens characterized by stunting and obesity. Infect Immun 1983; 39:410–422.
65. Kim YS, Carp RI, Callahan SM, Wisniewski HM. Scrapie-induced obesity in mice. J Infect Dis 1987; 156:402–405.

66. Gosztonyi G and Ludwig H. Borna disease: neuropathology and pathogenesis. Cur Topics in Microbiol Immunol 1995; 190:39–73.
67. Dhurandhar NV, Kulkarni PR, Ajinkya SM, Sherikar AA. Effect of adenovirus infection on adiposity in chickens. Veterinary Microbiol 1992; 31:101–107.
68. Dhurandhar NV, Kulkarni PR, Ajinkya SM, Sherikar AA, Atkinson RL. Association of adenovirus infection with human obesity. Obes Res 1997; 5:464–469.
69. Atkinson RL, Dhurandhar NV, Allison DB, Bowen RL, Israel BA, Albu JB, Augustus AS. Human adenovirus-36 is associated with increased body weight and paradoxical reduction of serum lipids. Int J Obesity, in press.
70. Keesey RE. A set point analysis of the regulation of body weight. In: AJ Stunkard, ed. Obesity. WB Saunders, Philadelphia, PA, 1980, pp. 144–165.
71. Harris RBS. Role of set-point theory in regulation of body weight. FASEB J 1990; 4:3310–3318.
72. Atkinson RL. Use of drugs in the treatment of obesity. Ann Rev Nutr 1997; 17:383–403.
73. Atkinson RL. Obesity surgery as a model for understanding the regulation of food intake and body weight. Am J Clin Nutr 1997; 66:184–185.

10 Medical Consequences of Obesity and Benefits of Weight Loss

Lalita Khaodhiar and George L. Blackburn

KEY POINTS

- Obese patients are at increased risk for developing numerous medical problems including insulin resistance and type 2 diabetes mellitus, hypertension, dyslipidemia, cardiovascular disease, stroke, sleep apnea, gallbladder disease, hyperuricemia and gout, osteoarthritis, and certain forms of cancers.
- Obesity and obesity-related disease accounts for significant mortality, particularly when the body mass index exceeds 30 kg/m^2.
- The association between type 2 diabetes mellitus with a cluster of disorders that includes obesity, hypertension, dyslipidemia, and atherosclerotic heart disease is known as Syndrome X or the insulin-resistance syndrome.
- Weight loss, even if moderate, can improve health status and lessen the incidence of obesity-related disease.

1. INTRODUCTION

Overweight and obesity have become epidemic in the United States and worldwide *(1)*. Data from the National Center for Health Statistics indicate that the prevalence of obesity, defined as a body mass index (BMI) of 30 kg/m^2 or more, increased from 12.8%in the years from 1976 to 1980, to 22.5% in the 1988 to1994 interval, to 30% in the 1999 and 2000 interval. Approximately 31% of US adults, about 59 million people, are considered obese, and more than 64% meet the criterion for overweight (BMI $\geq$25 kg/ m^2) *(2)*.

Obese patients are at increased risk for developing numerous medical problems including insulin resistance and type 2 diabetes mellitus (DM), hypertension, dyslipidemia, cardiovascular disease, stroke, sleep apnea, gallbladder disease, hyperuricemia and gout, osteoarthritis, and certain forms of cancers *(3–5)*. Excess body weight is also associated with substantial increases in cardiovascular and all-cause mortality. Each year, obesity and its complications results in 300,000 deaths *(6)* and estimated costs in excess of $100 billion. In 1995, obesity accounted for 11% of total national health expenditures and estimated direct medical costs of $52 billion *(7–9)*. Using data from the1994 National

From: *The Management of Eating Disorders and Obesity, Second Edition*
Edited by: D. J. Goldstein © Humana Press Inc., Totowa, NJ

Table 1
Chapter Overview

Health Institute Survey (NHIS), Wolf and Colditz *(8)* estimated the cost of lost productivity as a result of obesity at approx $3.9 billion, a figure that reflected 39.2 million days of missed work, as well as 239 million restricted-activity days, 89.5 million bed-days, and 62.6 million physician visits.

Ample evidence indicates that weight loss, even if moderate, can improve health status and lessen the incidence of obesity-related disease *(10–12)*. Studies show that a 10% decline in body weight reduces death rate by 280 per million and morbidity rates by 400 per million *(13,14)*. This chapter summarizes (Table 1) the medical consequences of obesity (Table 2) and benefits of weight loss. This information, which is important for patients to know, can be used to encourage weight loss for health benefits rather than often unrealistic cosmetic goals.

2. MORTALITY

Although, the relationship between body weight and mortality is still controversial *(15)*, it is generally accepted that overweight-related increased risk of death is modest until a BMI of 30 is reached, then increases thereafter. Obese adults have a 50 to 100% greater risk of premature death compared with those who have a BMI of 20 to 25 kg/m^2.

Table 2
Relative Risk of Health Problems Associated With Obesity

Obesity-associated conditions		
Greatly increased relative risk	Moderately increased relative risk	Slightly increased relative risk
(RR = >3)	(RR = 2 – 3)	(RR = >1 – <2)
• Diabetes mellitus • Insulin resistance • Hypertension • Dyslipidemia • Sleep apnea • Gallbladder disease	• Coronary heart disease • Osteoarthritis • Hyperuricemia and gout • Impaired fertility • Increased anesthetic risk • Low back pain	• Cancer (postmenopausal colon cancer, endometrial cancer, prostate cancer) • Reproductive hormone abnormalities • Polycystic ovary syndrome • Fetal defects from maternal obesity

Modified from ref. 4.

Important questions remain about optimal weight for longevity; the impact of age, race, and gender on the relationship between overweight and mortality; and the effects of smoking or concurrent disease in association with high mortality observed in lean people.

Most studies on the relationship between body weight and mortality support the hypothesis of a J- or U-shaped distribution, with increased risk among the very heavy or very lean (15–22). Several studies linking thinness to increased mortality have failed to exclude smokers and people with chronic disease; results are therefore questionable. Other research that excludes those groups suggests a positive correlation between mortality rate and body weight, with no excess risk among the lean (14,23).

The impact of age and race on the relationship between overweight and mortality is also controversial. The Department of Agriculture's most recent Dietary Guidelines for Americans (24) leave out age-specific recommendations (e.g., increased weight for height with advancing age) included in the 1990 version (25). The presumed reason is lack of sufficient supporting evidence for an age-specific recommendation. The American Cancer Society's Cancer Prevention Study suggests that the relative risk (RR) associated with higher body weight declines with age in adults older than 30 years (26). For example, an increment of 1 BMI unit was associated with a relative risk for death from cardiovascular disease (CVD) of 1.1 for 30- to 44-yr-old men compared with a relative risk of 1.03 in those aged 65–74; for women in the same age groups, the corresponding relative risks were 1.08 and 1.02.

Because the largest category in the Cancer Prevention study distribution was made up of those with a BMI of 32 kg/m^2 or more, the effect of age on excess mortality in those with higher BMI levels was unclear. Bender et al. (27) recently studied patients with mean BMI 36.6 kg/m^2 attending an obesity clinic. They found that risk of death increased with body weight, but that excess obesity-related mortality declined with age at all levels of obesity (i.e., no excess mortality was associated with a BMI of between 25 and 32 kg/m^2 in men or women aged 50 or older). This study's limitations included selection bias and insufficient information on putative confounders included in the analysis, such as smoking, alcohol consumption, medication, body fat distribution, obesity-associated disease, psychosocial status, and physical activity levels.

There are relatively few studies on effects of body weight on mortality in blacks, but evidence suggests that body weight may be a less important predictor of mortality in blacks than in whites, particularly among black women *(28)*. Findings from the American Cancer Society Prevention I Study indicate a significant association between ethnicity and BMI for both all-cause and CVD-related mortality in women *(29)*. BMI was associated with all-cause mortality in white women regardless of smoking status or education level, and in black women with a high school education. In black women with less than high school education, there was no significant association between BMI and all-cause mortality. Black women with a BMI of more than 35.9 kg/m^2, who had never smoked and had at least a high school education, had a 40% higher risk of all-cause mortality compared with black women at a normal BMI; white women with the same smoking history and education level had a 27.3% higher risk.

The Cancer Prevention Study II, a prospective study of more than 1 million adults in United States, examined the effects of age, race, gender, smoking status, and history of disease on the relation between BMI and overall mortality *(30)*. Data show that smoking status and preexisting disease significantly modified the association between BMI and the risk of death. In those who were healthy and had never smoked, the lowest mortality rate was found at a BMI of 23.5 to 24.9 kg/m^2 for men, and 22 to 23.4 kg/m^2 for women. At a BMI 40 kg/m^2 or more, relative risk of death was 2.58 for white men and 2 for white women (compared with white men with a BMI of 23.5 to 24.9 kg/m^2 and women with a BMI of 23.5 to 24.9 kg/m^2); the corresponding numbers for black men and women, 1.35 and 1.2, were not significant. A high BMI was most predictive of death from CVD, particularly in men (RR = 2.9). Obese men and women in all age groups had an increased risk of death.

In summary, data suggest an association between body weight and mortality that may vary according to age, race, gender, and the presence of concurrent disease.

3. MORBIDITY

3.1. Metabolic Syndrome (Syndrome X)

The association between type 2 DM with a cluster of disorders that includes obesity, hypertension, dyslipidemia, and atherosclerotic heart disease has long been recognized *(31,32)*. In the late 1980s, however, Reaven et al. suggested an underlying common cause (i.e., hyperinsulinemia resulting from insulin resistance). This cluster of disorders, known as "Syndrome X" or "the insulin-resistance syndrome," has since been widely studied to establish whether the coexisting conditions represented an as-yet-unexplained association of cardiovascular risk factors, or if insulin resistance was in fact the primary cause.

In 1998, the World Heath Organization (WHO) first proposed a unifying definition for the condition and called it "metabolic syndrome" instead of insulin-resistance syndrome *(33)*. This change was recommended because despite the relationship of metabolic syndrome to insulin resistance, insulin resistance was not a cause of all components of the syndrome. According to WHO criteria, patients with type 2 DM or impaired glucose tolerance or insulin resistance have the syndrome if they have at least two of the following four conditions; hypertension, dyslipidemia, obesity/abdominal obesity, and microalbuminuria (Table 3). Insulin resistance is defined as the lowest quartile of insulin-sensitivity measures (e.g., insulin-stimulated glucose uptake during euglycemic clamp), or highest quartile of fasting insulin or homeostasis model assessment.

Table 3
Metabolic Syndrome Proposed by the World Health Organization (33)

Diabetes or impaired glucose tolerance or insulin resistance with two
of the criteria below:

- Hypertension (antihypertensive treatment and/or blood pressure
  >160/90 mmHg)
- Dyslipidemia (triglyceride ≥1.7 mmol/L and/or HDL-C <0.9
  mmol/L in men, <1.0 mmol/L in women)
- Obesity/abdominal obesity (BMI ≥ 30 kg/m^2 and/or waist-hip ratio
  >0.9 in men and 0.85 in women)
- Microalbuminuria (overnight urinary excretion rate ≥ 20 μg/min)

HDL-C, high-density lipoprotein cholesterol; BMI, body mass index.

Table 4
Clinical Identification of the Metabolic Syndrome

- Abdominal obesity (waist circumference >102 cm [40 in] in men,
  >88 cm [35 in] in women)
- Hypertriglyceridemia (≥150 mg/dL)
- Low HDL-C (<40 mg/dL in men, <50 mg/dL in women)
- High blood pressure (≥130/85 mmHg)
- High fasting glucose (≥110 mg/dL)

HDL-C, high-density lipoprotein cholesterol.

3.1.1. DIAGNOSIS OF METABOLIC SYNDROME

Health care providers frequently see patients with multiple cardiac risk factors, but until recently, there were no clinically relevant or widely accepted diagnostic criteria for metabolic syndrome. The Third Report of the National Cholesterol Education Program Expert Panel on Detection, Evaluation, and Treatment of High Blood Cholesterol in Adults (Adult Treatment Panel III [ATP III]), released in 2001, changed this situation by underscoring the importance of the metabolic syndrome, and by providing a working definition of it *(34)*, that is, three or more of the criteria listed in Table 4. The US National Heart, Lung, and Blood Institute (NHLBI), the American Diabetes Association, the Center for the Disease Control, and other professional organizations have adopted this definition.

The ATP III panel did not find adequate evidence to recommend routine measurement of insulin resistance (e.g., plasma insulin), proinflammatory state (e.g., C-reactive protein), or prothrombotic state (e.g., fibrinogen) in clinical practice. It also noted that some men can develop multiple metabolic risk factors with only marginal increases in waist circumference (i.e., 94–102 cm) owing to a genetic predisposition to insulin resistance, and advised that such patients be treated the same as men with increased waist circumference.

3.1.2. Prevalence of Metabolic Syndrome

Metabolic syndrome, as defined by ATP III criteria, affects an estimated 24% of US adults (25% according to the WHO definition) *(35)*, or 47 million people *(36)*. This figure includes 10 to 15 million individuals with type 2 DM. Results from the third National Health and Nutrition Examination Study (NHANES III, 1988–1994) show that prevalence increases with age, rising from 7% in those aged 20 to 29 yr, to more than 40% in those over 60 yr of age. Mexican-Americans have the highest age-adjusted prevalence (32%). Overall, prevalence is similar for men and women. African-American women, however, have about 57% higher prevalence than African-American men, and Mexican-American women have about 26% higher prevalence than Mexican-American men.

3.1.3. Clinical Implication

Even in the absence of baseline coronary heart disease (CHD) and diabetes, individuals with metabolic syndrome have a markedly increased risk of CVD and all-cause mortality. The Kuopio Ischaemic Heart Disease Risk Factor Study tracked a cohort of 1209 Finnish men initially free of CHD, diabetes, or cancer over a mean follow-up of 11.4 yr *(37)*. In that study, 9–14% of the men had metabolic syndrome. The overall survival in those without metabolic syndrome was 90% compared with 79 to 83% for those with ATP III-defined metabolic syndrome, or 83 to 84% based on WHO criteria. After adjusting for conventional cardiovascular risk factors, men with ATP III-defined metabolic syndrome were 2.9 to 4.2 times more likely to die of CHD. Men with a WHO-defined metabolic syndrome were 2.9 to 3.3 times more likely to die of CHD. Metabolic syndrome accounted for an estimated 18% of the variance in cardiovascular risk.

3.1.3.1. Link to Non-Insulin Dependent Diabetes Mellitus

Several epidemiological studies have linked increased risk for non-insulin dependent (type 2) diabetes with higher BMIs. In the Nurses' Health Study *(38)*, greater risk of diabetes was observed with BMI as low as 22. Women with BMI in average range (24.0–24.9) had up to a fivefold elevated risk when compared with women with a BMI less than 22 kg/m^2. The risk of type 2 DM increased by more than 40-fold in those with a BMI over 31 kg/m^2. This relationship between BMI and diabetes was seen in black and white women and in those up to 69 yr of age. In addition, the study reported that changes in body weight during adulthood were a strong predictor of risk for diabetes. Women who gained 20 kg or more had a 12-fold increased risk compared with women whose weight changes were less than 5 kg. Conversely, a weight loss of 20 kg or more reduced the risk of diabetes by 87%.

The Professionals' Health Study, which includes more than 50,000 US male health professionals 40 to 75 yr of age, showed similar results. Relative risk of diabetes in men with a BMI of 35 kg/m^2 was 42 times higher than that in men with a BMI less than 23 kg/m^2 *(39)*. Men who gained at least 15 kg after age 21 had 3.4 times higher risk of diabetes than those who were within 2 kg of their weight at 21.

The association of higher BMI with increased risk of type 2 DM has been shown in diverse populations, including those with high and low rates of diabetes. Studies of the Pima Indian tribe *(40–42)*, with its very high prevalence of diabetes, show that the incidence of diabetes is strongly related to preexisting obesity with approx 0.8 cases per 1000 person-years for BMI less than 20 kg/m^2 compared with 72 cases per 1000 person-years for BMI over 40. Interestingly, diabetes was extremely rare in this tribe in the 1940s, when the diet consisted of complex carbohydrate with very low amounts of fat. Exposure of the Pima Indians to a more typical Western diet (i.e., high-calorie, high-fat) and a more sedentary lifestyle, has led to obesity and a prevalence of diabetes that exceeds 50% in adults.

Data suggest that obesity, particularly central (abdominal) obesity, causes insulin resistance, a state in which target organs are less able to respond to the metabolic effects of insulin (43). Insulin resistance is characterized by elevated serum insulin levels and a decreased ability to oxidize and store glucose. Insulin-resistant, non-diabetic obese subjects initially maintain euglycemia via a compensatory increase in insulin secretion. With time or further weight gain, particularly in genetic-susceptible patients, the β-cells are unable to sustain the degree of hyperinsulinemia, and hyperglycemia ensues.

Alterations of muscle fuel metabolism play a central role in obesity-related insulin resistance, although all other major glucose-regulatory tissues including liver, adipose tissue, and pancreas are affected. Evidence suggests that obesity-induced insulin resistance is mediated in part by high concentration of free fatty acid (FFA) and tumor necrosis factor (TNF)-α released by excess adipocytes. Elevated FFA causes hyperinsulinemia by inhibiting muscle glucose utilization, increasing hepatic glucose output, and stimulating insulin secretion from pancreatic β cells (44–46). Euglycemic hyperglycemic clamp studies demonstrate a 30 to 40% decrease in insulin sensitivity in patients who are 35 to 40% above their ideal body weight (47).

3.1.3.2. LINK TO CARDIOVASCULAR DISEASE

3.1.3.2.1. Hypertension

The association between obesity and hypertension is well documented. The NHANES III data show that in men as well as women, the prevalence of hypertension rises progressively with increased in BMI (48). In adults with BMI over 30 kg/m^2, the prevalence of high blood pressure (BP) is 38% in men and 32% in women; in those with BMI below 25 kg/m^2, it is 18% in men and 16% in women (with respective relative risks of 2.1 and 1.9). Data from the Nurses' Health Study indicate a similar relation between BMI and hypertension (49). Middle-age women with a BMI of at least 31 kg/m^2 had a 6.3 relative risk of hypertension compared with those with BMI below 20 kg/m^2.

Multivariate analysis showed that risk for hypertension rose 12% for every 1 kg/m^2 increase in BMI. Increases in risk were also seen with weight gain as small as 2.1 to 4.9 kg. Each 10 lb (4.5 kg) of weight gain increased the risk of hypertension by an estimated 20%. Women who gained more than 25 kg showed a fivefold increase in risk. Conversely those who lost more than 10 kg reduced their risk of hypertension by 26%. Similar findings from the large International Study of Salt (INTERSALT) showed that an additional 10 kg body weight was associated with increases in systolic (SBP) and diastolic BP (DBP) of 3.0 mmHg and 2.3 mmHg, respectively (50). Data from the Framingham Heart Study suggest that approx 65 to 75% of risk for hypertension can be directly attributed to excess weight (51).

Although the importance of obesity as a cause of hypertension is well recognized, the pathophysiological mechanisms that underlie their association are just starting to be understood (52). Obesity is associated with increases in regional blood flow, cardiac output, and arterial pressure. Although part of the increased cardiac output is the result of additional blood flow required by excess fat, blood flow to other tissues, such as the heart, kidneys, and skeletal muscle also increases. Vasodilation in these tissues appears to result from high metabolic rate and local accumulation of vasodilator metabolites *(53)*. The maintenance of hypervolemia in the present of hypertension implies a resetting of pressure natriuresis toward higher BP *(54)*. Obesity increases renal sodium reabsorption by activating renin-angiotensin and sympathetic nervous system *(55)*.

Hormones, such as leptin, that are secreted from adipose tissue may be partly responsible for sympathetic activation. Acute infusions of leptin increase renal sympathetic activity *(56)*. In addition, insulin may promulgate high BP. Insulin has been shown to increase renal tubular reabsorption of sodium and boosts intracellular stores of free calcium in the vascular smooth muscle cells, thereby increasing vascular tone *(57–59)*.

Prolonged obesity causes structural changes in the kidneys that eventually lead to a loss of nephron function, further increases in BP and severe renal disease in some cases.

Weight loss is associated with a decrease in BP in both hypertensive and nonhypertensive obese subjects. In general, weight loss of 1 kg lowers BP by 0.3 to 1 mmHg *(60—63)*. Weight-loss induced reduction in BP is explained partly by reduction in total blood volumes, cardiac output, and peripheral vascular resistance, improvement in insulin resistance, and a reduction in the activity of the sympathetic and ennin- angiotensin aldosterone system *(64)*.

3.1.3.2.2. Hyperlipidemia

Several deleterious changes in lipid metabolism are often seen in obese individuals. In general, obesity tends to elevate fasting plasma total cholesterol and triglycerides and reduce plasma high-density lipoprotein cholesterol (HDL-C) levels *(65)*. Plasma low-density lipoprotein cholesterol (LDL-C) levels are slightly elevated or normal, but small dense atherogenic LDL particles are usually increased, particularly in patients with insulin resistance associated with visceral adiposity *(66–68)*. The low HDL-C levels, high LDL-C to HDL-C ratio, and high proportion of small dense LDL particles put patients at greater risk for atherosclorosis *(69)*. Changes in plasma lipid levels observed in obesity are more closely correlated with the amount of visceral fat than total body fat.

Insulin resistance and hyperinsulinemia appear to be two important regulators of lipid metabolism disorders seen in abdominal obesity. There are also positive correlations between daily cholesterol production and both body fat and energy intake. Caloric restriction, on the other hand, reduces the activity of β-hydroxy-β-methylglutaryl-Co-A reductase *(70)*, the rate-limiting enzyme in cholesterol synthesis.

Central obesity and hyperinsulinemia may cause excess production of very low-density lipoprotein (VLDL), which is triglyceride-rich in the liver. Enhanced lipolytic activity of visceral adipocytes increases FFA flux to the liver and stimulates VLDL secretion *(71)*. Also, the activity of lipoprotein lipase, the enzyme that transforms triglyceride-rich chylomicrons to HDL, and VLDL to LDL, declines with insulin resistance *(72)*. These alterations in VLDL metabolism can lead to a slower VLDL clearance, a reduced HDL production and an increased in smaller, denser LDL particles *(65,68)*. In addition, obesity-related insulin resistance decreases affinity for the LDL receptor and may impair clearance of LDL particles *(73)*.

Table 5
Risk Factors for Coronary Heart Disease Associated With Obesity

- Hypertension
- Diabetes mellitus (type 2)
- Dyslipidemia (high TG, low HDL-C, small dense LDL-C)
- Hyperinsulinemia
- High levels of PAI-1
- Hyperviscosity
- Obstructive sleep apnea

TG, triglycerides; HDL-C, high-density lipoprotein cholesterol, LDL-C, low-density lipoprotein cholesterol; PAI-1, plasminogen activator inhibitor.

3.1.3.2.3. Coronary and Peripheral Vascular Diseases

Obesity is an important factor in the development of CVD, and is associated with excess morbidity and mortality from CHD *(74)*. Obesity is strongly associated with classic cardiovascular risk factors, such as hypertension, type 2 DM, low HDL-C, and high total cholesterol (Table 5). In addition, obstructive sleep apnea, hyperinsulinemia, and hemorheological (blood viscosity regulation) abnormalities including elevated plasma plasminogen activator inhibitor 1 (PAI-1) levels and high blood viscosity, may contribute to pathogenesis of coronary atherosclerosis in obese persons.

The association between obesity and CVD has been shown in several epidemiological studies. The Nurses' Health Study *(75)* demonstrated that moderately overweight women (BMI = 25–28.9 kg/m²) had an 80% greater risk than their lean counterparts of developing coronary artery disease (CAD). Even after adjusting for other cardiac risk factors such as smoking, hypertension, and diabetes, results showed that obesity was responsible for 40% of coronary events. The Framingham Study *(76)* reported that obese men had a 1.5 times higher risk of CHD than lean men, whereasd obese women had a 2.1 times greater CHD risk than their lean peers. The majority of obese men and women who developed CHD (56% of obese men and 62% of obese women) had clusters of two or more cardiac risk factors.

Insulin resistance also plays a major role in the development of CHD in obesity. The Quebec Cardiovascular Cohort, a 5-yr prospective study of more than 2000 men, clearly demonstrated that hyperinsulinemia is an independent risk factor for ischemic heart disease that cannot be explained by any concomitant dyslipidemia or hypertension *(77)*. The San Antonio Heart Study produced similar results *(78)*.

Hyperinsulinemia, through stimulation of arterial smooth muscle proliferation, has been implicated in the development of atherosclerotic plaque *(79,80)*. In dogs, insulin infusions have been shown to promote marked expansion of the intima and media of arterial walls. Degree of insulin resistance has been shown to be significantly correlated with CAD. Lean, nondiabetic normotensive patients with documented CAD also exhibit insulin resistance state *(81)*.

The association between insulin resistance and CVD may also be secondary to a hypercoaguable state. Several studies have shown that compared with non-obese controls, obese patients have higher plasma concentrations of all pro-thrombotic factors (fibrinogen, vonWillebrand factor, and factor VII) that have positive associations with central fat. Similarly, plasma concentrations of PAI-1 have been shown to be higher in obese patients as compared to non-obese controls and to be directly correlated with visceral fat *(82)*. Type I PAI-1 suppresses tissue plasminogen activator (tPA) inhibitor enzyme that converts plasminogen to plasmin, which in turn, degrades the fibrin polymers of clots. Therefore, high PAI-1 causes impaired fibrinolytic activity and increased in the extension of thrombosis *(83–86)*.

Fibrinogen may also play a role. Ample evidence indicates that elevated fibrinogen levels are a risk factor for CAD *(86,87)*. The Framingham Study followed 1315 healthy participants for a 12-yr period after measurement of their fibrinogen levels. Analysis showed a positive correlation between fibrinogen levels and the risk of developing CVD. This association persisted after multivariate analysis for other known cardiac risk factors, including BP, cholesterol level, smoking, and left ventricular hypertrophy.

3.2. Other Medical Complications

3.2.1. OSTEOARTHRITIS

Osteoarthritis (OA), one of the most common complications of obesity, accounts for substantial morbidity and disability in the elderly. It is the leading indication for more than 200,000 knee and hip replacement surgeries performed annually in the United States *(88,89)*. The link between obesity and OA is strong; and consistently demonstrated for knee OA. In contrast, epidemiological data linking obesity with OA of the hip have been inconsistent. Data from National Health and Nutrition Examination Survey (NHANES-I) showed that obesity was associated with bilateral, but not unilateral, hip OA *(90)*. Conversely, other studies from the United Kingdom *(91)*, Sweden *(92,93)*, Finland *(94)*, and the United States *(95)* reported a positive relation between obesity and hip OA. Indeed, growing evidence suggests negative effects of overweight and obesity on hip OA *(96)*.

OA of the hand has also been associated with increased weight. In middle-aged women, it was estimated that for every kilogram increases in body weight, the risk of OA of the knee and carpometacarpal joint of the hand increased by 9 to 13%. A recent study of the Finnish population indicated that BMI was a significant determinant for osteoarthritis of finger and distal interphalangeal joints *(97)*. Although OA of the knee is contributed by mechanical trauma associated with excess body weight, it is postulated that the arthritis of nonweight-bearing joints is probably the result of some systemic factor produced by fat cells, such as the cytokines interleukin (IL)-6, TNF-α, and leptin, that promotes cartilage breakdown or bone growth *(98,99)*.

Weight loss is associated with reduced risk of OA. In the Framingham Study *(100)*, a decrease of 2 or more BMI units (approx 5.1 kg) over 10 yr reduced the odds of developing OA of the knee by more than 50%; whereas, weight gain was associated with a slightly increased risk. The benefit of weight loss was also demonstrated in high-risk patients with a baseline BMI over 25 kg/m^2. McGoey et al. *(101)* found that weight reduction also improved symptoms in patients with established OA. In a group of 105 morbidly obese subjects who underwent gastric stapling, weight loss led to a significant decline in joint pain. After 1 yr, and a mean weight loss of 44 kg (96.8 lb), 89% of patients reported relief of lower back, hip, knee, ankle, and foot pain.

3.2.2. MALIGNANCY

A strong link exists between obesity and several types of cancer. The prospective American Cancer Society (ACS) Study *(102)*, which followed more than 750,000 men and women for 12 yr, found that cancer mortality ratios for men and women who were at least 40% overweight were 1.33 and 1.55, respectively. Overweight men had significantly higher mortality rates for colorectal and prostate cancers, whereas overweight women had significantly higher mortality rates for endometrial, gallbladder, cervical, ovarian, and breast cancers *(103)*. Although evidence implicating obesity as a risk factor for colon cancer in women remains inconclusive, more recent data suggest a similar relationship to that seen in men *(104–106)*. In NHANES-I, odds ratios for colon cancer ranged from 1.79 for BMIs of 22 to 24 kg/m^2 to 3.72 for BMIs of 28 to 30 kg/m^2 when compared with BMI of less than 22 kg/m^2 in both men and women *(105)*.

The relationship between obesity and breast cancer appears to depend on age at diagnosis. Data from the Nurses' Health Study showed that higher current BMI was associated with a lower incidence of breast cancer before menopause, but a slightly increased incidence after menopause *(107)*. Weight gain after age 18 was also only associated with postmenopausal breast cancer. This association was particularly strong in women who never used hormone replacement therapy. Women who gained more than 20 kg after age 18 doubled their risk of breast cancer.

Changes in the hormonal milieu are believed to be partly responsible for some of the relationship between weight and cancer. Specifically, obese women are exposed to chronically high estrogen levels. This heightened exposure is the result of the enzyme aromatase. Present in adipose cells, aromatase converts androstendione (produced by the adrenal gland) to estrone. Evidence indicates that this persistent stimulation of breast and endometrial tissue by estrogenic compounds creates a predisposition to malignant transformation *(108,109)*. Weight loss, however, may break this cycle by lowering aromatase levels, and thus, estrone production.

3.2.3. SLEEP APNEA

Obesity, especially upper body obesity, is the most important risk factor for obstructive sleep apnea (OSA) *(110,111)*. An increase of 1 standard deviation in any standard measure of body habitus is related to a threefold increase in the occurrence of OSA *(110)*. Up to 60 to 70% of OSA sufferers are obese; among the morbidly obese, OSA occurs at a 12- to 20-fold frequency *(112)*. Sleep studies on men and women with a mean BMI of 45.3 kg/m^2 and no sleep complaints, found that 40% of the men and 3% of the women had OSA severe enough for therapeutic intervention, compared with none of non-obese age-matched control *(113)*. An excessive amount of fat in the neck region is a main predisposing factor for upper airway narrowing and/or collapse.

The clinical characteristics of OSA are loud snoring, nocturnal hypoxia, frequent awakening, and daytime somnolence. Resulting disturbed and fragmented sleep may impair daytime functioning, possibly accounting for a sevenfold increase in automobile accidents. Other consequences of OSA include cognitive impairment, personality changes, systemic hypertension, cardiac arrhythmias, myocardial ischemia, stroke, obesity-hyperventilation syndrome, an extreme form of OSA characterized by awake respiratory failure, pulmonary hypertension and heart failure, and sudden death *(114,117)*.

3.2.4. GOUT

Many studies report positive correlations between serum uric acid levels and body weight *(118,119)*. Excess visceral fat is associated with abnormal uric acid metabolism including a decrease in renal uric acid clearance, and an increase in the urinary uric acid to creatinine ratio *(120)*. Hyperuricemia is frequently associated with a number of common metabolic disorders (e.g., hypertension, hyperlipidemia, obesity, and CHD). Nevertheless, there is scant evidence that uric acid acts as a causal factor in these settings *(121)*. Obesity and excessive weight gain are important risk factors for gout, particularly in adult men *(122,123)*.

3.2.5. GALLBLADDER DISEASE

Both cross-sectional *(124)* and longitudinal studies *(125)* have shown that increased body weight is associated with a greater incidence of gallbladder disease. Important risk factors for symptomatic gallstones include female gender (RR 8.8), obesity (BMI >30 kg/ m^2, RR 3.7), age over 50 (RR 2.5), and a positive history of previous cholecystectomy in a first-degree family member (RR 2.2) *(126)*. Data from the Nurses' Health Study showed that women with a BMI greater than 45 kg/m^2 had a sevenfold increased risk of gallstone compared with those with a BMI less than 24 kg/m^2. Incidence of gallstone was higher than 1% per year in women with a BMI over 30 kg/m^2, and up to 2% per year in those with a BMI equal to 45 kg/ m^2 or more *(125)*.

NHANES-III data show that risk of gallbladder disease differs substantially by gender. In men under 55 yr of age, weight gain produced a marked rise in prevalence of gallbladder disease; in older men, the association was weaker. In women, risk increased steadily with weight gain across all age group *(127)*. The usual gallstones that form in obese individuals are cholesterol stones that occur because of a cholesterol supersaturation of bile *(128)*. Although data are still controversial, gallbladder motor function may also be impaired in obese subjects *(129)*. Abnormal gallbladder contractility can lead to poor emptying and bile stasis.

3.3. Regional Fat Distribution

Regional fat distribution has become recognized as an important factor in determining health risk in obese individuals. Data from epidemiological and clinical studies have shown that excess abdominal fat is an independent predictor for CVD risk and mortality *(130–133)*. Risk factors include type 2 DM, impaired glucose tolerance, hypertension, dyslipidemia, and artherosclerosis of coronary, cerebral, and peripheral vessels. Data related to fat distribution, however, are not as extensive as for obesity *per se*.

The impact of regional fat distribution on health is related to both abdominal (upper body fat) and visceral fat located in the intra-abdominal cavity. One of the problems in performing studies on the effects of fat distribution and the impact of visceral fat has been measurement of fat distribution. In general, anthropometric measurements (waist circumference, waist-to-hip ratio [WHR], or skinfold thickness) have been used to estimate central or upper body obesity. These measurements are simple and convenient for epidemiological studies, and provide useful estimates of the proportion of abdominal fat; however, they do not distinguish between accumulations of deep abdominal (visceral) fat and subcutaneous abdominal fat. Imaging techniques such as computed tomography (CT) or magnetic resonance imaging, provide more accurate data, but are costly and not feasible for use in large studies. Because visceral fat is difficult to accurately measure, there are no data from large epidemiological study available on its health effects.

The impact of body fat distribution on mortality has been investigated in several epidemiologicla studies *(119,134–138)*. Results show that increased abdominal or upper body fat is associated with greater mortality independent of total degree of obesity in both men and women. Increased abdominal or visceral fat is also significantly related to CHD *(139)*, hypertension, and type 2 DM *(140)*. One study in adults 34 to 54 yr of age, reported that intra-abdominal adipose tissue, measured by CT, significantly predicted the levels of six metabolic risk factors: SBP, dBP, fasting blood glucose, serum HDL-C, serum triglyceride, and PAI-1 *(141)*.

In the Nurses' Health Study *(139)*, higher WHR and waist circumference were independently associated with a significantly increased age-adjusted risk of CHD. After adjusting for BMI and other cardiac risk factors, women with a WHR of 0.88 or higher had a relative risk of 3.25 for CHD compared with women with a WHR of less than 0.72. A waist circumference of 96.5 cm (38 in) or more was associated with a relative risk of 3.06. A similar association between abdominal obesity and increased risk for CHD was also reported in the Framingham Heart Study *(119)*, the Prospective Cardiovascular Munster (PROCAM) Study *(142)*, the Honolulu Heart Study *(136)*, the Paris Prospective Study *(138)*, and the Physicians' Health Study *(143)*. In four of these five studies, the association was independent of other CHD risk factors or BMI.

In the Honolulu Heart Study, central fat distribution, measured by subcutaneous skinfold thickness, was an independent risk factor for CHD in men. In the Paris Prospective Study, abdominal obesity was a better predictor of CHD than degree of obesity. Thus, central or abdominal fat mass distribution is an important risk factor for CHD, one that might be more important than degree of obesity alone. A number of studies have also reported that adipose tissue distribution is a risk factor for hypertension *(141,144–147)* and dyslipidemia (high concentrations of serum triglycerides and low concentrations of serum HDL-C) *(144,148,149)*. These associations, however, are weaker for women than they are for men.

Ample evidence shows that abdominal obesity is an important predictor of glucose intolerance and hyperinsulinemia in adults *(140,149–151)*. In obese individuals, increased WHR is correlated with decreased hepatic insulin extraction and a decline in metabolic clearance rate of insulin with regard to dyslipidemia. More peptides and nonpeptide compounds are produced and secreted in the visceral fat than in subcutaneous fat. Some of these compounds include adipose tissue lipoprotein lipase, cholesterylester transfer protein activity, PAI-1, TNF-α, and IL-6. The increased lipolytic activity in visceral fat results in higher FFA mobilization to the liver, increased gluconeogenesis and VLDL production, and decreased insulin sensitivity *(152)*. TNF-α and IL-6 also inhibit insulin receptor signaling, and block insulin action *(153–155)*.

The relationship between central obesity on gallbladder disease (Subheading 3.2.5.) has been documented *(129,156)*; likewise with cancer, although the data are not as complete. A majority of prospective studies show higher risk of breast cancer in obese postmenopausal women with upper abdominal adiposity than in those with overall adiposity *(157)*. In premenopausal women, however, the evidence is more limited and inconsistent *(158)*.

3.4. Benefits of Weight Loss

Weight reduction has been shown to improve obesity-related comorbid conditions, and have beneficial effects on cardiovascular risk factors (see Chapter 13). Modest weight loss as low as 5–10% has been associated with an improvement of fasting glycemia, BP, and plasma lipid profiles.

3.4.1. EFFECTS OF WEIGHT LOSS ON TYPE 2 DIABETES MELLITUS

Weight loss produced by diet and/or exercise improves insulin sensitivity and reduces blood glucose levels in both obese diabetic and non-diabetic individuals. Initiation of a hypocaloric diet frequently improves hyperglycemia, an outcome that suggests a beneficial effect from restricted caloric intake independent of weight loss. In a study of a very low-calorie diet in obese patients with type 2 DM, 87% of the reduction in plasma glucose levels was observed within the first 10 d of caloric restriction, whereas 60% of weight loss occurred between d 10 and 40 (159).

In another study, 93 obese patients with type 2 DM were assigned to either 1674 kJ/d (400 kcal) or 4185 kJ/d (1000 kcal) (160). At comparable degree of weight loss (11%), subjects on lower calorie diets had reduced fasting glucose levels (7.61 vs. 10.13 mmol/L) and improved insulin sensitivity. When subjects switched from 1674 kJ (400 kcal) to 4185 kJ (1000 kcal), glycemic control and insulin sensitivity worsened despite continued weight loss. Subjects on the 4185 kJ (1000 kcal) from the start of the study, however, showed further improvement in glycemic control and additional weight loss.

Moderate weight loss in obese patients with type 2 DM can significantly improve glycemic control, as shown by a reduction in HbA_1C levels; some patients are able to discontinue insulin or oral therapy. Depending on the level of weight maintenance, such improvements can last many years. One randomized, controlled study of diet and exercise in overweight African-Americans with type 2 DM, showed that at 6 mo, weight loss of 3% in the intervention group was accompanied by a reduction of HbA_1C by 2.4% (161). In another study of newly diagnosed diabetes, those who attended regular group education sessions run by nurses-specialists in diabetes and a dietitian, lost 5 kg more weight at 6 mo than those who had no structured education. Their HbA_1C was also 2% lower than that of subjects in the no-structured education group (162). Mancini et al.'s study on long-term effect of weight loss (163) found that patients who maintained reduction of at least 5% of initial body weight at 3 yr had lasting improvement of glycemic control, whereas those who maintained less than 5% had worsening glycemia.

Although diet and exercise are mainstays of treatment for type 2 DM, there are wide variations in patient response. A 48-mo retrospective study on 135 patients on diet therapy indicated that only 41% of those who lost at least 9.1 kg had plasma glucose concentration less than 10 mmol/L (164). Some of these individuals, however, decreased their plasma glucose levels after losing only 2.3 kg. Improvements in glycemic control occurred early in the course of weight loss; patients who remained hyperglycemic after reductions of 2.3 to 9.1 kg were unlikely to improve with additional weight loss.

These results might be due to relatively higher insulin resistance in patients who responded to diet therapy, and severe insulin deficiency in patients who did not. Other studies have shown that initial fasting plasma glucose is a strong predictor of response to diet therapy. The UK Prospective Diabetic Study found that patients with initial fasting blood glucose of 6 to 8 mmol/L (108–144 mg/dL) needed to lose 10 kg (16% of initial body weight) to achieve a normal fasting plasma glucose of less than 6 mmol/L; a weight loss of 26 kg (41% of initial body weight) was required in those with initial blood glucose greater than 14 mmol/L (252 mg/dL) *(165)*.

In addition to benefits of weight loss in diabetes treatment, recent studies have shown that modest weight reduction is effective in preventing type 2 DM. In the Finnish Diabetes Prevention Study, a diet and exercise program produced a 58% reduction in diabetes compared with control *(166,167)*. The US Diabetes Prevention Program, a randomized, clinical trial of more than 3200 overweight subjects at high risk for diabetes (i.e., impaired glucose tolerance) also showed a 58% reduction in diabetes from 11% per year in the control group to 4.8% per year in the lifestyle modification group, which lost 5 to 7% of initial body weight *(168–169)*.

In a majority of patients, gastric bypass surgery (*see* Chapter 20) can substantially control type 2 DM. In one large series, 608 morbidly obese patients underwent Roux-en-Y gastric bypass; prior to surgery, 165 patients had type 2 DM and 165 had impaired glucose tolerance (IGT) *(170171)*. Of those with diabetes, 121 of 146 patients (83%) maintained normal fasting blood glucose and HbA$_1$C levels at the end of follow-up (up to 14 yr), while 25 remained diabetic. Among patients with IGT, only two progressed to overt disease. Postoperatively, normalization of blood glucose was observed within a few days, before the occurrence of weight loss (which is probably owing to limitation of caloric intake). By the end of the first week, the majority of the patients were able to discontinue insulin or oral hypoglycemic drugs.

3.4.2. EFFECT OF WEIGHT LOSS ON BLOOD PRESSURE

Lifestyle modification, which includes diet intervention, physical activity, behavior therapy, or combination therapy can significantly reduce BP in hypertensive and nonhypertensive people with obesity. At 6 mo, the Trial of Antihypertensive Interventions and Management (TAIM) *(60,61)* reported a significant decrease in DBP of 11.6 mmHg in patients who lost 4.5 kg or more, compared with those who lost less than 2.5 kg, or those who treated with placebo. The effect was comparable to that produced by 25 mg chlorthalidone or 50 mg atenolol. Moreover, weight loss potentiated the effect of antihypertensive drugs.

In phase II of the TAIM, 587 patients with mild hypertension were followed for a mean of 4.5 yr. Of those receiving placebo, low dose diuretic, or β-blocker, a 2–3 kg weight loss reduced the need for additional antihypertensive medications by 23% *(172)*. A meta-analysis by MacMahon *(173)*, which included five randomized, controlled trials, supported the benefits of dietary intervention. Weight loss of 10 kg in hypertensive patients resulted in a reduction of 6.8 mmHg in SBP, and 3.4 mmHg in DBP. In the Dietary Intervention Study in Hypertension *(174)* and the Hypertension Control Program *(175)*, overweight patients with uncomplicated, well-controlled hypertension were withdrawn from drug treatment. Subsequent modest weight loss from diet therapy resulted in a significant reduction in the redevelopment of hypertension over 1 to 4 yr.

Weight loss is also effective in preventing hypertension in nonhypertensive, overweight individuals. Cutler reviewed four randomized, controlled trials in which 872 nonhypertensive adults and adolescents engaged in weight-loss programs using dietary intervention and/or exercise *(176)*. Weight loss of 1 kg in adults reduced both SBP and DBP by approx 0.45 mmHg; weight loss of 1 kg in adolescents resulted in a 5 mmHg reduction in BP. Modest weight reduction (mean 2.7 kg), in conjunction with low salt and alcohol intake and increased physical activity, reduced the 5-yr incidence of hypertension by 52% *(177)*. Data from the Trial of Hypertension Prevention Phase I (TOHP I) and Phase II (TOHP II), two large randomized,controlled trials, produced similar results. Modest weight loss by behavioral means in subjects with borderline hypertension (SBP <140 mmHg and DBP 83–89 mmHg) reduced the incidence of hypertension by 20 to 50% at 18 mo, and by 19% at 3 yr *(178,179)*.

Improvement in BP after bariatric surgery has been consistently reported. Foley et al. found that hypertension had resolved in 66% of 67 patients at the time of the last follow-up *(180)*. In another study, 45 morbidly obese patients with diastolic hypertension underwent gastric surgery; 12 mo later, hypertension had resolved in 22 of them (54%), and improvement was seen in 6 patients (15%) *(181)*. The resolution of hypertension depended on the severity of preoperative hypertension and the amount of postoperative weight loss. Patients who required no antihypertensive medications preoperatively, and those who lost more weight tended to do better regardless of preoperative weight.

3.4.3. EFFECT OF WEIGHT LOSS ON PLASMA LIPIDS

Modest weight loss, induced either by diet or exercise, is associated with increases in HDL-C and decreases in serum triglycerides, and serum total and LDL-C *(182)*. A meta-analysis by Dattilo and Kris-Etherton associated weight reduction with significant decreases in total cholesterol, LDL-C, VLDL, and triglycerides; during active weight loss, HDL increased by 0.007 mmol/L for every kilogram of weight loss *(183)*. The National Institutes of Health (NIH) and NHLBI reviewed 14 randomized controlled trials on the effect of weight loss induced by diet and/or physical activity on plasma lipid levels *(133)*. A 5 to13% weight loss in the intervention group was accompanied by changes of 0 to 18% in total cholesterol; –2 to –44% in triglycerides; –3 to –22% in LDL-C; and –7 to +27% in HDL-C.

Most of these trials lasted about 4 to 12 mo, excluding the period of acute caloric deprivation. Waki et al. *(184)* reported that the beneficial effect of weight loss continue for longer duration; healthy obese women who lost a mean of 16.7 kg had decreased serum total cholesterol, LDL-C and triglycerides; and increased HDL-C to total cholesterol ratio after 17 mo of follow-up.

Bariatric surgery normalized plasma triglycerides, increased plasma HDL-C levels, and reduced total cholesterol to HDL-C ratio in 42 morbidly obese patients within 6 mo of Roux-Y gastric bypass *(185,186)*. Despite some weight regain, the improved lipid profiles were sustained for 5 to 7 yr. Brolin *(187,188)*, Wolf *(189)*, and Cowen *(190)* found significant reduction in total triglycerides, total cholesterol, and increased in HDL-C levels within 6–12 mo of gastric surgery, with improvements sustained through 5 yr.

3.4.4. EFFECT OF WEIGHT LOSS ON CARDIOVASCULAR DISEASE

The beneficial effects of weight loss on cardiovascular risk factors are well established, but the effects of weight loss on the progression of CAD have not been wildly studied. Available data indicate that weight loss can help reduce cardiovascular events and cardiovascular mortality *(191)*. In the Lifestyle Heart Trial, patients with CAD were prescribed a lifestyle program including a low-fat vegetarian diet, exercise, stress-management training, smoking cessation, and group support *(192,193)*. The treatment group lost more weight and had a significant reduction in total cholesterol and LDL-C. Its members also showed significant regression in coronary lesions assessed by CT and quantitative angiography at 1 and 5 yr. In contrast, the control group showed no change in weight or lipid profiles and had progression of stenotic lesions. At 5 yr, the control group had suffered more than twice the number of cardiac events. Although one cannot conclude that weight loss *per se* causes regression in coronary artery lesions, the study proves that lifestyle modifications can have an impact on CHD.

4. CONCLUSION

There is clear evidence that obesity increases morbidity and mortality, and that weight loss improves obesity-related comorbid risk factors. In addition, central fat distribution is an important independent predictor of morbidity and mortality. Although the data on the relation of weight loss to all-cause or cardiovascular mortality are limited, available evidence suggests beneficial effects from intentional weight loss. Safe and effective diet, exercise, and lifestyle modifications are available to most patients. Although adverse effects of weight loss are not uncommon with medical treatment of obesity (e.g., VLCDs, medications, or gastric bypass surgery), they can usually be prevented or effectively treated, and do not contraindicate weight loss.

REFERENCES

1. World Health Organization. Obesity: Preventing and managing the global epidemic, Report of WHO Consultation on Obesity. June 3–5, 1997, Geneva, Switzerland, 1998.
2. National Center for Health Statistics. Prevalence of Overweight and Obesity Among Adults. 1999, 2000.
3. Pi-Sunyer FX. The medical risks of obesity. Obes Surg 2002; 12:6S–11S.
4. Bray GA. Health hazards associated with overweight. In: Bray GA, ed. Contemporary Diagnosis and Management of Obesity. Handbooks in Health Care Co., Newtown, PA, 1998, pp. 68–103.
5. Sjostrom LV. Mortality of severely obese subjects. Am J Clin Nutr. Feb 1992; 55:516S–523S.
6. McGinnis JM, Foege WH. Actual causes of death in the United States. JAMA 1993; 270:2207–2212.
7. Colditz GA. Economic costs of obesity and inactivity. Med Sci Sports Exerc 1999; 31:S663–667.
8. Wolf AM, Colditz GA. Current estimates of the economic cost of obesity in the United States. Obes Res 1998; 6:97–106.
9. Wolf AM, Colditz GA. Social and economic effects of body weight in the United States. Am J Clin Nutr 1996; 63:466S–469S.
10. Goldstein DJ. Beneficial health effects of modest weight loss. Int J Obes Relat Metab Disord 1992; 16:397–415.
11. Kanders BS, Blackburn GL. Health consequences of therapeutic weight loss: reducing primary risk factors. In: Wadden TA, Van Itallie TB, eds. The Treatment of the Seriously Obese Patient. Guilford, New York, NY, 1992, pp. 213–230.
12. Thomas PR. Weighing the Options, Criteria for Evaluating Weight Management Programs. National Academy Press, Washington, DC, 1995.
13. Manson JE, Faich GA. Pharmacotherapy for obesity — do the benefits outweigh the risks? N Engl J Med 1996; 335:659–660.
14. Manson JE, Willett WC, Stampfer MJ, et al. Body weight and mortality among women. N Engl J Med 1995; 333:677–685.
15. Troiano RP, Frongillo EA, Jr., Sobal J, Levitsky DA. The relationship between body weight and mortality: a quantitative analysis of combined information from existing studies. Int J Obes Relat Metab Disord 1996; 20:63–75.

16. Allison DB, Faith MS, Heo M, Kotler DP. Hypothesis concerning the U-shaped relation between body mass index and mortality. Am J Epidemiol 1997; 146:339–349.

17. Allison DB, Gallagher D, Heo M, Pi-Sunyer FX, Heymsfield SB. Body mass index and all-cause mortality among people age 70 and over: the Longitudinal Study of Aging. Int J Obes Relat Metab Disord 1997; 21:424–431.

18. Diehr P, Bild DE, Harris TB, Duxbury A, Siscovick D, Rossi M. Body mass index and mortality in nonsmoking older adults: the Cardiovascular Health Study. Am J Pub Health 1998; 88:623–629.

19. Folsom AR, Kaye SA, Sellers TA, et al. Body fat distribution and 5-year risk of death in older women. JAMA 1993; 269:483–487.

20. Lee IM, Manson JE. Body weight and mortality: what is the shape of the curve? Epidemiol 1998; 9:227–228.

21. Solomon CG, Manson JE. Obesity and mortality: a review of the epidemiologic data. Am J Clin Nutr 1997; 66:1044S–1050S.

22. Katzmarzyk PT, Craig CL, Bouchard C. Original article underweight, overweight and obesity: relationships with mortality in the 13-year follow-up of the Canada Fitness Survey. J Clin Epidemiol 2001; 54:916–920.

23. Lee IM, Manson JE, Hennekens CH, Paffenbarger RS, Jr. Body weight and mortality. A 27-year follow-up of middle-aged men. JAMA 1993; 270:2823–2828.

24. Dietary Guidelines for Americans. US Government Printing Office, Washington, DC, 1995.

25. Dietary Guidelines for Americans. US Government Printing Office, Washington, DC, 1990.

26. Stevens J, Cai J, Pamuk ER, Williamson DF, Thun MJ, Wood JL. The effect of age on the association between body-mass index and mortality. N Engl J Med 1998; 338:1–7.

27. Bender R, Jockel KH, Trautner C, Spraul M, Berger M. Effect of age on excess mortality in obesity. JAMA 1999; 281:1498–1504.

28. Stevens J, Keil JE, Rust PF, Tyroler HA, Davis CE, Gazes PC. Body mass index and body girths as predictors of mortality in black and white women. Arch Intern Med 1992; 152:1257–1262.

29. Stevens J, Plankey MW, Williamson DF, et al. The body mass index-mortality relationship in white and African American women. Obes Res 1998; 6:268–277.

30. Calle EE, Thun MJ, Petrelli JM, Rodriguez C, Heath CW, Jr. Body-mass index and mortality in a prospective cohort of U.S. adults. N Engl J Med 1999; 341:1097–1105.

31. Karam JH. Type II diabetes and syndrome X. Pathogenesis and glycemic management. Endocrinol Metab Clin North Am 1992; 21:329–350.

32. Reaven GM. Banting lecture 1988. Role of insulin resistance in human disease. Diabetes 1988; 37: 1595–1607.

33. Alberti KG, Zimmet PZ. Definition, diagnosis and classification of diabetes mellitus and its complications. Part 1: diagnosis and classification of diabetes mellitus provisional report of a WHO consultation. Diabet Med 1998; 15:539–553.

34. National Heart, Lung, and Blood Institute. Third Report of the Expert Panel on Detection, Evaluation, and Treatment of High Blood Cholesterol In Adults (Adult Treatment Panel III). National Cholesterol Education Program (NCEP), National Institutes of Health, Bethesda, MD, 2001. Available at Website: (http://www.nhlbi.nih.gov/ guidelines/cholesterol/ atp3_rpt.htm). Accessed August 15, 2002.

35. Ford ES, Giles WH. A comparison of the prevalence of the metabolic syndrome using two proposed definitions. Diabetes Care. 2003; 26:575–581.

36. Ford ES, Giles WH, Dietz WH. Prevalence of the metabolic syndrome among US adults: findings from the third National Health and Nutrition Examination Survey. JAMA 2002; 287:356–359.

37. Lakka HM, Laaksonen DE, Lakka TA, et al. The metabolic syndrome and total and cardiovascular disease mortality in middle-aged men. JAMA 2002; 288:2709–2716.

38. Colditz GA, Willett WC, Rotnitzky A, Manson JE. Weight gain as a risk factor for clinical diabetes mellitus in women. Ann Intern Med 1995; 122:481–486.

39. Chan JM, Rimm EB, Colditz GA, Stampfer MJ, Willett WC. Obesity, fat distribution, and weight gain as risk factors for clinical diabetes in men. Diabetes Care 1994; 17:961–969.

40. Knowler WC, Pettitt DJ, Saad MF, et al. Obesity in the Pima Indians: its magnitude and relationship with diabetes. Am J Clin Nutr 1991; 53:1543S–1551S.

41. Knowler WC, Saad MF, Pettitt DJ, Nelson RG, Bennett PH. Determinants of diabetes mellitus in the Pima Indians. Diabetes Care 1993; 16:216–227.
42. Knowler WC, Pettitt DJ, Saad MF, Bennett PH. Diabetes mellitus in the Pima Indians: incidence, risk factors and pathogenesis. Diabetes Metab Rev 1990;1–27.
43. Bonadonna RC, Groop L, Kraemer N, Ferrannini E, Del Prato S, DeFronzo RA. Obesity and insulin resistance in humans: a dose–response study. Metabolism 1990; 39:452–459.
44. Shulman GI. Cellular mechanisms of insulin resistance in humans. Am J Cardiol 1999; 84:3J–10J.
45. Yu C, Chen Y, Cline GW, et al. Mechanism by which fatty acids inhibit insulin activation of insulin receptor substrate-1 (IRS-1)-associated phosphatidylinositol 3-kinase activity in muscle. J Biol Chem 2002; 277: 50,230–50,236.
46. Boden G, Shulman GI. Free fatty acids in obesity and type 2 diabetes: defining their role in the development of insulin resistance and beta-cell dysfunction. Eur J Clin Invest 2002; 32:14–23.
47. Golay A, Defronzo RA, Thorin D, Jequier E, Felber JP. Glucose disposal in obese non-diabetic and diabetic type II patients. A study by indirect calorimetry and euglycemic insulin clamp. Diabete Metab 1988; 14:443–451.
48. Field AE, Byers T, Hunter DJ, et al. Weight cycling, weight gain, and risk of hypertension in women. Am J Epidemiol 1999;150:573–579.
49. Huang Z, Willett WC, Manson JE, et al. Body weight, weight change, and risk for hypertension in women. Ann Intern Med 1998;128:81–88.
50. Dyer AR, Elliott P. The INTERSALT study: relations of body mass index to blood pressure. INTERSALT Co-operative Research Group. J Hum Hypertens 1989; 3:299–308.
51. Garrison RJ, Kannel WB, Stokes J 3rd, Castelli WP. Incidence and precursors of hypertension in young adults: the Framingham Offspring Study. Prev Med 1987;16:235–251.
52. Hall JE, Kuo JJ, Da Silva AA, De Paula RB, Liu J, Tallam L. Obesity-associated hypertension and kidney disease. Curr Opin Nephrol Hypertens 2003;12:195–200.
53. Hall JE. The kidney, hypertension, and obesity. Hypertension 2003; 41:625–633.
54. Hall JE. Mechanisms of abnormal renal sodium handling in obesity hypertension. Am J Hypertens 1997; 10:49S–55S.
55. Reisin E. Sodium and obesity in the pathogenesis of hypertension. Am J Hypertens 1990; 3:164–167.
56. Hall JE, Hildebrandt DA, Kuo J. Obesity hypertension: role of leptin and sympathetic nervous system. Am J Hypertens 2001;14:103S–115S.
57. Skott P, Hother-Nielsen O, Bruun NE, et al. Effects of insulin on kidney function and sodium excretion in healthy subjects. Diabetologia 1989; 32:694–699.
58. Andersen UB, Skott P, Bruun NE, Dige-Petersen H, Ibsen H. Renal effects of hyperinsulinaemia in subjects with two hypertensive parents. Clin Sci (Lond) 1999; 97:681–687.
59. DeFronzo RA, Cooke CR, Andres R, Faloona GR, Davis PJ. The effect of insulin on renal handling of sodium, potassium, calcium, and phosphate in man. J Clin Invest 1975; 55:845–855.
60. Wassertheil-Smoller S, Oberman A, Blaufox MD, Davis B, Langford H. The Trial of Antihypertensive Interventions and Management (TAIM) Study. Final results with regard to blood pressure, cardiovascular risk, and quality of life. Am J Hypertens 1992; 5:37–44.
61. Wassertheil-Smoller S, Blaufox MD, Oberman AS, Langford HG, Davis BR, Wylie-Rosett J. The Trial of Antihypertensive Interventions and Management (TAIM) study. Adequate weight loss, alone and combined with drug therapy in the treatment of mild hypertension. Arch Intern Med 1992; 152:131–136.
62. Davis BR, Oberman A, Blaufox MD, et al. Effect of antihypertensive therapy on weight loss. The Trial of Antihypertensive Interventions and Management Research Group. Hypertension 1992; 19:393–399.
63. Reisin E, Tuck ML. Obesity-associated hypertension: hypothesized link between etiology and selection of therapy. Blood Press Monit 1999; 4:S23–26.
64. Reisin E. Weight reduction in the management of hypertension: epidemiologic and mechanistic evidence. Can J Physiol Pharmacol 1986; 64:818–824.
65. Despres JP. Dyslipidaemia and obesity. Baillieres Clin Endocrinol Metab 1994; 8:629–660.
66. Ruotolo G, Howard BV. Dyslipidemia of the metabolic syndrome. Curr Cardiol Rep 2002; 4:494–500.

67. Ravussin E, Klimes I, Sebokova E, Howard BV. Lipids and insulin resistance: what we've learned at the Fourth International Smolenice Symposium. Ann N Y Acad Sci 2002; 967:576–580.
68. Howard BV. Insulin resistance and lipid metabolism. Am J Cardiol 1999; 84:28J–32J.
69. Despres JP. The insulin resistance-dyslipidemic syndrome of visceral obesity: effect on patients' risk. Obes Res 1998; 6(Suppl 1):8S–17S.
70. Vaswani AN. Effect of weight reduction on circulating lipids: an integration of possible mechanisms. J Am Coll Nutr 1983; 2:123–132.
71. Frayn KN. Visceral fat and insulin resistance—causative or correlative? Br J Nutr 2000; 83(Suppl 1): S71–77.
72. Coppack SW, Evans RD, Fisher RM, et al. Adipose tissue metabolism in obesity: lipase action in vivo before and after a mixed meal. Metabolism 1992; 41:264–272.
73. Garg A. Insulin resistance in the pathogenesis of dyslipidemia. Diabetes Care 1996;19:387–389.
74. Garrison RJ, Higgins MW, Kannel WB. Obesity and coronary heart disease. Curr Opin Lipidol 1996; 7:199–202.
75. Manson JE, Colditz GA, Stampfer MJ, et al. A prospective study of obesity and risk of coronary heart disease in women. N Engl J Med 1990; 322:882–889.
76. Kannel WB, Wilson PW, Nam BH, D'Agostino RB. Risk stratification of obesity as a coronary risk factor. Am J Cardiol 2002; 90:697–701.
77. Despres JP, Lamarche B, Mauriege P, et al. Hyperinsulinemia as an independent risk factor for ischemic heart disease. N Engl J Med 1996; 334:952–957.
78. Ferrannini E, Muscelli E, Stern MP, Haffner SM. Differential impact of insulin and obesity on cardiovascular risk factors in non-diabetic subjects. Int J Obes Relat Metab Disord 1996; 20:7–14.
79. Pfeifle B, Ditschuneit H. Two separate receptors for insulin and insulinlike growth factors on arterial smooth muscle cells. Exp Clin Endocrinol 1983; 81:280–286.
80. Pfeifle B, Hamann H, Fussganger R, Ditschuneit H. Insulin as a growth regulator of arterial smooth muscle cells: effect of insulin of I.G.F.I. Diabete Metab 1987; 13:326–330.
81. Shinozaki K, Suzuki M, Ikebuchi M, Hara Y, Harano Y. Demonstration of insulin resistance in coronary artery disease documented with angiography. Diabetes Care 1996; 19:1–7.
82. De Pergola G, Pannacciulli N. Coagulation and fibrinolysis abnormalities in obesity. J Endocrinol Invest 2002; 25:899–904.
83. Alessi MC, Peiretti F, Morange P, Henry M, Nalbone G, Juhan-Vague I. Production of plasminogen activator inhibitor 1 by human adipose tissue: possible link between visceral fat accumulation and vascular disease. Diabetes 1997; 46:860–867.
84. Juhan-Vague I, Alessi MC. PAI-1, obesity, insulin resistance and risk of cardiovascular events. Thromb Haemost 1997; 78:656–660.
85. Juhan-Vague I, Morange P, Renucci JF, Alessi MC. Fibrinogen, obesity and insulin resistance. Blood Coagul Fibrinolysis 1999; 10:S25–28.
86. Kannel WB. Influence of fibrinogen on cardiovascular disease. Drugs 1997; 54:32–40.
87. Ford ES. The metabolic syndrome and C-reactive protein, fibrinogen, and leukocyte count: findings from the Third National Health and Nutrition Examination Survey. Atherosclerosis 2003; 168:351–358.
88. Harris WH, Sledge CB. Total hip and total knee replacement (2). N Engl J Med 1990; 323:801–807.
89. Harris WH, Sledge CB. Total hip and total knee replacement (1). N Engl J Med 1990; 323:725–731.
90. Tepper S, Hochberg MC. Factors associated with hip osteoarthritis: data from the First National Health and Nutrition Examination Survey (NHANES-I). Am J Epidemiol 1993; 137:1081–1088.
91. Cooper C, Inskip H, Croft P, et al. Individual risk factors for hip osteoarthritis: obesity, hip injury, and physical activity. Am J Epidemiol 1998; 147:516–522.
92. Vingard E, Alfredsson L, Malchau H. Lifestyle factors and hip arthrosis. A case referent study of body mass index, smoking and hormone therapy in 503 Swedish women. Acta Orthop Scand 1997; 68: 216–220.
93. Vingard E. Overweight predisposes to coxarthrosis. Body-mass index studied in 239 males with hip arthroplasty. Acta Orthop Scand 1991; 62:106–109.
94. Heliovaara M, Makela M, Impivaara O, Knekt P, Aromaa A, Sievers K. Association of overweight, trauma and workload with coxarthrosis. A health survey of 7,217 persons. Acta Orthop Scand 1993; 64:513–518.

95. Oliveria SA, Felson DT, Cirillo PA, Reed JI, Walker AM. Body weight, body mass index, and incident symptomatic osteoarthritis of the hand, hip, and knee. Epidemiology 1999; 10:161–166.
96. Gelber AC. Obesity and hip osteoarthritis: the weight of the evidence is increasing. Am J Med 2003; 114:158–159.
97. Haara MM, Manninen P, Kroger H, et al. Osteoarthritis of finger joints in Finns aged 30 or over: prevalence, determinants, and association with mortality. Ann Rheum Dis 2003; 62:151–158.
98. Felson DT. Weight and osteoarthritis. J Rheumatol Suppl 1995; 43:7–9.
99. Felson DT. Weight and osteoarthritis. Am J Clin Nutr 1996; 63:430S–432S.
100. Felson DT, Zhang Y, Anthony JM, Naimark A, Anderson JJ. Weight loss reduces the risk for symptomatic knee osteoarthritis in women. The Framingham Study. Ann Intern Med 1992; 116: 535–539.
101. McGoey BV, Deitel M, Saplys RJ, Kliman ME. Effect of weight loss on musculoskeletal pain in the morbidly obese. J Bone Joint Surg Br 1990; 72:322–323.
102. Garfinkel L. Overweight and mortality. Cancer 1986; 58:1826–1829.
103. Garfinkel L. Overweight and cancer. Ann Intern Med 1985; 103:1034–1036.
104. Martinez ME, Giovannucci E, Spiegelman D, Hunter DJ, Willett WC, Colditz GA. Leisure-time physical activity, body size, and colon cancer in women. Nurses' Health Study Research Group. J Natl Cancer Inst 1997; 89:948–955.
105. Ford ES. Body mass index and colon cancer in a national sample of adult US men and women. Am J Epidemiol 1999; 150:390–398.
106. Caan BJ, Coates AO, Slattery ML, Potter JD, Quesenberry CP, Jr., Edwards SM. Body size and the risk of colon cancer in a large case-control study. Int J Obes Relat Metab Disord 1998; 22:178–184.
107. Huang Z, Hankinson SE, Colditz GA, et al. Dual effects of weight and weight gain on breast cancer risk. JAMA 1997; 278:1407–1411.
108. Hulka BS, Liu ET, Lininger RA. Steroid hormones and risk of breast cancer. Cancer 1994; 74:1111–1124.
109. Hulka BS. Epidemiology of susceptibility to breast cancer. Prog Clin Biol Res 1996; 395:159–174.
110. Young T, Palta M, Dempsey J, Skatrud J, Weber S, Badr S. The occurrence of sleep-disordered breathing among middle-aged adults. N Engl J Med 1993; 328:1230–1235.
111. Partinen M, Telakivi T. Epidemiology of obstructive sleep apnea syndrome. Sleep 1992; 15:S1–4.
112. Sugerman HJ, Fairman RP, Baron PL, Kwentus JA. Gastric surgery for respiratory insufficiency of obesity. Chest 1986; 90:81–86.
113. Vgontzas AN, Tan TL, Bixler EO, Martin LF, Shubert D, Kales A. Sleep apnea and sleep disruption in obese patients. Arch Intern Med 1994;154:1705–1711.
114. Strohl KP, Redline S. Recognition of obstructive sleep apnea. Am J Respir Crit Care Med 1996; 154: 279–289.
115. Strollo PJ, Jr., Rogers RM. Obstructive sleep apnea. N Engl J Med 1996; 334:99–104.
116. Grunstein RR, Wilcox I. Sleep-disordered breathing and obesity. Baillieres Clin Endocrinol Metab 1994; 8:601–628.
117. Grunstein R. Obstructive sleep apnoea as a risk factor for hypertension. J Sleep Res 1995; 4:166–170.
118. Loenen HM, Eshuis H, Lowik MR, et al. Serum uric acid correlates in elderly men and women with special reference to body composition and dietary intake (Dutch Nutrition Surveillance System). J Clin Epidemiol 1990; 43:1297–1303.
119. Higgins M, Kannel W, Garrison R, Pinsky J, Stokes J, 3rd. Hazards of obesity—the Framingham experience. Acta Med Scand Suppl 1988; 723:23–36.
120. Takahashi S, Yamamoto T, Tsutsumi Z, Moriwaki Y, Yamakita J, Higashino K. Close correlation between visceral fat accumulation and uric acid metabolism in healthy men. Metabolism 1997; 46:1162–1165.
121. Johnson RJ, Kivlighn SD, Kim YG, Suga S, Fogo AB. Reappraisal of the pathogenesis and consequences of hyperuricemia in hypertension, cardiovascular disease, and renal disease. Am J Kidney Dis 1999; 33:225–234.
122. Lin KC, Lin HY, Chou P. The interaction between uric acid level and other risk factors on the development of gout among asymptomatic hyperuricemic men in a prospective study. J Rheumatol 2000; 27:1501–1505.

123. Roubenoff R, Klag MJ, Mead LA, Liang KY, Seidler AJ, Hochberg MC. Incidence and risk factors for gout in white men. JAMA 1991; 266:3004–3007.

124. Torgerson JS, Lindroos AK, Naslund I, Peltonen M. Gallstones, gallbladder disease, and pancreatitis: cross-sectional and 2-year data from the Swedish Obese Subjects (SOS) and SOS reference studies. Am J Gastroenterol 2003; 98:1032–1041.

125. Stampfer MJ, Maclure KM, Colditz GA, Manson JE, Willett WC. Risk of symptomatic gallstones in women with severe obesity. Am J Clin Nutr 1992; 55:652–658.

126. Nakeeb A, Comuzzie AG, Martin L, et al. Gallstones: genetics versus environment. Ann Surg 2002; 235:842–849.

127. Must A, Spadano J, Coakley EH, Field AE, Colditz G, Dietz WH. The disease burden associated with overweight and obesity. JAMA 1999; 282:1523–1529.

128. Strasberg SM. The pathogenesis of cholesterol gallstones a review. J Gastrointest Surg 1998; 2:109–125.

129. Petroni ML. Review article: gall-bladder motor function in obesity. Aliment Pharmacol Ther 2000; 14:48–50.

130. Bray GA. Clinical evaluation of the obese patient. Baillieres Best Pract Res Clin Endocrinol Metab 1999; 13:71–92.

131. Bray GA, Ryan DH. Clinical evaluation of the overweight patient. Endocrine 2000; 13:167–186.

132. Pi-Sunyer FX. Weight loss and mortality in type 2 diabetes. Diabetes Care 2000; 23:1451–1452.

133. Clinical guidelines on the identification, evaluation, and treatment of overweight and obesity in adults: executive summary. Expert Panel on the Identification, Evaluation, and Treatment of Overweight in Adults. Am J Clin Nutr 1998; 68:899–917.

134. Lapidus L, Bengtsson C, Larsson B, Pennert K, Rybo E, Sjostrom L. Distribution of adipose tissue and risk of cardiovascular disease and death: a 12 year follow up of participants in the population study of women in Gothenburg, Sweden. Br Med J (Clin Res Ed) 1984; 289:1257–1261.

135. Larsson B, Svardsudd K, Welin L, Wilhelmsen L, Bjorntorp P, Tibblin G. Abdominal adipose tissue distribution, obesity, and risk of cardiovascular disease and death: 13 year follow up of participants in the study of men born in 1913. Br Med J (Clin Res Ed) 1984; 288:1401–1404.

136. Donahue RP, Abbott RD, Bloom E, Reed DM, Yano K. Central obesity and coronary heart disease in men. Lancet 1987; 1:821–824.

137. Casassus P, Fontbonne A, Thibult N, et al. Upper-body fat distribution: a hyperinsulinemia-independent predictor of coronary heart disease mortality. The Paris Prospective Study. Arterioscler Thromb 1992; 12:1387–1392.

138. Ducimetiere P, Richard JL. The relationship between subsets of anthropometric upper versus lower body measurements and coronary heart disease risk in middle-aged men. The Paris Prospective Study. I. Int J Obes 1989; 13:111–121.

139. Rexrode KM, Carey VJ, Hennekens CH, et al. Abdominal adiposity and coronary heart disease in women. JAMA 1998; 280:1843–1848.

140. Lamarche B. Abdominal obesity and its metabolic complications: implications for the risk of ischaemic heart disease. Coron Artery Dis 1998; 9:473–481.

141. Von Eyben FE, Mouritsen E, Holm J, et al. Intra-abdominal obesity and metabolic risk factors: a study of young adults (*). Int J Obes Relat Metab Disord 2003; 27:941–949.

142. Megnien JL, Denarie N, Cocaul M, Simon A, Levenson J. Predictive value of waist-to-hip ratio on cardiovascular risk events. Int J Obes Relat Metab Disord. 1999; 23:90–97.

143. Rexrode KM, Buring JE, Manson JE. Abdominal and total adiposity and risk of coronary heart disease in men. Int J Obes Relat Metab Disord 2001; 25:1047–1056.

144. Lerario AC, Bosco A, Rocha M, et al. Risk factors in obese women, with particular reference to visceral fat component. Diabetes Metab 1997;23:68–74.

145. Kanai H, Matsuzawa Y, Kotani K, et al. Close correlation of intra-abdominal fat accumulation to hypertension in obese women. Hypertension 1990; 16:484–490.

146. Faria AN, Ribeiro Filho FF, Gouveia Ferreira SR, Zanella MT. Impact of visceral fat on blood pressure and insulin sensitivity in hypertensive obese women. Obes Res 2002; 10:1203–1206.

147. Folsom AR, Prineas RJ, Kaye SA, Munger RG. Incidence of hypertension and stroke in relation to body fat distribution and other risk factors in older women. Stroke 1990; 21:701–706.

148. Pouliot MC, Despres JP, Nadeau A, et al. Visceral obesity in men. Associations with glucose tolerance, plasma insulin, and lipoprotein levels. Diabetes 1992; 41:826–834.

149. Despres JP. Abdominal obesity as important component of insulin-resistance syndrome. Nutrition 1993; 9:452–459.

150. Kuo CS, Hwu CM, Chiang SC, et al. Waist circumference predicts insulin resistance in offspring of diabetic patients. Diabetes Nutr Metab 2002; 15:101–108.

151. Weyer C, Foley JE, Bogardus C, Tataranni PA, Pratley RE. Enlarged subcutaneous abdominal adipocyte size, but not obesity itself, predicts type II diabetes independent of insulin resistance. Diabetologia 2000; 43:1498–1506.

152. Wajchenberg BL. Subcutaneous and visceral adipose tissue: their relation to the metabolic syndrome. Endocr Rev 2000; 21:697–738.

153. Hube F, Hauner H. The role of TNF-alpha in human adipose tissue: prevention of weight gain at the expense of insulin resistance? Horm Metab Res 1999; 31:626–631.

154. Lofgren P, van Harmelen V, Reynisdottir S, et al. Secretion of tumor necrosis factor-alpha shows a strong relationship to insulin-stimulated glucose transport in human adipose tissue. Diabetes 2000; 49(5):688–692.

155. Bastard JP, Maachi M, Van Nhieu JT, et al. Adipose tissue IL-6 content correlates with resistance to insulin activation of glucose uptake both in vivo and in vitro. J Clin Endocrinol Metab 2002; 87:2084–2089.

156. Hendel HW, Hojgaard L, Andersen T, et al. Fasting gall bladder volume and lithogenicity in relation to glucose tolerance, total and intra-abdominal fat masses in obese non-diabetic subjects. Int J Obes Relat Metab Disord 1998; 22:294–302.

157. Stoll BA. Obesity and breast cancer. Int J Obes Relat Metab Disord 1996; 20:389–392.

158. Stoll BA. Upper abdominal obesity, insulin resistance and breast cancer risk. Int J Obes Relat Metab Disord 2002; 26:747–753.

159. Henry RR, Wiest-Kent TA, Scheaffer L, Kolterman OG, Olefsky JM. Metabolic consequences of very-low-calorie diet therapy in obese non-insulin-dependent diabetic and nondiabetic subjects. Diabetes 1986; 35:155–164.

160. Wing RR, Blair EH, Bononi P, Marcus MD, Watanabe R, Bergman RN. Caloric restriction per se is a significant factor in improvements in glycemic control and insulin sensitivity during weight loss in obese NIDDM patients. Diabetes Care 1994; 17:30–36.

161. Agurs-Collins TD, Kumanyika SK, Ten Have TR, Adams-Campbell LL. A randomized controlled trial of weight reduction and exercise for diabetes management in older African-American subjects. Diabetes Care 1997; 20:1503–1511.

162. Heller SR, Clarke P, Daly H, et al. Group education for obese patients with type 2 diabetes: greater success at less cost. Diabet Med 1988; 5:552–556.

163. Mancini M, Di Biase G, Contaldo F, Fischetti A, Grasso L, Mattioli PL. Medical complications of severe obesity: importance of treatment by very-low-calorie diets: intermediate and long-term effects. Int J Obes 1981; 5:341–352.

164. Watts NB, Spanheimer RG, DiGirolamo M, et al. Prediction of glucose response to weight loss in patients with non-insulin-dependent diabetes mellitus. Arch Intern Med 1990; 150:803–806.

165. UKPDS Group. UK Prospective Diabetes Study 7: response of fasting plasma glucose to diet therapy in newly presenting type II diabetic patients. Metabolism 1990; 39:905–912.

166. Tuomilehto J, Lindstrom J, Eriksson JG, et al. Prevention of type 2 diabetes mellitus by changes in lifestyle among subjects with impaired glucose tolerance. N Engl J Med 2001; 344:1343–1350.

167. Uusitupa M, Louheranta A, Lindstrom J, et al. The Finnish Diabetes Prevention Study. Br J Nutr 2000; 83:S137–142.

168. Molitch ME, Fujimoto W, Hamman RF, Knowler WC. The diabetes prevention program and its global implications. J Am Soc Nephrol 2003; 14:S103–107.

169. Knowler WC, Barrett-Connor E, Fowler SE, et al. Reduction in the incidence of type 2 diabetes with lifestyle intervention or metformin. N Engl J Med 2002; 346:393–403.

170. Pories WJ, MacDonald KG, Jr., Morgan EJ, et al. Surgical treatment of obesity and its effect on diabetes: 10-y follow-up. Am J Clin Nutr. Feb 1992;55:582S–585S.

171. Pories WJ, Swanson MS, MacDonald KG, et al. Who would have thought it? An operation proves to be the most effective therapy for adult-onset diabetes mellitus. Ann Surg 1995; 222:339–350.

172. Davis BR, Blaufox MD, Oberman A, et al. Reduction in long-term antihypertensive medication requirements. Effects of weight reduction by dietary intervention in overweight persons with mild hypertension. Arch Intern Med 1993; 153:1773–1782.

173. MacMahon S, Cutler J, Brittain E, Higgins M. Obesity and hypertension: epidemiological and clinical issues. Eur Heart J 1987; 8:57–70.

174. Langford HG, Blaufox MD, Oberman A, et al. Dietary therapy slows the return of hypertension after stopping prolonged medication. JAMA 1985; 253:657–664.

175. Stamler R, Stamler J, Grimm R, et al. Nutritional therapy for high blood pressure. Final report of a four-year randomized controlled trial—the Hypertension Control Program. JAMA 1987; 257:1484–1491.

176. Cutler JA. Randomized clinical trials of weight reduction in nonhypertensive persons. Ann Epidemiol 1991; 1:363–370.

177. Stamler R, Stamler J, Gosch FC, et al. Primary prevention of hypertension by nutritional-hygienic means. Final report of a randomized, controlled trial. JAMA 1989; 262:1801–1807.

178. Effects of weight loss and sodium reduction intervention on blood pressure and hypertension incidence in overweight people with high-normal blood pressure. The Trials of Hypertension Prevention, phase II. The Trials of Hypertension Prevention Collaborative Research Group. Arch Intern Med 1997; 157: 657–667.

179. Stevens VJ, Corrigan SA, Obarzanek E, et al. Weight loss intervention in phase 1 of the Trials of Hypertension Prevention. The TOHP Collaborative Research Group. Arch Intern Med 1993; 153: 849–858.

180. Foley EF, Benotti PN, Borlase BC, Hollingshead J, Blackburn GL. Impact of gastric restrictive surgery on hypertension in the morbidly obese. Am J Surg 1992; 163:294–297.

181. Carson JL, Ruddy ME, Duff AE, Holmes NJ, Cody RP, Brolin RE. The effect of gastric bypass surgery on hypertension in morbidly obese patients. Arch Intern Med 1994; 154:193–200.

182. Pi-Sunyer FX. Short-term medical benefits and adverse effects of weight loss. Ann Intern Med 1993; 119:722–726.

183. Dattilo AM, Kris-Etherton PM. Effects of weight reduction on blood lipids and lipoproteins: a meta-analysis. Am J Clin Nutr 1992; 56:320–328.

184. Waki M, Heshka S, Heymsfield SB. Long-term serum lipid lowering, behavior modification, and weight loss in obese women. Nutrition 1993; 9:23–28.

185. Gleysteen JJ, Barboriak JJ, Sasse EA. Sustained coronary-risk-factor reduction after gastric bypass for morbid obesity. Am J Clin Nutr 1990; 51:774–778.

186. Gleysteen JJ. Results of surgery: long-term effects on hyperlipidemia. Am J Clin Nutr 1992; 55: 591S–593S.

187. Brolin RE, Bradley LJ, Wilson AC, Cody RP. Lipid risk profile and weight stability after gastric restrictive operations for morbid obesity. J Gastrointest Surg 2000; 4:464–469.

188. Brolin RE, Kenler HA, Wilson AC, Kuo PT, Cody RP. Serum lipids after gastric bypass surgery for morbid obesity. Int J Obes 1990; 14:939–950.

189. Wolf AM, Beisiegel U, Kortner B, Kuhlmann HW. Does gastric restriction surgery reduce the risks of metabolic diseases? Obes Surg 1998; 8:9–13.

190. Cowan GS, Jr., Buffington CK. Significant changes in blood pressure, glucose, and lipids with gastric bypass surgery. World J Surg 1998; 22:987–992.

191. Van Gaal LF, Wauters MA, De Leeuw IH. The beneficial effects of modest weight loss on cardiovascular risk factors. Int J Obes Relat Metab Disord 1997; 21:S5–9.

192. Ornish D, Scherwitz LW, Billings JH, et al. Intensive lifestyle changes for reversal of coronary heart disease. JAMA 1998; 280:2001–2007.

193. Ornish D, Brown SE, Scherwitz LW, et al. Can lifestyle changes reverse coronary heart disease? The Lifestyle Heart Trial. Lancet 1990; 336:129–133.

11 Obese Patients With Binge-Eating Disorder

Marsha D. Marcus and Michele D. Levine

KEY POINTS

- Binge-eating disorder is characterized by regular episodes of binge eating (the ingestion of large amounts of food with an associated sense of loss of control over when, what, or the amount one is eating) without the regular compensatory behaviors (purging, fasting, or excessive exercise) Binge-eating episodes are associated with rapid eating, eating until uncomfortably full, eating large amounts when one is not hungry, eating alone because of embarrassment over the amount eaten, and feelings of disgust, depression, or guilt after overeating.
- Binge-eating disorder, a relatively recently defined entity, is a distinct entity and disordered eating is associated with psychiatric comorbidity.
- Treatment should be of an eating disorder. Cognitive behavioral, interpersonal, and dialectical behavior therapy can be effective.
- Therapy proceeds through three stages over months.
- Pharmacotherapy, particularly with antidepressants, is useful.
- Additional research is needed to develop more effective therapies.

1. INTRODUCTION

A substantial literature focuses on the subgroup of obese individuals who have persistent and frequent problems with binge eating *(1–3)*. Initially, research evidence suggested that binge eating was associated with attrition and poorer outcome in obesity treatment programs *(3,4)*, although subsequent investigations have disproved the notion that obesity treatment is contraindicated for patients with binge-eating disorder (BED) *(5–10)*. Nonetheless, questions of how to best treat this group of patients remain. In this chapter, we discuss binge eating among obese individuals, examine findings that relate to its treatment in overweight patients, and provide recommendations for practitioners (*see* Table 1).

1.1. Background

Although the phenomenon of binge eating as a problem in obesity first was described in the late 1950s *(11)*, binge eating began to receive systematic attention only in the 1980s

From: *The Management of Eating Disorders and Obesity, Second Edition*
Edited by: D. J. Goldstein © Humana Press Inc., Totowa, NJ

Table 1
Chapter Overview

(12,13). Robert Spitzer and colleagues proposed diagnostic criteria for BED that were subsequently evaluated in two field trials *(14,15)*. The Spitzer et al. investigations led to the inclusion of BED in the fourth edition of the Diagnostic and Statistical Manual of the American Psychiatric Association (DSM-IV) as a proposed diagnostic category requiring further study *(16)*. Controversy about the utility and validity of the specific criteria for a diagnosis of BED persist, but most investigators agree that aberrant overeating among obese individuals is associated with significant morbidity and presents a challenge for treating clinicians.

1.2. Diagnosis

BED is characterized by regular episodes of binge eating (the ingestion of large amounts of food with an associated sense of loss of control over when, what, or the amount one is eating) without the regular compensatory behaviors (purging, fasting, or excessive exercise) that are seen in bulimia nervosa *(16)*. Binge episodes are associated with rapid eating, eating until uncomfortably full, eating large amounts when one is not hungry, eating alone because of embarrassment over the amount eaten, and feelings of disgust, depression, or guilt after overeating *(16)*.

1.3. Epidemiology

BED is common among individuals seeking treatment for obesity, and affects as many as 30% of these individuals *(14)*, but is much less common in the general population. Available evidence indicates that BED occurs in 1–2% *(17,18)* of the population, but in as many as 4–8% of obese individuals *(17,18)*. BED occurs in women and men in a ratio of about 3:2; however, men and women with BED do not differ in eating-disorder psychopathology or age of onset *(19)*. The prevalence of binge eating in minority women is similar to *(17,18)* or higher than *(20,21)* the prevalence of binge eating in Caucasian women. In summary, although additional epidemiological research is needed, available evidence suggests that BED is more common than bulimia nervosa, and the population with BED is more diverse in terms of gender and ethnicity than is the population with bulimia nervosa *(22)*.

2. DIFFERENCES BETWEEN OBESE INDIVIDUALS WITH AND WITHOUT BED

Although there is a strong association between severity of binge eating and degree of obesity *(14,15,23,24)* several lines of evidence demonstrate the differences between overweight individuals with and without BED, and confirm that individuals with BED comprise a distinct subgroup of the obese population *(24)*.

2.1. Eating-Disorder Symptoms

First, when compared with equally overweight individuals without binge-eating problems, patients with BED report considerably less control over eating, more fear of weight gain, preoccupation with food, and body dissatisfaction *(25)*. BED patients also report less eating restraint *(26)*, less self-esteem, and more sadness *(27)* than do overweight individuals who do not binge eat. Indeed, obese patients with BED report levels of eating-disorder symptomatology that are comparable to those of normal-weight patients with bulimia nervosa *(28)* and in laboratory settings, react to negative mood by overeating *(29)*. Compared to patients with bulimia nervosa, however, patients with BED do not report elevated levels of dietary restraint *(30)*, that is, they often do not succeed in limiting calorie intake between binge episodes, and they do not report overvalued ideas about the importance of extreme thinness *(28)*.

Second, laboratory data confirm that compared to their equally overweight peers, patients with BED ingest more calories both at regular meals, and when directed to eat as much as possible *(31–35)*. Findings from studies that have utilized food diaries also have indicated that patients with BED report higher calorie intakes than non-binge eaters on both binge days and non-binge days *(36)*. Thus, it appears that patients with BED tend to overeat both during and between episodes of binge eating.

Third, BED patients have a strong desire to lose weight and continually struggle to gain control over their eating *(4)*. Perhaps because individuals with BED report periods of marked dyscontrol over eating, they also report earlier onset of obesity, more frequent episodes of dieting, marked weight fluctuations, and more severe obesity than those without binge-eating problems *(24,37)*. The clinical picture in BED is often one of numerous periods of relative control over eating, or weight loss during periods of successful calorie restriction, and periods characterized by binge eating, overeating, and weight gain *(1)*. In summary, it is hard to overestimate the distress associated with BED.

2.2. Psychiatric Comorbidity

Patients with BED also endorse high levels of psychiatric symptomatology, particularly depression and anxiety *(38,39)* and have high rates of diagnosable psychiatric disorder *(40)*. For example, when compared with weight-matched individuals without binge-eating problems, individuals with BED report significantly higher lifetime prevalence rates of major depressive disorder and anxiety disorders *(40–44)*. Individuals with BED also have considerably higher rates of personality disorders than overweight individuals without an eating disorder *(40,44,45)*, and the presence of a personality disorder has been related to more severe eating-disorder psychopathology *(43)*. Thus, among individuals with BED, psychiatric symptomatology appears to be related to disordered eating rather than to obesity itself *(46)*.

3. PYCHOSOCIAL TREATMENT FOR BED

Because investigations comparing obese binge eaters and non-binge eaters consistently have confirmed that the groups differ markedly, and because patients with BED resemble other eating-disordered patients, treatments found to be efficacious in the treatment of other eating disorders, particularly bulimia nervosa, have been utilized in the treatment of BED. Data from randomized clinical trials have shown that cognitive–behavior therapy (CBT) and interpersonal therapy (IPT) significantly affect eating-disordered behavior in patients with BED. In addition, the use of dialectical behavior therapy (DBT) and an extension of CBT known as appetite awareness training have begun to receive support in the treatment of BED.

3.1. Cognitive–Behavior Therapy

CBT is the most well-studied psychosocial treatment for BED. The cognitive–behavioral model of binge eating posits that maladaptive beliefs and attitudes about eating, shape, and weight perpetuate a cycle of efforts to diet, repeated disruptions of dietary restraint, and aberrant overeating *(47)*. This model is supported by a substantial body of work that has shown that habitual dietary restraint (i.e., stringent rules related to the control of calorie intake despite physiological pressures to eat) is associated with a vulnerability to periodic over-ingestion of food *(48,49)*.

Data from numerous controlled trials of the treatment of bulimia nervosa have shown that CBT is more effective than waiting list or no-treatment control groups *(50–55)*, whose binge eating frequency tends to remain stable or increase over time *(25)*. Because of its efficacy in the treatment of bulimia nervosa, CBT has been adapted for the treatment of BED *(56,57)*. Modifications of CBT for BED include adding a program of regular exercise, targeting overeating as well as the tendency to restrict dietary intake and promoting acceptance of a larger-than-average body size *(1,56)*. There is considerable evidence that CBT is effective in ameliorating binge eating and eating-disorder psychopathology in patients with BED with reductions ranging from 40 to 90% *(10)*.

Treatment consists of approx 22, 60-min sessions over a 6-mo period and has been delivered in both group and individual formats. Although there have been no controlled trials comparing the outcome of individual vs group therapy in patients with BED, a trial comparing group and individual treatment for bulimia nervosa, found no difference in the outcome of group or individual CBT *(58)*. Thus, the decision to use one or the other format should be dictated by clinician preference and practical considerations.

Table 2
Cognitive–Behavior Therapy for Binge-Eating Disorder

Phase 1:Treatment initiation (eight weekly sessions)

Goals: 1. Provide information about binge eating and obesity
      2. Disrupt disordered eating patterns and regain control over eating
      3. Initiate exercise program

Tools: 1. Self-monitoring
        • Record all foods and beverages ingested
        • Note all episodes of binge eating
        • Record thoughts and feelings before, during, and after eating
      2. Identification and practice of alternative behaviors
      3. Goal setting
      4. Stimulus control techniques (e.g., not buying high-risk foods)

Phase 2:Cognitive restructuring (eight weekly sessions)

Goals: 1. Identification and modification of maladaptive thoughts and beliefs
      2. Learn and practice problem-solving skills

Phase 3:Termination and maintenance of change (six sessions over 2 mo)

Goals: 1. Promote body acceptance
        • Identify positive role models
        • Encourage body enjoyment (e.g., exercise)
        • Decrease social avoidance due to body size
      2. Development of maintenance plan
        • Anticipate future difficulties and identify high-risk situations

The primary goal of CBT is the amelioration of binge eating and the maladaptive thoughts and beliefs that accompany disordered eating. Treatment is semistructured, problem-oriented and present-focused. The patient assumes primary responsibility for change, and the therapist provides information, guidance, and support. As in the treatment of bulimia nervosa, patients with BED are told that the primary goal of treatment is the normalization of eating. It is important to note that CBT treatment may not lead to weight loss. Although some patients may lose weight with abstinence from binge eating *(5,59)*, initial investigations have shown that elimination of binge episodes does not, on average, lead to weight loss *(7,60)*. More recent studies, however, suggest that abstinence from binge eating is associated with small but significant decreases in body weight *(61,62)*.

Patients with BED have difficulties in moderating food intake in combination with maladaptive beliefs about dieting, shape, and weight. That is, they may have forbidden foods and stringent beliefs about restricting *(13)*, coupled with an inability to actually restrict intake. Accordingly, patients with BED are instructed that normalization of eating involves learning to say "no" to food (i.e., to binge eating, overeating, and chaotic eating), as well as learning to say "yes" to food (i.e., to healthful and moderate consumption of all foods). Three stages of treatment (Table 2) can be distinguished as described here.

3.1.1. FIRST PHASE OF TREATMENT

The first phase of treatment consists of eight weekly sessions. The goals of the first stage are to provide information about binge eating and obesity, disrupt the disordered eating pattern and regain control over eating, and begin a regular program of exercise. Patients are provided with information about the nature of disordered eating, weight regulation, and the importance of a pattern of regular and healthful eating. The role of unrealistically strict dieting in perpetuating binge eating is emphasized and principles of sound nutrition are introduced. As in the treatment of bulimia nervosa, patients are told that maladaptive thoughts about dieting, shape, and weight play a critical role in maintaining eating problems. In BED, however, it is often the contrast between maladaptive thoughts and stringent beliefs (e.g., "I should never eat more than 1200 cal/d."), and actual eating behavior (e.g., daily intake in excess of 2500 cal) that contributes to feelings of shame and hopelessness and perpetuates disordered eating.

A variety of behavioral strategies are utilized to help patients establish normal eating, but the introduction of self-monitoring is of particular importance. Patients are taught to record all food and beverages ingested and to indicate which eating episodes were felt to be binges. They also record time of eating, place where the food was consumed, and the thoughts and feelings before, during, and after eating. Diaries are used to identify the specific context of binge behavior and to examine the functions of binges, as well as the factors serving to maintain binge eating. The therapist and patient then work together to identify alternative behaviors or solutions. Self-monitoring, stimulus-control techniques, reasonable goal-setting, and feedback are utilized to help each patient manage his or her eating behavior.

Finally, exercise is introduced as both a tool to self-manage tension and stress and as a critical tool for long-term weight management (63). Patients are directed to begin a regular program of walking (bicycling or swimming may be substituted for patients who cannot walk), and provided with stepwise goals for increasing exercise up to 45 min three to five times a week. The recommendations for physical activity are consistent with those made by the Centers for Disease Control and Prevention and the American College of Sports Medicine for all Americans (64).

3.1.2. SECOND PHASE OF TREATMENT

The second phase of treatment also consists of eight weekly sessions. It is more cognitively oriented; and a major goal is to identify and modify maladaptive thoughts and beliefs that perpetuate the eating problem. Dysfunctional beliefs among patients with BED are often associated with obesity and include acceptance of negative societal attitudes about obese individuals (e.g., large people have no self-discipline), belief in the necessity of stringent dieting to control weight, and extreme body image disparagement (e.g., obese individuals are disgusting). During the second phase of treatment, patients are also taught problem-solving techniques in order to better cope with life circumstances and moods that lead to binge eating.

3.1.3. THIRD PHASE OF TREATMENT

During the final six sessions of treatment, termination is anticipated and maintenance of change is emphasized. Patients are encouraged to take the initiative for structuring the content of the sessions, and to continue problem solving and cognitive restructuring as the therapist fades his or her involvement. In this phase, there is also an emphasis on working to help the patient to accept a larger-than-average body size. The goal is to promote recognition that a larger body can be both attractive and healthy (an ongoing emphasis on physical activity is also helpful in promoting body acceptance). Patients are encouraged to dress well at their current size in order to promote feelings of self-confidence, to identify attractive large individuals as positive role models, and to identify and enjoy positive aspects of their bodies. Therapists also work to help patients identify social situations that they have avoided because of body size, and focus on decreasing weight-related social anxiety.

Finally, patients are taught to anticipate future difficulties, particularly at stressful times, and are helped to develop a maintenance plan to be consulted if eating problems recur. Following Marlatt and Gordon *(63)*, patients are taught relapse-prevention techniques designed to aid in identifying and avoiding high-risk situations, and for minimizing consequences of setbacks (i.e., an immediate return to normal eating coupled with an avoidance of negative thoughts). Patients are taught to view setbacks as an opportunity to learn more about their eating behavior with a view toward preventing future problems.

3.2. Interpersonal Therapy

Another short-term psychotherapy, IPT *(65)* has been shown to be effective in the treatment of individuals with BED. As has been the case with CBT, favorable findings regarding the use of IPT in the treatment of bulimia nervosa *(52,53)* have led to its adaptation for use in the treatment of BED *(66)*. The rationale for the use of IPT in the treatment of disordered eating is that interpersonal factors appear to play a major role in its maintenance, and that improvement in interpersonal functioning will lead to the amelioration of aberrant eating behavior. Thus, an initial goal of treatment is to identify interpersonal issues that affect self-esteem, mood, and the onset and maintenance of the eating problem. Within this framework, IPT proceeds as it is utilized in the treatment of depression; that is, the treatment focuses on the interpersonal context, not the eating disorder.

Initial reports *(60)* have shown that IPT delivered in a group format is as effective as CBT in reducing binge eating in patients with BED both at posttreatment and 1-yr follow-up. More recently, Wilfley and colleagues *(62)* compared the outcome of overweight individuals with BED who received group IPT to those treated with group CBT. Both treatments were associated with significant improvements in binge eating, associated eating-disorder psychopathology, psychiatric symptoms, and self-esteem. Changes in binge eating, dietary restraint, and thoughts about shape and weight also were maintained during a 1-yr follow-up period. Thus, CBT and IPT appear to be equally effective in the treatment of BED, although the mechanisms by which they promote changes in eating behavior differ.

3.3. Dialectical Behavior Therapy

DBT, developed by Marsha Linehan *(67)*, was originally designed for the treatment of individuals with borderline personality disorder and self-injurious behaviors. Because it has been efficacious in the management of these difficult conditions *(68,69)*, researchers have begun to explore the application of DBT to other refractory or chronic conditions including eating disorders. Telch and colleagues *(70–72)* adapted DBT for use as a group treatment among individuals with BED, and have found it to be effective in decreasing binge-eating behavior and maladaptive attitudes about eating, shape, and weight.

For example, in one study *(73)*, 89% of the women with BED who completed the 20-wk DBT group treatment were abstinent from binge eating compared to only 13% of those in a waiting list control group. More than half of the women who received DBT maintained their binge-eating abstinence in the 6 mo following the end of treatment. Although those treated with DBT did not report improvements in mood or depressive symptoms compared to those on a waiting list, none of the patients dropped out of the DBT treatment *(74)*. Thus, DBT appears to be a promising alternative to IPT and CBT for the treatment of BED.

3.4. Appetite Awareness Training

Another psychosocial treatment for BED that has received research attention involves an extension of the principles in CBT, called appetite awareness training (AAT). Developed by Linda Craighead *(75)*, AAT is based on the assumption that individuals with BED have become desensitized to internal appetitive cues. Treatment is designed to teach individuals to recognize and respond to sensations of moderate hunger and satiety. Like CBT, AAT emphasizes pyschoeducation and self-monitoring. However, in AAT the behavioral targets are eating in response to moderate hunger and stopping eating when moderately full.

In a randomized trial of AAT, college women with BED who received 8 wk of AAT had significantly fewer episodes of binge eating and overeating than did those assigned to a waiting list *(75)*. However, urges to eat when hungry and reports of inappropriate eating restraint did not change with treatment. Additional research is needed to document the utility of AAT and compare AAT to other psychosocial approaches to the treatment of BED.

3.5. Self-Help Programs

A final approach to treatment that has received recent attention for individuals with BED is the use of self-help interventions. In 1995, Fairburn *(76)* published a cognitive–behavioral self-help program for binge eating. Using this manual, several studies have evaluated the efficacy and effectiveness of self-help treatment for BED *(77,78)*. Consistently, self-help, with or without input from a facilitator, has been associated with improvements in binge-eating behaviors *(77–80)*.

For example, Carter and Fairburn *(79)* assigned 72 women to a pure self-help (PSH) condition, a guided self-help (GSH) condition, or a waiting list. During a 12-wk program, women in the GSH group received six to eight brief (25-min) sessions with a facilitator who, although familiar with the self-help manual, was not a specialist in treating disordered eating. Those in the PSH group received the self-help materials in the mail. Women who completed either of the self-help programs reported significantly less binge eating posttreatment than did those in the waiting list group. Moreover, decreases in the frequency of binge eating were maintained during a 6-mo follow-up period. However, it is not known if improvements consequent to self-help are sustained over longer periods, or which individuals will benefit most from minimal intervention.

In summary, the majority of the research on psychosocial treatments for BED has supported two manualized approaches, CBT and IPT. In addition, DBT, AAT, and self-help programs show promise as alternative treatments for BED. Although BED can be a chronic and fluctuating disorder, available data suggest that treatment is associated with sustained improvements in binge eating and related psychopathology *(61,81)*. To date, however, none of these psychotherapeutic approaches have consistently been associated with significant weight loss. For example, over a 6-yr period, although most women experienced significant improvements in binge eating, there were only small changes in body weight over time *(81)*.

Because the majority of individuals with BED are also overweight and because obesity is associated with significant medical and psychosocial consequences, weight loss is a potentially important outcome in the treatment of BED.

4. WEIGHT-LOSS PROGRAMS

Almost all BED patients want to lose weight, and are concerned about obesity. There is considerable evidence, however, that weight lost through dieting is frequently regained and sustained weight change involves a permanent modification of eating and exercise patterns *(82)*. It is precisely these sustained changes that patients with BED typically have been unable to accomplish. Finally, there is concern that dieting or repeated bouts of weight loss and regain may be demoralizing and thus particularly deleterious for individuals with BED.

Recent studies have documented that, in contrast to earlier reports *(1)*, calorie restriction and weight loss do not exacerbate binge eating in BED patients *(5–9,83,84)*. Indeed, participation in weight-control programs appears to improve binge eating and mood in BED patients *(7)*. Moreover, weight regain in patients with BED does not appear to be associated with worsening of mood or binge eating *(7)*, and it has been shown that concerns about the potentially deleterious effects of dieting *(82)* or weight cycling *(85)* should not deter obese individuals from weight-control efforts. Finally, although obesity is associated with increased risks for heart disease, diabetes, and other diseases, it is not necessary to achieve large weight losses to improve risk factors. There is substantial evidence that sustained weight losses of about 10% of initial body weight can lead to significant improvements in modifiable risk factors such as lipids and blood sugar levels *(86)* (*see* Chapter 10).

Moreover, a study at our center *(7)* provides strong evidence that weight-control treatment does not harm individuals with BED. We directly compared CBT for binge eating and behavioral weight control in the treatment of BED. In this study, 115 obese women with BED were randomized to 6 mo of individual CBT for binge eating, 6 mo of individual standard behavioral weight control with moderate calorie restriction (1200–1500 cal/d), or a 6-mo delayed-treatment control group. Attrition from the treatment program was approx 30%, but drop-outs were evenly distributed between treatments. Posttreatment and 1-yr follow-up assessments indicated that, for individuals who completed treatment, CBT and behavioral weight control were equally effective in ameliorating binge eating and associated eating-disorder psychopathology in patients with BED. In contrast, however, those who received behavioral weight control lost significant amounts of weight (an average of 21.6 lb at the completion of treatment). At 1-yr follow-up, weight-control patients had regained a significant amount of weight, although overall weight loss remained significant (an average of 13.2 lb).

5. PHARMACOTHERAPY OF BED

5.1. Antidepressant Treatment

Because of their efficacy in ameliorating binge-eating and purge behaviors in bulimia nervosa *(87),* antidepressants have been studied in the treatment of BED. Research comparing tricyclyic antidepressants, such as desipramine *(87)* and imipramine (e.g., refs. 55,88) with placebo showed greater reductions in binge eating among obese binge eaters treated with the drug than with a placebo. Venlafaxine, a novel antidepressant agent, has shown promise in an uncontrolled trial *(89).* Finally, numerous trials have demonstrated that selective serotonin reuptake inhibitors (SSRIs) are useful in the treatment of BED.

For example, in a double-blind trial *(90),* fluvoxamine (50–300 mg/d for 9 wk) was significantly superior to placebo in reducing binge eating in patients with BED. Similarly, sertraline *(91)* and fluoxetine *(92)* have been associated with significantly greater reductions in binge eating than placebo. Moreover, short-term antidepressant treatment also has been associated with weight loss among obese binge eaters *(41,89,90–92).* Recently, a group of investigators *(93)* synthesized the available studies of SSRIs in the management of BED, and concluded that the effects of SSRIs on BED were clinically significant and comparable to their effects on major depressive disorders.

Thus, short-term investigations have shown that antidepressant treatment is associated with moderate reductions in binge eating in patients with BED. Antidepressant treatment also may be useful in treating depression associated with BED, although most studies have not shown significant effects of antidepressant treatment on depressive symptoms in BED patients *(5,41,87).* In contrast, deZwaan and colleagues *(94)* evaluated obese binge and non-binge eaters treated with dietary management or CBT, and either fluvoxamine (100 mg/d) or placebo and found fluvoxamine treatment to be more effective than placebo in reducing depressive symptoms among binge eaters. Thus, the utility of antidepressant treatment for depression in BED deserves further investigation. It is possible that long-term antidepressant treatment may help break the cycle of negative mood, binge eating, and weight gain that characterizes BED. Approximately half of BED patients report a lifetime history of major depressive disorder *(44,95),* and individuals seeking treatment report significant depressive symptomatology *(7,38,39).* Obese individuals may be especially likely to report weight gain and decreases in activity when depressed *(96).* Furthermore, weight gained during episodes of depression can be considerable; for example, in one study, the average weight gain during a depressive episode was more than 17 lb *(97).* The tendency to gain or lose weight during depression is consistent across episodes *(96),* and because depression is often recurrent, it is easy to see that weight gain associated with mood disorder can contribute to obesity in BED patients. Antidepressant treatment also may enhance dietary restraint *(98)* or improve compliance with a weight-loss program *(5,41).* Thus, it seems possible that longer term antidepressant treatment may be useful for some patients with BED.

5.2. Opioid Antagonists

In a laboratory study, Drewnowski et al. *(99)* showed that the opiate blocker, naloxone, suppressed the intake of high-fat, sweet foods in obese binge eaters, but not obese non-binge eaters. These investigators reasoned that opiate blockade reduces food reward, and may thus ameliorate the heightened preference for sweet, high-density foods among binge eaters. However, in an 8-wk double-blind trial of naltrexone (100–150 mg/d) vs placebo *(90)*, drug treatment did not lead to differential reductions in binge eating or weight among obese binge eaters. Although additional research with opioid agents might enhance our understanding of the neurobiology of binge eating, available data do not support their use in the treatment of BED.

5.3 Anorexic Agents

In 1996, the National Task Force on the Prevention and Treatment of Obesity concluded that pharmacotherapy for the management of obesity is justified in carefully selected cases, but that the long-term use of anorexic agents should be monitored carefully *(100)*. The specific utility of anorexic agents in the treatment of BED has been investigated in a few studies. Early research found that obese binge eaters treated with the serotoneric agent, D-fenfluramine, experienced a significantly greater reduction in binge eating than did those given placebo, although at a 4-mo follow-up assessment, binge frequency no longer differed between placebo- and drug-treated subjects *(101)*. However, because of the association between the longer term use of D-fenfluramine *(102)* and fenfluramine with serious pulmonary and cardiac problems *(102,103)*, these medications have since been withdrawn from the market.

Currently, two anorexic agents, sibutramine and orlistat, have been approved for long-term use in the treatment of obesity (*see* Chapter 16), and sibutramine has been investigated in the treatment of BED. In an open-label trial *(104)*, 10 obese women with BED were treated with sibutramine for 3 mo. On average, binge eating and body weight decreased at posttreatment and subjects reported decreases in depressive symptomatology. Additionally, Devlin and colleagues *(105)* found that the combination of phentermine and fluoxetine in conjunction with CBT resulted in decreased binge eating. However, women tended to resume binge eating and gain weight following the end of either or both medication and CBT treatment.

5.4. Topiramate

Studies of anticonvulsants in the treatment of bipolar disorder and impulse-control problems showed that topiramate was associated with weight loss as well as improvements in clinical status. Subsequently, topiramate has been used in the management of BED. A recent study has demonstrated the potential utility of topiramate *(106)* in the treatment of BED. Sixty-one overweight individuals with BED were randomly assigned to receive topiramate or placebo. At the end of a 14-wk treatment period, those who had received topiramate had significantly greater reductions in binge eating as well as weight.

In a recent review, Carter et al. *(93)* suggest that antidepressant medications might be a first-line option for patients with a history of mood disorder, and that it is reasonable to utilize an SSRI because these are best established in the treatment of BED, and have favorable side-effect profiles. They suggest consideration of a topiramate trial for patients with mood lability or bipolar disorder, and finally the use of venlafaxine or sibutramine for those who fail to respond to adequate trials of other agents.

5.5. Combined Treatments

Wonderlich and colleagues *(10)* recently summarized results of studies that have combined psychotherapy and medication, the most rigorous of which are ongoing. Several studies have documented that medication did not enhance reductions in binge eating when added to CBT *(107–109)*. However, as noted earlier, antidepressant medication may enhance weight loss in combination with CBT or behavioral weight control.

In summary, evidence related to the use of medication in the treatment of BED suggests that antidepressants may be efficacious in decreasing binge eating and weight among individuals with BED. However, pharmacotherapy does not appear to increase the effectiveness of psychotherapy for BED, and additional well-designed trials with longer periods of treatment and follow-up and are needed *(93)*. In addition, there are few data bearing on the use of anorexic agents in treating BED, and careful consideration of the risk–benefit ratio on a patient-by-patient basis is indicated until more information is available. Thus, the use of drugs should be considered as one aspect of either weight-control or eating-disorder treatment *(100)*.

6. SELECTION OF TREATMENT FOR SPECIFIC PATIENTS

In summary, available evidence has shown that a variety of psychosocial and pharmacological interventions as well as weight loss programs can help individuals with BED regain control over eating and reduce eating-disorder psychopathology. However, no available treatment approach is effective for all patients, and there are some important individual differences that may guide the selection of treatments.

For example, there is preliminary evidence that earlier-onset binge eaters may have a more severe variant of eating disorder *(110)*. Individuals who participated in the treatment study at our center were stratified into two groups, those who reported onset of binge eating by age 18, and those who first had binge-eating problems after age 18. Results indicated that those in the earlier-onset group had an early onset of obesity and dieting, higher levels of eating-disorder psychopathology, and were more likely to report a lifetime history of bulimia nervosa and mood disorder. Although it is not known whether such factors reflect differing etiologies or response to treatment, such findings may have implications for management (e.g., it may be that early-onset patients will benefit from antidepressant treatment).

Future research may provide both treatment alternatives and data that will be useful in decision making for individual patients. Until there is such information, individual clinicians and patients must decide on a course of treatment that may include psychosocial treatment, a weight-loss program, and/or adjunctive drug treatment. For patients with mild disorder or those with no previous treatment, a short course of self-help might be indicated. Decisions must be based on careful assessment of individual cases by the clinician or treatment team, and thorough discussion of the pros and cons of available treatment options with each patient.

6.1. Eating Disorder and Obesity History

A history of early onset of binge eating or obesity in combination with numerous bouts of weight loss and regain over time suggest a course of CBT or IPT to treat the eating disorder. Weight-loss programs for these patients may be indicated after CBT, but careful consideration of the risks and benefits of such an endeavor is recommended. It is important for each individual to evaluate the likelihood that he or she will be able to sustain lifelong changes in eating and exercise, as well as the consequences of weight regain on sense of well-being. Some patients report that they no longer wish to diet because of repeated failures to sustain improvements. In these instances, eating-disorder treatment is clearly the treatment of choice, and patients can be reassured that significant improvements in the aberrant eating and eating-disorder psychopathology associated with BED can be obtained without weight loss.

Anecdotal clinical evidence has indicated that patients who report adult onset of binge eating and obesity, and do not have a history of marked weight fluctuations, may be likelier to benefit from a weight-control approach. Again, in the absence of research support, a decision to focus on treatment of obesity in a patient with BED should be made only after discussion of all treatment options.

6.2. Psychiatric Status

Given the high psychiatric comorbidity in BED, a careful psychiatric assessment is important for all patients who seek treatment. Although mild or even moderate depression or anxiety is likely to improve during BED treatment, the presence of marked or severe current illness suggests primary treatment of the mood or anxiety disorder prior to treatment for BED. Similarly, the presence of personality disorders characterized by emotional, dramatic, or impulsive behavior appears to be related to more severe levels of binge eating among patients with BED seeking treatment, although it is not predictive of treatment outcome *(43)*. Finally, patients with comorbid psychiatric disorder may be particularly likely to benefit from adjunctive pharmacotherapy that targets the psychiatric symptomatology.

6.3. Available Resources

Clinicians trained in the use of CBT or IPT for eating disorders are likely to be found in most metropolitan areas, but may not be available in smaller cities or rural areas. Some insurance plans may pay for obesity treatment where there is a clear medical indication (e.g., hypertension or other cardiovascular risk), and may not pay for eating-disorder treatment. Thus, treatment decisions may need to be made on the basis of pragmatic factors such as clinician availability or patient insurance plan.

7. CONCLUSION

In summary, BED is a chronic disorder with a fluctuating course that is common among obese individuals who seek treatment. Patients with BED differ in robust ways from obese individuals without binge-eating problems in weight and eating history, eating behavior, and psychiatric profile. Nevertheless, available research indicates that most BED patients can be helped with either weight control or eating-disorder treatment, and that the benefits of either approach are apparent for at least 1 yr posttreatment. Pharmacotherapy also is helpful, at least in the short term, and additional studies are needed to determine the optimal duration of treatment and how to effectively combine pharmacotherapy with psychosocial interventions. Finally, more research is necessary to improve outcome and to provide strategies for long-term management of these patients.

REFERENCES

1. Marcus MD. Binge-eating in obesity. In: Fairburn CG, Wilson GT, eds. Binge-Eating: Nature, Assessment, and Treatment. Guilford, New York, NY, 1993, pp. 77–96.
2. Walsh BT. The current status of binge eating disorder. Int J of Eat Disord 2003; 34(Suppl):S1.

3. Yanovski SZ. Binge eating disorder: Current knowledge and future directions. Obes Res 1993; 1:306–324.
4. Marcus MD, Wing RR, Hopkins J. Obese binge eaters affect, cognitions, and response to behavioral weight control. J Consul Clin Psychol 1988; 56:433–439.
5. Agras WS, Telch CF, Arnow B, et al. Weight loss, cognitive-behavioral, and desipramine treatments in binge eating disorder: an additive design. Behavior Therapy 1994; 25:225–238.
6. LaPorte DJ. Treatment response in obese binge-eaters: preliminary results using a very low calorie diet (VLCD) and behavior therapy. Addict Behav 1992; 17:247–257.
7. Marcus MD, Wing RR, Fairburn CG. Cognitive treatment of binge-eating v. behavioral weight control in the treatment of binge eating disorder. Ann Behav Med 1995; 17:S909.
8. Telch CF, Agras WS. The effects of a very low calorie diet on binge-eating. Behavior Therapy 1993; 24:177–193.
9. Wadden TA, Foster GD, Letizia KA. Response of obese binge eaters to treatment by behavioral therapy combined with very low calorie diet. J Consult Clin Psychol 1992; 60:808–811.
10. Wonderlich SA, de Zwaan M, Mitchell JE, Peterson C, Crow S. Psychological and dietary treatments of binge eating disorder: Conceptual implications. Int J Eat Disord 2003; 34(Suppl):S58–S73.
11. Stunkard AJ. Eating patterns and obesity. Psychiatr Q 1959; 33:284–292.
12. Gormally J, Black S, Daston S, Rardin D. The assessment of binge-eating severity among obese persons. Addict Behav 1982; 7:47–55.
13. Marcus MD, Wing RR, Lamparski DM. Binge-eating and dietary restraint in obese patients. Addict Behav 1985; 10:163–168.
14. Spitzer RL, Devlin M, Walsh BT, et al. Binge eating disorder: a multisite field trial of the diagnostic criteria. Int J Eat Disord 1992; 11:191–203.
15. Spitzer RL, Yanovski S, Wadden T, et al. Binge eating disorder: its further validation in a multisite study. Int J Eat Disord 1993; 13:137–153.
16. American Psychiatric Association. Diagnostic and Statistical Manual of Mental Disorders, 4th Ed. American Psychiatric Association, Washington, DC, 1994.
17. Bruce B, Agras WS. Binge-eating in females: a population-based investigation. Int J Eat Disord 1992; 12:365–373.
18. Smith DE, Marcus MD, Lewis CE, Fitzgibbon M, Schreiner P. Prevalence of binge eating disorder, obesity, and depression in a biracial cohort of young adults. Ann Behav Med 1998; 20:227–232.
19. Barry DT, Grilo CM, Masheb RM. Gender differences in patients with binge eating disorder. Int J Eat Disord 2002; 31:63–70.
20. Fitzgibbon ML, Spring B, Avellone ME, Blackman LR, Pingitore R, Stolley MR. Correlates of binge-eating in Hispanic, black, and white women. Int J Eat Disord 1998; 24:43–52.
21. Striegel-Moore RH, Wilfley DE, Pike KM, Dohm FA, Fairburn CG. Recurrent binge-eating in black American women. Arch Fam Med 2000; 9:83–87.
22. Striegel-Moore RH, Franko DL. Epidemiology of binge eating disorder. Int J Eat Disord 2003; 34(Suppl):S19–S29.
23. Telch CF, Agras WS, Rossiter EM. Binge-eating increases with increasing adiposity. Int J Eat Disord 1988; 7:115–119.
24. Wilfley DE, Wilson GT, Agras WS. The clinical significance of binge eating disorder. Int J Eat Disord 2003; 34(Suppl):S96–S106.
25. Wilson GT, Nonas CA, Rosenblum GD. Assessment of binge-eating in obese patients. Int J Eat Disord 1993; 1:25–33.
26. Masheb RM, Grilo CM. Binge eating disorder: a need for additional diagnostic criteria. Compr Psychiatry 2000; 41:159–162.
27. Striegel-Moore RH, Wilson GT, Wilfley DE, Elder KA, Brownell KD. Binge-eating in an obese community sample. Int J Eat Disord 1998; 23:27–37.
28. Marcus MD, Smith D, Santelli R, Kaye W. Characterization of eating disordered behavior in obese binge eaters. Int J Eat Disord 1992; 12:249–255.
29. Agras WS, Telch CF. The effects of caloric deprivation and negative affect on binge-eating in obese binge eating disordered women. Behavior Therapy 1998; 29:491–503.
30. Wilfley DE, Schwartz MB, Spurrell EB, Fairburn CG. Using the Eating Disorder Examination to identify the specific psychopathology of binge eating disorder. Int J Eat Disord 2000; 27:259–269.

31. Cooke EA, Guss JL, Kissileff HR, Devlin MJ, Walsh T. Patterns of food selection during binges in women with binge eating disorder. Int J Eat Disord 1997; 22:187–193.
32. Guss JL, Kissileff HR, Devlin MJ, Zimmerli E, Walsh BT. Binge size increases with body mass index in women with binge eating disorder. Obes Res 2002; 10:1021–1029.
33. Guss JL, Kissileff HR, Walsh BT, Devlin MJ. Binge-eating behavior in patients with eating disorders. Obes Res 1994; 2:355–363.
34. Walsh BT, Boudreau G. Laboratory studies of binge eating disorder. Int J Eat Disord 2003; 34(Suppl): S30–S38.
35. Yanovski SZ, Leet M, Yanovski JA, et al. Food selection and intake of obese women with binge eating disorder. Am J Clin Nutr 1992; 56:975–980.
36. Yanovski SZ, Sebring NG. Recorded food intake of obese women with binge eating disorder before and after weight loss. Int J Eat Disord 1994; 15:135–150.
37. Grissett NI, Fitzgibbon ML. The clinical significance of binge-eating in an obese population: Support for BED and questions regarding its criteria. Addict Behav 1996; 21:57–66.
38. Antony MM, Johnson WG, Carr-Nangle RE, Abel JL. Psychopathology correlates of binge-eating and binge eating disorder. Compr Psychiatry 1994; 35:386–392.
39. de Zwaan M, Mitchell JE, Seim HC, et al. Eating related and general psychopathology in obese females with binge eating disorder. Int J Eat Disord 1994; 15:43–52.
40. Telch CF, Stice E. Psychiatric comorbidity in women with binge eating disorder: prevalence rates from a non-treatment-seeking sample. J Consult Clin Psychol 1998; 66:768–776.
41. Marcus MD, Wing RR, Ewing L, Kern E, McDermott M, Gooding W. A double blind, placebo-controlled trial of fluoxetine plus behavior modification in the treatment of obese binge-eaters and non-binge-eaters. Am J Psychiatry 1990; 147:876–881.
42. Specker S, de Zwaan M, Raymond N, Mitchell J. Psychopathology in subgroups of obese women with and without binge eating disorder. Compr Psychiatry 1994; 35:185–190.
43. Wilfley DE, Friedman MA, Dounchis JZ, Stein RI, Welch RR, Ball SA. Comorbid psychopathology in binge eating disorder: relation to eating disorder severity at baseline and following treatment. J Consult Clin Psychol 2000; 68:641–649.
44. Yonovski SZ, Nelson JE, Dubbert BK, Spitzer RL. Association of binge eating disorder and psychiatric comorbidity in obese subjects. Am J Psychiatry 1993;150: 1472–1479.
45. Sansone RA, Sansone LA, Mossis BS. Prevalence of borderline personality symptoms in two groups of obese subjects. Am J Psychiatry 1996; 154:117–117.
46. Telch CF, Agras WS. Obesity, binge-eating and psychopathology: are they related? Int J Eat Disord 1994; 15:53–61.
47. Fairburn CG. Cognitive-behavioral treatment for bulimia. In: Garner DM, Garfinkel PE, eds. Handbook of Psychotherapy for Anorexia Nervosa and Bulimia. Guilford, New York, NY, 1985, pp. 160–192.
48. Polivy J. Perception of calories and the regulation of intake in restrained and unrestrained subjects. Addict Behav 1976; 1:237–243.
49. Ruderman AJ. Dysphoric mood and overeating: a test of restraint theory's disinhibition hypothesis. J Abnorm Psychol 1985; 94:78–85.
50. Agras WS, Rossiter EM, Arnow B, et al. Pharmacological and cognitive behavioral treatment for bulimia nervosa: A controlled comparison. Am J Psychiatry 1992; 149:82–87.
51. Agras WS, Schneider JA, Arnow B, Raeburn SD, Telch CF. Cognitive-behavioral and response-prevention treatments for bulimia nervosa. J Consult Clin Psychol 1989; 57:215–221.
52. Fairburn CJ, Jones R, Peveler RC, et al. Three psychological treatments for bulimia nervosa. Arch Gen Psychiatry 1991; 48:463–468.
53. Fairburn CJ, Jones RC, Peveler RC, Hope RA, O'Connor ME. Psychotherapy and bulimia nervosa: longer-term effects of interpersonal psychotherapy behaviour therapy, and cognitive behaviour therapy. Arch Gen Psychiatry 1993; 50:419–428.
54. Garner DM, Rockert W, Davis R, Garner MV, Olmstead MP, Eagle M. Comparison of cognitive–behavioral and supportive expressive therapy for bulimia nervosa. Am J Psychiatry 1993; 150:37–47.
55. Mitchell JE, Pyle RL, Eckert ED, Hatsukami D, Pomeroy C, Zimmerman R. A comparison study of antidepressants and structured intensive group psychotherapy in the treatment of bulimia nervosa. Arch Gen Psychiatry 1990; 47:149–157.

56. Fairburn CG, Marcus MD, Wilson GT. Cognitive-behavioral treatment for binge-eating and bulimia nervosa: a comprehensive treatment manual. In: Fairburn CG, Wilson GT, eds. Binge-Eating Nature, Assessment, and Treatment. Guilford, New York, NY, 1993, pp. 361–404.
57. Marcus MD. Adapting treatment for patients with binge eating disorder. In: Garner DM, Garfinkel PE, eds. Handbook for Eating Disorders, 2nd Ed. Guilford, New York, NY, 1997, pp. 484–493.
58. Chen E, Touyz SW, Beumont PJV, et al. Comparison of group and individual cognitive–behavioral therapy for patients with bulimia nervosa. Int J Eat Disord 2003; 33:241–254.
59. Smith DE, Marcus MD, Kaye W. Cognitive–behavioral treatment of obese binge eaters. Int J Eat Disord 1992; 12:257–262.
60. Wilfley DE, Agras WS, Telch CF, et al. Group cognitive–behavioral therapy and group interpersonal psychotherapy for the nonpurging bulimic individual: a controlled comparison. J Consult Clin Psychol 1993; 61:296–305.
61. Agras WS, Telch CF, Arnow B, Eldredge K, Marnell M. One-year follow-up of cognitive–behavioral therapy for obese individuals with binge eating disorder. J Consult Clin Psychol 1997; 65:343–347.
62. Wilfley DE, Welch RR, Stein RI, et al. A randomized comparison of group cognitive-behavioral therapy and group interpersonal psychotherapy for the treatment of overweight individuals with binge eating disorder. Arch Gen Psychiatry 2002; 59:713–721.
63. Marlatt GA, Gordon JR. Relapse Prevention. Guilford, New York, NY, 1985.
64. Pate RR, Pratt M, Blair SN, et al. Physical activity and public health. A recommendation from the Centers for Disease Control and Prevention and the American College of Sports Medicine. JAMA 1995; 273: 402–407.
65. Klerman GL, Weissman MM, Rounsaville BJ, et al. Interpersonal Psychotherapy of Depression.Basic Books, New York, NY, 1984.
66. Wilfley DE, Frank MA, Welch R, Spurrell EB, Rounsaville BJ. Adapting interpersonal psychotherapy to a group format (IPT-G) for binge eating disorder: toward a model for adapting empirically supported treatments. Psychotherapy Research 1998; 8:379–391.
67. Linehan MM. Cognitive–Behavioral Treatment of Borderline Personality Disorder. Guilford, New York, NY, 1993.
68. Linehan MM, Armstrong HE, Suarez A, Allmon D, Heard HL. Cognitive–behavioral treatment of chronically parasuicidal borderline patients. Arch Gen Psychiatry 1991; 48:1060–1064.
69. Linehan MM, Heard HL, Armstring HE. Naturalistic follow-up of a behavioral treatment for chronically parasuicidal borderline patients. Arch Gen Psychiatry 1993; 50:971–974.
70. Telch CF, Agras WS, Linehan MM. Group dialectical behavior therapy for binge eating disorder: a preliminary, uncontrolled trial. Behavior Therapy 2000; 31:569–582.
71. Telch CF, Agras WS, Linehan MM. Dialectical behavior therapy for binge eating disorder. J Consult Clin Psychol 2001; 69:1061–1065.
72. Wiser S, Telch CF. Dialectical behavior therapy for binge eating disorder. J Clin Psychol 1999; 55: 755–768.
73. Telch CF, Agras WS, Linehan MM. Dialectical behavior therapy for binge eating disorder. J Consult Clin Psychol 2001; 69:1061–1065.
74. Safer DL, Telch CF, Agras WS. Dialectical behavior therapy adapted for bulimia: a case report. Int J Eat Disord 2001; 30:101–106.
75. Allen HN, Craighead LW. Appetite monitoring in the treatment of binge eating disorder. Behavior Therapy 1999; 30:253–272.
76. Fairburn CG. Overcoming Binge-Eating. Guilford, New York, NY, 1995.
77. Loeb KL, Wilson GT, Gilbert JS, Labouvie E. Guided and unguided self-help for binge-eating. Behav Res and Ther 2000; 38:25–272.
78. Wells AM, Garvin V, Dohm F-A, Streigel-Moore RH. Telephone-based guided self-help for binge eating disorder: A feasibility study. Int J Eat Disord 1997; 21:341–346.
79. Carter JC, Fairburn CG. Cognitive-behavioral self-help for binge eating disorder: A controlled effectiveness study. J Consult Clin Psychol 1998; 66:616–623.
80. Peterson CB, Mitchell JE, Engbloom S, Nugent S, Mussell MP, Miller JP. Group cognitive-behavioral treatment of binge eating disorder: a comparison of therapist-led versus self-help formats. Int J Eat Disord 1998; 24:125–136.

81. Fichter MM, Quadflieg N, Gnutzmann A. Binge eating disorder: treatment outcome over a 6-year course. J Psychosom Res 1998; 44:385–405.

82. French SA, Jeffery R. W. Consequences of dieting to lose weight: effects on physical and mental health. Health Psychol 1994; 13:195–212.

83. de Zwaan M, Mitchell JE, Mussell MP, et al. Short-term cognitive behavioral treatment does not improve outcome on a comprehensive very-low-calorie diet program in obese women with binge eating disorder, in press.

84. Raymond NC, de Zwaan M, Mitchell JE, Ackard D, Thuras P. Effect of a very low calorie diet on the diagnostic category of individuals with binge eating disorder. Int J Eat Disord 2002; 31:49–56.

85. National Task Force on the Prevention and Treatment of Obesity. Weight cycling. JAMA 1994; 272: 1196–1202.

86. Atkinson RL. Proposed standards for judging the success of the treatment of obesity. Ann Int Med 1993; 119:677–680.

87. McCann UD, Agras WS. Successful treatment of nonpurging bulimia nervosa with desipramine: a double blind, placebo-controlled study. Am J Psychiatry 1990; 147:1509–1513.

88. Laederach-Hofmann K, Graf C, Horber F, et al. Imipramine and diet counseling with psychological support in the treatment of obese binge eaters: a randomized, placebo-controlled double-blind study. Int J Eat Disord 1999; 26:231–244.

89. Malhotra S, King KH, Welge JA, Brusman-Lovins L, McElroy SL. Venlafaxine treatment of binge eating disorder associated with obesity: a series of 35 patients. J Clin Psychiatry 2002; 63:802–806.

90. Hudson JI, McElroy SL, Raymond NC, et al. Fluvoxamine in the treatment of binge eating disorder: a multicenter placebo-controlled, double-blind trial. Am J Psychiatry 1998; 155:1756–1762.

91. McElroy SL, Casuto LS, Nelson EB, et al. Placebo-controlled trial of sertraline in the treatment of binge eating disorder. Am J Psychiatry 2000; 157:1004–1006.

92. Arnold LM, McElroy SL, Hudson JI, Welge JA, Bennett AJ, Keck PE, Jr. A placebo-controlled, randomized trial of fluoxetine in the treatment of binge eating disorder. J Clin Psychiatry 2002; 63: 1028–1033.

93. Carter WP, Hudson JI, Lalonde JK, Pindyck L, McElroy SL, Pope HG Jr. Pharmacologic treatment of binge eating disorder. Int J Eat Disord 2003; 34(Suppl):S74–S88.

94. de Zwaan M, Nutzinger DO, Schoenbeck G. Binge-eating in overweight women. Compr Psychiatry 1992; 33:256–261.

95. Marcus MD, Wing RR, Ewing L, Kern E, Gooding W, McDermott M. Psychiatric disorders among obese binge eaters. Int J Eat Disord 1990; 9:69–77.

96. Stunkard A, Fernstrom M, Price A, Frank E, Kupfer D. Direction of weight change in recurrent depression. Arch Gen Psychiatry 1990; 47:857–860.

97. Weissenburger J, Rush A, Gilles DE, Stunkard AJ. Weight change in depression. Psychiatry Res 1986; 17:275–283.

98. Craighead LW, Agras WS. Mechanisms of action in cognitive–behavioral and pharmacological interventions for obesity and bulimia nervosa. J Consult Clin Psychol 1991; 59:115–125.

99. Drewnowski A, Krahn DD, Demitrack MA, Nairn K, Gosnell BA. Naloxone, an opiate blocker, reduces the consumption of sweet high-fat foods in obese and lean female binge eaters. Am J Clin Nutr 1995; 61:1206–1212.

100. National Task Force on the Prevention and Treatment of Obesity. Long-term pharmacotherapy in the management of obesity. JAMA 1996; 276:1907–1915.

101. Stunkard A, Berkowitz R, Tanrikut C, Reiss E, Young L. D-Fenfluramine treatment of binge eating disorder. Am J Psychiatry 1996; 153:1455–1459.

102. Gardin JM, Schumacher D, Constantine G, Davis KD, Leung C, Reid C. Valvular abnormalities and cardiovascular status following exposure to dexfenfluramine or phentermine/fenfluramine. JAMA 2000; 283:1703–1709.

103. Connolly HM, Crary JL, McGoon MD, et al. Valvular heart disease associated with fenfluramine-phentermine. N Engl J Med 1997; 337:581–588.

104. Appolinario JC, Godoy-Matos A, Fontenelle LF, et al. An open-label trial of sibutramine in obese patients with binge eating disorder. J Clin Psychiatry 2002; 63:28–30.

105. Devlin MJ, Goldfein JA, Carino JS, Wolk SL. Open treatment of overweight binge eaters with phentermine and fluoxetine as an adjunct to cognitive–behavioral therapy. Int J Eat Disord 2000; 28:325–332.
106. McElroy SL, Arnold LM, Shapira NA, et al. Topiramate in the treatment of binge eating disorder associated with obesity: A randomized, placebo-controlled trial. Am J Psychiatry 2003; 160:255–261.
107. Devlin M. Psychotherapy and medication for binge eating disorder. Proceedings of the International Conference on Eating Disorders, 2002.
108. Grilo CM, Masheb RM, Heninger G, Wilson GT. Psychotherapy and medication for binge eating disorder. Proceedings of the International Conference on Eating Disorders, 2002.
109. Ricca V, Mannucci E, Mezzani B, et al. Fluoxetine and fluvoxamine combined with individual cognitive-behaviour therapy in binge eating disorder: a one-year follow-up study. Psychother Psychosom 2001; 70:298–306.
110. Marcus MD, Moulton MM, Greeno CG. Binge-eating onset in obese patients with binge eating disorder. Addict Behav 1995; 20:747–756.

12 Overview and the Future of Obesity Treatment

Lisa Terre, Walker S. C. Poston II, and John P. Foreyt

KEY POINTS

- Obesity is a chronic, incurable condition, with significant health, economic, and personal costs.
- Obesity requires long-term management similar to diabetes and hypertension.
- Existing treatment includes counseling, modification of diet, increasing activity, pharmacotherapy, and surgery. New treatments are under investigation.
- Prevention of obesity and an emphasis on environmental change requires greater attention.
- Researchers and health care providers need to help patients become more aware of the positive outcomes associated with healthful lifestyles, regardless of the impact on weight.

1. INTRODUCTION

This chapter addresses the future of obesity treatment. To provide a foundation for discussing the future, we begin with a brief background on the importance of obesity treatment and review of current interventions. We then examine issues and controversies that we believe will affect the future of obesity treatment including the relevance of body mass index (BMI) to healthy weight, the impact of short-term weight changes and normalization of comorbid conditions on long-term health, the cost-effectiveness and feasibility of continuous care to improve weight-loss maintenance, the shift toward more comprehensive health models in obesity treatment, and promising directions in the prevention of obesity. Table 1 overviews the organization of the chapter.

1.1. Social, Economic, and Personal Costs of Obesity

Obesity is epidemic in the United States. Currently, nearly 65% of American adults are classified as overweight (BMI ≥ 25) and 30.5% of these meet the criterion for obesity

From: *The Management of Eating Disorders and Obesity, Second Edition*
Edited by: D. J. Goldstein © Humana Press Inc., Totowa, NJ

Table 1
Chapter Overview

(BMI ≥30) *(1)*. In terms of gender, the 1999–2000 age-adjusted obesity prevalence is 27.5% for men and 33.4% for women, which represents a 7.6% increase (7.3% for men, 8% for women) over 1988–1994 figures *(1)*. For African-American women, the picture is more alarming, as nearly 50% meet the current definition for obesity after adjustment for age, which represents an 11.5% increase *(1)*.

Obesity is associated with increased risk for numerous medical problems and health hazards, including hypertension, dyslipidemia, coronary heart disease, type 2 diabetes, gallbladder disease, sleep apnea, osteoarthritis, and various forms of cancer *(2–8)* *(see* Chapter 10). For example, the prevalence of hypertension is 2.9 times greater among overweight adults compared to their non-overweight peers. Overweight women experience substantially greater risk for all-cause and some cause-specific mortality than leaner women *(9)*. The relative risks of death for women who never smoked and recently had stable weight were as follow: 1.6 (95% confidence interval [CI] = 1.1–2.5) for BMI = 27 to 28.9; 2.1 (95% CI = 1.4–3.2) for BMI = 29 to 31.9; and 2.2 (95% CI = 1.4–3.4) for BMI of 32 or more. These data indicate that heavier women have 60 to 120% greater risk for death than their leaner counterparts *(9)*. Although it is estimated that individuals with BMI of 30 or more are disproportionately represented in the 280,000 annual obesity-related deaths in the United States *(10)*, Solomon and colleagues *(7)* point out that "the preponderance of evidence suggests that even mild overweight is probably associated with some increase in mortality risk" (p. 9).

Obesity also is associated with increased health and socioeconomic costs. Wolf *(11)* recently overviewed the direct and indirect health care costs associated with obesity. Direct obesity-related medical outcomes include "the measures of preventive, diagnosis, and treatment services used in the intervention or treatment regimen (e.g., hospital care, physicians services, and medications)" (p. 58S). Indirect outcomes consist of "productivity changes related to illness and death" (p. 58S) such as days of work lost, restricted activity, and premature death *(11)*. Despite the variety of models for estimating costs associated with these outcomes, there is widespread consensus that the direct and indirect economic consequences of obesity are substantial *(11–16)*. For instance, it is estimated that approx 5 to 9% of US health care costs may be attributable to obesity and/or overweight *(12,16)* and that the treatment of associated conditions may translate to as much as $93 billion annually *(12)*. Based on a comparison of behavioral risk factors, Sturm *(15)* concluded that the medical expense burden associated with obesity even exceeds that of smoking, with obesity contributing to a 36% increase in inpatient and outpatient costs (vs 21% for smokers) and a 77% increase in medications (vs 28–30% for smokers).

The costs of obesity are not only economic. There also are social and personal tolls involved in the increasing prevalence of obesity, especially for women *(17)*. For instance, in a longitudinal study, women who had been overweight as adolescents completed fewer years of school, were less likely to be married, had lower household incomes, and had higher incidence of household poverty *(17)*. Results all were adjusted for baseline socioeconomic status and aptitude test scores. Individuals with obesity are significantly underrepresented in the top third of their high school class when compared to their lean counterparts even though there is no difference in their mean IQs or SAT scores *(18)*. In addition, obese adults tend to earn lower salaries and attain lower social status, regardless of their levels of education or intelligence test scores. Finally, obese individuals are subject to prejudice, discrimination, and intense stigmatization. Those who are severely obese experience greater risk for impaired psychosocial and physical functioning, which negatively impacts their quality of life *(19)*.

In summary, obesity extracts tremendous societal and personal costs in the forms of increased risk for disease and death, health care costs associated with the increased prevalence of comorbid conditions, as well as reduced social status, educational attainment, and employment opportunities. Given these significant costs and the fact that therapeutic weight loss produces short-term improvements in several important risk factors *(6,20,21)* (e.g., type 2 diabetes, dyslipidemia, and hypertension), it is not surprising that substantial efforts have been made to develop effective treatments for obesity.

2. OBESITY TREATMENT

2.1. Psychosocial and Lifestyle Interventions

Lifestyle and psychosocial treatments have their roots in behavior modification and include a multitude of techniques and approaches that focus on changing behaviors that are thought to contribute to or maintain obesity (*see* Chapter 14). Most of the various lifestyle approaches have several factors in common, including the use of self-monitoring and goal-setting, stimulus control and modification of eating style and habits, use of reinforcement for healthy behaviors, nutritional education and counseling, physical activity, and cognitive–behavior therapy interventions that focus on improving coping skills (e.g., cognitive restructuring, stress management and inoculation training, relaxation skills, and relapse-prevention training) *(22,23)*. Stunkard *(24)* categorizes these approaches as "conservative" treatments for obesity because they produce moderate weight losses, have minimal side effects, and are reversible (in contrast to surgery).

Using this categorization, conservative treatments are most useful (as a primary or adjunctive form of treatment) for patients with BMI less than 40 (25).

Lifestyle interventions are effective at producing gradual and moderate weight losses. Perri and Fuller (23) summarized the results of the last two decades of research on lifestyle interventions. Average weight loss across studies was 8.4 kg and attrition rates were generally low (16–18%). Lifestyle interventions lasted approx 20 wk and usually included multiple treatment interventions. Patients were able to maintain, on average, about two-thirds of their initial weight loss 9 to 10 mo after treatment termination.

Lifestyle interventions have not fared as well when long-term maintenance was assessed. In most studies with long-term follow-up, patients gradually return to baseline within a few years after treatment termination (22,26–28). Thus far, only the continuous-care model of lifestyle intervention (29), which views obesity as a chronic disease requiring continuous support or contact after the conclusion of formal treatment, has been found to produce significant maintenance (30). Patients treated with this approach (with extended therapist support as a constant) lost between 9.6 and 13.7 kg and maintained 60% or more of their initial weight loss 6 to 11 mo after the termination of the posttreatment care programs (31–33). In a replication of the continuous therapist support program, patients reported almost 100% maintenance of initial weight losses 12 mo after formal treatment termination and 9 mo after termination of the therapist-facilitated maintenance program (34).

2.2. Pharmacotherapy

Historically, pharmacological interventions for obesity have produced modest and temporary reductions in weight, but have been associated all too frequently with aversive side effects, health risks, and abuse potential with amphetamines and methamphetamines (35,36). For example, fenfluramine and dexfenfluramine were withdrawn from the market in 1997 based on concerns about possibly serious side effects including valvular heart disease and primary pulmonary hypertension (37–39). Progress in the development of new obesity drugs has been hindered by the unfortunate history of amphetamine abuse, by the perception that obesity is a disorder of willpower, and by the belief that drugs are not an appropriate treatment approach because they must be taken indefinitely (35). However, there is renewed interest in pharmacological approaches as a result of the recognition that obesity is a chronic disease that cannot be cured, but can be managed (40). Indeed, between 1996 and 1998 an estimated 4.6 million adults were prescribed obesity medications, one-fourth of whom (approx 1.2 million) may not have met National Institutes of Health indications for pharmacotherapy (41) (BMI $\geq$ 30 or $\geq$ 27 with obesity-relevant risk or disease) (41,42). Despite this current focus on pharmacotherapy, accumulated research findings make clear that a mix of pharmacological and behavioral approaches yields better treatment outcomes than solo pharmacotherapy (43–45). For instance, in a 1-yr randomized trial, Wadden and colleagues (46) found that pharmacotherapy alone was associated with a mean weight loss of 4.1% (±6.3%), compared with 10.8% (±10.3%) when pharmacotherapy was paired with group lifestyle modification (1200–1500 kcal/d diet), and 16.5% (±8.0%) when pharmacotherapy was added to lifestyle modification that included a portion controlled (1000 kcal/d) diet during the first 4 mo. Based on a meta-analysis of lifestyle treatments in randomized clinical trials of pharmacotherapies for obesity, Poston and colleagues (47) concluded "that lifestyle interventions, including the use of behavioral strategies, are important contributors to weight loss and should be included and documented [with greater regularity] in pharmacotherapy drug trials" (p. 559) *(47)*. This kind of treatment optimization also makes good economic sense. When compared to the pharmaceutical costs of treating obesity-related risk factors, weight losses of 8.2–10.6% of initial BMI have been shown to translate into an overall pharmaceutical cost savings *(48)*.

Currently, two drugs (orlistat and sibutramine) are approved for the extended management of obesity and the anti-obesity potential of several others is under investigation. (Chapter 16 reviews obesity pharmacotherapies in detail).

2.2.1. ORLISTAT

Research suggests that orlistat, a lipase inhibitor, may facilitate weight management and the reduction of some obesity-related medical risk factors (e.g., glycemic control, blood pressure, heart rate, lipid profiles) when coupled with a hypocaloric diet *(49–56)*. In one of the earliest 2-yr, placebo-controlled trials, Sjostrom and colleagues *(56)* reported that orlistat (120 mg/tid) in conjunction with a reasonable (i.e., 600 kcal/d deficit or weight maintenance) diet was associated with significantly more weight loss, less weight regain, and greater decrements in cardiovascular risk factors relative to placebo. Subsequent research has yielded comparable results. For instance, in another 2-yr controlled study *(57)*, treatment with orlistat plus an energy-controlled diet was associated with significant weight loss (8.76 ± 0.37 kg orlistat 120mg/tid vs 5.81 ± 0.67 kg placebo) and some reduced comorbidities. After treatment with 120mg/tid orlistat for 1 yr, weight regain during the subsequent year-long weight-maintenance period appeared to be dose-dependent. Patients (maintained on 120 mg/tid orlistat [yr 2]) regained less weight (3.2 ± 0.45 kg; 35.2% regain) than those maintained on 60 mg/tid orlistat (4.26 ± 0.57 kg; 51.3% regain). Both of these groups regained less than those initially treated with orlistat who were treated with placebo during maintenance (5.63 ± 0.42kg; 63.4% regain). Nearly 80% of orlistat-treated patients reported at least one transient gastrointestinal side effect (vs 59% of patients administered placebo). Similar weight loss and risk-reduction findings also have been reported in research focused on patients with type 2 diabetes as well as those with hypertension *(58–63)*. There are some empirically based indications that short-term treatment response (i.e., 12-wk weight loss of ≥5%) may be a particularly useful predictor of subsequent weight loss and reduction in associated comorbidities with orlistat *(64)*. Moreover, preliminary results *(65)* raise the possibility that the short-term use of orlistat may be well tolerated and potentially effective with adolescents when used in combination with a behavioral program. However, as McDuffie and colleagues acknowledge, these findings are based on a very small number of adolescents ($N = 20$) followed for a brief period (3 mo) without a placebo control. Therefore, at this time, it is not possible to draw firm conclusions about the advisability of orlistat use in younger populations.

2.2.2. SIBUTRAMINE

Sibutramine, a norepinephrine and serotonin reuptake inhibitor, was approved for obesity treatment in 1997. Clinical trials lasting from 12 to 52 wk have reported weight losses of 4.7–7.6 kg *(66,67)*. Weight losses tend to be dose-dependent *(68)*. Research suggests maintenance of these weight losses for up to 2 yr with 10–20 mg sibutramine per day when used in combination with dietary control *(69,70)*. Sibutramine-induced weight losses have been accompanied by favorable reductions in plasma triglycerides, total cholesterol, low-density lipoproteins, and waist-to-hip ratio *(71,72)*. Although increases in blood pressure and pulse have been noted *(72)*, McMahon and colleagues *(73)* concluded that sibutramine was effective and well tolerated in obese Caucasian and African-American patients with controlled hypertension during a 1-yr trial.

Interestingly, Wadden and colleagues *(74)* found that supplementing sibutramine with orlistat does not appear to significantly enhance weight loss over and above the effect associated with sibutramine only. Consistent with results previously reported in adults, a randomized controlled study with adolescents *(75)* found that the combination of sibutramine and a comprehensive behavioral program resulted in weight loss superior to that associated with behavioral treatment plus placebo (8.5 vs 4.0% mean reduction in BMI). Nevertheless, the study's authors currently advise against the clinical use of obesity medications for youth, given the paucity of extant safety and efficacy data for younger populations.

2.2.3. POTENTIAL NEW DRUGS

Stimulated by the generally modest weight losses and substantial posttreatment relapse rates associated with existing approaches *(76,77)*, the search for novel anti-obesity agents has continued. Based on emerging developments in endocrinology *(77–80)*, several new potential treatment targets recently have been identified. Although Chapter 16 discusses pharmacotherapy in detail, some of the more interesting candidates deserve brief mention. Among the most promising are antagonists of ghrelin, a peptide hormone that appears to stimulate appetite and also has been implicated in more extended weight-regulation mechanisms *(76,77,81,82)*. There is some indication that ghrelin may be involved in certain aspects of the complex compensatory processes (e.g., increased appetite, reduced metabolism) linked to weight regain following hypocaloric dieting *(76,77,82–84)*. For this reason, ongoing work to identify and test gherlin-blocking agents may advance progress on the development of new anti-obesity medications *(77,84)*.

Among the new drugs currently in clinical trials, two seem to hold preliminary promise: Axokine and Rimonabant *(77,84–87)*. Axokine, a genetically engineered recombinant human variant ciliary neurotrophic factor, was associated with superior weight loss compared with placebo with no evidence of immediate posttreatment weight rebound in a preliminary 12-wk multicenter trial *(88)*. Rimonabant, a cannabinoid blocker *(89)* reported to reduce food intake in animals *(85,86,90)*, currently is being tested in a phase 3 trial *(77)*.

2.3. Very Low-Calorie Diets

Very low-calorie diets (VLCDs; *see* Chapter 15) have less than 800 kcal/d with sufficient protein to promote rapid weight loss and the preservation of lean body mass *(23)*, VLCDs promote rapid weight losses of up to 20 kg after 12 to 16 wk *(91,92)*. Although VLCDs produce substantial short-term weight loss and improvement in obesity complications, long-term results are disappointing. Wadden and associates *(28,92)* reported that the majority of patients in randomized trials who receive VLCD treatment experience significant regain within the first 2 yr after treatment. VLCDs generally are not viewed as very cost-effective or practical for many obese patients because they require intensive medical monitoring, are associated with fairly rapid posttreatment weight regain, and have been linked to numerous problematic side effects *(23,92)*.

2.4. Surgery

Surgical procedures (*see* Chapter 20) are considered adjunctive treatment and generally are used with severely obese individuals whose lives are potentially threatened by their excess weight *(93)*. For many years, the most common surgical techniques were the vertical-banded gastroplasty and the gastric bypass. However, based on an accumulation of disappointing outcomes, gastroplasty is now less popular *(94)*. Indeed, Pope and colleagues *(95)* reported that from 1990 to 1997, gastric bypass increased from 52 to 84% of bariatric surgeries with an associated reduction in complications such as pulmonary emboli, early reoperation, and pulmonary complications. Nevertheless, some patients still suffer complications and side effects, such as nutritional deficiencies and "dumping" syndrome *(94,96)*. Overall, gastric bypass is associated with substantial weight loss, reductions in comorbidities, and fairly good weight loss maintenance *(94,96,97)*. Illustratively, results of an extended bariatric surgery follow-up *(98,99)* reported that surgically treated patients lost 28 (±15) kg after 2 yr and 20 (±16) kg after 8 yr compared to 0.5 (±8.9) kg at 2 yr and a weight gain of 0.7 (±12) kg for control patients. Although at 2 yr, these weight losses were linked to an amelioration of several obesity-related comorbidities, by yr 8 the treatment and control groups differed primarily in diabetes risk *(98,99)*. Findings such as these have led some recent reviewers *(100,101)* to discuss obesity surgery as a treatment for diabetes and to raise the possibility that the resulting diabetes control may be attributable to postsurgical physiological changes other than weight loss *per se*. Increasingly, gastric bypass is being performed laparoscopically with promising preliminary outcomes *(102,103)*. However, extensive surgical experience with the laparoscopic procedure is especially critical to patient outcome *(102,104–106)*. Research suggests that surgical treatment for severe obesity may be more cost-effective than either no treatment (when quality-adjusted life-years, life-years, and lifetime costs are taken into consideration) *(107)* or than VLCDs supplemented with behavior therapy and 1-yr maintenance program *(108)*. Yet, in terms of pharmaceutical costs only, the savings associated with reduced obesity-related risk factors may be offset by other postsurgical medication expenses (e.g., for pain, gastrointestinal complaints, vitamin deficiencies) *(109)*. Weight and risk-factor reductions notwithstanding, surgical approaches alone may not be associated with optimal long-term health behaviors. For instance, a longitudinal comparison of weight-maintenance behaviors among individuals who initially lost weight surgically vs nonsurgically and successfully maintained the loss *(110)* indicated that the former surgery patients reported consuming more dietary fat and participating in less exercise than their non-surgery counterparts.

3. ISSUES FOR THE FUTURE OF OBESITY TREATMENT

Obesity treatments are effective in producing short-term weight loss and reducing risks for complications associated with obesity *(23)*, but there are several important issues and limitations that need to be addressed in future obesity treatment research.

3.1. Issue 1: What Is a Healthy Weight?

The prevalence of obesity and overweight is increasing in the United States at a rapid rate, but the impact of the secular trends reflected in National Health and Nutrition Examination Survey 1999–2000 on the development of comorbid conditions currently is unclear *(1)*. As Flegal and colleagues *(1)* point out, although the prevalence of obesity and diabetes appear to have remained positively correlated, other obesity-related risk factors do not seem to have increased with population BMI *(1)*.

Although it is important to emphasize empirically derived cut-offs for research purposes, these population-based definitions may not readily translate into best practices for health care providers and their patients. Because morbidity and mortality ratios do not reflect direct risk to an individual *(5)*, it may be more beneficial for patients and health care providers to focus primarily on maintaining a "reasonable" weight" *(111)* and healthy lifestyle, including regular exercise, a low-fat diet, and normalized eating patterns *(22,112)*, rather than attempting to estimate risk based on BMI category. Finally, there is a need for more research assessing the potential psychological hazards of obesity treatment, and the benefit of broader outcome measures, such as dietary changes, psychosocial functioning, physical activity levels, and control or prevention of obesity-related complications.

3.2. Issue 2: Short-Term Weight Loss and Improved Health and Longevity

Obesity research has not shown that the short-term weight losses and improved metabolic functioning produced by current treatments lead to long-term improvements in health, quality of life, and longevity. Although there is little dispute about the short-term effects of moderate weight loss on improvements in hypertension, lipid levels, and insulin resistance *(6,20,21)*, there are few data to suggest that these benefits are long-standing, particularly because weight-loss maintenance is so difficult for most people *(113)*.

In terms of improved longevity, it is clear that there is a strong, positive relationship between BMI and risk for all-cause and some forms of cause-specific mortality *(7–9)* but it is unclear how much excess weight is dangerous, whether weight loss changes this risk in the long term *(114,115)*, and the extent to which ethnicity and gender moderate this relationship *(5,116)*. For example, a large cohort study found only minimal and nonsignificant increases in mortality risk associated with moderate degrees of obesity *(114)*. Relatedly, Andres and colleagues *(117)* concluded that mortality rates were lowest for adults who had gained moderate amounts of weight and highest for individuals who had lost weight or gained excessive weight. Likewise, results of an observational study of intentional weight loss and mortality among overweight individuals with diabetes *(118)* indicated a 25% reduced mortality among those reporting intentional weight loss, with the greatest benefits for those losing 10–15% of body weight and a slightly increased death risk for those with weight losses of 30% or more of initial weight. In contrast, when intentional weight loss was examined in a prospective cohort study with adult, middle-aged women, data suggested that intentional weight loss in women with obesity-related illnesses was associated with decreased risk for all-cause mortality proportionate to weight lost. Results were equivocal for healthy, middle-aged women *(119)*. Recent estimates of ethnic and gender differences in obesity-related years of life lost suggest that obesity may be associated with somewhat higher mortality risk for Caucasians (compared with African-Americans) and for men (relative to women) *(116)*. However, as noted by the National Task Force on the Prevention and Treatment of Obesity *(5)*, "although populations may differ in their health risk at a given BMI, such population differences are not necessarily relevant to individuals in clinical settings" (p. 902) *(5)*.

3.2.1. WEIGHT CYCLING

Although it is somewhat unclear whether weight loss confers long-term benefits, the impact of weight cycling is even less certain *(120)*. Weight cycling is a problem because so many individuals who try to lose weight, regardless of the method used, typically regain the lost weight over a period of several years *(22)*. Some data suggest that weight variability is associated with greater risk for cardiovascular disease and all-cause mortality in men *(121)*. Other studies have not found a relationship between weight fluctuation and mortality in healthy men who had never smoked. By contrast, men who smoked or had preexisting illness and whose weight fluctuated experienced greater risk for death *(122)*. The National Task Force on the Prevention and Treatment of Obesity summarized the issue by stating that "the currently available evidence is not sufficiently compelling to override the potential benefits of moderate weight loss in the severely obese" (p. 1201) *(123)*. It still is not clear whether weight cycling has any significant psychological side effects, such as depression resulting from repeated failed attempts at losing weight *(120–125)*. Clearly, the jury is still out on this controversial issue and it will remain a puzzle until we can more adequately study the effects of intentional long-term weight loss.

3.3. Issue 3: Weight Maintenance and Cost-Effectiveness

Long-term weight maintenance is a goal that current obesity treatments have not adequately met. This has led to the view that obesity is a chronic, incurable disease *(40)* and speculation that obesity may need to be viewed like type 2 diabetes, which requires treatment indefinitely *(126)*. Accordingly, obesity should require long-term management and obese patients should receive extended care. In recent years, this philosophy has stimulated an increased emphasis on evaluating the benefits of long-term pharmacotherapy and lifestyle interventions *(23,127–129)*. Given the effectiveness of the continuous-care model of lifestyle intervention, with a focus on long-term support and therapist contact *(31,34,128)*, as well as the effectiveness of continuous drug therapy *(23,129)*, it is likely that greater attention will be focused on longer-term approaches.

However, there are important barriers to long-term management, including the general lack of insurance reimbursement for obesity *(130)* (although the new health and behavior Current Procedural Terminology codes may provide a funding vehicle for some patients) *(131,132)* and the lack of data to support the cost-effectiveness and feasibility of continuous care *(130)*. There is a need for future research addressing the cost-effectiveness and feasibility of treating obesity continuously (and potentially preventing comorbid conditions) vs the direct and indirect costs of treating obesity complications as they arise. In addition, more research should focus on methods of implementing interventions at the lowest cost possible and evaluating which elements of multicomponent treatments are most effective for which patients *(47,77)*. Research in these areas might include studies on the cost-effectiveness and acceptability of interventions delivered by a variety of formats and change agents (e.g., Internet, paraprofessionals) for different patient groups *(133,134)*.

3.4. Issue 4: Environmental Intervention and Prevention

Unless current policies are reshaped toward an increased emphasis on prevention and health promotion *(112,135)*, Foreyt and Goodrick's *(136)* prediction that 100% of adults in the United States will be overweight by the year 2230 may become a reality. At the policy and environmental intervention level, there is an urgent need for a greater focus on the role of diet and sedentary lifestyle in the development and maintenance of obesity. Cross-sectional, migrant, and ecological studies have demonstrated the impact of increasing dietary fat on relative weight *(137–139)*. Because Americans eat substantial amounts of dietary fat and large portion sizes, more research on developing and implementing effective population and community nutritional interventions is essential *(139–141)*.

3.4.1. PHYSICAL ACTIVITY

The importance of regular physical activity deserves increased emphasis (*see* Chapter 13). Over the years, a variety of data sources have consistently indicated that only a minority of American women and men engage in regular, vigorous physical activity *(142–146)*. Moreover, of those attempting to lose or maintain weight, most report not meeting the national recommendations to follow a hypocaloric diet supplemented with at least 150 min of exercise per week *(142,147)*. Interestingly, research suggests that the majority of physicians do not routinely (e.g., in the context of annual medical examinations) encourage most patients to exercise, although they may be more likely to raise the issue with patients after weight and other risk-factor problems emerge *(148)*. Decreasing sedentary lifestyle and increasing physical activity of all Americans, including those who are obese, should be an important public health priority, given that regular physical activity is an important predictor of weight maintenance *(22,144,145,149,150)*. For instance, standing in stark contrast to the results cited here based on national probability samples of individuals making an effort to lose or maintain weight *(142,147)*, findings from the National Weight Control Registry *(30,151–153)* reveal that individuals who have successfully maintained weight loss of 13.6 kg or more for at least 1 yr reported considerable amounts of exercise (i.e., mean >2800 cal/wk expended) in conjunction with reduced calorie intake (i.e., <1400 kcal/d on average) *(30,151)*. As Wing and Hill *(153)* point out, "very few of these successful weight loss maintainers used diet alone to lose weight" (p. 327) *(153)*. There is a pressing need for more research on the development of cost-effective community intervention strategies to promote "active living" *(144–146,149,154)* and on the potential for "healthy" overweight, for example, individuals who are physically fit, but remain overweight *(5)*. For example, Barlow and colleagues *(155)* found that moderate and high-fit men, regardless of BMI, experienced significantly lower age-adjusted risk for all-cause mortality compared to sedentary or low-fit men.

3.4.2. TARGETED PREVENTION

Greater research and treatment emphasis should focus on targeted prevention programs for high-risk individuals and populations. For example, there are ample data linking perinatal risk factors (e.g. hyperinsulinism and maternal adiposity) and low infant birth weight to the development of type 2 diabetes, hypertension, hyperlipidemia, and coronary heart disease in adulthood *(138,156–158)*. These problems are particularly problematic for low-income and minority women because they experience a higher prevalence of overweight *(159)*. Future generations are potentially at risk for repetitive cycles of obesity and related health problems because of these perinatal risks. There is a need for research focused on developing targeted, safe, and effective treatment and prevention programs for at-risk pregnant women as this method of transmitting risk for obesity is potentially preventable and could reduce the prevalence of obesity and obesity-related disorders in future generations.

Finally, more resources should be directed at treating obese and overweight children in an effort to prevent adult obesity. Epstein and associates *(160)* reported long-term outcome data on treatment targeted at obese children. Ten years after treatment, more than 30% of the children had decreased their percentage overweight by 20% or more and 30% were no longer obese. Although this study requires replication, it highlights the promise of early intervention for preventing adult obesity.

4. CONCLUSION

What is the future for obesity treatment? We believe that treatment will be most fruitful when the health care community and the general public recognize obesity as a chronic, incurable condition, requiring long-term management similar to diabetes and hypertension. Many chronic diseases do not have cures, yet we do not view their long-term management as a failure, even though treatment withdrawal results in problem recurrence. In addition, we do not consider treatment a failure just because patients experience difficulty adhering to the regimen. Rather, we acknowledge that many health care problems require long-term management and focus on improving treatment adherence *(30,161,162)*. Kirschenbaum and Fitzgibbon *(162)* suggest that, owing to cognitive biases, more exacting standards may be applied to obesity treatment than to interventions for other chronic conditions. For instance, there is no expectation that patients with diabetes or severe hypertension will be "cured" after a brief medication trial and few would advocate the withdrawal of insulin or antihypertensive medication and dietary modification from a patient with diabetes or severe hypertension without appropriate weight loss. Yet, by contrast, relapse after short-term obesity treatment and/or difficulty adhering to a weight-loss regimen is more likely to be viewed as evidence of treatment failure *(161,162)*.

Because obesity is influenced by numerous biopsychosocial factors and is partially the result of a mismatch between modern lifestyle and the lifestyle in which humans evolved, simple solutions are inadequate to address this complicated problem. For example, the total fat intake in late paleolithic diets was estimated to be about 20% of calories from fat, compared to the current American diet, of about 34% of calories from fat *(163–165)*. Data from humans who continue to exist as hunter–gatherers, as well as anthropological data, suggest that humans were significantly more active, and their diets were less energy dense, higher in fiber, and lower in fat than current Western societies *(164)*. Given this disparity, we believe that research on the long-term management of obesity (e.g., the cost-effectiveness of long-term management compared with usual time-limited care), as well as genetic and metabolic studies (e.g., examining the complicated genetic, metabolic, and environmental interactions that play a role in the development and maintenance of obesity), should be given the highest priority.

The prevention of obesity and an emphasis on environmental change is another area that requires greater attention. For example, despite our knowledge about the role of dietary fat in childhood obesity, school lunch programs often provide significantly more fat than dietary guidelines suggest *(166)*. Chapman et al. *(167)* found that less than 5% of schools sampled offered lunches that came close to current dietary recommendations for fat. At a time when obesity is increasing among adults and children in the United States, it is ironic that fast-food companies provide lunches in schools and outlets in hospitals. There is even a fast-food restaurant in one of Houston's premier children's hospitals. It is imperative that population and community-based dietary programs focus on teaching children prudent exercise and dietary habits *(136)*.

More research and legislative support for potential environmental controls on obesity should be examined. Subsidizing fruits and vegetables, providing monetary incentives to food manufacturers to develop low-fat alternatives, increasing access to exercise facilities and designing health-enhancing communities based on "smart" urban planning are just a few approaches to providing external or environmental incentives for healthful lifestyles *(140,168–170)*. We must also begin to recognize the value of targeted interventions (e.g., obese children and obese pregnant women) and support their development and implementation.

Finally, the concept of "healthy" obesity (i.e., an individual who is obese yet exercises regularly and eats a healthful diet) deserves further study. Health care providers and researchers should not presume that obesity automatically is synonymous with poor health or increased mortality *(19,155,171)*. Many Americans, regardless of their weight status, engage in unhealthful behaviors *(142–146,165)*. Some obese individuals exercise regularly and eat a healthy diet, and still do not lose significant amounts of weight. Data suggest that obese individuals can improve their risk profiles with exercise and dietary change *(172,173)* and that improvements in lipid profiles often attributed to weight loss might also be due to changes in dietary composition *(172–174)*. It is important for researchers and health care providers to help patients become more aware of the positive outcomes associated with healthful lifestyles, regardless of the impact on weight *(46,175,176)*. We believe that these approaches are the future of obesity treatment.

ACKNOWLEDGMENTS

The authors wish to acknowledge that this work was partially supported by grants from the National Institute of Diabetes & Digestive & Kidney Diseases, DK058299 (Foreyt) and DK064284 (Poston).

REFERENCES

1. Flegal, KM, Carroll, MS, Ogden, CL, Johnson, CL. Prevalence and trends in obesity among US adults, 1999–2000. JAMA 2002; 288:1723–1727.
2. Denke MA, Sempos CT, Grundy SM. Excess body weight: an under-recognized contributor to dyslipidemia in White American women. Arch Intern Med 1994; 154:401–410.
3. Denke MA, Sempos CT, Grundy SM. Excess body weight: an under-recognized contributor to high blood cholesterol levels in White American women. Arch Intern Med 1993; 153:1093–1103.
4. MacMahon S, Cutler J, Brittain E, et al. Obesity and hypertension: epidemiological and clinical issues. Eur Heart J 1987; 8 (Suppl B):57–70.
5. National Task Force on the Prevention and Treatment of Obesity. Overweight, obesity, and health risk. Arch Intern Med 2000; 160:898–904.

6. Pi-Sunyer FX. Medical hazards of obesity. Ann Intern Med 1993;119:655–660.
7. Solomon CG, Willett WC, Manson JE. Body weight and mortality. In: VanItallie TB, Simonpoulos AP, eds. Obesity: New directions in assessment and management. Charles Press, Philadelphia, PA, 1995, pp. 1–11.
8. Troiano RP, Frongillo EA Jr, Sobal J, et al. The relationship between body weight and mortality: a quantitative analysis of combined information from existing studies. Int J Obes Relat Metab Disord 1996; 20:63–75.
9. Manson JE, Willett WC, Stampfer MJ, et al. Body weight and mortality among women. N Engl J Med 1995; 333:677–685.
10. Allison, DB, Fontaine, KR, Manson JE, et al. Annual deaths attributable to obesity in the United States. JAMA 1999; 282:1530–1538.
11. Wolf A. Economic outcomes of the obese patient. Obesity Res, 2002; 10:58S–62S.
12. Finkelstein E, Fiebelkorn I, Wang G. National medical spending attributable to overweight and obesity: how much, and who's paying? Health Affairs 2003; W3:219–226.
13. Pronk N, Goodman M, O'Connor P, Martinson B. Relationship between modifiable health risks and short-term health care charges. JAMA 1999; 282:2235–2239.
14. Sjöström L, Narbro, K, Sjöström D. Costs and benefits when treating obesity. Int J Obes Relat Metab Disord 1995; 19(Suppl 6):S9–S12.
15. Sturm R. The effects of obesity, smoking, and drinking on medical problems and costs. Health Affairs 2002; 21:245–253.
16. Thompson D, Wolf A. The medical-care cost burden of obesity. Obes Rev 2001; 2:189–197.
17. Gortmaker SL, Must A, Perrin JM, et al. Social and economic consequences of overweight in adolescence and young adulthood. N Engl J Med 1993; 329:1008–1012.
18. Enzi G. Socioeconomic consequences of obesity: the effect of obesity on the individual. Pharmaco Econom 1994; 5(Suppl 1):54–57.
19. Sarlio-Lähteenkorva S, Stunkard AJ, Rissanen A. Psychosocial factors and quality of life in obesity. Int J Obes Relat Metab Disord 1995; 19(Suppl 6):S1–S5.
20. Dattilo AM, Kris-Etherton PM. Effects of weight reduction on blood lipids and lipoproteins: a meta-analysis. Am J Clin Nutr 1992; 56:320–328.
21. Kanders BS, Blackburn GL. Reducing primary risk factors by therapeutic weight loss. In: Wadden TA, VanItallie TB, eds. Treatment of the seriously obese patient. Guilford, New York, NY, 1992, pp. 213–230.
22. Foreyt JP, Goodrick GK. Attributes of successful approaches to weight loss and control. Appl Prev Psychol 1994; 3:209–215.
23. Perri MG, Fuller PR. Success and failure in the treatment of obesity: where do we go from here? Medicine, Exercise, Nutrition, and Health 1995; 4:255–272.
24. Stunkard AJ. An overview of current treatments for obesity. In: Wadden TA, VanItallie TB, eds. Treatment of the seriously obese patient. Guilford, New York, NY, 1992, pp. 33–43.
25. Wadden TA, Brownell KD, Foster GD. Obesity: Responding to the global epidemic. J Consult Clin Psychol 2002; 70:510–525.
26. Kramer FM, Jeffery RW, Forster JL, et al. Long-term follow-up of behavioral treatment for obesity: patterns of weight gain among men and women. Int J Obes Relat Metab Disord 1989; 13:124–136.
27. Stalonas PM, Perri MG, Kerzner AB. Do behavioral treatments of obesity last? a five-year follow-up investigation. Addict Behav 1984; 9:175–184.
28. Wadden TA, Sternberg JA, Letizia KA, et al. Treatment of obesity by very low calorie diet, behavioral therapy, and their combination: a five-year perspective. Int J Obes Relat Metab Disord 1989; 13(Suppl 2):39–46.
29. Perri MG, Nezu AM, Viegener BJ. Improving the long-term management of obesity: theory, research, and clinical guidelines. Wiley, New York, NY, 1992, pp. 3–124.
30. Lee I, Blair S, Allison D, et al. Epidemiologic data on the relationships of caloric intake, energy balance, and weight gain over the life span with longevity and morbidity. Journals of Gerontology: SERIES A 2001; 56A:7–19.
31. Perri MG, Shapiro RM, Ludwig WW, et al. Maintenance strategies for the treatment of obesity: an evaluation of relapse prevention training and posttreatment contact by mail and telephone. J Consult Clin Psychol 1984; 52:404–413.

32. Perri MG, McAdoo, WG, McAllister DA, et al. Effects of peer support and therapist contact on long-term weight loss. J Consult Clin Psychol 1987; 55:615–617.

33. Perri MG, McAllister DA, Gange JJ, et al. Effects of four maintenance programs on the long-term management of obesity. J Consult Clin Psychol 1988; 56:529–534.

34. Baum JG, Clark HB, Sandler J. Preventing relapse in obesity through posttreatment maintenance systems: comparing the relative efficacy of two levels of therapist support. J Behav Med 1991; 14: 287–302.

35. Bray GA. Use and abuse of appetite-suppressant drugs in the treatment of obesity. Ann Intern Med 1993; 119:707–713.

36. Haddock C, Poston W, Dill P, Foreyt J, Ericsson M. Pharmacotherapy for obesity: a quantitative analysis of four decades of published randomized clinical trials. Int J Obes 2002; 26:262–273.

37. Abenhaim L, Moride Y, Brenot F, et al. Appetite-suppressant drugs and the risk of primary pulmonary hypertension. JAMA 1996; 335:609–616.

38. Centers for Disease Control (CDC).Cardiac valvulopathy associated with fenfluramine or dexfen-fluramine: U.S. Department of Health and Human Services Interim Public Health Recommendations, November 1997. MMWR 1997; 46:1061–1066.

39. Connolly HM, Crary JL, McGoon MD, et al. Valvular heart disease associated with fenfluramine–phentermine. N Engl J Med 1997; 337:581–588.

40. Stunkard AJ, Harris JR, Pederson NL, et al.The body mass of twins reared apart. N Engl J Med 1990; 322:1483–1487.

41. Kahn L, Serdula M, Bowman B, Williamson D. Use of prescription weight loss pills among U.S. adults in 1996–1998. Ann Intern Med 2001; 134:282–286.

42. National Institutes of Health (National Heart, Lung, and Blood Institute in cooperation with The National Institute of Diabetes and Digestive and Kidney Disease), Clinical guidelines on the identification, evaluation, and treatment of overweight and obesity in adults 1998. NIH Publication No. 98–4083. US Government Printing Office, Washington, DC.

43. Phelan S, Wadden T. Combining behavioral and pharmacological treatments for obesity. Obes Res 2002; 10:560–574.

44. Frost GL, Bovill-Taylor C, Carter L, et al. Intensive lifestyle intervention combined with the choice of pharmacotherapy improves weight loss and cardiac risk factors in the obese. J Hum Nutr Diet 2002; 15:287–295.

45. Finer N. Sibutramine: its mode of action and efficacy. Int J Obes Relat Metab Disord 2002; 26:S29–33.

46. Wadden T, Berkowitz R, Sarwer D, Prus-Wisniewski R. Benefits of lifestyle modification in the pharmacologic treatment of obesity. Arch Intern Med 2001; 161:218–227.

47. Poston W, Haddock C, Dill P, Thayer B, Foreyt J. Lifestyle treatments in randomized clinical trials of pharmacotherapies for obesity. Obes Res 2001; 9:552–563.

48. Greenway, FL, Ryan DH, Bray G, et al. Pharmaceutical cost savings of treating obesity with weight loss medications. Obes Res 1999; 7:523–531.

49. Drent ML, van der Veen EA. Lipase inhibition: a novel concept in the treatment of obesity. Int J Obes Relat Metab Disord 1993; 17:241–244.

50. Drent ML, Larsson I, William-Olsson T, et al. Orlistat (RO 18–0647), a lipase inhibitor, in the treatment of human obesity: a multiple dose study. Int J Obes Relat Metab Disord 1995; 19:221–226

51. Drent ML, van der Veen EA. First clinical studies with orlistat: a short review. Obes Res 1995; 3(Suppl 4):623S–625S.

52. Finer N, James W, Kopelman P, et al. One-year treatment of obesity: a randomized double-blind, placebo-controlled, multicentre study of orlistat, a gastrointestinal lipase inhibitor. Intern J Obes 2000; 24:306–313.

53. Heymsfield S, Segal K, Hauptman J, et al. Effects of weight loss with orlistat on glucose tolerance and progression to type 2 diabetes in obese adults. Arch Intern Med 2000; 160:1321–1326.

54. James W, Avenell A, Broom J, et al. A one-year trial to assess the value of orlistat in the management of obesity. Int J Obes Relat Metab Disord 1997; 21(Suppl 3):S24–S30.

55. Lindgarde F on behalf of the Orlistat Swedish Multimorbidity Study Group. The effect of orlistat on body weight and coronary heart disease risk profile in obese patients: the Swedish Multimorbidity Study. J Int Med 2000; 248:245–254.

56. Sjostrom L, Rissanen A, Andersen T, et al. Randomised placebo-controlled trial of orlistat for weight loss and prevention of weight regain in obese patients. Lancet 1998: 352:167– 172.

57. Davidson M, Hauptman J, DiGirolamo M, Foreyt J, et al. Weight control and risk factor reduction in obese subjects treated for 2 years with orlistat. JAMA 1999; 281:235–242.

58. Broom I, Wilding J, Stott P, Myers N. Randomised trial of the effect of orlistat on body weight and cardiovascular disease risk profile in obese patients: UK Multimorbidity Study. Int J Clin Pract 2002; 56:494–499.

59. Hanefeld M, Sachse G. Diabetes, The effects of orlistat on body weight and glycaemic control in overweight patients with type 2 diabetes: a randomized, placebo-controlled trial. Diab Obes Metab 2002; 4:415–423.

60. Kelley D, Bray G, Pi-Sunyer F, et al. Clinical efficacy of orlistat therapy in overweight and obese patients with type 2 diabetes: a 1 year randomized controlled trial. Diabetes Care 2002; 25:1033–1041.

61. Miles J, Leiter L, Hollander, P, et al. Effect of orlistat in overweight and obese patients with type 2 diabetes treated with metformin. Diabetes Care 2002; 25:1123–1128.

62. Sharma AM, Golay A. Effect of orlistat-induced weight loss on blood pressure and heart rate in obese patients with hypertension. J Hypertens 2002; 29:1873–1878.

63. Snider L, Malone M. Orlistat use in type 2 diabetes. Ann Pharmacother 2002; 36:1210–1218.

64. Rissanen A, Lean M, Rossner S, et al. Predictive value of early weight loss in obesity management with orlistat: an evidence-based assessment of prescribing guidelines. Int J Obes Relat Metab Dis 2003; 27: 103–109.

65. McDuffie J, Calis K, Uwaifo G, et al. Three-month tolerability of orlistat in adolescents with obesity-related co-morbid conditions. Obes Res 2002;10:642–650.

66. Ryan DH, Kaiser P, Bray GA. Sibutramine: a novel new agent for obesity treatment. Obes Res 1995; 3(Suppl 4):553S–559S.

67. Stock MJ. Sibutramine - A review of the pharmacology of a novel anti-obesity agent. Int J Obes Relat Metab Disord 1997; 21(Suppl 1):S25–S29.

68. Bray G, Greenway F. Current and potential drugs for treatment of obesity. Endocrine Reviews 1999; 20:805–875.

69. Apfelbaum M, Vague P, Ziegler O, et al. Long-term maintenance of weight loss after a very low calorie diet: a randomized blinded trial of the efficacy and tolerability of Sibutramine. Amer J Med 1999; 106: 179–184.

70. James WP, Astrup A, Finer N, et al. Effect of sibutramine on weight maintenance after weight loss: a randomized trial. Lancet 2000; 356:2119–2125.

71. Lean MEJ: Sibutramine—a review of clinical efficacy. Int J Obes Relat Metab Disord 1997; 21(Suppl 1): S30–S36.

72. Yanovski S, Yanovski, J. Drug therapy: obesity. N Engl J Med 2002; 346:591–602.

73. McMahon, F, Fujioka K, Singh, B, et al. Efficacy and safety of Sibutramine in obese white and African-American patients with hypertension: a 1-year, double blind placebo controlled, multicenter trial. Arch Int Med 2000; 160:2185–2191.

74. Wadden T, Berkowitz R, Womble L, et al. Effects of sibutramine plus orlistat in obese women following one year of treatment by sibutramine alone: a placebo-controlled trial. Obes Res 2000; 8: 431–437.

75. Berkowitz R, Wadden T, Tershakovec A, Cronquist J. Behavior therapy and sibutramine for the treatment of adolescent obesity. JAMA 2003; 289:1805–1812.

76. Cummings D, Shannon M. Roles for ghrelin in the regulation of appetite and body weight. Arch Surg 2003; 138:389–396.

77. Vastag B. Experimental drugs take aim at obesity. JAMA 2003; 289:1763–1764.

78. Bray G, Tartaglia L. Medicinal strategies in the treatment of obesity. Nature 2000; 404:672–677.

79. Schwartz M, Woods S, Porte D, et al. Central nervous system control of food intake. Nature 2000; 404: 661–671.

80. Woods S, Seeley R, Porte D, Schwartz M. Signals that regulate food intake and energy homeostasis. Science 1998; 280:1378–1383.

81. Kojima M, Hosoda H, Dte Y, et al. Ghrelin is a growth-hormone-releasing acylated peptide from stomach. Nature 1999; 402:656–660.

82. Weigle D, Cummings D, Newby P, et al. Roles of leptin and ghrelin in the loss of body weight caused by a low fat, high carbohydrate diet. J Clin Endocrinol Metab 2003; 88:1577–1586.

83. Nakazato M, Murakami N, Date, Y, et al. A role for ghrelin in the central regulation of feeding. Nature 2001; 409:194–198.

84. Weigle D. Pharmacological therapy of obesity: past, present, and future. J Clin Endocrinol Metab 2003; 88:2462–2469.

85. Bensaid M, Gary-Bobo M, Esclangon A, et al. The cannabinoid CB1 receptor antagonist SR141716 increases Acrp30 mRNA expression in adipose tissue of obese fa/fa rats and in cultured adipocyte cells. Molec Pharmacol 2003; 63:908–14.

86. Ravinet T, Arnone M, Delgorge C, et al. Anti-obesity effect of SR141716, a CB1 receptor antagonist, in diet-induced obese mice. Amer J Physiol-RegIntegrative Compar Physiol 2003; 284:R345–53.

87. Williams C, Kirkham T. Anandamide induces overeating: mediation by central cannabinoid (CB1) receptors. Psychopharmacol 1999; 143:315–317.

88. Ettinger M, Littlejohn T, Schwartz S, et al. Recombinant variant of ciliary neurotrophic factor for weight loss in obese adults: a randomized, dose-ranging study. JAMA 2003; 289:1826–1832.

89. Huestis M, Gorelick D, Heishman S, et al. Blockade of effects of smoked marijuana by the CB1-selective cannabinoid receptor antagonist SR141716. Arch Gen Psychiatry 2001; 58: 322–328.

90. Vickers S, Webster, L, Wyatt A, et al. Preferential effects of the cannabinoid CB-sub-1 receptor antaonist, SR 141716, on food intake and body weight gain of obese (fa/fa) compared to lean Zucker rats. Psychopharmacology 2003; 167:103–111.

91. National Task Force on the Prevention and Treatment of Obesity. Very low-calorie diets. JAMA 1993; 270:967–974.

92. Wadden TA, Bartlett SJ. Very low calorie diets: an overview and appraisal. In: Wadden TA, VanItallie TB, eds. Treatment of the seriously obese patient. Guilford, New York, NY, 1992, pp. 44–79.

93. Kral JG. Surgical treatment of obesity. In: Wadden TA, VanItallie TB, eds. Treatment of the seriously obese patient. Guilford, New York, NY, 1992, pp. 496–506.

94. Brolin R. Bariatric surgery and long-term control of morbid obesity. JAMA 2002; 288: 2793–2796.

95. Pope G, Birkmeyer J, Finlayson S. National trends in utilization and in-hospital outcomes of bariatric surgery. J Gastrointestinal Surg 2002; 6:855–860.

96. Benotti PN, Forse RA. The role of gastric surgery in the multidisciplinary management of severe obesity. Am J Surg 1995; 169:361–367.

97. WHO. Obesity Preventing and Managing the Global Epidemic. World Health Organization, Geneva, Switzerland, 1998.

98. Sjostrom C, Lissner L, Wedel H, Sjostrom L. Reduction in incidence of diabetes, hypertension and lipid disturbances after intentional weight loss induced by bariatric surgery: the SOS Intervention Study. Obesity Res 1999; 7:477–484.

99. Torgerson J, Sjostrom L. The Swedish Obese Subjects (SOS) Study-rationale and results. Int J Obes 2001; 25:S2–S4.

100. Greenway S, Greenway F, Klein S. Effects of obesity surgery on non-insulin-dependent diabetes mellitus. Arch Surg 2002; 137:1109–1117.

101. Rubino F, Gagner M. Potential of surgery for curing type 2 diabetes mellitus. Ann Surg 2002; 236: 554–559.

102. Lujan J, Hernandez, Q, Frutos M, et al. Laparoscopic gastric bypass in the treatment of morbid obesity: preliminary results of a new technique. Surgical Endoscopy 2002; 16:1658–1662.

103. Papasavas PK, Hayetian FD, Caushaj PF, et al. Outcome analysis of laparoscopic Roux-en-Y gastric bypass for morbid obesity: the first 116 cases. Surgical Endoscopy 2002; 16:1653–1657.

104. Gould, JC, Needleman BJ, Ellison EC, et al. Evolution of minimally invasive bariatric surgery. Surgery 2002; 132:565–571.

105. Dresel A, Kuhn JA. Establishing a laparoscopic gastric bypass program. Amer J Surg 2002; 184: 617–620.

106. Schauer P, Ikramuddin S, Hamad G, Gourash W. The learning curve for laparoscopic Roux-en-Y gastric bypass is 100 cases. Surg Endoscopy 2003; 17:212–215.

107. Craig BM, Tseng DS. Cost-effectiveness of gastric bypass for severe obesity. Amer J Med 2002; 113:491–498.

108. Martin LF, Tan TL, Horn JR, et al. Comparison of the costs associated with medical and surgical treatment of obesity. Surgery 1995; 118:599–607.

109. Narbro K, Goran A, Jonsson E, et al. Pharmaceutical costs in obese individuals: comparison with a randomly selected population sample and long-term changes after conventional and surgical treatment: the SOS intervention study. Arch Int Med 2002; 162:2061–2069.

110. Klem M, Wing R, Chang C, et al. A case-control study of successful maintenance of a substantial weight loss: individuals who lost weight through surgery versus those who lost weight through non-surgical means. Int J Obes Relat Metab Disord 2000; 24:573–579.

111. Brownell KD, Wadden TA. Etiology and treatment of obesity: understanding a serious, prevalent, and refractory disorder. J Consult Clin Psychol 1992; 60:505–517.

112. Foreyt JP, Poston WSC, Goodrick GK. Future directions in obesity and eating disorders. Addict Behav 1996; 21:767–778.

113. Institute of Medicine. Weighing the options: criteria for evaluating weight-management programs. National Academy Press, Washington, DC, 1995, pp. 37–63.

114. Bender R, Trautner C, Spraul M, et al. Assessment of excess mortality in obesity. Am J Epidemiol 1998; 147:42–48.

115. Williamson DF, Pamuk ER. The association between weight loss and increased longevity: a review of the evidence. Ann Intern Med 1993; 119:731–736.

116. Fontaine, K, Redden, D, Wang, C, et al. Years of life lost due to obesity. JAMA 2003; 289:187–193.

117. Andres R, Muller DC, Sorkin JD. Long-term effects of change in body weight on all-cause mortality: a review. Ann Intern Med 1993; 119:737–743.

118. Williamson, DF, Thompson, TJ, Thun, et al. Intentional weight loss and mortality among overweight individuals with diabetes. Diabetes Care 2000; 23:1499–1504.

119. Williamson DF, Pamuk ER, Thun M, et al. Prospective study of intentional weight loss and mortality in never-smoking overweight U.S. white women aged 40–64 years. Am J Epidemiol 1995; 141: 1128–1141.

120. Foster GD, Sarwer DB, Wadden TA. Psychological effects of weight cycling in obese persons: a review and research agenda. Obes Res 1997; 5:474–488.

121. Blair SN, Shaten J, Brownell K, et al. Body weight change, all-cause mortality, and cause-specific mortality in the Multiple Risk Factor Intervention Trial. Ann Intern Med 1993; 119:749–757.

122. Iribarren C, Sharp DS, Burchfiel CM, et al. Association of weight loss and weight fluctuation with mortality in Japanese American men. N Engl J Med 1995; 333:686–692.

123. National Task Force on the Prevention and Treatment of Obesity. Weight cycling. JAMA 1994; 272: 1196–1202.

124. Venditti EM, Wing RR, Jakicic JM, et al. Weight cycling, psychological health, and binge eating in obese women. J Consult Clin Psychol 1996; 64:400–405.

125. Foreyt JP, Brunner RL, Goodrick GK, et al. Psychological correlates of weight fluctuation. Int J Eat Disord 1995; 17:263–275.

126. Yanovski SZ. Are anorectic agents the "magic bullet" for obesity? Arch Fam Med 1993; 2:1025–1027.

127. Gullo SP. Food control training as a successor to dieting: a new model for weight management. In: VanItallie TB, Simonpoulos AP, eds. Obesity: new directions in assessment and management. Charles Press, Philadelphia, PA, 1995, pp. 153–171.

128. Perri MG. Improving maintenance of weight loss following treatment by diet and lifestyle modification. In: Wadden TA, VanItallie TB, eds. Treatment of the seriously obese patient. Guilford, New York, NY, 1992, pp. 456–477.

129. Guy-Grand B. Long-term pharmacological treatment of obesity. In: Wadden TA, VanItallie TB, eds. Treatment of the seriously obese patient. Guilford, New York, NY, 1992, pp. 478–495.

130. Institute of Medicine. Weighing the options: criteria for evaluating weight-management programs. National Academy Press, Washington, DC, 1995, pp. 152–170.

131. APA Practice Directorate. Website: (www.apa.org/practice/cpt 2002.html).

132. Kerns R. The new health and behavior assessment and intervention CPT codes: advancing the practice of clinical health psychology. Health Psychologist 2002; 24:10–11.

133. Klem M, Viteri J, Wing R. Primary prevention of weight gain for women aged 25–34: the acceptability of treatment formats. Int J Obes 2000; 24:219–225.

134. Tate D, Wing R, Winett R. Using internet technology to deliver a behavioral weight loss program. JAMA 2001; 285:1172–1177.

135. Fries JF, Koop, CE, Beadle CE, et al. Reducing health care costs by reducing the need and demand for medical services. N Engl J Med 1993; 329:321–325.

136. Foreyt JP, Goodrick GK. The ultimate triumph of obesity. Lancet 1995; 346:134–135.

137. Curb JD, Marcus EB. Body fat and obesity in Japanese Americans. Am J Clin Nutr 1991; 53:1552S–1555S.

138. James WPT. A public health approach to the problem of obesity. Int J Obes Relat Metab Disord 1995; 19(Suppl. 3):S37–S45.

139. Lissner L, Heitman BL. Dietary fat and obesity: evidence from epidemiology. Eur J Clin Nutr 1995; 49:79–90.

140. Battle EK, Brownell KD. Confronting a rising tide of eating disorders and obesity: treatment vs. prevention and policy. Addict Behav 1996; 21:755–765.

141. Institute of Medicine. Weighing the options: criteria for evaluating weight-management programs. National Academy Press, Washington, DC, 1995, pp. 102–117.

142. Mokdad A, Bowman B, Ford E, et al. The continuing epidemics of obesity and diabetes in the United States. JAMA 2001; 286:1195–2000.

143. Sherwood N, Jeffrey R. The behavioral determinants of exercise: implications for physical activity interventions. Annu Rev Nut 2000; 20:21–44.

144. US Department of Health and Human Services (USDHHS). Physical Activity and Health: a Report of the Surgeon General. National Center for Chronic Disease Prevention and Health Promotion, Centers for Disease Control and Prevention, Atlanta, GA, 1996.

145. USDHHS. Healthy People 2010. US Government Printing Office, Washington, DC, 2000. Available at Website: (www.healthypeople.gov).

146. USDHHS. Healthy people in healthy communities. Washington, DC: US Government Printing Office, 2001. Available at Website: (www.healthypeople.gov).

147. Serdula M, Mokdad A, Williamson D, et al. Prevalence of attempting weight loss and strategies for controlling weight, JAMA 1999; 282:1353–1358.

148. Wee C, McCarthy E, Davis R, Phillips R. Physician counseling about exercise. JAMA 1999; 282: 1583–1588.

149. Grilo CM. The role of physical activity in weight loss and weight loss management. Medicine, Exercise, Nutrition, And Health 1995; 4:60–76.

150. Klem ML, Wing RR, McGuire MT, et al. A descriptive study of individuals successful at long-term maintenance of substantial weight loss. Am J Clin Nutr 1997; 66:239–246.

151. Klem M. Successful losers: The habits of individuals who have maintained long-term weight loss. Minnesota Medicine 2000; 83:43–45.

152. McGuire M, Wing R, Klem M, et al. Long-term maintenance of weight loss: do people who lose weight through various weight loss methods use different behaviors to maintain their weight? Int J Obes Relat Metab Disord 1998; 22:572–577.

153. Wing R, Hill J. Successful weight loss maintenance. Ann Rev Nut 2001; 21:323–341.

154. Orleans C, Kraft K, Marx J, McGinnis J. Why are some neighborhoods active and others not? charting a new course for research on the policy and environmental determinants of physical activity. Ann Behav Med 2003; 25:77–79.

155. Barlow CE, Kohl HW, Gibbons LW, et al. Physical fitness, mortality, and obesity. Int J Obes Relat Metab Disord 1995; 19(Suppl 4):S41–S44.

156. Barker DJP, Hales CN, Fall CHD, et al. Type 2 (non-insulin-dependent) diabetes mellitus, hypertension, and hyperlipidaemia (syndrome X): relation to reduced fetal growth. Diabetologia 1993; 36: 62–67.

157. Dorner G, Plagemann A. Perinatal hyperinsulinism as a possible predisposing factor for diabetes mellitus, obesity, and enhanced cardiovascular risk in later life. Horm Metab Res 1994; 26:213–221.

158. Fall CH, Vijayakumar M, Barker DJ, et al. Weight in infancy and prevalence of coronary heart disease in adult life. BMJ 1995; 310:17–19.

159. Bowen DJ, Tomoyasu N, Cauce AM. The triple threat: a discussion of gender, class, and race differences in weight. Women Health 1991; 17:123–143.

160. Epstein LH, Valoski A, Wing RR, et al. Ten-year outcomes of behavioral family-based treatment for childhood obesity. Health Psychol 1994; 13:373–383.

161. Burke LE, Dunbar-Jacobs J. Adherence to medication, diet, and activity recommendations: from assessment to maintenance. J Cardiovasc Nurs 1995; 9:62–79.

162. Kirschenbaum DS, Fitzgibbon ML. Controversy about the treatment of obesity: criticisms or challenges? Behavior Therapy 1995; 26:43–68.

163. Anonymous. Daily dietary fat and total food-energy intakes—Third National Health and Nutrition Examination Survey, Phase 1, 1988–91. MMWR 1994; 43:116–124.

164. Burkitt DP, Eaton SB. Putting the wrong fuel in the tank. Nutrition 1989; 5:189–191.

165. Eaton SB. Humans, lipids and evolution. Lipids 1992; 27:814–820.

166. Whitaker RC, Wright JA, Finch AJ, et al. School lunch: a comparison of the fat and cholesterol content with dietary guidelines. J Pediatr 1993; 123:857–862.

167. Chapman N, Gordon AR, Burghardt JA. Factors affecting the fat content of National School Lunch Program lunches. Am J Clin Nutr 1995; 61(Suppl 1):199S–204S.

168. Jacobson MF, Brownell, KD. Small taxes on soft drinks and snack foods to promote health. Amer J Public Health 2000; 90:854–857.

169. Saelens B, Sallis J, Frank L. Environmental correlates of walking and cycling: findings from the transportation, urban design, and planning literature. Ann Behav Med 2003; 80–91.

170. Poston W, Haddock C, Hughey J, et al. (2002, April). Obesity and the environment: a tale of two Kansas cities. Presentation at the Society of Behavioral Medicine's Twenty-Third Annual Scientific Sessions, Washington, DC (Rapid Submission).

171. Goodman WC. The invisible woman: confronting weight prejudice in America. Carlsbad, CA: Gürze Books, 1995, pp. 18–45.

172. Andersen RE, Wadden TA, Bartlett SJ, et al. Relation of weight loss to changes in serum lipids and lipoproteins in obese women. Am J Clin Nutr 1995; 62:350–357.

173. Björntorp P. Evolution of the understanding of the role of exercise in obesity and its complications. Int J Obes Relat Metab Disord 1995; 19 (Suppl 4):S1–S4.

174. Wooley SC. Maelstrom revisited. Am Psychol 1995; 50:943–944.

175. Foreyt JP, Goodrick GK. Living without dieting. New York, NY: Warner Books, 1994, pp. 15–126.

176. O'Neil PM, Smith CF, Foster GD, Anderson DA. The perceived relative worth of reaching and maintaining goal weight. Int J Obes 2000; 24:1069–1076.

13 The Role of Physical Activity, Exercise, and Nutrition in the Treatment of Obesity

Edward T. Mannix, Helmut O. Steinberg, Stacey Faryna, Jodi Hazard, Reed J. Engel, and Michael F. Busk

KEY POINTS

- There are benefits of physical activity beyond weight control.
- Increasing physical activity has physical and psychological benefits. These include reduction of coronary heart disease risk factors, enhanced cardiovascular and respiratory function, and reduction of colon and breast cancer.
- The physician needs to be aware of strategies to encourage patients to increase their activity. Encouraging slow and steady progress is generally more effective than more rapid introduction to an exercise program.

1. INTRODUCTION

The increasing prevalence of obesity and overweight has caused many experts to declare that a "health care epidemic of being overweight and obese" is gripping our nation and becoming a significant health care problem. According to a published report cited by The National Institutes for Health (NIH) *(1)*, as of the late 1990s, more than half of the adults in the United States are overweight (body mass index [BMI] ≥ 25 kg/m^2, including those who are obese) and nearly one-quarter of US adults are obese (BMI ≥ 30 kg/m^2) *(2)*. Unfortunately, the prevalence of overweight and obesity has steadily increased in nearly all ethnic and racial groups over the latter portion of the 20th century, as a 3.2% increase in the prevalence of the overweight category occurred during the years 1960 through 1994, along with a 66.4% increase in the prevalence of obesity during the same time period *(2)*. Tragically, each year approx 280,000 adult deaths in the United States are attributed to obesity *(3)*, with a total annual cost of $99.2 billion in the year 1995 *(4)*.

Being overweight or obese can pose significant problems. Fortunately there are lifestyle changes that overweight and obese people can make which, over time, can result

From: *The Management of Eating Disorders and Obesity, Second Edition*
Edited by: D. J. Goldstein © Humana Press Inc., Totowa, NJ

Table 1
Chapter Overview

in significant weight loss and improvement in their general state of health and well-being. Many Americans have already incorporated an exercise routine into their daily schedules, but many others lead sedentary lifestyles, rarely engage in vigorous physical activity, and remain overweight. Most sedentary individuals are aware of the potential benefits that exercise has to offer, but still have not committed themselves to a more active lifestyle and a program of progressive weight loss. Implementation of such a plan can be accomplished in a stepwise progression. One of the first steps is to acquire knowledge of the benefits of regular exercise, beginning with a working definition of two key terms: physical activity and exercise. Physical activity is defined as "any bodily movement produced by skeletal muscles that results in energy expenditure." It is a global term, and generally includes activities performed at a moderate intensity such as walking, cycling for pleasure, mowing the lawn, gardening, dancing, raking leaves, and shoveling snow, to name a few. Exercise is an aspect of physical activity and is defined as "any planned, structured, and repetitive bodily movement done to improve or maintain one or more component of physical fitness." It includes but is not limited to vigorous and continuous activities such as jogging, swimming, and cycling (5).

There are conflicting reports in the literature regarding the amount and type of activity necessary to achieve health benefits. Most researchers have concluded that many of the benefits can be realized by individuals who expend at least 200 cal per day in either physical activity or exercise (6). A recommendation from the American College of Sports Medicine, the Centers for Disease Control, and the President's Council on Physical Fitness and Sports, and a consensus panel from the NIH have advised that all Americans should accumulate at least 30 min of moderate intensity physical activity or planned exercise on most days of the week to reap the benefits (7,8).

This chapter presents an overview of the role of physical activity, exercise, and nutrition in the treatment of obesity (Table 1) and will discuss the benefits of physical activity and exercise, individualizing an exercise program, identifying and overcoming barriers to exercise, and the role of proper nutrition.

2. THE BENEFITS OF PHYSICAL ACTIVITY AND EXERCISE

The benefits of physical activity and exercise include, but are not limited to, an increase in one's ability to deal with stress, increased energy to perform tasks of daily living, improved sleep, decreased body fat and blood pressure (BP), and an improved blood lipid profile. Many of these benefits have been known and professed for centuries. Maimonides declared in the 12th century that,"anyone who sits around idle and takes no exercise will be subject to physical discomforts and failing strength." The importance of an active body and mind was articulated by President John F. Kennedy: "We know what the Greeks knew: that intelligence and skill can only function at the peak of their capacity when the body is healthy and strong, and that hardy spirits and tough minds usually inhabit sound bodies" (9). Twenty-five years later an investigative team lead by Powell provided hard evidence that regular exercise results in physiological benefits, as an inverse relationship was found between physical activity and the risk of developing coronary artery disease in men (10), a finding corroborated by a meta-analysis (11). This benefit is not limited to men. By the end of the 20th century a large, prospective study of more than 120,000 female registered nurses (The Nurses' Health Study) presented evidence that regular, brisk walking and vigorous exercise are equally associated with a reduction in coronary events of women (12).

The regular performance of physical activity and exercise has many possible health benefits including the following:

1. An increased ability to perform physical activity and improvement of one's health.
2. A reduction in coronary heart disease (CHD) risk factors.
3. Improvement of cardiovascular and respiratory function.
4. Maintenance of basal metabolic rate.
5. A positive effect on food intake and appetite.
6. A reduction of certain cancers and osteoporosis
7. Enhanced psychological effects.

The health risks of a sedentary lifestyle and benefits of physical activity in the obese are similar to those listed for the general population; however, obesity magnifies many of the medical consequences of inactivity (i.e., hypertension, atherosclerosis, CHD, congestive heart failure, diabetes mellitus [DM], osteoarthritis, reduced pulmonary function) and the benefits of physical activity and exercise in obese individuals can be very significant. The following discussion focuses on the aforementioned benefits for both the general population and for the obese.

2.1. Increased Physical Activity and Improvement of One's Health

Numerous studies have been conducted to determine the importance of regular physical activity as a means of preventing disease. The significance of these investigations has grown as individuals have become increasingly sedentary and reliant on labor-saving devices. Evidence suggests that obesity is related more to reduced activity than to increased ingestion (13,14). From elevators and escalators, to home shopping and remote controls, such advances in our culture have created an environment where individuals have to consciously think about opportunities to integrate physical activity into their lives.

In 1949, Morris et al. were among the first to investigate the relationship between vocational and leisure-time physical activity and the risk of CHD. Their observations resulted in the finding that highly active conductors who climbed the stairs on London's double-decker buses were at lower risk for CHD than the more sedentary bus drivers (15). They also discovered that sedentary telephone operators and supervisors had higher rates of CHD than postal workers who delivered the mail on foot (15).

Such research served as the cornerstone for more sophisticated studies that have affirmed the relationship between the amount of activity (measured by caloric expenditure or minutes of physical activity) and death rate from CHD. A significantly lower mortality rate from CHD has been observed in studies of individuals who performed an average of 47 min of activity per day vs 15 min (16). Another study found that men who expended more than 2000 cal per week exercising experienced a lower death rate from CHD than those who expended less than 500 cal per week during activity (17). A prospective study by Blair and coworkers underscores the importance of regular exercise in decreasing mortality (18). In 9777 individuals observed over a 5-yr period, the highest age-adjusted all-cause death rate was noted in people who maintained sedentary lifestyles, whereas the lowest death rate was observed in those who were classified as physically fit over the span of the study. These findings were recently corroborated by another investigative team that found that older men (61–81 yr of age) who walked more than 2 miles per day had mortality rates nearly half that of older men who walked less than 1 mile per day (19). The large body of evidence linking increased physical activity with decreased morbidity and mortality spawned a set of recommendations published by the American Heart Association (13,20). Importantly, these benefits extend also to subjects with extremely high risk of cardiovascular disease owing to impaired glucose metabolism or other known risk factors (21,22). These recommendations emphasize the fact that regular exercise plays a vital role in primary and secondary prevention of cardiovascular disease. Without question, physical activity and exercise are powerful allies in protecting against heart disease and other lifestyle diseases for both the general and obese populations.

2.2. Reduction of Coronary Heart Disease Risk Factors

Physical activity and exercise influence a number of CHD risk factors including hypertension, lipoprotein profiles, inflammatory markers, obesity, glucose intolerance, and DM.

2.2.1. HYPERTENSION

Epidemiologists have found that physically active individuals have a lower prevalence of hypertension (23). For individuals with hypertension, regular, moderate physical activity decreases systolic BP up to 10 mmHg (24). This BP-lowering effect appears to be independent of weight loss (25–27). For individuals who are sedentary and obese, weight gain has been shown to correlate with the development of hypertension (28). When encouraging obese patients, physicians should refer to The Sixth Report of the Joint National Committee on Detection, Evaluation, and Treatment of High Blood Pressure which indicated that a weight loss as little as 10 lb has a BP-lowering effect for many individuals (29,30). The report incorporated aerobic activity as one of the lifestyle modifications for hypertension control and reduced overall cardiovascular risk.

2.2.2. LIPOPROTEIN PROFILES

Vigorous activity in endurance athletes has been associated with increased high-density lipoprotein cholesterol (HDL-C) (31). In prospective training studies of apparently healthy subjects (32) and obese individuals (33), endurance exercise has increased HDL-C levels. In addition, individuals who reduce their body fat through activity or weight loss have experienced increased HDL-C (34,35). Moreover, regular, moderate intensity exercise has a favorable impact on the HDL-C–low-density lipoprotein cholesterol (LDL-C) ratio (a significant factor in preventing CHD) in both obese and lean individuals (36). Dietary strategies have also been implemented to lower high levels of LDL-C, another CHD risk factor. One recent report noted that a widely accepted diet designed to reduce LDL was only successful if participants were engaged in regular, aerobic exercise during its administration (37). Also, physically active individuals appear to have lower triglyceride (TG) levels; and, sedentary individuals with high TGs have experienced up to a 20–40% reduction in plasma TGs during a controlled exercise program (33). A recent study comparing obese with non-obese patients has confirmed these benefits (38).

2.2.3. INFLAMMATORY MARKERS

Over the last several years, it has become clear that the classic cardiovascular risk factors explain only half of the mortality and morbidity observed. Clearly, other factors play a role. Recently, markers of inflammation such as C-reactive protein (CRP), fibrinogen, white blood cell count, tumor necrosis factor-α, and interleukins have been proposed to be related to the development of vascular disease. Interestingly, CRP is elevated in obesity (39), which may explain some of the excess mortality in this population. Exercise, even at moderate levels is associated with lower levels of CRP, white cell blood count, and fibrinogen (40), possibly contributing to the cardioprotective effects of exercise.

2.2.4. OBESITY

Without a doubt, one of the most common benefits exercise participants seek is weight loss and a reduction in body fat. Incorporating more activity into one's lifestyle and engaging in regular exercise increases overall energy expenditure and favorably impacts caloric balance. Increases in proportion of lean body mass have been noted in research studies in which the participants engaged in vigorous physical training performed consistently for 3 mo or more (41,42). Although there are conflicting literature reports, many indicate that regular physical activity reduces fat while preserving lean body mass (43–46).

Although weight loss and reduction of body fat are primary objectives of diet and exercise programs for obese individuals, maintenance of lower body weight following weight loss should be an important secondary objective. A meta-analysis of 493 studies published between 1969 and 1994, which reported weight loss in obese men and women, indicates that a typical 15-wk diet or diet plus exercise program produces an average weight loss of 11 kg, with a 6.6- and 8.6-kg maintained weight loss after 1 yr, respectively (47). It is clear that even successful weight-loss programs cannot guarantee that the new, lower weight will be maintained. A recent study of 77 obese women whose weight loss averaged between 13.5 and 17.3 kg over 48 wk of diet plus aerobic exercise, diet plus strength training, diet plus aerobic exercise and strength training, or diet alone may offer a solution to the problem of weight maintenance following weight loss (48). A 1 yr follow-up study of these women found that those who exercised regularly during the 4 mo preceding follow-up testing regained significantly less weight than those who did not exercise during the same time period. This report confirms the belief that regular exercise can help maintain weight loss in this population.

It is important to remind obese individuals who are frustrated about exercise and weight loss that, independent of weight loss, exercise can counteract many of the ill effects of obesity such as high BP and low cardiorespiratory function (49). In addition, even if no weight is lost, favorable body composition changes may be taking place.

2.2.5. GLUCOSE INTOLERANCE AND DIABETES MELLITUS

Regular vigorous exercise is associated with a decrease in plasma insulin levels. Although exercise shows little effect on glucose tolerance in subjects with normal glucose metabolism, exercise can drastically improve glucose tolerance in subjects with impaired fasting glucose or with diabetes. Hence, an increase in insulin sensitivity is noted regardless of a decrease in body fat (50). All of these effects work together in preventing and controlling diabetes, particularly non-insulin-dependent diabetes mellitus (NIDDM) (51), and even low levels of exercise can provide substantial protection from the development of NIDDM (52).

For the obese diabetic patient with insulin insensitivity, regular exercise may be an effective treatment. A study of obese subjects found an increase in insulin sensitivity the day following strenuous exercise; this effect lasted 4 to 6 d following exercise (53). This is an important effect of exercise, as increased insulin sensitivity will reduce the requirements for hypoglycemic medications. Another study involved six previously inactive moderately obese men with NIDDM who rode a cycle ergometer five times a week for 3 to 6 mo. Intravenous glucose tolerance increased, whereas serum insulin level was not increased, suggesting that insulin sensitivity increased. However, after 2 wk of inactivity, participants reverted to their pre-exercise status (54). Thus, maintenance of an exercise program is a critical component of managing NIDDM.

Two recent publications emphasize the importance of exercise in the treatment of obese individuals suffering from DM. One study documented the efficacy of short-term

(7 d) aerobic training in improving insulin sensitivity and glucose metabolism in 12 obese, hypertensive African-American women, a segment of our population that is known to have a higher prevalence of insulin resistance, obesity, and hypertension *(55)*. Results indicate that although there was no significant improvement in maximal O_2 consumption, body composition, or body weight, this short-term program aided in the treatment of the underlying disease process, as significant improvements in insulin sensitivity and glucose metabolism were observed. A second report in 13 sedentary, obese females examined the effects of long-term (32 wk), moderate intensity (50–55% of maximum heart rate), intermittent exercise (10 min, three times/d, 5 d/wk) on its ability to improve aerobic capacity, body composition, blood lipids, insulin sensitivity, and glucose metabolism *(56)*. Those subjects who were least fit and had the highest percentage of body fat at the beginning of the study had significant improvements in body weight, fat weight, maximal O_2 consumption, insulin levels, and insulin sensitivity by the end of the study. Again, these investigative reports uphold the axiom that exercise, even of short-term or of moderate intensity, can help in the treatment of obesity and DM.

2.3. Improvement of Cardiovascular and Respiratory Function

Individuals who participate regularly in continuous aerobic exercise often experience an improvement in cardiovascular and respiratory function, including increased ability to use oxygen efficiently, decreased resting heart rate, increased stroke volume, lower heart rate, and lower total peripheral vascular resistance at submaximal intensities *(57)*. This improvement in cardiovascular and respiratory function ultimately results in increased stamina and endurance. For the obese population, the combination of weight reduction and improved cardiovascular function may produce similar results *(58)*.

2.3.1. Exercise Tolerance

In the extremely obese individual, there is increased deposition of adipose tissue overlying the thoracic and abdominal cavity, resulting in reduced pulmonary function, particularly decreases in resting end-expiratory volumes. The functional residual capacity (FRC) and expiratory reserve volume (ERV) are both decreased in obese individuals, with preservation of the residual volume *(59)*. As the ERV decreases, abnormalities in the ventilation–perfusion distribution can occur secondary to the restricted lung mechanics seen with obesity, ultimately resulting in abnormalities in gas exchange. During exercise, these abnormalities are exacerbated, so that the slightest exertion may cause dyspnea in an extremely obese individual.

Although there is reduced FRC and ERV in the slightly or moderately obese individuals, there are no significant abnormalities in ventilation–perfusion distribution or gas exchange. Thus, the majority of these individuals may start an exercise program before losing a significant amount of weight without any negative consequences to their cardiorespiratory system. For those obese individuals who become so severely dyspneic that exercise tolerance is impaired, weight loss may be required before they are able to participate in vigorous exercise programs *(60)*. The ERV and FRC of the extremely obese individual has been shown to return to near normal after significant weight loss *(61)*. Interestingly, gas exchange does not improve until these individuals decrease their weight to within 30% in excess of their ideal body weight *(62)*.

2.3.2. SLEEP APNEA

As noted previously, various morphological and physiological changes occur in obese individuals that can alter lung function. Obesity-mediated changes in lung function result from alterations in mechanical, pulmonary, and central factors and can result in the development of obstructive sleep apnea (OSA).

Mechanical factors include the marked increase in abdominal contents of obese individuals that raises the diaphragm, making it less able to efficiently fill the lungs, increased chest wall weight that increases the inspiratory load, thus increasing the work of breathing, and fatty deposition within the diaphragm and intercostal muscles that decreases the contractile capability of these muscles and reduces the compliance of the chest wall, making it more difficult to ventilate the lungs. Alterations in pulmonary factors of obese individuals often result in the development of a restrictive pulmonary disease pattern, as evidenced by changes in spirometry, including decreases in forced vital capacity, residual lung volume, ERV, FRC, and maximum minute ventilation *(63)*. Finally, two key central factors that are often altered in the obese have negative affects on pulmonary function. These central factors include the mechanoreflex-mediated activity of dilator muscles and hypoglossal nucleus stimulation of genioglossus activity. As the number and/or magnitude of these factors increase, the potential for significant changes in pulmonary function and the development of OSA increases.

The apnea–hypopnea index (AHI), a ratio of the number of apnea and hypopnea episodes that occur per hour of sleep, is used to determine whether OSA is operative *(64)*. An AHI of 5 of more in patients with excessive daytime somnolence defines OSA. Approximately 4% of the male population between the ages of 30 to 60 yr old and 2% of the female population in the same age range have OSA. Risk factors for OSA include obesity, a large neck circumference, craniofacial abnormalities, hypothyroidism, and acromegaly. The differential diagnosis for OSA encompasses snoring, central sleep apnea, and other disorders that cause daytime somnolence, including insufficient sleep, circadian rhythm disturbance, narcolepsy, and periodic limb movement disorder. Diagnosis of OSA should be based on both symptoms and the magnitude of the patient's respiratory disturbances.

The potential consequences of OSA range from an impaired quality of life, to the development of cardiovascular disease, and in the worst cases, death. Impaired quality of life can be the result of snoring, fatigue, depression, nocturnal awakening, fear of dying, disruption in relationships and sex, and problems with obesity treatment. Two of the more common cardiovascular diseases that may develop as a result of OSA are hypertension and elevated pulmonary systolic pressure. Death from OSA can result from cardiovascular and cerebrovascular events. Interestingly, individuals with OSA have a threefold increase in death from motor vehicle accidents over those without OSA.

Treatment for OSA includes avoidance of sedatives (including benzodiazepines and alcohol) and a change to a lateral sleeping position. Use of a continuous positive airway pressure (CPAP) is immediately effective in decreasing somnolence and in improving quality of life, mood, and alertness. Oral appliances that advance the position of the jaw and tongue have been somewhat effective, but less successful than CPAP *(65)*. Serotonin reuptake inhibitors may benefit patients with mild OSA, as they improve breathing during non-rapid eye movement sleep *(66,67)*. Various surgical techniques have been employed to treat OSA, but because of uncertain effectiveness *(68)* and various complications, surgery should only be considered as a last resort for patients with the most severe forms of the disease.

Weight loss remains the most effective treatment for OSA. A 10% weight loss has been associated with significant improvements in the AHI score; however, attaining this weight loss entails delay and is not well maintained by most individuals (69). Obesity surgery (see Chapter 20) has been used with some success (70).

2.4. Maintenance of Basal Metabolic Rate, Potential Benefits of Strength Training

A significant portion of total caloric expenditure is due to the basal metabolic rate (BMR). An individual's BMR is related to both lean body mass and body fat, with a higher BMR seen in individuals with a higher proportion of lean body mass (71). Thus, one might expect that endurance-trained athletes with high fitness levels and decreased amounts of body fat would have an increased BMR. This notion has been supported by two studies (72,73), whereas another study failed to show a relationship between fitness level and BMR (74).

Significant reduction of body weight in obese individuals is a primary goal of treatment modalities for this population. This seemingly intuitive objective may have two potentially negative outcomes. First, when individuals strive to lose weight through caloric restriction alone, there is often a reduction in lean body mass and, consequently, a lower BMR (75). Second, reports indicate that maintenance of reduced body weight in obese subjects is often associated with compensatory changes in energy expenditure which counteract the maintenance of the newly achieved lower weight (76). Exercise, particularly when it includes strength training, may have a positive effect on preservation of lean body mass (36); however, it does not seem to prevent the decrease in BMR during weight loss, which appears to be related to the degree of caloric deprivation and rate of weight loss (76,77). Thus, even with the addition of exercise, those who severely restrict caloric intake and lose weight rapidly are likely to experience a decrease in BMR. Perhaps an approach consisting of moderate caloric restriction plus regular aerobic exercise and resistance training performed over prolonged time periods would have the desired effect.

2.5. Effect of Exercise on Food Intake and Appetite

There is considerable controversy regarding the effect of exercise on food intake and appetite. The results of studies examining increased physical activity and the effect on intake in the obese have been inconsistent. Two studies support the notion that exercise has no effect on food intake in the obese (78,79), whereas other research of documented weight loss provides evidence of decreased intake (80–82). Another study examining vigorous physical activity and food intake in the obese reported an increase in intake (83).

In the obese population, food-derived signals or sensory characteristics of the food may impact the amount and type of intake more than cues elicited from exercise. In short, the effect of exercise on food intake and appetite is a complex matter influenced by many variables, such as intensity and duration of exercise, as well as food appeal (84,85).

2.6. Reduction of Colon and Breast Cancer

Much is yet to be understood regarding the relationship between physical activity, exercise, and the prevention of certain cancers. It is estimated that 15–20% of all cancers in the United States are the result of excessive weight (body fat) *(86)*. In addition, obesity has been suggested as a greater risk for certain cancers (such as colon) *(85,87,88)*. For the obese individual, physical activity and exercise may reduce the risk through a decrease in body fat and weight. Specifically, there is evidence that consistent exercisers have increased protection from colon cancer. A recent review indicates that inactive individuals have 1.2 to 3.6 times the risk of colon cancer *(87,89)*. The reduced risk among regular exercisers is most often associated with a decrease in intestinal transit time.

The research encompassing breast cancer and physical activity is more controversial. However, a recent finding suggested that the amount of time spent in physical activity was a critical variable. The results indicated that sedentary women had 2.4 times the breast cancer risk than women who engaged in greater than 3.8 hr of exercise per week *(90)*. In addition, women who exercise more experience 30–40% less breast cancer *(91,92)*.

An increase in body fat may make finding lumps through breast self-examination more difficult for the obese population, potentially delaying diagnosis. An increase in physical activity may facilitate decreasing body fat, thus improving detection.

2.7. Enhanced Psychological Effects

Individuals contemplating the benefits of an active lifestyle often focus solely on reaping physical benefits, with little or no attention given to psychological benefits. Many of these psychological benefits produce an immediate sense of well-being, in contrast to physical benefits which often require more time and patience.

The primary mental benefit of exercise is an improved ability to manage stress *(93,94)*. A meta-analysis of 34 studies concluded that aerobically fit subjects exhibited a reduced psychosocial response to stress, regardless of the type of physiological or psychological measure used *(95)*. The preliminary explanation for this result was that exercise may serve as a catalyst to facilitate a more constructive response to stress and a coping strategy that decreases the physiological response to stress.

Improved self-esteem and self-concept are reported as psychological benefits of regular exercise among obese individuals *(96–98)*. Other possible effects of regular exercise among obese individuals include increased self-satisfaction and acceptance, improved self-perception, improved social interactions, and more balanced perspectives *(96–98)*.

The realization of the aforementioned psychological benefits of physical activity and exercise can be extremely beneficial for obese individuals desiring to lose weight. Research on dieting alone validates what many individuals have known for years. Restricting food intake results in depression, anxiety, fatigue, and irritability in half of all dieters *(99)*. For obese individuals with weight-loss goals, exercise can help reduce stress, and enhance self-esteem and self-concept (which is often profoundly reduced after years of obesity). The increased sense of personal control and mastery gained through exercise may have a positive influence on eating habits by cultivating a series of small successes.

Physicians and other health care professionals should convey the relationship between physical activity and improved psychological function to their patients. The ability of physical activity and exercise to elicit an immediate sense of well-being should be neither underestimated nor overlooked.

Table 2
Prior to Beginning an Exercise Program

1. Perform health status assessment
   a. Current health status examination
   b. Graded exercise test for patients with possible coronary heart disease
2. Perform individual fitness assessment
   a. Cardiovascular endurance
   b. Muscular strength
   c. Muscular endurance
   d. Body composition
   e. Flexibility
3. Assess patient's needs and interest
4. Goal-setting and program development
   a. Specific measurable attainable realistic time-based goals
      i. Consider National Institutes of Health consensus statement
      ii. Consider American College of Sports Medicine guidelines
      iii. Make modifications appropriate for degree of obesity
   b. Evaluate prior exercise history
5. Evaluate potential barriers to exercise

3. INDIVIDUALIZING AN EXERCISE PROGRAM

Obese individuals desiring to perform weight-bearing activity may have difficulty because of their excess body fat or excessive perceived exertion *(100)*. They may have adopted a sedentary lifestyle with subsequent loss of muscle tone, bone density, and an increased likelihood of future injury. A reasonable recommendation is to begin with non-weight-bearing activities (such as cycling), progress to lower impact weight-bearing activities (such as walking), and gradually incorporate a moderate resistance/strength training component into an exercise program to maintain and eventually increase muscle tone and bone density *(101,102)*.

Tailoring regular physical activity to an individual's needs, interests, and abilities rather than applying the more generic "get some exercise" solution, is more likely to be successful. This success brings an increase in the patient's ability to gain a degree of control over his or her own health, which becomes a powerful tool. Furthermore, when potential obstacles to maintaining an effective exercise program are recognized and accounted for, success (adherence to a program of regular exercise leading to improved health) is much more likely. A recent study supports the idea that tailoring a program to one's specific needs is productive, as it was reported that most patients will achieve greater weight loss if they are instructed to complete a home-based exercise program *(103)*.

3.1. Prior to Beginning an Exercise Program

Table 2 summarizes the tasks that should be performed prior to initiating an exercise program. Some of these are best performed by a physician, others by an exercise therapist or certified exercise trainer.

3.1.1. Current Health Status and Individual Health Assessment

Prior to beginning an exercise program, it is important for the individual to discuss with a health professional which types of health assessments and exercise programs are appropriate. Conversations should begin by focusing on the current health status of the individual in order to determine the individual's suitability for exercise. In some cases, a graded exercise test may be indicated if the patient is deemed to be at risk for CHD *(104)*. The health professional can then advise the client about appropriate, safe, and effective activities to incorporate into the program, seeking to avoid those activities that may be contraindicated owing to current health status.

An initial individual fitness assessment by a qualified exercise specialist is a desirable compliment to the discussion of current health status. Such an assessment provides valuable benchmark information from which future progress can be measured in cardiovascular endurance, muscular strength, muscular endurance, body composition (girth measurements may be most appropriate for an obese population), and flexibility.

A current health status review and initial individual fitness assessment will uncover the most obvious patient needs, such as weight control, BP management, and stress reduction. Discussion concerning which activities are best suited to accomplish these objectives should begin during the initial fitness assessment. Suggesting several cardiovascular-based options gives the individual the freedom to choose an enjoyable activity and enhances his or her ability to vary the routine, yet remain focused on goals.

3.1.2. Patient's Needs and Interests

Equally important to a consideration of patient needs is an accounting of patient interests. If an exercise prescription is given without first eliciting individual desires, the probability of compliance and eventual success will diminish because of a lack of patient input, choice, and program ownership. The health professional should delve into what the individual enjoys so that the suggested activities are not perceived as boring or, in the worst-case scenario, punishment. Taking an exercise history may eliminate unpopular, frustrating, and/or painful activities. Having determined and discussed the patient's current health status, fitness level, activity needs, and interests, the health professional is ready to recommend an exercise program.

3.2. Goal-Setting and Program Development

The first step in any serious endeavor involves the setting of appropriate goals. Incorporating physical activity and exercise into one's lifestyle is no different. Some individuals may aspire to embark on an exercise program that will result in their being mistaken for a body builder. Others may just say they want to "get back into shape." The problem with these goals is that they set individuals up for failure. Rare is the individual who can realistically and safely reach and maintain the physique of a professional body builder. Likewise, the "get back into shape" objective is vague and can go unfulfilled because no parameters are established to show if and when the goal has been realized. When goals remain out of reach or are too vague, progress toward them is certainly impaired, often creating a disparity between actual and expected outcomes *(105)* and eventually resulting in abandonment of the initial goal of loosing weight and improving health.

3.2.1. S.M.A.R.T. Goals

An effective tool that the health professional can use to decrease this disparity between outcomes is to assist the individual with setting goals that are Specific, Measurable, Attainable, Realistic, and Time-based (S.M.A.R.T.). An example of a S.M.A.R.T. goal would be a plan to lose 20 lb in 20 wk by emphasizing both prudent eating habits (i.e., 55–65% carbohydrate, 15% protein, and 20–30% fat) and regular exercise (i.e., three to five sessions per week, 20–60 min per session, at an appropriate target; *see* Subheading 5.).

The health professional should encourage the individual to take an active role in setting his or her own long-term outcome goals, with short-term goals serving as milestones of progress toward the ultimate objective. The role of the health professional here is two-fold: to ensure that proper goals are set and to provide the appropriate knowledge and guidance so that the patient understands how to reach these goals by developing a program of activity that is safe, effective, and enjoyable. Equipped with information regarding current health status, fitness level, needs, interests, and exercise history, the exercise prescription and goals can and should be modified to meet these patient-specific considerations.

3.2.2. NIH Consensus Statement

Many potential exercisers think that they must perform vigorous physical activity in order to bring about significant weight loss and health gains. Subsequently, many Americans fail to start or to maintain an exercise program. Owing in part to these misperceptions, the NIH issued a Consensus Development Conference Statement that recommends "that children and adults should set a long-term goal to accumulate at least 30 min or more of moderate-intensity physical activity on most, or preferably all, days of the week. Intermittent or shorter bouts of activity (at least 10 min), including occupational, non-occupational, or tasks of daily living, also have similar cardiovascular and health benefits if performed at a level of moderate intensity (such as brisk walking) and accumulate to 30 min per day" *(8)*. This statement effectively makes guidelines for an exercise program appear less rigid and may serve as a more realistic starting point for previously sedentary individuals.

3.2.3. American College of Sports Medicine Guidelines

Additionally, a widely recognized set of general exercise guidelines developed by the American College of Sports Medicine (ACSM) *(104)* includes recommendations for frequency, intensity, duration, mode, and rate of progression (Table 3). With the ultimate goal of maximizing caloric expenditure and combating obesity, the ACSM recommends exercising 5 to 7 d each week, 40 to 60 min per session, at an intensity between 40 and 70% of one's VO_2 max, using low-impact modes of activity (e.g., walking, biking, or swimming) and focusing on increasing duration rather than intensity as the program progresses.

3.2.4 Modifications for the Obese Population

Still, the sedentary individual may not be ready for even 20 min a day, most days of the week. Therefore, it is essential to constantly encourage and focus on progression. One way to achieve this and to increase compliance at the beginning of a program is to alert

Table 3
American College of Sports Medicine General Exercise Guidelines

	Recommendation
1. Frequency of exercise	Three to five exercise sessions per week
2. Intensity of exercise	50–85% of maximal oxygen uptake (VO_2 max) or heart rate reserve (HRR). (Note: because not all patients undergo graded exercise tests, and most will not know or comprehend VO_2 max, HRR may be a more useful tool; *see* Fig. 1.)
3. Duration of exercise	20–60 min of continuous activity
4. Mode of exercise	Aerobic, rhythmic activities involving large muscle groups (i.e., walking, swimming, cycling, rowing, and stairclimbing)
5. Rate of progression	
Initial stage	Wk 1–5, three exercise sessions per week, 40–70% of HRR, 12–20 min per session
Improvement stage	Wk 6–27, –three to five exercise sessions per week, 70–85% of HRR, 20–30 min per session
Maintenance stage	Wk 28+, three exercise sessions per week, 70–85% of HRR, 30–45 min per session

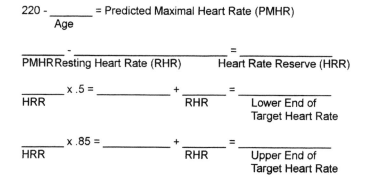

Fig. 1. Formula for estimating target heart rate (using heart rate reserve).

the patient to the fact that even intermittent and shorter duration bouts of exercise performed on any given day (i.e., three 10-min bouts) can accumulate and have the same desired affect as one 30-min session. With continued support and encouragement, patients can achieve a gradual increase in time spent exercising per session.

Another concern for beginning exercisers revolves around exercise intensity. As an alternative to pulse-taking and measured heart rates, patients can also ensure moderate intensity by utilizing either the Talk Test or the Rating of Perceived Exertion (RPE). The Talk Test emphasizes exercising at a level in which it is possible to converse without being short of breath. Table 4 illustrates the RPE scales (original and revised) in which exercisers rate the difficulty of exertion (*106*). Moderate intensity exercisers should attempt to stay in the 12–14 (somewhat hard–original scale) or 3–5 (somewhat strong–revised scale) range on these continuums during activity. Individuals may find the revised RPE scale easier to comprehend.

Table 4
Borg Rating of Perceived Exertion Scales

	Original		Revised
6		0	Nothing at all
7	Very, very light	0.5	Very, very weak
8		1	Very weak
9	Very light	2	Weak
10		3	Moderate
11	Fairly light	4	Somewhat strong
12		5	Strong
13	Somewhat hard	6	
14		7	Very strong
15	Hard	8	
16		9	
17	Very hard	10	Very, very strong
18		•	Maximal
19	Very, very hard		
20			

The types of physical activities suggested are as important as the other components of an exercise program. Important activity selection considerations include safety, enjoyment, effectiveness, and accessibility. Table 5, adapted by Buskirk *(60)*, lists activities of various aerobic quality and their respective caloric expenditure values for a 10-min time period. Cardiovascular-based activities (as opposed to strengthening/ toning exercises) should be emphasized first because of their more direct effect on caloric expenditure. Non-weight-bearing and nonimpact modes of cardiovascular activity are important to consider because of reduced risk of musculoskeletal injuries. For many, walking should be encouraged because no special equipment is required (except for proper shoes), and it can easily be incorporated into the daily routine. Regardless of which activities the individual chooses, the health professional should be sure to encourage a variety of exercises (cross-training) to decrease the chance of overuse injury and/or mental burnout.

Finally, no exercise program recommendation would be complete without an explanation of the reasons for proper warm-up and cool-down. If the patient understands that warming up decreases early muscle stiffness and the likelihood of injury, the individual is more apt to comply. An effective warm-up period of 5 to 10 min should consist of very low intensity exercise that slowly mimics the chosen form of activity. This is followed by 10 to 15 min of stretching of the affected muscle groups. The cool-down, on the other hand, helps to prevent postexercise dizziness, caused by pooling of blood in the extremities, and lessens the likelihood of delayed onset muscle soreness that so frequently plagues those just getting started in an exercise program. On completion of exercise, the individual should remain active at a low intensity until the heart rate approaches or falls below 100 beats per minute. Postexercise stretching of the muscles used in the activity (holding each stretch 10–30 s) not only helps decrease muscle stiffness, but also promotes flexibility.

By assessing the patient's health and assisting with the setting of realistic exercise program goals and guidelines, the health professional can increase the odds of success for anyone who has decided to lose weight and improve their quality of life using exercise as a means to an end.

Table 5
Calories Expended During 10 Min of Various Physical Activities [a]

Activity	Body weight in kg (lb)	Calories expended in 10 min				
		56.8 125	68 150	80 175	91 200	113.6 250
Sitting quietly		10	12	14	16	20
Domestic housework		34	41	47	53	68
Walking downstairs		56	67	78	88	111
Walking upstairs		146	175	202	229	288
Walking (2 mph) [b]		29	35	40	46	58
Walking (4 mph)		52	62	72	81	102
Jogging (5.5 mph)		90	108	125	142	178
Running (7 mph)		118	141	164	187	232
Cycling (5.5 mph)		42	50	58	67	83
Cycling (13 mph)		89	107	124	142	178
Mowing grass (power)		34	41	47	53	67
Mowing grass (manual)		38	45	52	58	74
Chopping wood		60	73	84	96	121
Bowling (nonstop)		56	67	78	90	111
Dancing (moderate)		35	42	48	55	69
Dancing (vigorous)		48	57	66	75	94
Golfing (walk)		33	40	48	55	68
Skiing (cross-country)		98	117	138	158	194
Swimming (moderate crawl)		40	48	56	63	80

[a] Approximate values for activities that can be undertaken by many obese individuals. Values will vary with rate of exercise and efficiency with which the activity is performed. Interposition and extrapolation can be used for subject's actual weight (Adapted from ref. *60*, with permission from Lippincott, Williams & Wilkins.)

[b] Conversion factor mph to km • hr^{-1}: multiply by 1.6093.

4. IDENTIFYING AND OVERCOMING BARRIERS TO EXERCISE

Just as individuals vary in their health needs and interests, they adjust their actual and perceived abilities to accomplish their goals. Exercise excuses may signal uncertainty about whether physical activity is worth the time and effort and/or frustration over previous unsuccessful attempts. The health professional can assist the patient in gaining insight into the value of physical activity by asking the individual to consider and focus on the potential benefits to be derived from such an endeavor. For the obese patient these benefits may include both physical and psychological improvements (*see* Subheading 2.). An individual's concern regarding lack of desired results from earlier exercise programs is best handled by a discussion of inefficiencies of previous programs and starting anew armed with the proper knowledge (i.e., goals and guidelines) to make it work. A reminder that it took some time to gain weight and/or become out of shape, and that some results may be slow to realize, is prudent. Impatience and faulty expectations are the seeds of doubt that allow other obstacles to present themselves.

Table 6
Barriers to Exercise

Exercise programs may be difficult to start and/or maintain owing to a lack of the following:

• Time	• Convenience
• Support	• Enjoyment
• Self-esteem/confidence	• Program direction
• Knowledge regarding exercise (myths)	• Being injured/illness-free
• Energy	• Program success

There is no way to remove all roadblocks to physical activity before they appear. A survey of nonexercisers regarding reasons for their inactive lifestyle is likely to yield a wide range of responses from "too tired" to "bad knees." Table 6 lists some of the more frequent barriers to exercise. The health professional can play a critical role in the exercise program start-up and maintenance process by helping the patient identify the potential obstacles to success, and then assisting him or her with viable options to overcome those roadblocks. Table 7 lists 10 common barriers and possible solutions.

Anticipating and preparing for obstacles to regular exercise improves the odds of success. However, barriers to physical activity are varied and unpredictable. Thus, barriers need to be reassessed periodically. Occasional crises and relapses should be expected, but not considered failures. Resume and/or modify activity as soon as each situation allows. The best advice is to be flexible, patient, and persistent.

Regular physical activity is an essential part of any weight-management plan. Health improvements can be realized and maintained if consideration is given to individual needs and interests, as well as the setting of appropriate goals and exercise program guidelines. A discussion of potential roadblocks and options to overcome those barriers increases the probability that the aforementioned plans are carried out and the objectives met. In short, physical activity and exercise play a large role in the treatment of obesity. But without proper eating habits, physical activity, and exercise, patients may never reach their full potential.

5. THE ROLE OF PROPER NUTRITION

Proper nutrition is vital for sustaining life, preventing chronic disease, and treating and managing many medical conditions including obesity. Health care providers need to be at the forefront of providing appropriate education, support, and referrals to specialists to help overweight patients. Long-term nutrition, activity, behavioral, and lifestyle modification should be emphasized for effective weight loss and long-term weight management.

There are a multitude of fad and commercial diets available that promote quick weight loss. However, most of these diets are typically difficult to maintain, lack important nutrients, may be unhealthy and potentially harmful, and are not specific to an individual's nutritional, energy, or lifestyle needs. Unfortunately, long-term outcome data show that most people who lose weight regain the weight lost within 5 yr *(107)*. Reported weight losses that remain after 4 to 5 yr are about 3 to 6% of initial body weight *(108)*.

Table 7
Patient's Barriers to Exercise and Possible Solutions

Barrier	Solutions:
1. *No time* to exercise because of work and/or family obligations.	Exercise and socializing need not be mutually exclusive. Try exercising with family, friends, and coworkers to accomplish multiple objectives; schedule exercise into the day like any other appointment or meeting; exercise first thing in the morning before the day becomes too busy or fatigue becomes a factor.
2. *Not convenient* because of lack of fitness center, frequent travel, or vacation.	Because exercise minutes can have an accumulated effect, seek opportunities to incorporate physical activity into the daily routine. For example, take the stairs instead of the elevator or park further away from a destination; select health clubs that are on the way to and from work; choose activities like walking that can be done almost anytime or anywhere; inquire about workout facilities and/or nearby parks when making hotel arrangements.
3. *Lack of support* or too many distractions to stay committed.	The buddy system is very effective in keeping exercisers on track. Join a group or find a friend with similar goals; make an agreement to exercise. This helps to keep both parties honest when other options or diversions arise.
4. *Boredom/lack of enjoyment* makes exercise undesirable and easy to put off.	Make it fun! Read, listen to music/books on tape, watch TV or movies; change scenery and/or vary the routine; engage in conversation to pass the time.
5. *Embarrassment* from being out of shape, exercising in front of others, and/or not hav -ing or being able to wear the right clothes.	Remind yourself for whom you're doing this: you. Don't worry about competing with others, but instead concentrate on your goals. Find a friend with similar objectives for mutual encouragement; wear comfortable clothes; exercise at times when the fitness center is less busy if privacy is still an issue.
6. *Lack of direction* or structure in the exercise program.	Don't hesitate to seek assistance from qualified health professionals regarding exercise program development (goals and guidelines). After all, it is their job and there are no stupid questions where your health and fitness are concerned; check back with the exercise specialist periodically to update your goals and program as needed.
7 *"No pain, no gain"* (and other myths) make exercise less than appealing.	Again, discuss concerns and questions with a health professional to clear up misperceptions regarding exercise. For example, as stated earlier, even moderate intensity exercise can yield positive health results. In other words, it doesn't have to hurt to be effective.
8. *Injury and/or illness* won't allow for the development of a regular exercise program.	Listen to your body and if frequent or chronic injuries occur, seek assistance from your physician or sports medicine specialist; vary the exercise routine to avoid overuse injuries; verify that the proper technique is being used during exercise; replace shoes if excessively worn; examine your daily lifestyle –(i.e., sleep habits, physical and/or mental work environment, and diet patterns) for clues to possible causes of the problem(s).
9. *Not a priority:* too lazy and/or tired to exercise.	List the potential benefits to be gained from exercise and post them to remind you of your goals; low energy may be a sign that stamina needs improvement. Exercising may decrease early or chronic fatigue and permit even more daily activity; keep a bag packed with exercise clothes by the door ready for the next day.
10. *Lack of success* in previous attempts, resulting in dissatisfaction and disenchantment with physical activity.	Consult a health professional regarding the setting and updating of appropriate goals, exercise guidelines, and program development; start slowly and increase activity gradually; keep an exercise log to review your accomplishments; seek periodic health and fitness assessments to measure progress; be patient, as results may take time to realize.

This reiterates that physicians should not only emphasize the health benefits of marginal weight loss but also the necessity for long-term weight maintenance of weight loss, prevention of weight gain, and sustaining an active, nutritious, health-conscience lifestyle. Overweight patients need to transition from the strict diet notion to recognizing that they have choices, can eat a variety of foods, feel satisfied, continue to dine out, and still experience weight loss without unreasonably strict dieting.

Diet remains the foundation of weight-loss therapy for the obese adult because caloric restriction (via dietary modification) produces far greater energy deficit than exercise alone. Most overweight patients will express that they know what to eat and they are experts at dieting, but most really do not understand the principles promoting a calorie deficit that results in weight loss. A starting point for initiating dietary changes would be basic patient education on calorie balance and caloric density of foods to promote weight loss.

5.1. Answers to Important Questions

It might be prudent to start by defining specific terms and concepts. The following questions and answers are offered for your consideration:

Question: What is a calorie?

Answer: A calorie is a unit used to express the heat or energy value of foods. Calories come from carbohydrates, proteins, fats, and alcohol (a form of carbohydrate) *(109)*.

Question: What is the caloric density of nutrients?

Answer: Carbohydrates contain 4 cal/g, fat contains 9 cal/g, protein contains 4 cal/g, and alcohol contains 7 cal/g. Calories are not only a unit of energy available to the body (via intake) but also a measure of energy that the body uses (expenditure). Overweight individuals need to become aware of the calories they consume and the calories they burn or use through their daily activities and exercise to be more effective at achieving caloric balance and weight loss. Caloric balance refers to the difference between caloric intake and caloric expenditure *(104)*.

Question: How does a person's weight change?

Answer: If caloric intake is greater than the expenditure, the result will be weight gain. If caloric intake is suppressed and the caloric expenditure exceeds caloric intake, then body weight is lost. If caloric intake equals the expenditure, the result will be weight maintenance.

Question: What does it take to lose 1 lb of fat?

Answer: One pound of fat is equivalent to approx 3500 cal of stored energy *(104)*. Weight loss is a process requiring patience and determination. Individuals can lose weight by consuming fewer calories and/or increasing their physical activity. It is best to combine both practices. In order to lose 1 lb of fat, one must create a 3500-calorie deficit. A 500-calorie deficit per d will yield 1 lb of fat loss per wk. Instructing patients on opportunities to control their caloric intake and increase their expenditure through activity can help them understand the calorie balance and weight-loss principles. The following example demonstrates this principle. A woman ate an English muffin instead of a Danish, thereby saving 300 cal. The same woman walked 2 miles, thus expending 200 calories. On this d, the woman created a 500-calorie deficit from her usual daily caloric balance. If these dietary and activity modifications and other behaviors are established and maintained over a period of time, the calorie deficit will accumulate and the result will provide the desired weight loss. A 500-calorie deficit every day for 1 wk will result in a 3500-cal deficit and yield a 1-lb fat loss at the end of the week. Patients need to be reminded of the little dietary and activity changes that can yield big results in weight loss.

Question: How many calories do individuals need in a day?

Answer: Individuals' caloric needs vary and depend on body weight, amount of body fat and muscle mass, level of physical activity, genetic factors, medical conditions, and need for weight gain, maintenance, or loss. Caloric needs can be calculated in a variety of ways. A quick method of estimating caloric needs is by multiplying body weight by a set number based on weight status and activity level. For example, total daily energy needs based on weight and activity level can be arrived at by adhering to the following guidelines. For overweight individuals who are

- sedentary, 20–25 cal/kg body weight
- moderately active, 30 cal/kg
- active, 35 cal/kg.

For normal weight individuals who are

- sedentary, 30 cal/kg
- moderately active, 35cal/kg
- active, 40 cal/kg *(110)*.

Example: A 45-yr-old woman who is 5'4" and weighs 196 lb (89 kg) is considered obese. She has a sedentary job, typing at a computer, and does not partake in any structured exercise. She is classified as being sedentary. To determine her caloric needs multiply her weight of 89 kg × 20 to 25 calories/kg, which equals 1780 to 2225 cal.

- Her energy needs are 1780 to 2225 cal/d to maintain her current weight status.

In order to promote weight loss, an individually designed meal plan (diet prescription) that takes into account the patient's weight status should be designed to promote a deficit of 500 to 1000 cal/d to facilitate a healthy, safe weight loss of 1 to 2 lb per wk *(111)*.

Because a physician's time with patients may be limited and there is an inability to address all dietary and weight-management issues, referring overweight patients to a registered dietitian can be of value and provide a more comprehensive approach to facilitating weight loss. A registered dietitian is skilled at assessing a patient's usual dietary and caloric intake and daily expenditure along with determining appropriate, realistic, and more defined calorie goals, providing individualized meal plans, and resources to guide the patient in establishing new, healthier eating and activity habits. The following information on various calorie levels of diets can assist you when patients inquire about diets or when you need to initiate a discussion on various dietary options for weight loss.

Question: Which diets and calorie ranges are most effective?

Answer: The calorie-reduced diet or balanced deficit diet.

A calorie-reduced diet is designed to promote a 500 to1000 cal deficit daily from a patient's estimated energy expenditure. This type of diet was provided in the example previously described in which a 500 to 1000 cal deficit per d would promote a 1- to 2-lb weight loss per wk. These diets generally provide 1200 or more calories/d and can be nutritionally adequate and should include servings from the five major food groups *(112)*. Calorie-reduced diets focus on portion control, counting calories, dietary balance, and limiting fat to 25 to 30% of the total calories. Patients must recognize the importance of reducing calories and not just fat intake or minimal weight loss will occur *(111)*. Many people attempt a calorie-reduced diet on their own, lose weight slowly and healthfully, and may need little or no medical supervision while on this diet.

Question: Now that I have achieved my weight loss goal, am I done?

Answer: Overweight is a chronic condition. After initial weight loss, patients who were overweight tend to gradually regain weight as they gradually return to their prior behaviors. As a consequence, weight maintenance requires continuing efforts to maintain the new behaviors, including improved dietary habits and increased activity and exercise that were required to lose weight initially.

5.2. The Low-Calorie Diet

Low-calorie diets provide approx 800–1200 cal/d *(113)*. These diets may include regular foods, whereas others may incorporate fortified meal replacements. Low-calorie diets may include but are not limited to low-fat/high-carbohydrate, high-protein/low-carbohydrate, portion controlled, specific patterns, and restriction of one type of food or food groups *(113)*. A multivitamin and mineral supplement is warranted to meet the nutritional needs of the patient and to provide replacements for the micronutrients lacking in the low-calorie diet. Combined intervention of a low-calorie diet, increased physical activity, and behavior therapy provides the most successful therapy for weight loss and weight maintenance. Low-calorie diets can decrease one's weight by an average of 8% over 3 to 12 mo of treatment *(111)*. Behavioral counseling, group support, nutrition and exercise education, and medical management should be part of the treatment protocol for patients on a low-calorie diet program for long-term weight-maintenance success.

5.3. The Very Low-Calorie Diet

Very low-calorie diets (VLCDs) provide approx 400 to 800 cal/d and are protein-sparing modified fasts *(114)*. The VLCD (*see* Chapter 15) is often consumed in a liquid, high-protein, low-carbohydrate form. These diets promote rapid weight loss and should only be used with obese clients and are contraindicated for patients with renal, hepatic disease, psychological disturbances, insulin-dependent diabetes, alcoholism, cardiac disease, and cholecystitis *(115)*. Patients should be informed of the risks associated with the VLCD and that even though most patients will experience significant weight losses, their chances for long-term maintenance of the weight loss is unlikely *(116)*. A skilled physician specializing in treatment of obesity should medically monitor patients frequently and review laboratory tests and medical changes weekly. Treatment with this restrictive calorie level should not exceed 12 to 16 wk and must include a period of 4 to 6 wk of gradual refeeding and reintroduction of solid foods and carbohydrates *(114,117)*. Psychological counseling, group support, nutrition and exercise education, and medical management along with long-term weight-maintenance support should be part of the treatment protocol for patients on a VLCD program.

5.4. Achieving Success

When patients decide to lose weight, both physician and patient must be realistic in their weight loss expectations and focus on long-term behavior, dietary, and activity modification. A reasonable, initial goal for weight loss is a reduction of 10% body weight from baseline weight over 6 mo of therapy *(111)*. There will be many issues to address with your patients such as one's readiness for commitment to weight loss, motivation for losing weight, potential barriers to success, such as time and financial constraints, and physical or psychological issues, current or lack of knowledge, and support system *(114)*. These issues should guide your approach and rapport with the overweight patient and help you define whether you should counsel the patient by recommending simple dietary or activity modifications or refer to a registered dietitian or comprehensive weight-management program. Having educational materials on nutrition, activity and weight management to provide to the patient along with referral to proper ancillary staff and effective programs will demonstrate your concern regarding the patient's weight and health. There are many resources available to physicians and the overweight patient, such as registered dietitians specializing in obesity treatment, calorie counters, food and activity diaries, American Diabetes Association Exchange Lists for Weight Management, low-fat, low-calorie cookbooks, self-help books, reputable nutrition and weight management websites (*see* Chapter 23), comprehensive clinical weight management programs, commercial weight loss programs, local hospitals, fitness facilities, state health departments, and national health agencies.

Weight loss provides many health benefits. However, the emphasis should no longer be on weight loss solely, but should also focus on long-term maintenance of weight loss. At this time, a successful program is one that succeeds in helping patients maintain a weight loss of at least 5% or 6 kg of body weight long term *(118)*. Physicians can instill motivation and knowledge so overweight patients feel empowered to apply knowledge learned about proper nutrition and weight-management principles, self-control strategies, behavioral modification, and activity. Physicians should help patients succeed with initial weight loss and help them to maintain successful behaviors to maintain weight loss over a long period of time.

6. CONCLUSION

The health benefits of exercise include reduction in CHD risk factors, improved cardiovascular and respiratory function, reduced colon cancer risk, and enhanced psychological well-being.

The first stage in the health professional's role in treating obesity through physical activity, exercise, and proper nutrition is to explain the benefits of an active lifestyle. Knowledge alone, however, is not likely to lead to permanent lifestyle change. The second stage should focus on individualizing an exercise and nutrition program to meet the person's needs and interests. Roadblocks to positive behavior change can be avoided through a discussion of potential barriers. A combination of regular physical activity and sound eating habits is essential to enhance the chances for achieving a healthful weight. Most importantly, individuals should be encouraged to view physical activity and dietary modifications as a permanent lifestyle behavior, a lifetime goal, not a 12-wk project. The recommendation to "be a tortoise, not a hare" will allow a modest, consistent effort over a long time and will yield satisfying results for those who stay the course.

ACKNOWLEDGMENTS

We wish to acknowledge Jerry Taylor, president of The National Institute for Fitness and Sport for his leadership, vision, and continued support.

REFERENCES

1. NIH (NIDDK). Statistics related to overweight and obesity. Publication no. 96-4158. Website: (http://www.niddk.nih.gov/health/nutrit/pubs/statobes.htm).
2. Flegal KM, Carroll MD, Kuczmarski RJ, Johnson CL. Overweight and obesity in the United States: prevalence and trends. Int J Obes 1998; 22:39–47.
3. Allison DB, Fontaine KR, et al. Annual deaths attributable to obesity in the United States. JAMA 1999; 282:1530–1538.
4. Wolf AM, Colditz GA. Current estimates of the economic cost of obesity in the United States. Obes Res 1998; 6:97–106.
5. Caspersen CJ, Powell KE, Christenson GM. Physical activity, exercise, and physical fitness. Public Health Rep 1985; 100:126–131.
6. Pate RR, Pratt M, Blair SN, et al. Physical activity and public health: a recommendation from the Centers for Disease Control and Prevention and the American College of Sports Medicine. JAMA 1995; 273:402–407.
7. American College of Sports Medicine, U.S. Centers for Disease Control and Prevention, in cooperation with the President's Council on Physical Fitness and Sports. Experts release new recommendation to fight America's epidemic of physical inactivity. News Release 1993.
8. National Institutes of Health Consensus Development Conference Statement. Physical Activity and Cardiovascular Health, 1995.
9. Kennedy JF. The soft American. Sports Illustrated 1960; 13.
10. Powell KE, Thompson PD, Caspersen CJ, Kendricks JS. Physical activity and the incidence of coronary heart disease. Ann Rev Public Health 1987; 8:253–287.
11. Berlin JA, Colditz GA. A meta-analysis of physical activity in the prevention of coronary heart disease. Am J Epidemiol 1990; 132:612–628.
12. Manson JE, Hu FB, Rich-Edwards JW, Colditz GA, Stampfer MJ, Willet WC, Speizer FE, Hennekens CH. A prospective study of walking as compared with vigorous exercise in the prevention of coronary heart disease in women. N Engl J Med 1999; 341:650–658.
13. Hill J.O., Wyatt HR, Reed GW, Peters JC. Obesity and the environment: where do we go from here? Science 2003; 299:853–855.
14. Bar-Or O, Foreyt J, Bouchard C, Brownell KD, Dietz WH, Ravussin E, Salbe AD, Schwenger S, St. Jeor S, Torun B. Physical activity, genetic, and nutritional considerations in childhood weight management. Med Sci Sports Exercise 1998; 30:2–10.
15. Morris JN, Heady JA, Raffle PAB, Roberts CG, Parks JW. Coronary heart disease and physical activity of work. Lancet 1953; 2:1053–1057,1111–1120.
16. Leon AS, Connet J, Jacobs DR, Rauramaa R. Leisure-time physical activity levels and risk of coronary heart disease and death: the multiple risk factor intervention trial. JAMA 1987; 258:2388–2395.
17. Paffenbarger RS, Hyde RT, Wing AL, Hsieh C-C. Physical activity, all-cause mortality, and longevity of college alumni. N Engl J Med 1986; 314:605–613.
18. Blair SN, Kohl HW, Barlow CE, Paffenbarger RS, Gibbons LW, Macera CA. Changes in physical fitness and all-cause mortality: a prospective study of healthy men. JAMA 1995; 273:1093–1098.
19. Hakim AA, Petrovitch H, Burchfiel CM, Ross W, Rodriguez BL, White LR, Yano K, Curb JD, Abbott RD. Effects of walking on mortality among nonsmoking retired men. N Eng J Med 1998; 338: 94–99.
20. Fletcher GF, Balady G, Blair SN, Blumenthal J, Caspersen C, Chaitman B, Epstein S, Froelicher ES, Froelicher VF, Pina IL, Pollock ML. Statement on exercise: benefits and recommendation for physical activity programs for all Americans. Circulation 1996; 94:857–862.
21. Galgali G, Beaglehole R, Scragg R, Tobias M. Potential for prevention of premature death and disease in New Zealand. N Z Med J 1998; 111:7–10.

22. Eriksson KF, Lindgarde F. No excess 12-year mortality in men with impaired glucose tolerance who participated in the Malmo Preventive Trial with diet and exercise. Diabetologia 1998; 41:1010–1016.

23. Blair SN, Goodyear NN, Gibbons LW, Cooper KH. Physical fitness and incidence of hypertension in healthy normotensive men and women. JAMA 1984; 252:487–490.

24. Physical exercise in the management of hypertension: a consensus statement by the World Hypertension League. J Hypertens 1991; 9:283–287.

25. Steffen PR, Sherwood A, Gullette EC, Georgiades A, Hinderliter A, Blumenthal JA. Effects of exercise and weight loss on blood pressure during daily life. Med Sci Sports Exerc 2001; 33:1635–1640.

26. Hagberg JM, Park JJ, Brown MD. The role of exercise training in the treatment of hypertension: an update. Sports Med 2000; 30:193–206.

27. Arroll B, Beaglehole R. Does physical activity lower blood pressure?: A critical review of the clinical trials. J Clin Epidemiol 1992; 45:439–447.

28. Kannel WB, Brand N, Skinner JJ, Dawber TR, McNamara P. The relation of adiposity to blood pressure and development of hypertension: the Framingham Study. Ann Intern Med 1967; 67:48–59.

29. The sixth report of the Joint National Committee on prevention, detection, evaluation, and treatment of high blood pressure. Arch Intern Med 1997; 157:2413–2446.

30. The Fifth Report of the Joint National Committee on Detection, Evaluation, and Treatment of High Blood Pressure (JNC–V). Arch Intern Med 1993; 153:154–183.

31. Laporte RE, Adams LL, Savage DD, Brenes G, Dearwater S, Cook T. The spectrum of physical activity, cardiovascular disease, and health: an epidemiologic perspective. Am J Epidemiol 1984; 120:507–517.

32. Kiens B, Jorgensen I, Lewis S, et al. Increased plasma HDL-cholesterol and apo A-I in sedentary middle aged men after physical conditioning. Eur J Clin Invest 1980; 10:203–209.

33. Hanefeld M, Leonhardt W, Julius U, et al. Effects of exercise on hyperlipidemia in obesity. In: Bjorntorp P, Jairella M, Howard AN, eds. Recent Advances in Obesity Research: Third International Congress on Obesity. John Liebe, London, UK, 1981, pp. 348–353.

34. Goldberg L, Elliot DL. The effects of physical activity on lipid and lipoprotein levels. Med Clin North Am 1985; 69:41–55.

35. Tran ZV, Weltman A. Differential effects of exercise on serum lipid and lipoprotein levels seen with changes in body weight: a meta-analysis. JAMA 1985; 254:919–924.

36. Lewis S, Haskell WL, Wood PD, Manoogian N, Bailey JE, Pereira MB. Effects of physical activity on weight reduction in obese middle-aged women. Am J Clin Nutr 1976; 29:151–156.

37. Stefanick ML, Mackey S, Sheehan M, Ellsworth N, Haskell WL, Wood PD. Effects of diet and exercise in men and postmenopausal women with low levels of HDL cholesterol and high levels of LDL cholesterol. N Eng J Med 1998; 339:12–20.

38. Lavie CJ, Milani RV. Effects of cardiac rehabilitation, exercise training, and weight reduction on exercise capacity, coronary risk factors, behavioral characteristics, and quality of life in obese coronary patients. Am J Cardiol 1997; 79:397–401.

39. Forouhi NG, Sattar N, McKeigue PM. Relation of C-reactive protein to body fat distribution and features of the metabolic syndrome in Europeans and South Asians. Int J Obes Relat Metab Disord 2001; 25:1327–1331.

40. Pitsavos C, Chrysohoou C, Panagiotakos DB, et al.. Association of leisure-time physical activity on inflammation markers (C-reactive protein, white cell blood count, serum amyloid A, and fibrinogen) in healthy subjects (from the ATTICA study). Am J Cardiol 2003; 91:368–370.

41. Bjorntorp P, DeJounge K, Krotkiewski M, Sullivan L, Sjostrom L, Stenberg J. Physical training in human obesity. III: effects of long-term physical training on body composition. Metabolism 1973; 22:1467–1474.

42. Lampman RM, Schteingart DE. Moderate and extreme obesity. In: Franklin BA, Gordon S, Timmis GC, eds. Exercise in Modern Medicine. Williams and Wilkins, Baltimore, MD, 1989, pp. 156–174.

43. Weltman A, Mattler S, Stamford BA. Caloric restriction and/or mild exercise: effects on serum lipids and body composition. Am J Clin Nutr 1980; 33:1002–1009.

44. Pavlou KN, Steffe WP, Lerman RH, Burrows BA. Effects of dieting and exercise on lean body mass, oxygen uptake, and strength. Med Sci Sports Exerc 1985; 17:466–471.

45. Hill JO, Sparling PB, Shields TW, Heller PA. Effects of exercise and food restriction on body composition and metabolic rate in obese women. Am J Clin Nutr 1987; 46:622–630.
46. Pritchard JE, Nowson CA, Wark JD. A worksite program for overweight middle-aged men achieves lesser weight loss with exercise than with dietary change. J Am Diet Assoc 1997; 97:583.
47. Miller WC, Koceja DM, Hamilton EJ. A meta-analysis of the past 25 years of weight loss research using diet, exercise or diet plus exercise intervention. Int J Obes Relat Metab Disord 1997; 21: 941–947.
48. Wadden TA, Vogt RA, Foster GD, Anderson DA. Exercise and the maintenance of weight loss: 1-year follow-up of a controlled clinical trial. J Consult Clin Psychol 1998; 66:429–433.
49. Brownell KD, Grilo GM. Weight management. In: American College of Sports Medicine's Resource Manual for the Guidelines for Exercise Testing and Prescription, 2nd Ed. Lea and Febiger, Philadelphia, PA, 1993, pp. 458–459.
50. Bjorntorp P, De Jounge K, Sjostrom L, Sullivan L. The effect of physical training on insulin production in obesity. Metabolism 1970; 19:631–638.
51. Knowler WC, Barrett-Connor E, Fowler SE, Hamman RF, Lachin JM, Walker EA, Nathan DM. Reduction in the incidence of type 2 diabetes with lifestyle intervention or metformin. N Engl J Med 2002; 346:393–403.
52. Hu G, Qiao Q, Silventoinen K, Eriksson JG, Jousilahti P, Lindstrom J, Valle TT, Nissinen A, Toumilehto J. Occupational, commuting, and leisure-time physical activity in relation to risk for type 2 diabetes in middle-aged Finnish men and women. Diabetologia 2003; 46:322–329.
53. Fahlen M, Stenberg J, Bjorntorp P. Insulin secretion in obesity after exercise. Diabetologia 1972; 8: 141–144.
54. Ruderman NB, Ganda OP, Johansen K. The effect of physical training on glucose tolerance and plasma lipids in maturity-onset diabetes. Diabetes 1979; 28(Suppl 1): 89.
55. Brown MD, Moore GE, Korytkowski MT, McCole SD, Hagberg JM. Improvement of insulin sensitivity by short-term exercise training in hypertensive African American women. Hypertension 1997; 30:1549–1553.
56. Snyder KA, Donnelly JE, Jabobsen DJ, Hertner G, Jakicic JM. The effects of long-term, moderate intensity, intermittent exercise an aerobic capacity, body composition, blood lipids, insulin and glucose in overweight females. Int J Obes Relat Metab Disord 1997; 21:1180–1189.
57. Smith ML, Mitchell JH. Cardiorespiratory adaptations to exercise training. In: American College of Sports Medicine's Resource Manual for the Guidelines for Exercise Testing and Prescription, 2nd Ed. Lea and Febiger, Philadelphia, PA, 1993, pp. 75–81.
58. Lampman RM, Schteingart DE, Fossi MI. Exercise as a partial therapy for the extremely obese. Med Sci Sports Exerc 1986; 18:19–24.
59. Buskirk ER, Barlett HL. Pulmonary function and obesity. In: Tobia RB, Mehlman MA, eds. Advances in Modern Human Nutrition. Pathotox, Park Forest South, IL, 1980, pp. 211–224.
60. Buskirk ER. Obesity. In: Skinner JS, ed. Exercise Testing and Exercise Prescription for Special Cases: Theoretical Basis and Clinical Application, 2nd Ed. Lea and Febiger, Philadelphia, PA, 1993, pp. 191–193, p. 200.
61. Emirgil C, Sobel BJ. The effects of weight reduction on pulmonary function and sensitivity of the respiratory center in obesity. Am Rev Respir Dis 1973; 108:831–842.
62. Farebrother MJB, McHardy GJR, Munro JF. Relation between pulmonary gas exchange and closing volume before and after substantial weight loss in obese subjects. Br Med J 1974; 3:391–393.
63. Legere BM, Kavuru MS. Pulmonary function in obesity. Respir Care 2000; 45:967–968.
64. Flemons WW. Clinical practice. Obstructive sleep apnea. N Engl J Med. 2002; 347:498–504.
65. Ferguson KA, Ono T, Lowe AA, Keenan SP, Fleetham JA. A randomized crossover study of an oral appliance vs. nasal-continuous positive airway pressure in the treatment of mild–moderate obstructive sleep apnea. Chest 1996; 109:1269–1275.
66. Hanzel DA, Proia NG, Hudgel DW. Response of obstructive sleep apnea to fluoxetine and protriptyline. Chest 1991; 100:416–421.
67. Berry RB, Yamaura EM, Gill K, Reist C. Acute effects of paroxetine on genioglossus activity in obstructive sleep apnea. Sleep 1999; 22:1087–1092.
68. Bridgman SA, Dunn KM. Cochrane Database. Syst Rev 2000; 2:CD001004.

69. Peppard PE, Young T, Palta M, Dempsey J, Skatrud J. Longitudinal study of moderate weight change and sleep-disordered breathing. JAMA 2000;284:15–21.

70. Sugerman HJ, Fairman RP, Sood RK, Engle K, Wolfe L, Kellum JM. Long-term effects of gastric surgery for treating respiratory insufficiency of obesity. Am J Clin Nutr 1992; 55:597S–601S.

71. Elliot DL, Goldberg L. Exercise and obesity. In: Goldberg L, Elliott DL eds. Exercise for Prevention and Treatment of Illness. F.A. Davis, Philadelphia, PA, 1994, pp. 212–213.

72. Poehlman ET, Melby CL, Badylak SF. Resting metabolic rate and postprandial thermogenesis in highly trained and untrained males. Am J Clin Nutr 1988; 47:793–798.

73. Poehlman ET, Melby CL, Badylak SF, Calles J. Aerobic fitness and resting energy expenditure in young adult males. Metabolism 1989; 38:85–90.

74. Hill JO, Heymsfield SB, McMannus C, DiGirolamo M. Meal size and thermic response to food in male subjects as a function of maximum aerobic capacity. Metabolism 1984; 33:743–749.

75. Bray G. Effect of caloric restriction on energy expenditure in obese subjects. Lancet 1969; 2:397–398.

76. Leibel RL, Rosenbaum M, Hirsch J. Changes in energy expenditure resulting from altered body weight. N Eng J Med 1995; 332:621–628.

77. Saris WH. The role of exercise in the dietary treatment of obesity. Int J Obes 1993; 17(Suppl 1):S17–S21.

78. Geliebter A, Maher MM, Gerace L, Gutin B, Heymsfield SB, Hashim SA. Effects of strength or aerobic training on body composition, resting metabolic rate, and peak oxygen consumption in obese dieting subjects. Am J Clin Nutr 1997; 66:557–63.

79. Dempsey JA. Anthropometrical observations on obese and non-obese young men undergoing a program of vigorous physical exercise. Res Quarterly 1964; 35:275–287.

80. Dudleston AK, Benniou M. Effect of diet and/or exercise on obese college women. J Am Diet Assn 1970; 56:126–129.

81. Oscai LB, Williams BT. Effect of exercise on overweight middle-aged males. J Am Geriatr Soc 1968; 16:794–797.

82. Boileau RA, Buskirk ER, Horstman DH, Mendez J, Nicholas WC. Body compositional changes in obese and lean med during physical conditioning. Med Sci Sports 1971; 3:183–189.

83. Westerterp-Plantenga MS, Verwegen CR, Ijedema MJ, Wijckmans NE, Saris WH. Acute effects of exercise or sauna on appetite in obese and nonobese men. Physiol Behav 1997; 62:1345–1354.

84. Leon AS, Conrad J, Hunninghake DB, Serfass R. Effects of a vigorous walking program on body composition and lipid metabolism of obese young men. Am J Clin Nutr 1979; 33:1776–1787.

85. Pi-Sunyer FX. Effect of exercise on food intake. In: Hirsch J, Van Itallie TB, eds. Recent Advances in Obesity Research, Vol. 4. John Libbey, London, UK, 1985.

86. Calle EE, Rodriguez C, Walker-Thurmond K, Thun MJ. Overweight, obesity, and mortality from cancer in a prospectively studied cohort of U.S. adults. N Engl J Med 2003; 348:1625–1638.

87. Physical Activity and Fitness Research Digest. Physical activity and cancer 1995; 2:1–6.

88. Murphy TK, Calle EE, Rodriguez C, Kahn HS, Thun MJ. Body mass index and colon cancer mortality in a large prospective study. Am J Epidemiol 2000; 152:847–854.

89. Lew EA, Garfinkel L. Variations in mortality by weight among 750,000 men and women. J Chron Dis 1979; 32:563–576.

90. Bernstein L. Henderson BE, Hanisch R, Sullivan-Halley J, Ross RK. Physical exercise and reduced risk of breast cancer in young women. J Natl Cancer Inst 1994; 86: 1403–1408.

91. Gilliland FD, Li YF, Baumgartner K, Crumley D, Samet JM. Physical activity and breast cancer risk in hispanic and non-hispanic white women. Am J Epidemiol 2001; 154:442–450.

92. Friedenreich CM, Courneya KS, Bryant HE. Influence of physical activity in different age and life periods on the risk of breast cancer. Epidemiol 2001; 12:604–612.

93. Sinyor D, Schwartz SG, Peronnet F, Brisson G, Seraganian P. Aerobic fitness level and reactivity to psychosocial stress: physiological, biochemical and subjective measures. Psychosomat Med 1983; 45: 205–217.

94. Keller S, Seraganian P. Physical fitness level and automatic reactivity to psychosocial stress. J of Psychosomat Res 1984; 28:279–287.

95. Tucker LA, Cole GE, Friedman GM. Physical fitness: a buffer against stress. Percep Mot Skill 1986; 63:955–961.

 96. Crews DJ, Landers, DM. A meta-analytic review of aerobic fitness and reactivity to psychosocial stressors. Med Sci Sports Exerc 1987; 19:S114–120.
 97. Brownell KD, Stunkard AJ. Physical activity in the development and control of obesity. In Stunkard AJ, ed. Obesity. WB Saunders, Philadelphia, PA, 1980, pp. 300–324.
 98. Horton ES. The role of exercise in the prevention and treatment of obesity. In: Bray GA, ed. Obesity in Perspective, Vol. 2, Part 1. DHEW Publication No. [NIH]75—708). US Government Printing Office, Washington, DC, 1975, pp. 62–66.
 99. Mahoney KB. Adipose cellularity as a predictor of responsiveness to treatment of obesity. PhD dissertation. Pennsylvania State University, University Park, PA, 1977.
100. Wilson GT, Brownell KD. Behavior therapy for obesity: an evaluation of treatment outcome. Adv Behav Res Ther 1980; 3:49–86.
101. Mattsson E, Larsson UE, Rossner S. Is walking for exercise too exhausting for obese women? Int J Obes Rel Metab Disorders 1997; 21:380–386.
102. Rikli RE, McManis BG. Effects of exercise on bone mineral content in post menopausal women. Res Quart Exerc Sport 1990; 61:243.
103. Perri MG, Martin AD, Leermakers EA, Sears SF, Notelovitz M. Effects of group-versus home-based exercise in the treatment of obesity. J Consult Clin Psychol 1997; 65:278–285.
104. American College of Sports Medicine. ACSM's Guidelines for Exercise Testing and Prescription, 6th Ed. Lippincott, Williams and Wilkins, Philadelphia, PA, 2000, pp. 12–26,153–175, 211, 214–216.
105. Foster GD, Wadden TA, Phelan S, Sarwer DB, David B, Sanderson RS. Obese patients' perceptions of treatment outcomes and the factors that influence them. Arch Intern Med 2001; 161:2133–2139.
106. Borg GAV. Psychophysical bases of perceived exertion. Med Sci Sports Exerc 1982; 14:377–381.
107. Wadden TA, Sternberg JA, Letizia KA, Stunkard AJ, Foster GD. Treatment of obesity by very low calorie diet, behavior therapy, and their combination: a five year perspective. Int J Obes 1989; 13: S39–46.
108. Anderson JW, Hontz EC, Frederich RC, Wood CL. Long-term weight-loss maintenance: a meta analysis of US studies. Am J Clin Nutr 2001; 74:579–584.
109. American Dietetic Association. American Diabetes Assoc. Exchange Lists for Weight Management. American Dietetic Association, Chicago, IL, 2003, p. 40
110. Manual of Clinical Dietetics, 5th Ed. American Dietetic Association, Chicago, IL, 1996, p. 17.
111. NIH Clinical Guidelines on the Identification, Evaluation, and Treatment of Overweight and Obesity in Adult—the Evidence Report. Publication no. 98-4083. National Heart, Lung, and Blood Institute, Bethesda, MD, 1998; pp. 75, 95.
112. Institute of Medicine. Weighing the Options, Criteria for Evaluating Weight-Management Programs. National Academy Press, Washington, DC, 1995; p. 81, pp. 108–109.
113. Bray GA. Contemporary diagnosis and management of obesity. Handbooks in Healthcare, Newtown, PA, 1998, pp. 219–223.
114. American Dietetic Association. Position of the American Dietetic Association: Weight Management. JADA 2002; 102:1150.
115. Wadden T, Itallie T, Blackburn G. Responsible and irresponsible use of very low calorie diets in treatment of obesity. JAMA 1990; 263:83–85.
116. National Task Force on the Prevention and Treatment of Obesity, National Institutes of Health. Very low-calorie diets. JAMA 1993; 119:688–698.
117. ADA. Manual of Clinical Dietetics, 6th Ed. American Dietetic Association, Chicago, IL, 2000, p. 374.
118. NIH Clinical Guidelines on the Identification, Evaluation, and Treatment of Overweight and Obesity in Adult–the Evidence Report. Obes Res 1998; 6:111S.

14 Lifestyle Modification in the Treatment of Obesity

Anthony N. Fabricatore and Thomas A. Wadden

KEY POINTS

- Lifestyle modification techniques are being extended and applied in new ways.
- The first step in lifestyle modification is a behavioral assessment. This is summarized as BEST: *b*iological, *e*nvironmental, *s*ocial-psychological, and *t*emporal factors as they relate to weight control.
- Goals and options need to be determined
- Lifestyle modification involves behavior therapy, dietary intervention, and increasing activity.
- Behavior therapy consists of self-monitoring, stimulus control, problem solving, slowing the rate of eating, and cognitive restructuring.
- Weight loss achieved with lifestyle modification is associated with significant reductions in health risks.

1. INTRODUCTION

The World Health Organization has labeled obesity a global epidemic *(1)*. In the United States, the prevalence of obesity (body mass index [BMI] ≥ 30 kg/m^2) doubled from 15% in 1980 to 30% in 2000 *(2)*. Despite the recent discovery of genetic factors that regulate body weight, an increase of this magnitude cannot be attributed to changes in our genes. The eating and activity habits of Americans have changed significantly during that time period and are the more likely culprits behind the nation's fattening. Some have labeled ours a "toxic environment," characterized by heavily advertised and readily available high-calorie foods, large portion sizes, and technological advances that implicitly discourage physical activity *(3)*.

A variety of weight-loss options are available for overweight and obese persons. The National Heart, Lung, and Blood Institute (NHLBI), in conjunction with the North American Association for the Study of Obesity (NAASO), has recommended that all individuals begin with a program of lifestyle modification, consisting of behavior

From: *The Management of Eating Disorders and Obesity, Second Edition*
Edited by: D. J. Goldstein © Humana Press Inc., Totowa, NJ

Table 1
Chapter Overview

therapy, diet, and exercise *(4)*. This chapter discusses the goals and methods of lifestyle modification, its short- and long-term results, and recent efforts to maximize its success (Table 1). First, we briefly review the rationale and guidelines for conducting a brief behavioral assessment of individuals who seek weight reduction.

2. BEHAVIORAL ASSESSMENT

Results of a comprehensive behavioral evaluation guide the selection of appropriate goals and interventions. During this assessment, which requires about 1 hr, the clinician

Table 2
Comprehensive Behavioral Assessment (BEST)

B	*Biological factors: Helps in setting reasonable goal weight*	
	• Family history	• Onset of obesity
	• Weights at 5-yr intervals	• Dieting history
E	*Environmental influences*	
	• Eating habits	• Physical activity
S	*Social/psychological status*	
	• Mood	• Daily functioning
	• Coping resources	• Quality of life
T	*Temporal factors*	
	• Motivating factors	• Life stressors

evaluates *B*iological, *E*nvironmental, *S*ocial/psychological, and *T*emporal factors as they relate to weight control. The evaluation permits the selection of the most appropriate treatment plan for the particular individual. Hence, this process is summarized by the acronym BEST Treatment (*see* Table 2). A more detailed description of the evaluation is available elsewhere *(5)*. The assessment is best conducted by a mental health professional, although it can be completed by physicians, nurses, or dietitians who have access to psychiatric consultation when needed.

2.1. B: Biological Factors

Individuals with a biological predisposition to obesity may be "fighting an uphill battle" in trying to lose weight. Childhood/adolescent onset of obesity, a positive family history of this disorder, and a marked history of weight loss and regain (i.e., weight cycling) suggest a genetic predisposition. Other physical factors, including the use of steroidal medications and the presence of hypothyroidism or polycystic ovarian syndrome, also may contribute to an individual's weight problem.

Knowledge of these biological factors, in conjunction with body weights at various milestones, is useful for selecting weight-loss goals. Patients lose weight with lifestyle modification, but rarely achieve the goal weights they desire *(6)*. As a rule, the goal weight should be no lower than the lowest weight since age 21 that the patient has maintained for 1 yr or more without illness or dieting. In most cases, patients will be fortunate to lose 10 to 15% of their initial weight.

2.2. E: Environmental Influences

George Bray succinctly summarized the roles of nature and nurture in the development of obesity, noting "genes load the gun, the environment pulls the trigger" *(7)*. Thus, the behavioral assessment also includes an evaluation of environmental factors, which include patients' eating and activity habits.

Eating habits are best assessed by having patients record their food and beverage intake for several days before the interview *(5)*. The goal is to determine the general composition of the diet, the approximate calorie content, and the individual's pattern of eating. Patients should be instructed to consume their usual diet, although some dietary restraint may occur as a result of recording.

Binge-eating disorder (*see* Chapter 11) occurs in about 2% of the general population, but in approx 30% of obese individuals who seek weight reduction *(8)*. This disorder should be assessed by asking whether patients have occasions on which they eat, in a brief period of time, large amounts of food (i.e., which would be considered large by others) and feel out of control while doing so *(8)*. Two questionnaires also may be used to assess binge eating *(9,10)*. Binge eating can be treated by methods including cognitive–behavioral therapy that specifically targets that behavior *(11)* or antidepressant medications *(12)*. Binge eating is associated with significant mood disturbances and other psychopathology *(13)*. Obese binge eaters, therefore, may require more structure and emotional support during weight loss than do obese non-binge eaters. Treatment of binge eating, however, does not appear to be a necessary precursor to success in a behavioral weight-loss program. Gladis et al.*(14)* reported that binge eaters lost more weight in their lifestyle modification program than did non-binge eaters.

The patient's level of physical activity also should be assessed. Clinicians can obtain a complete picture by inquiring not only about programmed activity (i.e., participation in recreational sports or "working out") but also about daily lifestyle activity (i.e., walking and stair use). A pedometer is an inexpensive device that registers the number of steps walked in a day and provides a useful estimate of patients' lifestyle activity. Many obese individuals state that they are unable to complete programmed exercise as a result of weight-related complications, including severe pain in weight-bearing joints and shortness of breath. They also may express frustration because previous attempts to increase activity did not result in significant weight reductions. Clinicians should meet patients' reports with empathy and educate them about the relative contributions of reduced energy intake and increased energy expenditure to weight control.

Patients often describe their eating and exercise habits with shame or embarrassment. Their distress should be greeted with reassurance that they can learn new eating and exercise behaviors. The most challenging cases are those in which patients report exemplary eating and activity habits and yet are substantially overweight. Assessment of resting energy expenditure is useful in such cases to verify the patient's report of low energy intake.

2.3. S: Social/Psychological Status

Obese persons seeking weight-loss therapy report greater psychological distress than comparably obese persons who do not seek treatment *(15)*. Estimates of the prevalence of depressive disorders among treatment-seeking obese individuals range from a modest 9.2% to a full 47.5% *(13)*. Major depression and related disturbances require separate treatment. Care must be taken to distinguish clinically significant pathology from periodic sadness and stress reactions. Thus, the practitioner should inquire about not only the patient's mood, but also the extent to which symptoms interfere with family, social, and occupational functioning and the individual's enjoyment of activities. Patient self-rated tests, such as the Beck Depression Inventory, Second Edition *(16)*, provide an excellent method of screening. Clinicians should be aware, however, that scores on depression scales may be inflated because of the presence of obesity-related conditions. For example, patients may report sleep disturbances or fatigue, which are both symptoms of depression but may be better accounted for by sleep apnea.

In addition to mood, it is important to assess patients' health-related quality of life. Numerous studies have shown that obese individuals experience limitations in their physical or social functioning, despite having normal mental health *(17–18)*. Assessment of quality of life may reveal areas for intervention, independent of weight loss.

2.4. T: Temporal Factors

Most patients who seek weight reduction have been overweight for years. Thus, practitioners should seek to understand why the patient has decided to lose weight at this time *(5)*. The prompt is often a source of distress (e.g., a doctor's warning, a spouse's "nagging") and may be important for gauging the patient's motivation to lose weight. The discovery of a weight-related illness (e.g., diabetes, hypertension) is likely to be a stronger motivator than is the insistence of friends or family members that the patient "really should lose some weight."

Patient and provider also should determine whether it is a favorable time to attempt weight loss. Losing weight takes time and effort. Thus, the patient should be relatively free of major life stressors for the next few months. One study found that the higher the stress level (i.e., new job, financial problems, family illness, etc.), the greater the likelihood of attrition from therapy *(19)*. During difficult times, patients should strive to maintain their weight (i.e., neither gaining nor losing) and begin treatment when their level of stress becomes more manageable.

3. TREATMENT

Obese individuals frequently enter weight-loss therapy with hopes of losing 25% or more of their initial weight and improving their lives socially, emotionally, or professionally. The behavioral assessment should conclude with a discussion of patients' goals and the extent to which these goals are realistic.

3.1. Goals

We usually assess desired changes in four areas: weight, health and mobility, appearance and body image, and social life and self-esteem. Based on findings discussed later in this chapter, we suggest that patients expect a weight loss of approx 8–10% of initial weight when treated by lifestyle modification and 10–15% when treated by this therapy combined with medication *(20,21)*. These losses are usually far smaller than those desired by significantly obese persons, who maintain their high expectations despite education about the biological and behavioral mechanisms that render their "dream weights" difficult to attain *(22)*. Although most individuals experience improvements in mood with weight loss *(14,23)*, patients who hope to resolve psychosocial problems through weight loss should be encouraged to take additional steps to meet their goals (e.g., psychotherapy or pharmacotherapy for depression, couples therapy for marital distress).

3.2. Options

The patient's BMI and the medical need for weight reduction—as judged by the presence of comorbid conditions or other risk factors—are key determinants in selecting

Table 3
A Guide to Selecting Treatment

Treatment	BMI category				
	25–26.9	27–29.9	30–34.9	35–39.9	≥40
Diet, physical activity, and behavior therapy	WC	WC	+	+	+
Pharmacotherapy		WC	+	+	+
Surgery				WC	

WC, With comorbidities.

Note. Prevention of weight gain with lifestyle therapy is indicated in any patient with a BMI ≥25 kg/m², even without comorbidities, whereas weight loss is not necessarily recommended for those with a BMI of 25–29.9 kg/m² or a high waist circumference unless they have two or more comorbidities. Combined therapy with a low-calorie diet, increased physical activity, and behavior therapy provide the most successful intervention for weight loss and weight maintenance. Consider pharmacotherapy only if a patient has not lost 1 lb/wk after 6 mo of combined lifestyle therapy. The + represents the use of indicated treatment regardless of comorbidities. (Reprinted from ref. *4*.)

the most appropriate weight-loss option. Table 3 presents a conceptual scheme for selecting treatment. According to NHLBI/NAASO treatment guidelines *(4)*, all persons with a BMI ≥30 kg/m² should first be treated by a comprehensive lifestyle modification program. Those unsuccessful with this approach may be treated, in addition, by pharmacotherapy *(see* Chapter 16). Extremely obese patients, with a BMI ≥40 kg/m² (or ≥35 kg/m² plus two or more comorbidities), have the option of bariatric surgery *(see* Chapter 20).

4. LIFESTYLE MODIFICATION

Lifestyle modification is comprised of behavior therapy, dietary intervention, and physical activity. Each of these three components is described below. As is seen here, behavior therapy provides a set of principles and techniques for adopting different diet and activity regimens.

4.1. Behavior Therapy

Behavioral treatment examines not only eating and exercise behaviors but also the antecedents and consequences of these behaviors. Once antecedents of problem behaviors (e.g., overeating) are identified, steps are taken to control or modify those events. For example, a man who consistently snacks on high-calorie foods while watching television would be encouraged to confine his eating to the kitchen, thereby extinguishing the association between the television and snacking. Consequences are assessed to determine the function of behaviors. Behaviors that are reinforced (with pleasant consequences or the removal of unpleasant consequences) are more likely to be repeated than are behaviors that are punished (with unpleasant consequences).

For instance, a woman who attempts to increase from no activity to 300 min/wk of vigorous exercise, is likely to experience physical exhaustion and soreness. Such consequences would make her less likely to continue to exercise. If she had begun her activity regimen more modestly (e.g., walking 10 min/d, 5 d/wk), she might feel successful and, thus, be motivated to continue exercising. A pilot study suggested that increasing patients' focus on the consequences of their behavioral choices may be beneficial in long-term weight control *(24)*.

Behavior therapy has been distilled into several principal components. Brownell has presented the principles and techniques of behavior therapy in a user-friendly format, the LEARN Program for Weight Management 2000 *(25)*. This program is often used as a treatment manual in clinical trials. We review some of the key elements of this treatment here.

4.1.1. SELF-MONITORING

Self-monitoring is perhaps the single most important element of behavior therapy for obesity. Patients keep extensive records of their food intake, physical activity, and weight throughout treatment. In the initial weeks, they record daily the types, amounts, and caloric values of foods eaten. Armed with this information, they try to reduce hidden sources of fat and sugar from their diet and, thus, decrease their energy intake by approx 500–1000 kcal/d. Record-keeping is increased over time to include information about times, places, and feelings associated with eating. These more detailed records often reveal patterns of which patients were not previously aware. A patient might discover, for instance, that her "picking" and "tasting" while preparing meals added several hundred calories to her daily intake. Another might find that he ends meals with dessert, even if he is not hungry. Patterns are analyzed to determine the precipitants of inappropriate eating and to plan interventions. Several correlational studies have shown that self-monitoring is associated with successful long-term weight control *(26)*.

4.1.2. STIMULUS CONTROL

Self-monitoring informs the process of stimulus control, which is another important element of behavioral weight reduction. Patients are shown how to modify their environment so that it is conducive to eating less (and more healthfully) and exercising more. This requires collaboration and creativity on the parts of the patient and practitioner. For instance, a patient may decide to drive a different route to work if her current travel takes her past a tempting fast-food restaurant or donut shop. Controlling environmental stimuli may be as simple as clearing the freezer of ice cream or moving the bag of potato chips from the counter to the cupboard. "Out of sight, out of mouth," is one of the most obvious benefits of stimulus control.

4.1.3. PROBLEM SOLVING

Patients in behavior therapy are instructed in a step-by-step approach to overcoming obstacles to weight-loss goals *(27)*. The first step is to define the problem in detail, identifying the chain of events that led to it. Next, patients brainstorm possible solutions to the problem, weigh the pros and cons of each alternative, and select the most appropriate strategy. The final steps involve implementing a solution and evaluating the result. Problem solving is taught as a dynamic process, and thus, individuals are encouraged to repeat the above steps until they obtain a satisfactory outcome. Effective problem solving correlates positively with the maintenance of weight loss *(28)*.

4.1.4. SLOWING THE RATE OF EATING

Eating slowly may increase enjoyment of food, improve satiety, and reduce intake. Consider, for example, a man who tends to finish his meals well before the others at his table. He finds that he takes a second helping and continues to eat until the slowest eater at the table has finished. Eating quickly has allowed him to consume extra calories with little additional enjoyment. When he paces himself with a slower eater, he discovers that he tastes and appreciates his food more and that he becomes sated with less food. Typical strategies for slowing the rate of eating include putting down utensils between bites, pausing during meals, and chewing food thoroughly before swallowing (25). Spiegel et al. (29) found that patients who ate more slowly lost larger amounts of weight.

4.1.5. COGNITIVE RESTRUCTURING

Negative thoughts can undermine dieters. Such thoughts typically fall into one of three categories: (a) the impossibility of successful weight control, (b) unrealistic eating and weight loss goals, and (c) self-criticism in response to perceived dietary lapses (25,30). Patients are taught to identify their negative thoughts (through self-monitoring) and then challenge and correct them with more rational, reality-based thoughts.

Cognitive restructuring is a common component of the behavioral treatment of obesity. Some researchers place primary importance on the correction of negative thoughts in weight reduction (31). Cognitive therapy has proven effective in the treatments of depression (32), bulimia nervosa (11), and other psychiatric conditions (33). Its efficacy, however, with obesity has not been adequately demonstrated.

4.2. Dietary Interventions

Dietary interventions for obesity are designed to induce a negative energy balance (i.e., calories ingested less than calories expended) by reducing daily calorie intake below energy requirements. Those requirements vary by gender, weight, and level of physical activity such that men, heavier individuals, and those who are more active have greater energy needs. Regardless of an individual patient's requirements, greater deficits result in greater weight losses. Deficits of 500–1000 kcal/d can be expected to produce reductions of 0.5 to 1 kg/wk. Accordingly, the NHLBI/NAASO guidelines recommend low-calorie diets (LCDs) of 1000–1200 kcal/d for most overweight women and 1200–1600 kcal/d for overweight men (and heavier or more active women) (4).

There are many ways to achieve negative energy balance through manipulating calorie intake and macronutrient balance. Several popular dietary approaches are described here. Regardless of the approach taken, careful self-monitoring of intake is crucial to the success of LCDs. Obese individuals underestimate their calorie intake by 30 to 50% (34). Thus, patients must be instructed in reading food labels, measuring portion sizes, and recording intake as soon as possible after eating.

4.2.1. BALANCED-DEFICIT DIETS

A balanced-deficit diet (BDD) provides a healthy distribution of macronutrients, while reducing calorie intake below daily energy requirements. One such diet, taken from the NHLBI/NAASO guidelines (4), can be found in Table 4. For patients who are averse to figuring what percentage of calories come from which macronutrient category, the Food Guide Pyramid (35) is a convenient guideline for consuming a BDD (see Fig. 1). Patients have the option of monitoring their calorie intake, fat intake, servings from the Food Guide Pyramid, or some combination of these.

Table 4
Low-Calorie Step I Diet

Nutrient	Recommended Intake
Calories	Approximately 500 to 1000 kcal/d reduction from usual intake
Total fat	30% or less of total calories
Saturated fatty acids	8–10% of total calories
Monounsaturated fatty acids	Up to 15% of total calories
Polyunsaturated fatty acids	Up to 10% of total calories
Cholesterol	<300 mg/d
Protein	Approximately15% of total calories
Carbohydrate	55% or more of total calories
Sodium chloride	No more than 100 mmol/d (~2.4 g of sodium or ~6 g of sodium chloride
Calcium	1000–1500 mg/d
Fiber	20–30 g/d

Reprinted from ref. *4*.

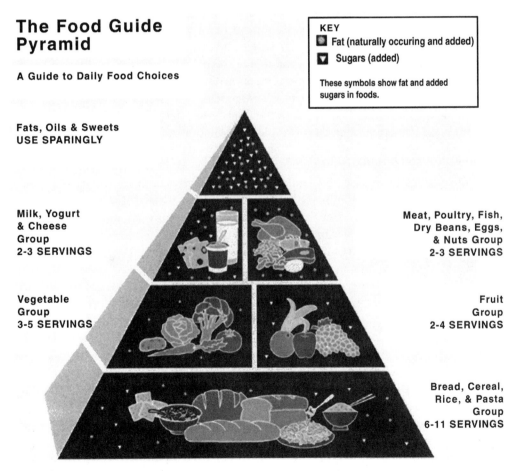

The Food Guide Pyramid

A Guide to Daily Food Choices

KEY
⬛ Fat (naturally occuring and added)
🔻 Sugars (added)

These symbols show fat and added sugars in foods.

Fats, Oils & Sweets
USE SPARINGLY

Milk, Yogurt & Cheese Group
2-3 SERVINGS

Meat, Poultry, Fish, Dry Beans, Eggs, & Nuts Group
2-3 SERVINGS

Vegetable Group
3-5 SERVINGS

Fruit Group
2-4 SERVINGS

Bread, Cereal, Rice, & Pasta Group
6-11 SERVINGS

Fig. 1. The Food Guide Pyramid. (Reprinted from the US Department of Agriculture and the US Department of Health and Human Services .)

4.2.2. Low-Energy Density Diets

The energy density of a food is a function of its calorie content and weight. Foods that contain fewer calories per gram are considered to be lower in energy density. Energy density is an important concept, given findings that people tend to eat the same amount (i.e., weight or volume) of food each day, regardless of its macronutrient composition *(36)*. Laboratory studies have shown that people consume approx 20 to 50% fewer calories when given a low- as compared to a high-energy density diet, even if palatability and macronutrient composition are equivalent *(37–39)*. Individuals can consume a diet lower in energy density and lower in calories by increasing the water and fiber content of foods *(36)*.

4.2.3. Low-Carbohydrate Diets

Low-carbohydrate diets (e.g., the Atkins' Diet *[40]*) have been popular for many years (*see* Chapter 19). Such diets encourage their adherents to restrict intake of carbohydrate (to ≤20 g/d initially), while consuming a large percentage of daily calories from protein and fat. Many experts have expressed concern about the health consequences of consuming a diet that provides more fat and cholesterol than is typically recommended *(41)*.

Four randomized, controlled trials now have compared the effects of low-carbohydrate with low-fat diets *(42–45)*. Results from these studies showed that individuals achieved similar or greater reductions in weight and cardiovascular risk factors with low-carbohydrate, as compared with low-fat diets. The mechanisms that accounted for the greater weight losses and health improvements with the low-carbohydrate diets are not clear. Given the popularity of this approach, more research is needed to discover not only the mechanisms of weight loss, but also the long-term safety and efficacy of following a diet higher in fat and protein than is typically recommended.

4.2.4. Improving Dietary Adherence

Recent studies have assessed strategies for improving both short- and long-term adherence to dietary interventions. Chief among these are the use of specific meal plans (with and without food provision) and the use of portion-controlled meal replacements. Both strategies involve increasing the structure of the dietary plan, reducing the effort required for adherence, and eliminating much of the decision making, temptation, and guesswork involved in making healthy food choices.

Jeffery et al. *(46)* found that providing patients foods for five breakfasts and five dinners per wk produced better weight loss over 18 mo than an isocaloric diet of self-selected foods. Wing, Jeffery, and colleagues *(47)* then compared weight loss among groups who received standard behavioral treatment plus (1) no additional structure, (2) structured meal plans and grocery lists, (3) meal plans with food provided at reduced cost, and (4) meal plans with free food provision. Although the calorie goals were equivalent across groups, participants in group 2, 3, and 4 lost significantly more weight after 6 mo of treatment and maintained greater losses at 18 mo follow-up than did those in group 1. There were no differences in weight loss or maintenance among groups 2, 3, and 4. This finding indicates that specifying what foods and what amounts patients should eat improves weight loss, but that providing the food has no additional effect.

Liquid meal replacements are another means of increasing the structure of a dietary plan. Ditschuneit et al. *(48)* randomized patients to receive a self-selected diet of conventional foods or a diet in which they replaced two meals and two snacks a day with calorie-controlled shakes and snack bars. Both diets were designed to provide 1200–1500 kcal/d. After 3 mo, those who consumed the meal replacements lost more than five times as much weight as did those who followed the diet of conventional foods (mean ± SD = 7.8 ± 0.5% vs 1.5 ± 0.4%, respectively). Heymsfield et al. *(49)* conducted a meta-analysis of six randomized, controlled trials (including Ditschuneit et al.*[48]*) and found that participants who received meal replacements lost an average 2.54 kg and 2.43 kg more at 3 mo and 1 yr, respectively, than did those who received conventional LCDs. Furthermore, there were significantly fewer dropouts across studies among those assigned to receive meal replacements.

Meal replacements may also facilitate the maintenance of weight loss. Patients in the Ditschuneit study who continued to replace one meal and one snack per day maintained a weight loss of 8.4 ± 0.8% at 51 mo *(50)*. Controlled, randomized trials are needed to assess the long-term benefits of meal replacements.

4.3. Physical Activity

The third component of lifestyle modification is increasing physical activity *(see* Chapter 13). Exercise is beneficial because it creates greater caloric deficits and spares fat-free mass during weight loss *(51)*. Physical fitness also reduces the risk of cardiovascular disease independent of body fatness *(52)*.

Patients should be aware, however, that increasing exercise without reducing energy intake is unlikely to induce significant weight loss. For example, most people can burn 0.5 kg of fat by eating 500 fewer calories/d for 1 wk. To lose the same 0.5 kg of fat with exercise, most people will need to walk 35 miles (at a brisk pace, to boot).

4.3.1. PROGRAMMED VS LIFESTYLE ACTIVITY

Individuals can increase their energy expenditure in two ways: programmed and lifestyle activity. Programmed activity (e.g., walking, biking, swimming) is typically planned and completed in a discrete period of time (i.e., 30–60 min) at a relatively high intensity (i.e., 60–80% of maximum heart rate). Lifestyle activity, by contrast, involves increasing energy expenditure while completing everyday tasks. For example, patients may increase their lifestyle activity by choosing distant parking spots, taking stairs rather than elevators, and even by throwing out the remote control for the television. Andersen and colleagues *(53)* compared the effects of programmed and lifestyle activity among women. They found that both types of activity, when combined with a 1200 kcal/d diet, produced a loss of approx 8 kg in 16 wk. There was a trend ($p = 0.06$) for lifestyle activity to be associated with less weight regain than programmed exercise 1 yr after treatment (0.1 kg vs 1.6 kg, respectively). Results of this study await replication in a larger sample that includes men.

4.3.2. LONG- VS SHORT-BOUT ACTIVITY

Jakicic and colleagues *(54,55)* investigated the effects of prescribing exercise in multiple short bouts, as compared with a single long bout. All patients were instructed to exercise for 20–40 min/d. Those who were encouraged to complete their activity in multiple 10-min bouts exercised on more days over 20 wk than did patients who were instructed to exercise in a single bout (87.3 ± 29.5 d and 69.1 ± 28.9 d, respectively) *(54)*.

There was a trend ($p = 0.07$) toward greater weight loss among those in the short-bout group (8.9 ± 5.3 kg vs 6.4 ± 4.5 kg). At 18 mo, however, Jakicic et al. observed no differences in weight loss, adherence, or cardiovascular fitness between short- and long-bout exercisers *(55)*.

4.3.3. Improving Exercise Adherence

Researchers have studied whether increasing the structure of physical activity *(56,57)* or providing incentives *(57)* is associated with better adherence and greater weight losses. Perri and colleagues *(56)* randomized obese participants to receive 12 mo of lifestyle modification that included on-site supervised exercise or a comparable program of home-based activity. They found during the first 6 mo that the two groups exercised approx the same number of minutes per wk (107–120 min) and lost comparable amounts of weight (10.6–10.9 kg). At 15 mo, however, those who exercised at home had greater weight losses than those who exercised on site (–11.9 ± 9.1 kg and –9.2 ± 8.2 kg, respectively). The greater weight loss in the at-home group appeared to result from greater exercise adherence. Wing et al. *(57)* found that pairing participants with a "personal trainer" (who met participants at home or work and led them on a walk), in addition to having three supervised activity sessions per week, did not improve weight loss over the supervised activity sessions alone. In another study, Wing and colleagues *(57)* provided 24 wk of lifestyle modification and three supervised exercise sessions per wk. Additionally, patients were randomized to receive either no incentives, or to be eligible for a lottery drawing that rewarded more frequent attendance at exercise sessions. The two groups did not differ at the 24-wk assessment in weight loss or minutes of physical activity.

Contrary to findings that imposing structure on LCDs is beneficial, increasing the structure of physical activity does not appear to improve adherence or weight loss. In fact, less-structured exercise plans (e.g., lifestyle vs programmed and home-based vs supervised) appear to be more conducive to long-term success *(53,56,57)*. With less structure comes a reduction in exercise-related demands and barriers (e.g., time, travel, getting dressed). Further research will determine whether any externally focused interventions can improve motivation, thereby facilitating adherence.

5. STRUCTURE AND RESULTS OF LIFESTYLE MODIFICATION

5.1. Treatment Delivery

Lifestyle modification programs typically require weekly meetings for 16 to 26 wk. Patients are given a treatment manual that provides weekly readings and homework assignments for adopting new behaviors. The first phase of treatment is often followed by a period of every-other-week meetings aimed at maintaining the behavioral changes achieved during the first 4 to 6 mo of treatment.

Treatment is typically delivered to groups of 10 to 20 people in sessions lasting 60 to 90 min. Individual treatment allows the therapist to spend more time analyzing patients' eating and exercise habits, but produces smaller weight losses than group intervention. In a study conducted by Renjilian and colleagues *(58)*, patients who expressed a preference for either group or individual treatment were randomized to receive either their preferred or nonpreferred treatment modality. Thus, the four conditions were: preferred group and received group, preferred individual and received group, preferred individual and received individual, and preferred group and received individual. Whether patients received their preferred or nonpreferred modality did not affect weight loss outcomes. Those who received group treatment—regardless of their preference–lost significantly more weight after 26 wk of treatment (11.0 ± 4.8 kg) than did those who received individual counseling (9.1 ± 3.7 kg).

5.2. Results

The short-term results of lifestyle modification are relatively consistent across studies. Approximately 80% of enrollees complete 6 mo of treatment *(59)*. Patients lose, on average, 8 to 10% of their initial weight *(60)*. Without further treatment, they regain approx one-third of the lost weight within 1 yr and return to their pretreatment weights within 3 to 5 yr *(60)*. Obesity must, therefore, be conceptualized and treated as a chronic condition. Antihypertensive therapy is rarely discontinued when a patient's blood pressure is stabilized; continued treatment is necessary to maintain control over the patient's hypertension. Likewise, weight-loss therapy is most effective when care is extended beyond the acute treatment phase.

Perri et al. *(61)* provided empirical evidence for the benefits of continuing care. Their patients received 20 weekly lifestyle modification sessions, followed by a 52-wk period in which participants were randomly assigned to no additional treatment or twice-monthly therapist contacts. Patients who received extended contact maintained, at 18 mo follow-up, 87% of their end-of-treatment weight loss. By contrast, patients who had no additional contact maintained only 33% of their original reduction. These findings indicate that continued care is critical to the maintenance of treatment effects. It appears to provide patients the support and motivation to continue to exercise regularly and consume a LCD.

The most successful weight losers—regardless of their weight-loss strategies—are eligible to enter the National Weight Control Registry (NWCR) *(62)*. NWCR members have maintained an average loss of approx 30 kg for nearly 6 yr and have become a valuable resource for those seeking the secrets to weight maintenance. NWCR members practice many of the behaviors recommended in lifestyle modification treatment. Specifically, registrants report eating a low-fat diet, exercising regularly, and continuing to monitor their weight and food intake *(63,64)*.

6. LIFESTYLE MODIFICATION AND COMMERCIAL WEIGHT-LOSS PROGRAMS

All of the clinical trials of lifestyle modification reviewed in this chapter were conducted in university-based weight-loss centers. The large majority of obese and overweight individuals attempting to lose weight, however, are not treated at academic centers. They are more likely to use do-it-yourself strategies or to enroll in a commercial weight-loss program. Several programs (e.g., Weight Watchers, Jenny Craig, L.A. Weight Loss) have incorporated the principles of lifestyle modification in their interventions. These may include self-monitoring of energy intake and expenditure, the use of structured meal plans, or regular treatment visits (in group or individual format).

Among commercial weight-loss programs, Weight Watchers has undergone the most thorough empirical examination. Lowe et al. *(65)* randomly assigned participants to a 4-wk Weight Watchers program or to a wait-list control group. The wait-list controls were instructed to use any weight-loss method they desired, other than formal programs.

At the end of 4 wk, the Weight Watchers group lost significantly more weight than the control group (1.9 kg vs 0.8 kg, respectively). Those in the Weight Watchers group also reported greater improvements in quality of life, even after controlling for the amount of weight lost.

Heshka and colleagues *(66,67)* conducted a long-term study that illustrated the effectiveness of Weight Watchers. Participants were randomized to receive a 2-yr trial of Weight Watchers (at no cost) or a self-help program that consisted of two 20-min nutrition sessions and the provision of written resources. Two-year retention was good in both conditions (Weight Watchers = 71%, self-help = 75%). Using last-observation-carried-forward analyses, Heshka et al. found that participants assigned to Weight Watchers had greater weight losses at 6 mo (4.8 kg vs 1.4 kg), 1 yr (4.3 kg vs 1.3 kg), and 2 yr (2.9 kg vs 0.2 kg) than those in the self-help group.

Weight Watchers participants are encouraged to set goal weights that fall between a BMI of 20 and 25 kg/m². (Higher goal weights may be selected for heavier participants by their physicians.) Lowe et al. *(68)* surveyed a national sample of successful Weight Watchers participants 5 yr after reaching their goal. Nearly 19% of participants maintained a 10% reduction from initial weight, 42.6% maintained a 5% loss, and 70.3% remained below their initial weight. These results are encouraging but clearly from a very select subsample of the program's most successful participants.

7. NEW DIRECTIONS AND GOALS FOR LIFESTYLE MODIFICATION

Researchers have begun investigating the effects of several additions to traditional lifestyle modification, as well as alternative methods of delivering treatment. These new directions, including the recruitment of participants in "teams," the use of motivational interviewing, and the use of technology to provide lifestyle modification are discussed here. The chapter concludes with a discussion of the benefits of lifestyle modification in reducing obesity-related morbidity.

7.1. Social Support

As discussed previously, lifestyle modification produces larger weight losses when it is delivered in groups than in individual sessions *(58)*. Recent studies have investigated the components of social support that improve treatment. Wing and Jeffery *(69)* recruited participants either alone or in teams of four (i.e., with three family members or friends). Participants were randomized to receive a 4-mo trial of lifestyle modification with or without additional social support strategies (e.g., sitting with team members, intragroup activities, intergroup competitions), followed by a 6-mo maintenance program. Those who were recruited in teams and received a social support intervention had significantly higher retention than each of the other three groups: (1) recruited alone with standard treatment, (2) recruited alone with standard treatment plus social support, or (3) recruited in teams with standard treatment. An intent-to-treat analysis revealed a main effect for recruitment strategy. Participants recruited in teams had a significantly greater weight loss at 10 mo (7.7 kg) than did those recruited alone (4.3 kg). Weight loss did not differ as a function of whether participants received (6.2 kg) or did not receive (5.6 kg) the additional social support intervention. Naturally occurring, but not facilitated social support, appears to improve weight loss among participants in lifestyle modification.

Enrolling teams of participants into lifestyle modification is worthy of further research. Wing and Jeffery's *(69)* findings have yet to be replicated. Furthermore, these authors found no weight-loss differences among groups at 16 mo (i.e., 6 mo after completing the maintenance program). It appears that natural social support systems do not inoculate dieters against weight regain. Future research is necessary to discover whether extended contact with the treatment center delays regain among participants who enter lifestyle modification with a group of family members or friends.

7.2. Motivational Interviewing

Although the benefits of weight loss are often clear to patients (e.g., improving health, mobility, quality of life, and appearance), the drawbacks (e.g., the tedium of measuring portions and keeping food records, restricting intake of many palatable foods) may be even more salient. Not surprisingly, participation in lifestyle modification frequently results in ambivalence. Motivational interviewing (MI) is a directive, yet client-centered approach to behavior change that acknowledges and targets participants' ambivalence about making desired changes *(70)*. The approach was developed for the treatment of substance dependence, but can be readily applied to interventions for other behavioral disorders.

Smith and colleagues *(71)* conducted a pilot investigation, in women with type 2 diabetes, of a 16-wk lifestyle modification program, with or without the addition of three individual MI sessions. Those who received the MI intervention displayed significantly greater attendance and adherence (i.e., completing food records, monitoring blood glucose) than those in the standard lifestyle group. There were not, however, significant differences in weight loss between the two groups (MI = 5.5 ± 3.9 kg, standard = 4.5 ± 2.2 kg).

The small sample size (*n* = 22), short duration of treatment, and lack of follow-up in this study *(71)* may account for the lack of differences in weight loss between groups. The increased attendance and adherence among patients who received the three MI sessions is promising. Including MI sessions in long-term maintenance programs may be particularly beneficial, given that participants' motivation to adhere to diet and exercise regimens appear to decline over time. Additional research is needed to determine the value of MI in lifestyle modification.

7.3. Technology in Lifestyle Modification

Investigators are now examining the Internet as a medium for delivering behavioral programs for the induction and maintenance of weight loss (*see* Chapter 23). Initial results have been promising. Tate and colleagues *(72,73)* conducted two randomized, controlled trials of Internet-based weight-loss interventions. In the first *(72)*, participants received a 6-mo trial of Internet-based education or Internet-based behavior therapy. Both treatments included one in-person session in which participants were instructed in behavioral weight-control methods and encouraged to self-monitor their eating and exercise behavior. Participants in both groups also received instructions for logging in to a website that directed them to various Internet resources on diet, exercise, self-monitoring, and other elements of lifestyle modification. Those who received behavior therapy, in addition, were instructed to submit weekly records of weight, calorie and fat intake, and physical activity, along with any questions. A therapist sent participants weekly feedback and behavior therapy lessons via e-mail. Finally, those in the behavior therapy group had access to an electronic bulletin board, through which they could contact other participants. Internet-based behavior therapy produced larger weight losses than the education program at 3 mo (3.2 kg and 1 kg, respectively) and 6 mo (2.9 kg and 1.3 kg, respectively).

The second study by Tate and colleagues (73) was similar, but the duration was longer (1 yr), the sample included patients at risk of developing type 2 diabetes, and the control treatment was more comprehensive. Participants were randomized to a basic Internet group or to a behavioral e-counseling group. The basic Internet intervention consisted of one in-person session, the recommendation to self-monitor, access to a message board and a website with weight-loss tutorials and links that were updated weekly, and weekly reminders to submit weights. The behavioral e-counseling intervention, additionally, consisted of weekly submission of self-monitoring records, questions or comments for a therapist, and e-mail responses from a therapist. After 12 mo of treatment, the basic Internet and behavioral e-counseling groups lost 2.0 kg and 4.4 kg, respectively. The difference between groups was significant ($p = 0.04$).

In both studies by Tate et al. (72,73), the weight losses produced by Internet-based behavior therapy were approximately half the size of those resulting from traditional lifestyle modification provided on site. A possible mechanism suppressing weight losses, suggested by Tate and colleagues, was poor treatment adherence. Behavior therapy participants in the first study submitted an average of 13.7 weekly self-monitoring diaries over the course of 24 wk. As in traditional lifestyle modification, the completion of food records was a strong predictor of weight loss in participants in the Internet-based behavior therapy group ($r = -0.50$). Perhaps participants felt less accountability in this intervention, given the interpersonal distance that characterizes Internet-based communication. It is also possible that participants who seek Internet-based interventions differ on important variables from those who seek in-person treatment.

Harvey-Berino and colleagues (74) compared on-site and Internet-based weight-maintenance programs. All participants received 6 mo of on-site lifestyle modification and were randomly assigned to receive one of three maintenance programs. The first group received frequent on-site support (i.e., twice-monthly group meetings for 52 wk). The second group was provided minimal in-person support (i.e., monthly group meetings for 26 wk, followed by 26 wk of no meetings). The third group received Internet support (i.e., twice-monthly "chat" sessions with other participants and a therapist for 52 wk). Weight losses were equivalent across groups at the end of the 6-mo program (8, 11, and 9.8 kg, respectively). At the end of the 12-mo maintenance period, however, participants in the Internet support group maintained a significantly smaller weight loss (5.7 kg) than participants in the minimal or frequent in-person support groups (10.4 kg for both).

Internet-based behavior therapy is in its infancy. Early studies have produced modest results, and future research may discover ways of maximizing the induction and maintenance of weight loss. Given the health benefits of modest weight loss, described next, even small improvements in the effectiveness of Internet-based behavior therapy may be sufficient to provide a useful tool for reducing the social and economic costs of obesity-related health complications.

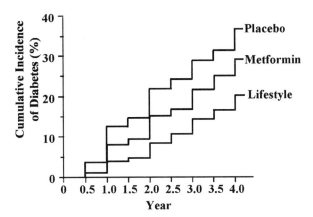

Fig. 2. Cumulative incidence of diabetes for participants in the Diabetes Prevention Program. The diagnosis of diabetes was based on the criteria of the American Diabetes Association. The incidence of diabetes differed significantly among the three groups ($p \leq 0.001$ for each comparison). (Reprinted with permission ref. *76*.)

8. HEALTH BENEFITS OF MODEST WEIGHT LOSS

Recent studies indicate that a 5 to 10% weight reduction is associated with significant improvements in blood pressure, cholesterol, and glycemic control *(75)* (*see* Chapter 10). The extent to which these short-term health benefits translate to long-term reductions in obesity-related morbidity and mortality is the subject of two recent studies and one ongoing investigation.

The Diabetes Prevention Program (DPP) *(76)* was a randomized, controlled trial that compared the effectiveness of placebo, metformin (Glucophage, 850 mg/BID), and lifestyle modification in preventing the onset of type 2 diabetes among 3200 overweight individuals with impaired glucose tolerance. The lifestyle modification intervention was designed to induce a loss of 7% of initial weight and to increase physical activity to at least 150 min/wk. Participants in the lifestyle modification condition obtained a maximum weight loss of approx 7 kg and maintained a loss of approx 4 kg at yr 4 of the trial. Figure 2 displays the results. Lifestyle modification significantly reduced the risk of developing type 2 diabetes by 58% and 31%, compared with placebo and metformin, respectively.

A similar trial was conducted in Finland *(77)*. Five hundred twenty-two overweight adults with impaired glucose tolerance were randomized to receive an individualized program of diet and exercise, or verbal instruction and a two-page leaflet about diet and exercise. Those who received the weight loss treatment lost 4.3 ± 5.1 kg at 1 yr and 3.5 ± 5.5 kg at 2 yr. By comparison, participants in the control group lost 0.8 ± 3.7 kg and 0.8 ± 4.4 at 1 and 2 yr, respectively. As in the DPP, the weight-loss intervention reduced the risk of developing diabetes by 58%. These two studies provide the strongest evidence to date of the health benefits of modest weight loss.

A follow-up trial is currently being conducted to determine whether modest weight loss ($\geq 7\%$) and increased physical activity (≥ 175 min/wk) will decrease mortality from heart attack and stroke in persons who already have type 2 diabetes. The Look AHEAD study is the first randomized, prospective trial to examine this issue *(78)*.

9. CONCLUSION

This is an exciting time in obesity research. Although the principles of behavior therapy have not changed substantially over the years, researchers are investigating different means of applying these principles. Scientists are also discovering that lifestyle modification can produce benefits that extend beyond mere weight loss to significant reductions in health risks. Lifestyle modification will likely occupy a prominent role in future efforts both to prevent and treat obesity.

ACKNOWLEDGMENTS

Preparation of this chapter was supported, in part, by a Mid-Career Patient-Oriented Research Award, by grant 1-U01-DK57135 from the National Institute of Diabetes and Digestive and Kidney Diseases, and by an unrestricted educational grant from Abbott Laboratories. The authors gratefully acknowledge the contributions of Inessa Manevich to the preparation of this chapter.

REFERENCES

1. World Health Organization. Obesity: Preventing and Managing the Global Epidemic. World Health Organization, Geneva, Switzerland, 1998.
2. Flegal KM, Carroll MD, Ogden CL, Johnson CL. Prevalence and trends in obesity among US adults, 1999–2000. JAMA 2002; 288:1723–1727.
3. Horgen KB, Brownell KD. Confronting the toxic environment: Environmental, public health actions in a world crisis. In: Wadden TA, Stunkard AJ, eds. Handbook of Obesity Treatment. Guilford, New York, NY, 2002, pp. 95–106.
4. National Heart, Lung and Blood Institute and North American Association for the Study of Obesity. Practical Guide to the Identification, Evaluation, and Treatment of Overweight and Obesity in Adults. National Institutes of Health, Bethesda, MD, 2000.
5. Wadden TA, Phelan SP. Behavioral assessment of the obese patient. In: Wadden TA, Stunkard AJ, eds. Handbook of Obesity Treatment. Guilford, New York, NY, 2002, pp. 186–226.
6. Foster GD, Wadden TA, Vogt RA, Brewer G. What is a reasonable weight loss? Patients' expectations and evaluations of obesity treatment outcomes. J Consult Clin Psychol 1997; 65:79–85.
7. Bray GA. What causes overweight? Nature versus nurture. In: Bray GA, ed. Contemporary Diagnosis and Management of Obesity. Handbooks in Health Care, Newtown, PA, 1998, pp. 35–67.
8. Spitzer RL, Devlin M, Walsh TB, et al. Binge eating disorder: A multisite field trial of the diagnostic criteria. Int J Eat Disord 1992; 11:191–203.
9. Yanovski SZ. Binge eating disorder: current knowledge and future directions. Obes Res 1993; 1:306–324.
10. Fairburn CG, Beglin SJ. Assessment of eating disorders: Interview or self-report questionnaire? Int J Eat Disord 1994; 16:363–370.
11. Fairburn CG, Wilson GT. Binge Eating: Nature, Assessment and Treatment. Guilford, New York, NY, 1993.
12. Arnold LM, McElroy SL, Hudson JI, Welge JA, Bennett AJ, Keck PE. A placebo-controlled, randomized trial of fluoxetine in the treatment of binge-eating disorder. J Clin Psychiatry 2002; 63:1028–1033.
13. Wadden TA, Womble LG, Stunkard AJ, Anderson DA. Psychosocial consequences of obesity and weight loss. In: Wadden TA, Stunkard AJ, eds. Handbook of Obesity Treatment. Guilford, New York, NY, 2002, pp. 144–169.
14. Gladis MM, Wadden TA, Foster GD, Vogt RA, Wingate BJ. A comparison of two approaches to the assessment of binge eating in obesity. Int J Eat Disord 1998; 23:17–26.
15. Fitzgibbon ML, Stolley MR, Kirschenbaum DS. Obese people who seek treatment have different characteristics than those who do not seek treatment. Health Psychol 1993; 12:342–345.
16. Beck AT, Steer RA, Brown GK. Manual for Beck Depression Inventory—II. Psychological Corporation, San Antonio, TX, 1996.

17. Doll HA, Petersen SEK, Stewart-Brown SL. Obesity and physical and emotional well-being: associations between body mass index, chronic illness, and the physical and mental components of the SF-36 questionnaire. Obes Res 2000; 8:160–170.
18. Kolotkin RL, Meter K, Williams GR. Quality of life and obesity. Obesity Reviews 2001; 2:219–229.
19. Wadden TA, Letizia KA: Predictors of attrition and weight loss in persons treated by moderate and severe caloric restriction, In: Wadden TA, VanItallie TB, eds. Treatment of the Seriously Obese Patient. Guilford, New York, NY, 1992, pp. 383–410.
20. Wadden TA, Steen SN. Improving the maintenance of weight loss: the ten percent solution. In: Angel A, Anderson H, Bouchard C, Lau D, Leiter L, Mendelson R, eds. Progress in Obesity Research: VII. John Libbey, 1996, London, UK, pp. 745–750.
21. Wadden TA, Berkowitz RI, Sarwer DB, Prus-Wisniewski R, Steinberg C. Benefits of lifestyle modification in the pharmacologic treatment of obesity: a randomized trial. Arch Intern Med 2001; 161:218–227.
22. Wadden TA, Womble LG, Sarwer DB, Berkowitz RI, Clark VL, Foster GD. Great expectations: "I'm losing 25% of my weight no matter what you say." J Consult Clin Psychol 2003; 71:1084–1089.
23. French S, Jeffery RW. The consequences of dieting to lose weight: effects on physical and mental health. Health Psychol 1994; 13:195–212.
24. Sbrocco T, Nedegaard R, Stone JM, Lewis EL. Behavioral choice treatment promotes continuing weight loss: preliminary results of a cognitive–behavioral decision-based treatment for obesity. J Consult Clin Psychol 1999; 67:260–266.
25. Brownell KD. The LEARN Program for Weight Management 2000. American Health Publishing, Dallas, TX, 2000.
26. Wadden TA. Characteristics of successful weight loss maintainers. In: Allison DB, Pi-Sunyer FX, eds. Obesity Treatment: Establishing Goals, Improving Outcomes, and Reviewing the Research Agenda. Plenum Press, New York, NY, 1995, pp. 103–111.
27. Black DR. A minimal intervention program and a problem-solving program for weight control. Cog Ther Res 1987; 11:107–120.
28. Kayman S, Bruvold W, Stern JS. Maintenance and relapse after weight loss in women: Behavioral aspects. Am J Clin Nutr 1990; 52:800–807.
29. Spiegel T, Wadden TA, Foster GD. Objective measurement of eating rate during behavioral treatment of obesity. Behav Ther 1991; 22:61–67.
30. Wadden TA, Foster GD. Behavioral assessment and treatment of markedly obese patients. In: Wadden TA, VanItallie TB, eds. Treatment of the Seriously Obese Patient. Guilford, New York, NY, 1992, pp. 290–330.
31. Cooper Z, Fairburn CG, Hawker DM. Cognitive–Behavioral Treatment of Obesity. Guilford, New York, NY, 2003.
32. Beck AT, Rush A, Shaw B, Emery G. Cognitive Therapy of Depression. Guilford, New York, NY, 1979.
33. Beck AT, Emery G, Greenberg R. Anxiety Disorders and Phobias: a Cognitive Perspective. Basic Books, New York, NY, 1985.
34. Lichtman SW, Pisarka K, Berman ER, et al. Discrepancy between self-reported and actual caloric intake and exercise in obese subjects. N Engl J Med 1992; 327:1893–1898.
35. United States Department of Agriculture. USDA's Food Guide Pyramid. USDA Human Nutrition Service, Washington, DC, 1992
36. Rolls BJ, Barnett RA. Volumetrics. HarperCollins, New York, NY, 2000.
37. Duncan KH, Bacon JA, Weinsier RL. The effects of high and low energy density diets on satiety, energy intake, and eating time of obese and nonobese individuals. Am J Clin Nutr 1983; 37:763–767.
38. Bell EA, Rolls BJ. Energy density of foods affects energy intake across multiple levels of fat content in lean and obese women. Am J Clin Nutr 2001; 73:1010–1018.
39. Kral TV, Roe LS, Rolls BJ. Does nutrition information about the energy density of meals affect food intake in normal-weight women? Appetite 2002; 39:137–145.
40. Atkins RC. Dr. Atkins' New Diet Revolution. Avon Books, New York, NY, 1998.
41. Blackburn GL, Phillips JC, Morreale S. Physician's guide to popular low-carbohydrate weight-loss diets. Cleveland Clin J of Med 2001;.68:761–774.
42. Brehm BJ, Seeley RJ, Daniels SR, D'Alessio DA. A randomized trial comparing a very low carbohydrate diet and a calorie-restricted low fat diet on body weight and cardiovascular risk factors in healthy women. J Clin Endocrin Metab 2003; 88:1617–1623.

43. Foster GD, Wyatt HR, Hill JO, et al. A randomized trial of a low-carbohydrate diet for obesity. New Engl J Med 2003; 348:2082–2090.

44. Samaha FF, Iqbal N, Seshadri P, et al. A low-carbohydrate as compared with a low-fat diet in severe obesity. New Engl J Med 2003; 348:2074–2081.

45. Sondike SB, Cooperman N, Jacobson MS. Effects of a low-carbohydrate diet on weight loss and cardiovascular risk factors in overweight adolescents. J Pediatr 2003;142:253–258.

46. Jeffery RW, Wing RR, Thorson C, et al. Strengthening behavioral interventions for weight loss: A randomized trial of food provision and monetary incentives. J Consult Clin Psychol 1993; 61:1038–1045.

47. Wing RR, Jeffery RW, Burton LR, Thorson C, Nissinoff K, Baxter JE. Food provision vs. structured meal plans in the behavioral treatment of obesity. J Consult Clin Psychol 1996; 20:56–62.

48. Ditschuneit HH, Flechtner-Mors M, Johnson TD, Adler G. Metabolic and weight loss effects of long-term dietary intervention in obese subjects. Am J Clin Nutr 1999; 69:198–204.

49. Heymsfeld SB, van Mierlo CA, van der Knaap HC, Heo M, Frier HI. Weight management using a meal replacement strategy: meta and pooling analysis from six studies. Int J Obes 2003; 27:537–549.

50. Flechtner-Mors M, Ditschuneit HH, Johnson TD, Suchard M, Adler G. Metabolic and weight loss effects of long-term intervention in obese patients: Four-year results. Obes Res 2000; 8:399–402.

51. Bouchard C, Depres JP, Tremblay A. Exercise and obesity. Obes Res 1993; 1:133–147.

52. Lee CD, Blair SN, Jackson AS. Cardiorespiratory fitness, body composition, and all-cause and cardiovascular disease mortality in men. Am J Clin Nutr 1999; 69:373–380.

53. Andersen RE, Wadden TA, Bartlett SJ, Zemel BS, Verde TJ, Franckowiak SC. Effects of lifestyle activity vs. structured aerobic exercise in obese women: a randomized trial. JAMA 1999; 281:335–340.

54. Jakicic JM, Butler BA, Robertson RJ. Prescribing exercise in multiple short bouts versus one continuous bout: effects on adherence, cardiorespiratory fitness, and weight loss in overweight women. Int J Obes 1995; 19:382–387.

55. Jakicic JM, Winters C, Lang W, Wing RR. Effects of intermittent exercise and use of home exercise equipment on adherence, weight loss, and fitness in overweight women: a randomized trial. JAMA 1999; 16:1554–1560.

56. Perri MG, Martin AD, Leermakers EA, Sears SF. Effects of group- versus home-based exercise training in healthy older men and women. J Consult Clin Psychol 1997; 65:278–285.

57. Wing RR, Jeffery RW, Pronk N, Hellerstedt WL. Effects of a personal trainer and financial incentives on exercise adherence in overweight women in a behavioral weight loss program. Obes Res 1996; 4: 457–462.

58. Renjilian DA, Perri MG, Nezu AM, Mckelvey WF, Shermer.R.L., Anton SD. Individual vs. group therapy for obesity: effects of matching participants to their treatment preference. J Consult Clin Psychol 2001; 69:717–721.

59. Wadden TA, Foster GD. Behavioral treatment of obesity. Med Clin N Amer 2000; 84:441–461.

60. Wilson GT, Brownell KD. Behavioral treatment for obesity. In: Fairburn CG, Brownell KD, eds. Eating Disorders and Obesity. Guilford, New York, NY, 2002, pp. 524–533.

61. Perri MG, McAllister DA, Gange JJ, Jordan RC, McAdoo WG, Nezu AM. Effects of four maintenance programs on the long-term management of obesity. J Consult Clin Psychol 1988; 56:529–534.

62. Klem ML, Wing RR, McGuire MT, Seagle HM, Hill JO. A descriptive study of individuals successful at long-term maintenance of substantial weight loss. Am J Clin Nutr 1997; 66:239–246.

63. McGuire MT, Wing RR, Klem ML, Lang W, Hill JO. What predicts weight regain in a group of successful weight losers? J Consult Clin Psychol 1999; 67:177–185.

64. Wing RR, Hill JO. Successful weight loss maintenance. Ann Rev Nutr 2001; 21:323–341.

65. Lowe MR, Miller-Kovach K, Frye N, Phelan S. An initial evaluation of a commercial weight loss program: Short-term effects on weight, eating behavior, and mood. Obes Res 1999; 7:51–59.

66. Heshka S, Greenway F, Anderson JW, et al: Self-help weight loss versus a structured commerical program after 26 weeks: A randomized controlled study. Am J Med 2000; 109:282–285.

67. Heshka S, Anderson JW, Atkinson RL, et al. Weight loss with self-help compared with a structured commercial program. JAMA 2003; 289:1792–1798.

68. Lowe MR, Miller-Kovach K, Phelan S. Weight-loss maintenance in overweight individuals one to five years following successful completion of a commercial weight loss program. Int J Obes 2001; 25: 325–331.

69. Wing RR, Jeffery RW. Benefits of recruiting participants with friends and increasing social support for weight loss and maintenance. J Consult Clin Psychol 1999; 67:132–138.
70. Miller WR, Rollnick S. Motivational Interviewing: Preparing People for Change. Guilford, New York, NY, 2002:
71. Smith DE, Heckemeyer CM, Kratt PP, Mason DA. Motivational interviewing to improve adherence to a behavioral weight-control program for older obese women with NIDDM: a pilot study. Diabetes Care 1997; 20:52–54.
72. Tate DF, Wing RR, Winett RA. Using internet technology to deliver a behavioral weight loss program. JAMA 2001; 285:1172–1177.
73. Tate DF, Jackvony EH, Wing RR. Effects of internet behavioral counseling on weight loss in adults at risk for type 2 diabetes. JAMA 2003; 289:1833–1836.
74. Harvey-Berino J, Pintauro S, Buzzell P, et al. Does using the Internet facilitate the maintenance of weight loss? Int J Obes 2002; 26:1254–1260.
75. Blackburn GL. Effect of degree of weight loss on health benefits. Obes Res 1995; 3:211S–216S.
76. Diabetes Prevention Program Research Group. Reduction in the incidence of type 2 diabetes with lifestyle intervention or metformin. New Engl J Med 2002; 346:393–403.
77. Tuomilehto J, Lindström J, Eriksson JG, et al. Prevention of type 2 diabetes mellitus by changes in lifestyle among subjects with impaired glucose tolerance. New Engl J Med 2001; 344:1343–1350.
78. Look AHEAD Research Group. Look AHEAD (Action for Health in Diabetes): design and methods for a clinical trial of weight loss for the prevention of cardiovascular disease in type 2 diabetes. Controlled Clinical Trials 2003; 24:610–628.

15 Very Low-Calorie Diets

Stephen D. Phinney

KEY POINTS

- Very low-calorie diets are potentially safe and very useful in the treatment of obesity.
- The physician should understand the nutritional constituents of the very low-calorie diet and be aware of potential medical complications.
- Very low-calorie diets require close monitoring and should always be followed by a credible and sustained weight-maintenance program.

1. INTRODUCTION

Very low-calorie diets (VLCDs) have a history of cyclic popularity. Although a VLCD can be a very effective tool for the rapid mobilization of body fat, both the margin of safety and the efficacy of this class of diet are limited by their inherent calorie restriction. The result is a potent weight-management tool that requires close medical monitoring for adequate safe use. This chapter defines the nutrient range of VLCDs, their history, composition, indications, contraindications, effects, side effects, and the appropriate context for their safe use (Table 1).

2. DEFINITION

VLCDs, also referred to as supplemented fasting, by convention are diets that provide between 300 and 800 kcal per day. All VLCDs provide enough protein to meaningfully reduce lean tissue wasting, essential minerals and vitamins, and varying amounts of carbohydrates and fats. Although some early VLCDs provided as little as 35 g of protein and 300 kcal, in the last 20 yr most commercial formulations have provided at least 50 g of protein and ranged in daily energy intake between 400 and 600 kcal.

There are two general classes of VLCD: one consisting of common foods with dietary supplements of minerals and vitamins; the other consisting of a defined formula providing all nutrients as a beverage taken three to five times per day. The common food VLCD consists mostly of lean meat, fish, and poultry, whereas the formula VLCD usually requires the addition of carbohydrate as sugar or modified starch for the sake of palatability. The meat-based VLCD provides a modest dose of fat inherent in the food choices, whereas fat is not always provided in the defined formula diets.

From: *The Management of Eating Disorders and Obesity, Second Edition*
Edited by: D. J. Goldstein © Humana Press Inc., Totowa, NJ

Table 1
Chapter Overview

1. Introduction
2. Definition
3. History of the VLCD
4. Composition
    4.1. Carbohydrate
    4.2. Sodium, Potassium, and Trace Minerals
    4.3. Fat
5. Indications
6. Contraindications
7. Effects
    7.1. Weight
    7.2. Obesity-Associated Conditions
8. Side Effects
9. Context of Safe Use
10. Conclusion

Depending on the nutrients provided, VLCDs have a varying impact on starvation metabolism. Those providing less than 50 g of carbohydrate per day result in a state of nutritional ketosis (defined as serum β-hydroxybutyrate >0.5 mM). Depending on physical activity level, VLCDs exceeding 50 g of carbohydrate per day usually result in ketone levels below this threshold. The presence of ketosis during a VLCD has an impact on both the benefits and side effects anticipated during the diet.

3. HISTORY OF THE VLCD

The medical use of low-carbohydrate weight-loss diets dates back more than a century. In the 1930s, a food VLCD providing 50 g of protein in less than 400 kcal/d was demonstrated to reduce weight by more than 20 lb *(1)*. In this same time period, however, some physicians also advocated total fasting supplemented only by noncaloric fluids. In the post-World War II period, metabolic studies demonstrated that total fasting resulted in unacceptable losses of lean tissue and organ function, even in severely obese humans *(2)*. Among other concerns with total fasting, electrolyte imbalances and loss of cardiac function led physicians to abandon starvation as a therapeutic tool. This insight into the differentiation of lean tissue and body fat losses directed research attention to the development of rapid weight-loss diets that preserved lean tissue.

This interest in functional tissue preservation resulted in a series of studies demonstrating rapid outpatient weight loss without apparent cardiac harm *(3–5)*. The studies by Apfelbaum *(3)* and Genuth et al. *(4)* used defined amounts of purified protein plus minerals and vitamins with protein intakes ranging from 50 to 70 g/d. The study by Bistrian et al. *(5)* resulted in a recommendation that protein intake be based on the gender and stature of the patient, providing protein at 1.5 g/d/kg of ideal body weight. This translates into protein intakes varying in the range of 80 to 120 g/d for typical adults—substantially greater than that provided by most defined formulations of the time. In comparative studies, this higher protein intake has been demonstrated to be more efficacious in maintaining nitrogen balance *(6)* and physical performance *(7)*.

A watershed event in the history of VLCDs was the publication of a book *The Last Chance Diet* in 1976, which advocated an unmonitored 300 kcal/d diet consisting of hydrolyzed collagen. This "liquid protein diet" was notably deficient in both the major and trace minerals, and resulting cardiac dysrhythmias were responsible for the reported deaths of more than 50 people in the United States *(8)*. Most of these deaths occurred in people taking the hydrolyzed collagen as their sole source of energy for more than 2 mo. Electrocardiogram (EKG) findings in affected people who came to medical attention included low QRS-complex voltage and a prolonged QTc interval. At autopsy, cardiac atrophy was commonly noted *(9)*.

Although there were questions raised at the time about the inherent safety of ketogenic weight-loss diets, subsequent human studies demonstrated that cardiac rhythm disturbances and EKG changes could be prevented with adequate mineral and trace mineral supplementation of a ketogenic VLCD *(10,11)*. In addition, it was demonstrated that submaximal exercise performance was unimpaired after 6 wk and 25 lb of weight loss with a properly formulated common food *(12)* or formula *(13)* VLCD.

This unfortunate set of events surrounding the "liquid protein diet" serves to underscore the tenuous nutritional adequacy when total energy intake is restricted in the VLCD range. However, the subsequent research also documented that a properly formulated and monitored VLCD can be both safe and effective in preserving lean body mass and physical function across major weight loss.

4. COMPOSITION

4.1. Carbohydrate

As demonstrated by the "liquid protein diet" debacle, a VLCD requires many more nutrients than just protein to be safe and effective. The optimum protein content remains a point of debate, with some advocates claiming that added carbohydrate enhances the protein-sparing effects of a lower protein intake *(14)*. This claim was supported by the often quoted study by DeHaven et al.; however, this study was flawed by depriving one group of essential electrolytes. Subsequent studies have shown that providing protein at 1.5 g/kg reference body weight, as opposed to lower doses ranging from 0.8 to 1.1 g/kg, yields superior functional results across major weight loss *(6,7)*.

The inclusion of carbohydrate in a VLCD remains a topic of debate. There is no absolute human metabolic requirement for carbohydrate. Its inclusion reduces the degree of ketosis, and with it the amount of sodium necessary to maintain euvolemia (*see* Subheading 4.2.). Given, however, that the 2 to 3 g/d of sodium necessary to maintain euvolemia during ketosis is itself a relatively low salt intake, the anti-natriuretic effects of adding carbohydrate to a VLCD represents no real advantage. In addition, the published evidence does not support the claim that carbohydrate improves the protein-sparing effect of a VLCD over that achieved with an equivalent amount of additional protein. In the end, the primary driving force for the addition of carbohydrate to a VLCD is the simple reality that it improves the palatability of a defined formula (i.e., the popular "shake" mixtures used in lieu of food). It is thus likely that carbohydrate will continue to be used in defined formula VLCDs, and not be included in the food-based versions.

4.2. Sodium, Potassium, and Trace Minerals

A characteristic inherent to ketogenic diets is enhanced renal sodium clearance (natriuresis), that appears to result from increased renal tubular production of prostaglandin E_2. This is the cause of the early rapid weight loss owing to fluid mobilization in the first 1 to 2 wk of a VLCD, but it can also lead to hypovolemia, dizziness, and syncope if the VLCD is not supplemented with a modicum of sodium. In addition, prolonged hypovolemia induces an aldosterone response that leads to chronic potassium wasting with symptoms of weakness, muscle cramps, and dysrhythmias. Thus, a minimum of 2 to 3 g/d of sodium and 2 g/d of potassium are obligate components of a properly formulated VLCD.

The specific requirements for the other major minerals, calcium, phosphorus, and magnesium during a VLCD have not been carefully studied. Clinical experience dictates that the current daily reference intake (DRI) values are probably adequate. These are usually provided in current commercial VLCD formulations, but they require additional supplementation with calcium and magnesium during a food-based VLCD. This is also true for vitamins and trace minerals, with a standard multivitamin with trace minerals formulated against the DRI values providing adequate intakes of these essential nutrients.

4.3. Fats

An early concern with VLCDs was their lack of adequate essential fatty acids when used for prolonged periods. In the current era in developed countries where our basic diet is heavily laden with vegetable oils rich in linoleic acid, however, adipose tissue provides a fully adequate reserve for the ω-6 essential fatty acids, even after major weight loss *(15)*. However rapid weight loss depletes adipose tissue of its more limited reserves of ω-3 fats *(16)*. Given the propensity for the ω-3 fatty acid precursor α-linolenic acid to be β-oxidized during calorie restriction, however, it is not clear that supplementation with this ω-3 fatty acid has any net benefit during a VLCD *(17)*.

Another role of dietary fat during a VLCD is to maintain normal functional stimulation of the gallbladder. A daily intake of 20 g of fat will elicit a cholecystokinin response and gallbladder contraction, causing it to empty both bile acids and cholesterol into the upper gastrointestinal tract. We now know that rapid mobilization of adipose triglyceride (TG) during a VLCD is accompanied by mobilization of cholesterol dissolved in the adipose lipid stores, and that this occurs at a rate of about 300 mg/d *(18)*. This egress of a substantial pool of cholesterol via the gallbladder, accompanied by a lack of contractile stimulation of this organ, is likely the cause of frequent cholelithiasis seen with very low-fat VLCDs *(19)*.

The inclusion of fat in a VLCD is therefore primarily in the interest of maintaining normal gallbladder function, as ω-6 essential fatty acid status is not a problem and depletion of ω-3 fats is difficult to prevent. With a food-based VLCD, cold-water ocean fish containing a moderate amount of fat that is naturally rich in the ω-3 class may be beneficial, but repletion of the body's ω-3 content in adipose reserves is best achieved with a subsequent maintenance diet rich in these essential fatty acids (provided as fish, dark green vegetables, and selected nuts and grains).

5. INDICATIONS

The decision of whether the use of a VLCD is warranted for a particular patient revolves around the balance of the small risks associated with this very restricted diet compared to that individual's risks associated with excess body fat. With a well-formulated diet and appropriate medical monitoring (discussed in Subheading 9), the risks inherent in a VLCD are low, and its use therefore needs not be unduly restricted. In the past, arbitrary convention dictated that, to be a candidate for VLCD, a patient needed to be more than 20% above reference body weight (which translates to a body mass index [BMI] >27). With the increased awareness of the interaction between obesity and co-morbidity conditions like type 2 diabetes and hypertension, employing a VLCD for individuals with BMIs as low as 25 plus at least one comorbidity is reasonable.

Also important in determining appropriate use of a VLCD is the context in which the diet is used. Although this type of diet can be a very effective tool to induce rapid weight loss, VLCDs used in isolation have been documented to have little lasting effect on a person's weight over a period of years (20). Thus, some form of ongoing maintenance therapy, be it behavioral/group support or pharmacotherapy, should be anticipated before undertaking the expense, rigor, and small risks associated with a VLCD. Despite the well-intentioned patient and physician/therapist assumption that the weight-reduced obese patient will be motivated to self-regulate his or her weight, such that the reduced weight induced by a VLCD will be maintained, history shows that this rarely occurs. In the end, a VLCD does nothing to change the underlying biology that led to the initial weight accumulation and the typical patient resumes pre-VLCD metabolic set and/or eating behaviors.

6. CONTRAINDICATIONS

Medical conditions that contraindicate use of a VLCD include type-1 diabetes or any history of diabetic ketoacidosis, symptomatic cerebrovascular disease, myocardial infarction within the prior 6 mo, unstable angina, active life-threatening malignancy, and significantly impaired liver function (e.g., serum albumin <32 g/L) or renal function (e.g., serum creatinine >20 mg/L). In addition, patients who are unable to comprehend the need for close diet adherence and medical monitoring should be excluded, as should those with a history of poorly controlled eating disorders, such as anorexia nervosa or bulimia nervosa.

7. EFFECTS

7.1. Weight

With initiation of a VLCD, prompt and frequently marked weight loss occurs. The onset within a few days of the natriuresis of fasting and mobilization of liver and muscle glycogen with its associated intracellular water can result in up to 10 lb of total weight loss in the first wk. Along with this major fluid egress in the first wk, the actual adipose tissue loss may total 2 to 3 lb, plus 1 or 2 lb of lean body mass as the body adapts to the developing nutritional ketosis. By the end of wk 2 of a VLCD, the patient's fluid and electrolyte status stabilizes and, given adequate protein and minerals, the loss of lean body mass ceases. From that time on, the average weekly weight loss ranges from 1.5 lb/wk for the shorter person with little activity to 3 lb/week for a taller and more active person.

The total weight loss achievable with a VLCD varies greatly depending on a number of factors such as initial weight, the degree of support provided to the patient, and the duration of diet use. If used for sustained periods of 4 to 5 mo, a majority of appropriately selected patients will adhere to a VLCD and achieve mean losses in the 50 to 60 lb range *(21)*. Interestingly, if the VLCD is interrupted even briefly during a major weight-loss effort, resumption of the diet proves to be very difficult for unknown reasons *(22)*.

Most patients on a VLCD report a reduced perceived need to eat within the first week or two of the diet. This effect usually persists for a number of months as long as the diet-induced nutritional ketosis is not interrupted by increased carbohydrate. This effect has been difficult to quantify using an objective metric, owing in part to the variable perceptions of patients. Some report it as decreased hunger, whereas others note that hunger persists, but that they are better able to resist it.

7.2. Obesity-Associated Conditions

A number of medical conditions improve markedly upon initiation of a VLCD (*see* Chapter 10). Type 2 diabetes usually responds with marked improvement in blood sugar, often requiring early reduction or cessation of injected insulin or oral agents. Analogously, patients with hypertension experience prompt improvement in blood pressure requiring withdrawal of medication. This is especially true of patients taking diuretics, for whom reduction in dosage or cessation is usually necessary in the first week of the diet.

Among the blood lipids, the most consistent response is seen in the serum TGs, which demonstrate a sharp and sustained decline in most patients. The typical response of serum cholesterol to a VLCD is an initial decline in total cholesterol, coming mostly from a reduction in the low-density lipoprotein (LDL) fraction. This reduction in serum cholesterol usually persists for the first 2 to 3 mo of a VLCD. However, when a patient's weight loss exceeds 30 lb, continuation of the VLCD is often accompanied by a rise in the LDL cholesterol, sometimes to the point that the total cholesterol exceeds the patient's initial value *(18)*. This hypercholesterolemic response to major weight loss is the result of resident cholesterol being mobilized out of the shrinking adipose TG pool. This effect is transient, ceasing when the patient's weight stabilizes after completion of the VLCD. Because the transient elevation is driven by existing cholesterol coming from adipose stores, Z-hydroxy-Z-CoA reductase inhibitors are relatively ineffective against this mechanism.

In light of the recent interest in low-grade inflammation associated with both heart disease *(23)* and obesity *(24)*, the effect of a ketogenic diet on biomarkers of inflammation is worth noting. In one study in healthy male athletes given a weight-maintaining ketogenic diet, the total white blood cell count declined 15% in 4 wk *(25)*. A comparative study of the Atkins diet vs a balanced weight-loss regimen demonstrated decreases in serum amyloid A and serum C-reactive protein with the ketogenic diet *(26)*. Although weight loss itself has the potential to reduce inflammatory mediators such as tumor necrosis factor-α and leptin produced in adipose tissue, carbohydrate-restricted diets appear to have both independent and more pronounced effects on this class of disease biomarkers.

8. SIDE EFFECTS

There are two groupings of VLCD side effects, based on when they occur during the VLCD. Those that occur initially during adaptation to carbohydrate restriction and nutritional ketosis are either transient or respond promptly to intervention. The most common among these is the combination of weakness, fatigue, and lightheadedness.

Although there is a modest reduction in peak aerobic performance in the first week or two of a VLCD *(12)*, orthostatic symptoms (noted in Subheading 4.2.) occurring during normal daily activities are the result of the combination of diet-induced natriuresis and an inadequate sodium intake. Thus, these symptoms can be prevented by the routine addition of 2 to 3 g/d of sodium (taken as bouillon) in all patients not requiring continued diuretic medication, along with attention to adequate dietary potassium.

Most patients starting on a VLCD also note greater sensitivity to cold, and this is associated with a 10% reduction in resting metabolic rate *(13)*. This is the result of the severe energy restriction, and returns to normal when the VLCD is stopped. This effect of the VLCD on resting metabolism is not reversed with exercise *(13)* and cannot be safely overcome with the addition of exogenous thyroid hormone.

Constipation can also occur during a VLCD. This is owing in part to the low fiber content of many formulations, but it is usually exacerbated by dehydration. If increasing fluid intake to a minimum of 2 L/d does not resolve it, then a carbohydrate-free fiber supplement can be used.

Muscle cramps sometimes occur either early or late in treatment with a VLCD. They are more common in people with a history of diuretic medication use or prior heavy ethanol consumption. In almost all cases, they respond promptly to supplementation with 200 mEq/d of slow-release magnesium chloride, suggesting prior depletion of this essential mineral as the root cause.

In patients with a history of gout, an attack of this acute arthritis can be induced during initiation of the VLCD. The mechanism for this effect of ketogenic diets is the competition between β-hydroxybutyrate and uric acid for excretion in the renal tubule. This process induces a transient rise in serum uric acid in the first few weeks of a VLCD, during which time those patients prone to gout are at risk of an attack. With the subsequent adaptation to nutritional ketosis, however, the renal handling of uric acid returns to normal and the risk of an acute attack subsides. This can be managed by prophylaxis with allopurinol in selected patients with a history of gout, or by treatment of the acute event with a nonsteroidal anti-inflammatory drug (NSAID).

As noted previously, the gallbladder experiences an increased flux of cholesterol during rapid weight loss (*see* Subheading 4.3.). This is best managed by maintaining enough daily fat intake (>20 g/d) to prevent cholestasis. Given the typical patient's net oxidation of 150 to 200 g/d of body fat, this modest dietary fat intake does not significantly impact the rate of weight loss. In addition, patients deemed high risk because of prior history of or existing gallstones can be treated prophylactically with ursodeoxycholic acid *(28)*.

Late-onset side effects can include dry skin, hair loss, and loss of normal menstrual cycles in women. All of these are self-limited and can be treated symptomatically or by physician reassurance, and they routinely resolve when the VLCD is stopped.

9. CONTEXT OF SAFE USE

Because of the narrow margin of nutrient adequacy caused by the severe energy restriction of a VLCD, this type of diet should only be employed in the context of careful patient screening and monitoring by an experienced physician. Initial patient screening should evaluate the patient for the presence of exclusion criteria. This evaluation requires a medical history, physical examination, EKG, blood chemistries, and a complete blood count.

Routine monitoring should include weekly weight and blood pressure determinations and assessment for subjective side effects. Blood chemistries should be repeated monthly, or more frequently, if abnormalities are identified in electrolytes or organ function.

Although slow weight loss may be to the result of nonadherence to the VLCD, it can also occur transiently owing to exercise-induced muscle soreness or fluid retention associated with concurrent NSAID use. After the first week, weight loss exceeding an average of 3 lb/wk is a medical concern, and warrants evaluation of potential inappropriate diuretic use or nonconsumption of the VLCD. Patients need to understand that speeding weight loss by not consuming the prescribed nutrients sacrifices lean body mass and function, putting both their health and their potential to subsequently maintain the loss at risk.

10. CONCLUSION

A VLCD is potentially a safe and very useful tool in the treatment of obesity. But just as an engine is of little value as transportation unless it is incorporated into a complete automobile, a VLCD by itself cannot be regarded as effective therapy. Its value in treatment of obesity is thus highly context-dependent. Its use requires close monitoring, and it should always be followed by a credible and sustained weight-maintenance program. Further progress in understanding the biology underlying excess adipose tissue accumulation should lead to effective and safe methods to suppress weight regain, at which time the VLCD will be a useful first step in the long-term treatment of the severely obese.

REFERENCES

1. Evans FA, Strang JM. The treatment of obesity with low calorie diets. JAMA 1931; 97:1063–1069.
2. Cahill GF. Starvation in man. N Engl J Med 1970; 282:668–675.
3. Apfelbaum M. The effects of very restrictive high protein diets. Clin Endocrinol Metab 1976; 5:417–430.
4. Genuth SM, Castro JH, Vertes V. Weight reduction in obesity by outpatient semi-starvation. JAMA 1974; 230:987–991.
5. Bistrian BR, Winterer J, Blackburn GL, Young V, Sherman M. Effect of a protein-sparing diet and brief fast on nitrogen metabolism in mildly obese subjects. J Lab Clin Med 1977; 89:1030–1035.
6. Hoffer LJ, Bistrian BR, Young VR, Blackburn GL, Matthews DE. Metabolic effects of very low calorie weight reduction diets. J Clin Invest 1984; 73:750–758.
7. Davis PG, Phinney SD. Differential effects of two very low calorie diets on aerobic and anaerobic performance. Int J Ob 1990; 14:779–787.
8. Sours HE, Fratelli VP, Brand CD, Feldman RA, Forbes AL, Swanson RC, Paris AL. Sudden death associated with very low calorie weight reduction regimens. Am J Clin Nutr 1981; 34:453–461.
9. Brown JM, Yetter JF Spicer MJ, Jones JD. Cardiac complications of a protein sparing modified fast. JAMA 1978; 240:120–122.
10. Amatruda JM, Biddle TL, Patton ML, Lockwood DH. Vigorous supplementation of a hypocaloric diet prevents cardiac arrhythmias and mineral depletion. Am J Med 1983; 74:1016–1022.
11. Phinney SD, Bistrian BR, Kosinski E, et al. Normal cardiac rhythm during hypocaloric diets of varying carbohydrate content. Arch Int Med 1983; 143:2258–2261.
12. Phinney SD, Horton ES, Sims EAH, Hanson JS, Danforth E Jr, LaGrange BM. Capacity for moderate exercise in obese subjects after adaptation to a hypocaloric ketogenic diet. J Clin Invest 1980; 66: 1152–1161.
13. Phinney SD, LaGrange BM, O'Connell M, Danforth E Jr. Effects of aerobic exercise on energy expenditure and nitrogen balance during very low calorie dieting. Metabolism 1988; 37:758–765.
14. DeHaven J, Sherwin R, Hendler R, Felig P. Nitrogen and sodium balance and sympathetic nervous system activity in obese subjects treated with a low calorie protein or mixed diet. N Engl J Med 1980; 302:477–482.

15. Phinney SD, Tang AB, Johnson SB, Holman RT. Reduced adipose 18:3ω3 with weight loss by very low calorie dieting. Lipids 1990; 25:798–806.
16. Kunesova M, Phinney S, Hainer V, et al. Serum and adipose fatty acids in female obese identical twins—one year weight Reduction. Proc NY Acad Sci 2002; 967:214–218.
17. Tang AB, Nishimura KY, Phinney SD. Preferential reduction in adipose tissue α-linolenic acid (18:3ω3) during very low calorie dieting despite supplementation with 3ω3. Lipids 1994; 28:987–993.
18. Phinney SD, Tang AB, Waggoner CR, Tesanos-Pinto R, Davis P. The transient hypercholesterolemia of major weight loss. Am J Clin Nutr 1991; 53:1404–1410.
19. Liddle RA, Goldstein RB, Saxton J. Gallstone formation during weight reduction dieting. Arch Int Med 1989; 149:1750–1753.
20. Very low-calorie diets. National Task Force on the Prevention and Treatment of Obesity, National Institutes of Health. JAMA 1993; 270:967–974.
21. Palgi A, Read JL, Greenberg I, Hoefer MA, Bistrian BR, Blackburn GL. Multidisciplinary treatment of obesity with a protein-sparing modified fast: results in 668 outpatients. Am J Public Health 1985; 75: 1190–1194.
22. Smith DE, Wing RR. Diminished weight loss and behavioral compliance during repeated diets in obese patients with type II diabetes. Health Psychol 1991; 10:378–383.
23. Ridker PM, Rifai N, Rose L, Buring JE, Cook NR. Comparison of C-reactive protein and low-density lipoprotein cholesterol levels in the prediction of first cardiovascular events. N Engl J Med 2002; 347: 1557–1565.
24. M. Visser, LM. Bouter, GM. McQuillan, Wener MH, Harris TB. Elevated C-reactive protein levels in overweight and obese adults JAMA 1999; 282:2131–2135.
25. Phinney SD. The eucaloric ketogenic diet: the human metabolic response with rest and exercise. PhD thesis. MIT, Cambridge, MA, 1980.
26. O'Brien KD, Brehm BJ, Seeley RJ. Greater reduction in inflammatory markers with a low carbohydrate diet than with a calorically matched low fat diet. Abstract no.: 117597. Presented at American Heart Association's Scientific Sessions, November 19, 2002.
27. Shiffman ML, Kaplan GD, Brinkman-Kaplan V, Vickers FF. Prophylaxis against gallstone formation with ursodeoxycholic acid in patients participating in a very-low-calorie diet program. Ann Intern Med 1995; 122:899–905.

16   Pharmacotherapy of Obesity

George A. Bray

KEY POINTS

- Patients with body mass index (BMI) of 30 kg/m^2 or more or no less than 27 kg/m^2 with a cormorbid condition are potential candidates for pharmacotherapy.
- Drugs to treat obesity can be divided into three groups: those that reduce food intake, those that alter metabolism, and those that increase thermogenesis.
- Present obesity pharmacotherapies result in modest weight loss on average.
- Patients who are motivated to undertake concurrent lifestyle change may receive health benefits from the additional weight loss that accompanies medication use.

1. INTRODUCTION

Medicating for treatment of obesity can be a useful adjunct to diet and exercise and can help selected patients achieve and maintain meaningful weight loss. A report from the Heart, Lung and Blood Institute of the National Institutes of Health entitled *Clinical Guidelines on the Identification, Evaluation, and Treatment of Overweight and Obesity in Adults—The Evidence Report (1)* emphasizes the need for physicians to address obesity in their patients. This report sanctions the clinical use of weight loss drugs approved by the US Food and Drug Administration (FDA) for long-term use as part of a concomitant lifestyle-modification program. Appropriate patients include those who have been unsuccessful in previous weight-loss attempts and whose BMI exceeds 27 kg/m^2 who have associated conditions such as diabetes, hypertension, or dyslipidemia, or whose BMI exceeds 30 kg/m^2. Still, for many physicians, treatment of obesity is not a routine part of their clinical practices, in part because of the stigma associated with medication usage.

Drug treatment for obesity has been tarnished by a number of unfortunate problems *(2)*. Since the introduction of thyroid hormone to treat obesity in 1893, almost every drug that has been tried in obese patients has lead to undesirable outcomes that have resulted in their termination. Thus, caution must be used in accepting any new drugs for treatment of obesity, unless the safety profile would make it acceptable for almost everyone (*see* Chapter 24).

From: *The Management of Eating Disorders and Obesity, Second Edition*
Edited by: D. J. Goldstein © Humana Press Inc., Totowa, NJ

Table 1
Chapter Overview

An additional serious negative aspect to the use of drug treatment for obesity is the negative halo spread by the addictive properties of amphetamine *(3)*. Amphetamine stands for α-methyl-phenethylamine. It is indicated for narcolepsy and attention deficit disorder, but it is also addictive. It reduces food intake, but it is not recommended for obesity management. The addictiveness of amphetamine is probably related to its effects on dopaminergic neurotransmission. On the other hand, its anorectic effects appear to result from modulation of noradrenergic neurotransmission. Drugs such as phentermine, diethylpropion, fenfluramine, sibutramine, and the antidepressant venlafaxine are all β-phenethylamines. Phentermine and diethylpropion are sympathomimetic amines, like amphetamine, but differ from amphetamine in having little or no effect on dopamine release or reuptake at the synapse. Abuse of either phentermine or diethylpropion is rare *(2)*. Fenfluramine is also a β-phenethylamine, but it has no effect on reuptake or release of either norepinephrine or dopamine in the brain. Fenfluramine is a potent serotonin releaser and it inhibits monoamine reuptake; its effect on dopamine is minimal and it partially inhibits serotonin reuptake. There have been no reports of addiction to fenflur-amine. Sibutramine has no evident abuse potential *(4)*. Thus, derivatives of β-phen-ethylamine have a wide range of pharmacologic effects and highly variable potential for abuse. However, if examined uncritically, they could all be lumped with "amphetamine" and carry its negative halo. It is thus misleading to use "amphetamine-like" in reference to appetite-suppressant β-phenethylamine drugs except amphetamine and methamphetamine because of the negative linguistic images and inaccurate linguistic content.

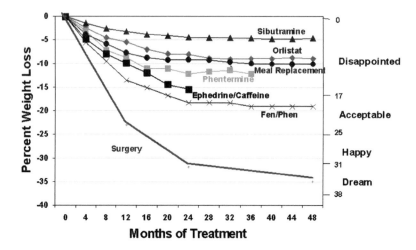

Fig. 1. Relation of plateaued weight during treatment for obesity and participant expectations in a weight-loss program. The left-hand ordinate shows the percent weight loss for each treatment. The right-hand ordinate shows the cut points for weight-loss expectations for each category. Only surgical treatment *(17)* produced a "dream" level of weight loss. The combination of fenfluramine and phentermine *(2,3)* produced acceptable weight loss, but the other treatments, including ephedrine combined with caffeine *(16)*, phentermine *(14)*, meal replacement *(13)*, orlistat *(12)*, and sibutramine *(11)* left patients disappointed.

A third issue surrounding drug treatment of obesity is the negative attitude that results when patients relapse after successful treatment. The perception arises that the drugs are ineffective because weight regain occurs when drug treatment is stopped *(5)*. Cure for obesity is rare, and treatment is thus aimed at palliation. As clinicians, we do not expect to cure such diseases as hypertension or hypercholesterolemia with medications. Rather, we expect to palliate them. When the medications for any of these diseases are discontinued, we expect the disease to recur. This means that medications only work when used. The same arguments apply to medications used to treat overweight. It is a chronic, incurable disease for which drugs only work when used.

Reports of valvular heart disease associated with the use of fenfluramine, dexfenfluramine, and phentermine have provided the most recent ammunition for those who disapprove of treating obesity with medications *(6–8)*. This is an example of the "law of unintended consequences." The reports of valvulopathy in patients treated with fenfluramine or dexfenfluramine were totally unexpected. Thankfully, the extent of the problem has not proven to be as great as first suspected *(8)*. It is now recognized that risk for valvulopathy associated with fenfluramine is associated with duration of exposure to the medication *(8)* and that the lesions are likely to remit off medication *(9,10)*. The finding, however, will add caution when any future drugs are marketed to treat obesity and will provide support for those who believe drug treatment of obesity is inappropriate and risky.

The final issue to address is the plateau of weight that occurs with all treatments for obesity *(11–17)*. Figure 1 shows the weight loss that can be achieved by various treatments in relation to the expectations of patients when they enter treatment. At the beginning of treatment a weight loss of less than 15% is considered unsatisfactory by most obese patients *(18)*. This is a discrepancy in the amount of weight loss that is cosmetically desired and the amount of weight loss that will produce health benefits. Yet the reality is that none of the treatments, except gastric bypass (*see* Chapter 20) *(17)*, produce a consistent weight loss of more than15%. When weight loss plateaus at a level above their desired cosmetic goal, patients usually blame the treatment. The perceived loss of effectiveness often leads patients to terminate treatment with the inevitable slow regain of the weight that had been lost.

In weighing the options regarding treatments for obesity, physicians must be cognizant of these barriers to success. It is against these limitations that we review currently available medications (*see* Table 1).

2. MECHANISMS FOR DRUG TREATMENT OF OBESITY

Obesity results from an imbalance between energy intake (EI) and energy expenditure (EE). Drugs can shift this balance in a favorable way by reducing food intake (EI), altering metabolism, and/or by increasing EE. These three mechanisms will be used to classify the drugs used for treating obesity *(2,19)*.

2.1. Reducing Food Intake

2.1.1. Neurotransmitters in the Central Nervous System

2.1.1.1. Monoamines and Amino Acids

2.1.1.1.1. Norepinephrine

A number of monoamines and neuropeptides are known to modulate food intake. Both noradrenergic receptors and serotonergic receptors have served as the site for clinically useful drugs to decrease food intake *(2,15)* (Table 2). Activation of the α_1- and β_2-adrenoceptors decreases food intake. On the other hand, activation of the α_2-adrenoceptor in experimental animals increases food intake. Direct agonists and drugs that release norepinephrine (NE) or block NE reuptake at the neuronal junction can activate one or more of these receptors depending on where the NE is released. Phenylpropanolamine (PPA) is an α_1-agonist formerly used for weight loss, that decreases food intake by acting on α_1-adrenergic receptors in the paraventricular nucleus (PVN). The weight gain, seen in patients treated with α_1-adrenergic antagonists for hypertension or prostatic hypertrophy, indicates that the α_1-adrenoceptor is clinically important in regulation of body weight. Stimulation of the β_2-adrenoceptor by NE or agonists like terbutaline, clenbuterol, or salbutamol reduces food intake. The weight gain in patients treated with some β_2-adrenergic antagonists also indicates that this is a clinically important receptor for regulation of body weight.

2.1.1.1.2. Serotonin

The serotonin receptor system consists of seven families of receptors. Stimulation of receptors in the hydroxytryptamine 5-HT$_1$ and 5-HT$_2$ families produces the major effects on feeding. Activation of the 5-HT$_{1A}$ receptor increases food intake but this acute effect is rapidly downregulated and is not clinically significant in control of body weight. Activation of the 5-HT$_{2C}$ and possibly 5-HT$_{1B}$ receptor decreases food intake. Direct agonists, such as quipazine, or drugs that block serotonin reuptake, such as fluoxetine,

Table 2
Mechanisms That Reduce Food Intake

System	Mechanism	Example
Noradrenergic	α_1-Agonist	Phenylpropanolamine
	α_2-Antagonist	Yohimbine
	β_2-Agonist	Clenbuterol
	Stimulate norepinephrine release	Phentermine
	Block norepinephrine reuptake	Mazindol
Serotonergic	5-HT$_{1B}$ or 5-HT$_{1C}$ Agonist	Metergoline
	Stimulates 5-HT release	Fenfluramine
	Serotonin reuptake inhibitor	Fluoxetine
Dopaminergic	D-2 Agonist	Apomorphine
Mixed monoaminergic	Norepinephrine, serotonin, and dopamine reuptake inhibitor	Buproprion Sibutramine
Histaminergic	H-1 Antagonist	Chlorpheniramine

sertraline, or fenfluramine, will reduce food intake by acting on these receptors or by providing the serotonin that modulates these receptors.

2.1.1.1.3. Amino Acids

Several amino acids act as neurotransmitters within the central nervous system (CNS). From the perspective of this chapter, γ-aminobutyric acid (GABA) is the most important. This amino acid binds to two different receptors, one that is coupled to a chloride channel and the other generates cyclic nucleotides. The GABA$_A$ receptor is a pentameric structure that also has binding sites for the benzodiazepines. GABA$_A$ can increase or decrease food intake, depending on the brain-stem site of action. This receptor may be the site for modulation of several drugs that increase or decrease food intake.

2.1.1.1.4. Cannabinoids

Some of the cannabinoids isolated from the cannabis species (marijuana) reduce food intake by acting on central receptors (*see* Subheading 3.4.2.).

2.1.1.2. CNS PEPTIDES

2.1.1.2.1. Neuropeptide Y

Neuropeptide Y (NPY), a 36 amino acid peptide that is widely distributed in the CNS, is one of the most potent activators of the hunger system. The peptide involved in feeding is produced in the arcuate nucleus and is released to activate NPY receptors in the PVN. There are four receptors (1, 2, 4 and 5) for this peptide; and both Y-1 and Y-5 have been implicated in feeding.

2.1.1.2.2. Melanocortin Modulators

Proopiomelanocortin is a large peptide precursor formed during posttranslational processing of several biologically active peptides, including adrenocorticotrophic hormone, lipotropin, and α-melanocyte stimulating hormones (α-MSH. α-MSH released in the brain reduces food intake through interaction with melanocortin receptors 3 and 4.

A naturally occurring antagonist to α-MSH, agouti-related peptide (AGRP) is a biological inhibitor of α-MSH. Overexpression of AGRP through genetic engineering produces obesity in animals.

2.1.1.3. GASTROINTESTINAL PEPTIDES

2.1.1.3.1. Ghrelin

Ghrelin is a 28 amino acid peptide with an octanoyl linkage. It is released from the stomach and is the natural agonist for the growth hormone secreteagogue receptor. It is a potent stimulator of food intake in experimental animals and humans.

2.1.1.3.2. Amylin

Amylin is co-secreted with insulin from the β-cell of the pancreas. In experimental animals exendin, an analogue of amylin, was shown to reduce food intake.

2.1.1.3.3. Polypeptide YY

Polypeptide YY (PYY) (3-36) is named because of the tyrosine amino acids at each end of the peptide chain. PYY is released from the gastrointestinal (GI) track and reduces food intake in experimental animals and in human beings.

2.1.1.3.4. Cholecystokinin

Cholecystokinin was one of the earliest GI peptides to be isolated and was one of the first to be shown to affect feeding. Acting through cholecystokinin receptor A, this peptide produces dose-dependent decreases in food intake in experimental animals and human beings.

2.1.1.3.5. Glucagon-Like Peptide-1

The precursor of glucagon can be processed into several forms, including the 9-36 amino acid derivative called glucagon-like peptide-1. When administered to human beings, this peptide will reduce food intake and stimulate insulin release from the β-cell of the pancreas.

2.1.1.4. ADIPOSE TISSUE

2.1.1.4.1. Leptin

Leptin, isolated by molecular cloning in 1994 (20), changed the biological understanding of food intake. This large peptide is formed primarily in adipose tissue where it is released into the circulation in direct relation to the amount of fat tissue in the body. It acts on receptors in the brain to reduce food intake and to stimulate the sympathetic nervous system.

2.2. Altering Metabolism

Excess fat is the visible sign of obesity. Metabolic strategies have been directed at pre-absorptive and postabsorptive mechanisms for modifying fat or carbohydrate absorption or metabolism. Preabsorptive mechanisms that influence digestion and absorption of macronutrients provide the mechanism of action for orlistat, a drug that inhibits intestinal digestion of fat and lowers body weight. The second strategy is to affect intermediary metabolism. Enhancing lipolysis, inhibiting lipogenesis, and affecting fat distribution between subcutaneous and visceral sites are strategies that can be developed (2,21).

Table 3
Drugs Approved by the US Food and Drug Administration for Treatment of Obesity

Drug	Trade names	Dosage	DEA schedule	Cost per day
Pancreatic lipase inhbitor approved for long-term use				
Orlistat	Xenical	120 mg tid before meals	—	$3.56/d
Norepinephrine-serotonin reuptake inhibitor approved for long-term use				
Sibutramine	Meridia	5–15 mg/d	IV	
	Reductil			$2.98–$3.68
Noradrenergic drugs approved for short-term use				
Diethylpropion	Tenuate	25 mg tid	IV	$1.27–$ 1.52
	Tepanil			
	Tenuate Dospan	75 mg q AM		
Phentermine	Adipex	15–37.5 mg/d	IV	$0.67–$1.60
	Fastin			
	Oby-Cap	15–30 mg/d		
	Ionamin slow			
	release			$1.75–$2.01
Benzphetamine	Didrex	25–50 mg tid	III	$1.19–$2.38
Phendimetrazine	Bontril	17.5–70 mg tid	III	$1.20–$5.25
	Plegine			
	Prelu-2	105 mg qd.		
	X-Trozine			

DEA, Drug Enforcement Agency.

2.3. Increasing Energy Expenditure

Increasing EE through exercise would be an ideal approach to treating obesity. Drugs that have the same physiological thermogenic consequences as exercise could provide a useful pharmaceutical alternative for treating this intractable problem *(2,20)*.

3. DRUGS THAT REDUCE FOOD INTAKE

Table 3 summarizes the effects of a number of drugs that are currently available in the United States to treat obesity *(2,21)*. They are discussed in more detail in this section.

3.1. Sympathomimetic Drugs Approved by the FDA to Treat Obesity

3.1.1. Pharmacology

The sympathomimetic drugs are grouped together because they can increase blood pressure (BP) and, in part, act like NE. Drugs in this group work by a variety of mechanisms including the release of NE from synaptic granules (benzphetamine, phendimetrazine, phentermine, and diethylpropion), the blockade of NE reuptake (mazindol), or blockade of reuptake of both NE and 5-HT (sibutramine).

All of these drugs are absorbed orally and reach peak blood concentrations within a short time. The half-life in blood is also short for all except the two pharmacologically active metabolites of sibutramine, which have a long half-life *(2)*. Although the two metabolites of sibutramine are active, this is not true for the metabolites of other drugs in this group. Liver metabolism inactivates a large fraction of these drugs before excretion. Side effects include dry mouth, constipation, and insomnia. Food intake is suppressed either by delaying the onset of a meal or by producing early satiety. Sibutramine and mazindol have both been shown to increase thermogenesis *(23–26)*.

3.1.2. EFFICACY

The criterion used by the FDA for the efficacy of appetite-suppressing drugs is demonstration in randomized double-blind placebo-controlled clinical trials of statistically significant weight loss that is 5% below the placebo group *(2)*. A decrease in weight that is 10% below baseline and significantly greater than placebo is the major criterion for the European Committee on Proprietary Medicinal Products. Clinical trials of sympathomimetic drugs done before 1975 were generally short term because it was widely believed that short-term treatment would "cure obesity" *(2,27)*. This was unfounded optimism, but because the trials were of short duration, and often crossover in design, they provided little long-term data. In this review, we focus on longer-term trials lasting 24 wk or more and only those trials in which there is an adequate control group.

3.1.2.1. PHENTERMINE, DIETHYLPROPION, BENZPHETAMINE, AND PHENDIMETRAZINE

Table 4 provides a summary of the long-term clinical trials on the first generation of sympathomimetic drugs *(2,19,28–33)*. The best and one of the longest of these clinical trials lasted 36 wk and compared placebo treatment with continuous phentermine or intermittent phentermine (Fig. 2) *(14)*. Both continuous and intermittent phentermine therapy produced more weight loss than did placebo. In the drug-free periods, the patients treated intermittently slowed their weight loss only to lose more rapidly when the drug was reinstituted.

The US Drug Enforcement Agency classifies phentermine and diethylpropion as schedule IV drugs and benzphetamine and phendimetrazine as schedule III drugs. This regulatory classification indicates the government's belief that they have the potential for abuse, although this potential appears to be very low. Phentermine and diethylpropion are only approved for a "few weeks" use, which is usually interpreted as up to 12 wk. Weight loss with phentermine and diethylpropion persists for the duration of treatment, suggesting that tolerance does not develop to these drugs. If tolerance were to develop, the drugs would be expected to lose their effectiveness or require increased amounts of drug for patients to maintain weight loss. This does not occur. Of the agents in this group, phentermine is prescribed most frequently in the United States, probably because it is inexpensive, since it is no longer protected by patents. Phentermine is not available in Europe. A recent review in a prestigious journal *(34)* recommends obtaining written informed consent if phentermine is prescribed for longer than 12 wk, because this is off-label usage and there are too few published reports on the use of phentermine for long-term use.

3.1.2.2. SIBUTRAMINE

In contrast to the sympathomimetic drugs in Table 4, sibutramine has been extensively evaluated in several multicenter trials lasting 6 to 24 mo that are summarized in Table 5 *(11,35–47)*. In a clinical trial lasting 8 wk, sibutramine produced a dose-dependent weight loss with doses of 5 and 20 mg/d *(48)*. Several long-term, randomized,

Table 4
Long-Term Studies With Noradrenergic Drugs

Year (reference)	No. of subjects Start P	Start D	Complete P	Complete D	Dose (mg/d)	Duration of study (weeks)	Initial weight (kg) P	D	Weight loss (kg) P	D	Weight loss (%) P	D	Comments
Diethylpropion													
1965 (28)	16	16	6	5	75	52	78.8	80.7	−10.5	−8.9	−13.3	−11.0	Medication given on alternate months
1973 (29)	10	10	6	10	75	24	84.5	92.3	−2.5	−11.7	−2.8	−12.3	
Phentermine													
1968 (14)	36	36	25	17	30	36	92.3	94.1	−4.8	−12.2	−5.9	−15	Continuous Rx group (top) lost as much as intermittent therapy (bottom)
	36	22						97.3		−13.0		−16	
1974 (30)	35	35	29	30	30	14	87.0	85.1	−1.8	−7.3	−2.1	−8.5	1000 kcal/d diet
1977 (31)	11	11	11	11	30	16	84.1	85.0	−2.9	−7.8	−3.4	−9.2	Obese diabetics
1977 (32)	35	36	32	34	30	24	N/A	N/A	−1.5	−5.3	N/A	N/A	Obese diabetics; Diet, biguanide or insulin
1981 (33)	15	15	11	11	30	24	73.6	73.6	−4.5	−6.3	−9.2	−12.6	Elderly with osteoarthritis
1984 (3)	20	20	10	14	30 (resin)	20	N/A	N/A	−4.4	−10.0	N/A	N/A	Four-arm trial: placebo; fenfluramine (F); phentermine (P); and F + P

P, placebo-treated patients; D, drug-treated patients.
No baseline weights were given

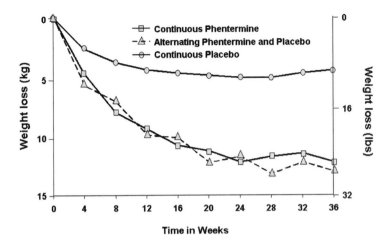

Fig. 2. Comparison of weight loss with continuous and intermittent therapy using phentermine *(14)*. Overweight patients were randomized to perceive either placebo or one of two dosing regimens with phentermine. One regimen provided 15 mg/d each morning for 9 mo and the other provided 15 mg/d for 1 mo and then 1 mo of no treatment. (From ref. *14*. Reprinted with permission from the BMJ Publishing Group.)

placebo-controlled, double-blind clinical trials have been conducted in men and women of all ethnic groups with ages ranging from 18 to 65 yr and with a BMI between 27 kg/m^2 and 40 kg/m^2. In a 6-mo dose-ranging study of 1047 patients, 67% achieved a 5% weight loss and 35% lost 10% or more. Data from this multicenter trial is shown in Fig. 3 *(36)*. There is a clear dose-response in this 24-wk trial, and regain of weight occurred when the drug was stopped, indicating that the drug remained effective when used. Nearly two-thirds of the patients treated with sibutramine lost more than 5% of their body weight from baseline and nearly one-third lost more than 10%. In a study of patients who were randomized to 10 mg/d of sibutramine or placebo, and behavioral program after initially losing weight after a very low-calorie diet, sibutramine produced additional weight loss (16% from baseline at 1 yr), whereas the placebo-treated patients regained weight *(37)*.

A number of observations about sibutramine can be drawn from the Sibutramine Trial of Obesity Reduction and Maintenance (STORM) trial *(39)*, but the effect of sibutramine in aiding weight maintenance is most persuasive. Seven centers participated in the STORM trial in which patients were initially treated open-label with 10 mg/d of sibutra-mine for 6 mo (Fig. 4). Those patients who lost more than 5% (and 77% of enrolled patients met this goal) were then randomized two-thirds to sibutramine and one-third to placebo. During the 18-mo double-blind portion of the trial, the placebo-treated patients steadily regained weight, maintaining only 20% of their weight loss at the end of the trial. In contrast, the subjects treated with sibutramine maintained their weight for 12 mo and then regained an average of only 2 kg, thus maintaining 80% of their initial weight loss after 2 yr *(39)*. Despite that sibutramine-treated patients had lost several kilograms more than the placebo-treated patients at the end of the 18 mo of controlled observation, the mean BP of the sibutramine-treated patients was still higher than that of placebo-treated patients.

Table 5
Clinical Trials With Sibutramine

Year (reference)	No. of subjects Start P	Start D	Complete P	Complete D	Dose (mg/d)	Duration of study (weeks)	Initial weight (kg) P	D	Weight loss (kg) P	D	Weight loss (%) P	D	Comments
1991 (48)	20	20	19	19	—	8	97		-1.4		-1.3		Dose-ranging phase II
	20	20	18	18	5			97.9		-2.9		-3.0	
	20	20	18	18	20			102.4		-5.0		-5.1	
1996 (35)	24	24	23	23		24	92.0		-0.75		-0.77		Part of multicenter study. Data on completing women.
	24	24	21	21	1			95.8		-2.96		-3.20	
	25	25	24	24	5			90.9		-2.87		-0.07	
	25	25	22	22	10			87.2		-6.19		-6.91	
	25	25	20	20	15			89.7		-6.89		-7.77	
	24	24	22	22	20			90.9		-7.30		-8.06	
	26	26	23	23	30			91.4		-8.24		-9.17	
1999 (36)	148	148	87	87	0	24	95		-1.3		-1.2		Multicenter phase III trial
	149	149	95	95	1			94		-2.4		-2.7	
	151	151	107	107	5			94		-3.7		-3.9	
	150	150	99	99	10			91		-5.7		-6.1	
	152	152	98	98	15			93		-7.0		-7.4	
	146	146	96	96	20			93		-8.2		-8.8	
	151	151	101	101	30			95		-9.0		-9.4	
1999 (37)	181	82	48	60	10	52	97.7	95.7	+0.2	-6.1	+0.2	-6.4	Multicenter Wt loss ≥6 kg after 4 wk VLCD were randomized
2000 (49)	44	47	40	43	15	12	82.5	84.6	-0.1	-2.4	-0.5		Multicenter trial in diabetics
2000 (44)	86	89	61	60	5–20	24	98.2	99.3	-0.4	-3.7		-4.5	Multicenter trial in diabetics
2000 (38)	54	55	44	40	10	26	86.4	87.5	-4.6	-8.8	-4.8	-9.9	Body mass index >30 kg/m². Diet 30 kcal/kg of ideal body weight
2000 (47)	74	150	69	142	5–20	52	95.5	97.0	-0.5	-4.4	-0.7	-4.7	Multicenter trial in hypertensives on calcium channel blockers
2000 (39)	115	232	57	204	10–20	78	102.1	102.3	-4.7	-10.2	-4.4	-10.0	Multicenter trial in subjects who lost ≥5% on 10 mg sibutramine in 6 mo
2001 (51)	32	29	55	55	5–20	12	95.9	94.2	-0.3	-4.2	-0.4	-4.5	Multicenter trial in hypertensives on β-blockers

P, placebo-treated patients; D, drug-treated patients.

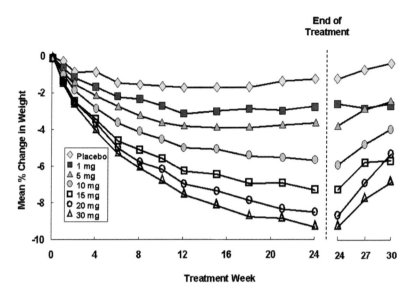

Fig. 3. Dose-related weight loss with sibutramine. A total of 1047 patients were randomly assigned to receive placebo or one of six doses of sibutramine in a double-blind fashion for 6 mo. By the end of the trial, weight loss had plateaued for most doses. When the drug was discontinued at 6 mo, weight was regained, indicating that the drug remained effective during treatment. (From ref. *36*. Reprinted with permission from the North American Association for the Study of Obesity.)

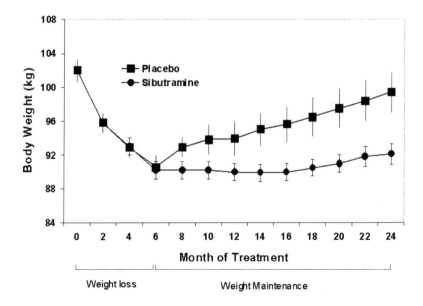

Fig. 4. Sibutramine Trial of Obesity Reduction and Maintenance (STORM) *(39)*. Patients were initially enrolled in an open-label fashion and treated with 10 mg/d of sibutramine for 6 mo. Those who lost more than 5% were then randomized two-thirds to sibutramine and one-third to placebo. Placebo-treated patients steadily regained weight, maintaining only 20% of their weight loss at the end of the trial, whereas subjects treated with sibutramine maintained their weight for 12 mo and then regained an average of only 2 kg. (From ref. *39*. Reprinted with permission from Elsevier.)

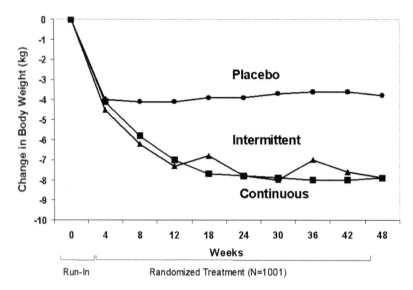

Fig. 5. Intermittent and continuous treatment with sibutramine *(43)*. Patients who had lost 2% or 2 kg after 4 wks of treatment with 15 mg/d of sibutramine were randomized to placebo as continued sibutramine vs sibutramine prescribed intermittently (wk 1–12, 19–30, and 37–48). Both sibutramine treatment regimens gave equivalent results and were significantly better than placebo. (From ref. *43*. Copyright © 2001. American Medical Association. All rights reserved.)

Sibutramine, given continuously for 1 yr, has been compared to placebo and sibutramine given intermittently *(43)*. In this study (Fig. 5), patients who had lost 2% or 2 kg after 4 wk of treatment with sibutramine (15 mg/d) were randomized to placebo, continued sibutramine or sibutramine prescribed intermittently (wk 1–12, 19–30, and 37–48). Both sibutramine treatment regimens gave equal results and were significantly better than placebo. As illustrated in Fig. 5, the effect of stopping sibutramine results in small increases in weight, which is then reversed when the medication is restarted.

Four clinical trials document sibutramine use in patients with diabetes. One was for 12 wk *(49)* and the other three were for 24 wk *(43–45)* (Table 5). In the 12-wk trial, diabetic patients treated with sibutramine (15 mg/d) lost 2.4 kg (2.8%) compared to 0.1 kg (0.12%) in the placebo group *(49)*. In this study, hemoglobin (Hb)A1c fell –0.3% in the drug-treated group and remained stable in the placebo-treated group. In the study by Gokcel et al. *(45)*, 60 female patients who had poorly controlled glucose levels (HbA1c >8%) on maximal doses of sulfonylureas and metformin were randomly assigned to sibutramine 10 mg twice daily or placebo. The weight loss at 24 wk was –9.6 kg in the sibutramine-treated patients and –0.9 kg in those on placebo. The improvements in glycemic control were equally striking. In the sibutramine-treated patients, HbA1c fell –2.73% compared with –0.53% with the placebo. Insulin levels fell –5.66 U/mL compared with –0.68 for placebo and fasting glucose fell –124.88 mg/mL compared with –15.76 mg/mL for placebo. Although the weight loss in most studies of patients with diabetes does not appear as great as in nondiabetic patients, all of the studies found that the percentage of patients who achieved weight loss of at least 5% from baseline was significantly greater than placebo. In all studies, the degree of weight loss corresponds to the degree of improvement in glycemic control.

Two trials have been reported using sibutramine to treat hypertensive patients over 1 yr *(11,47)* (Table 5), and two additional studies provide data on 12 wk of treatment *(50,51)*. In all instances, the weight-loss pattern favors sibutramine. However, except for one study *(51)*, mean weight loss, although favorable, was associated with mean BP increases. In a 3-mo trial, all patients were receiving β-blockers with or without thiazides for their hypertension *(50)*. The sibutramine-treated patients lost –4.2 kg (4.5%), compared to a loss of –0.3 kg (0.3%) in the placebo-treated group. Mean supine and standing diastolic (DBP) and systolic BP (SBP) were not significantly different between drug-treated and placebo-treated patients. Heart rate, however, increased 5.6 ± 8.3 (M ± SD) beats per minute (bpm) in the sibutramine-treated patients as compared to an increase in heart rate of +2.2 ± 6.4 (M ± SD) bpm in the placebo group. McMahon et al. *(11)* reported a 52-wk trial in hypertensive patients whose BP was controlled with calcium channel blockers with or without β-blockers or thiazides (Table 5). Sibutramine doses were increased from 5 to 20 mg/d during the first 6 wk. Weight loss was significantly greater in the sibutramine-treated patients, averaging –4.4 kg (4.7%) as compared with –0.5 kg (0.7%) in the placebo-treated group. DBP decreased –1.3 mmHg in the placebo-treated group and increased by 2.0 mmHg in the sibutramine-treated group. The SBP increased 1.5 mmHg in the placebo-treated group and by 2.7 in the sibutramine-treated group. Heart rate was unchanged in the placebo-treated patients, and increased 4.9 bpm in the sibutramine-treated patients *(11)*. One small study in eight obese men demonstrated that an aerobic exercise program mitigated the adverse BP effects of sibutramine *(52)*.

Because the dose of sibutramine influences the amount of weight loss with the drug *(35,36)*, the intensity of the behavioral component is also likely to have an effect. This is readily demonstrated in a study by Wadden (53). With minimal behavioral intervention, the weight loss in that study was about 5 kg over 12 mo. When group counseling to produce behavior modification was added to sibutramine, the weight loss increased to 10 kg, and when a structured meal plan using meal replacements was added to the medication and behavior plan, the weight loss increased further to 15 kg *(53)*. This indicates that the amount of weight loss observed during pharmacotherapy is, in part, the result of the intensity of the behavioral approach.

Sibutramine is available in 5-, 10-, and 15-mg strengths; 10 mg/d as a single daily dose is the recommended starting dosage with titration up or down based on response. Doses larger than 15 mg/d are not recommended by the FDA. The chance of achieving meaningful weight loss can be determined by the response to treatment in the first 4 wk. In one large trial *(36)* of the patients who lost 2 kg (4 lb) in the first 4 wk of treatment, 60% achieved a weight loss of more than 5%, compared to less than 10% of those who did not lose 2 kg (4 lb) in 4 wk *(36)*. Except for BP, weight loss with sibutramine is associated with improvement in profiles of cardiovascular risk factors. Combining data from 11 studies on sibutramine showed a weight-related reduction in triglyceride (TG), total cholesterol, and low-density lipoprotein cholesterol (LDL-C) and a weight loss related rise in high-density lipoprotein cholesterol (HDL-C) that was related to the magnitude of the weight loss *(54)*.

3.1.3. SAFETY

The side-effect profile for sympathomimetic drugs is similar *(2)*. They produce insomnia, dry mouth, asthenia, and constipation. The sympathomimetic drugs phentermine, diethylpropion, benzphetamine and phendimetrazine have very little abuse potential as assessed by the low rate of reinforcement when the drugs are self-injected intravenously to test animals *(2)*. In this same paradigm, neither PPA nor fenfluramine showed any reinforcing effects and no clinical data show any abuse potential for either of these drugs. Sibutramine, likewise, has no abuse potential *(4)*, but it is nonetheless a schedule IV drug.

Sympathomimetic drugs can increase BP. PPA is a β_1-agonist and at doses of 75 mg or more it can increase BP. PPA has been associated with hemorrhagic stroke in women *(55)*. In December 2000, the FDA removed PPA from cold remedies and weight-loss products because of the alleged relation to the development of hemorrhagic strokes *(55)*. PPA has also been reported in association with cardiomyopathy.

There are two issues to consider regarding BP management and sibutramine use. The first is the development of clinically significant BP elevations. Individual BP responses to sibutramine are quite variable. From the studies reviewed, withdrawals for clinically significant BP increase are usually 2 to 5% of participants in the trial. Higher doses tend to produce higher withdrawal rates *(36)*, thus lower doses are preferred. The other issue with BP increases is the small mean increase of 2 to 4 mmHg in SBP and DBP that occurs in sibutramine-treated patients vs controls. Weight loss is usually associated with improvement in risk factors for cardiovascular disease (BP, lipids, measures of glycemic control). If sibutraminehas mixed effects on risk factors, with improvement in some (lipids, glycemic control) but slight worsening of others, then the prescribing physician must use judgment in the decision to continue sibutramine.

Managing potential increases in BP should be a part of the sibutramine treatment plan. Evaluation of BP 2 to 4 wk after starting sibutramine is recommended. The initial dose is usually 10 mg/d. About 5% of patients who take sibutramine will have unacceptable increases in BP and for them, the medication should be stopped. If the BP is less than 135/80 and there has been less than 10 mmHg systolic and 5 mmHg diastolic increase from baseline, continued use of medication is acceptable. If patients have acceptable weight loss in the first month of treatment (4 lb in 4 wk), the BP response should then be a part of the decision to continue treatment.

Sibutramine should not be used in patients with a history of coronary artery disease, congestive heart failure, cardiac arrhythmias, or stroke. There should be a 2-wk interval between termination of monoamine oxidase inhibitors and beginning sibutramine and sibutramine should not be used with selective serotonin reuptake inhibitors. Because sibutramine is metabolized by the cytochrome P_{450} enzyme system (isozyme CYP3A4) when drugs like erythromycin and ketoconazole are taken, there may be competition for this enzymatic pathway and prolonged metabolism can result.

3.2. Sympathomimetic Drugs Not Approved by the FDA to Treat Obesity

3.2.1. BUPROPION

Bupropion, a drug approved by the FDA for treatment of depression, produces weight loss *(56)*. It is a relative of diethylpropion, an approved drug for treating obesity (*see* Subheading 3.1.1.). It is an inhibitor of NE, serotonin, and dopamine reuptake, but is thought to produce weight loss through modulating the action of NE *(56)*. A 6 -mo randomized, double-blind, placebo-controlled trial *(56)* with a 6-moh blinded extension where all patients received active medication has compared two doses of bupropion against placebo. Both doses of medication produced significantly more weight loss than placebo. During the 6-mo extension, the weight loss was largely maintained. Buprop-ion has not been given approval by the FDA for weight loss.

3.3. Serotonergic Drugs

No drugs working by this mechanism are currently approved by the FDA to treat obesity. Serotonergic drugs that act on specific serotonin receptors (5-HT$_{1B}$ or 5-HT$_{2C}$) reduce food intake and specifically reduce fat intake. Several drugs that influence serotonin release (fenfluramine and dexfenfluramine) or serotonin reuptake (fluoxetine and sertraline) have been used in obese patients. The clinical trial data are reviewed in detail elsewhere *(2,57)*.

3.4. Other Drugs in Clinical Trial

3.4.1. TOPIRAMATE

Topiramate (TPM) is a neurotherapeutic agent approved for treatment of epilepsy, both as monotherapy and in combination with other anti-epileptic drugs. TPM is a carbonic anhydrase inhibitor that also affects the GABA$_A$ receptor. In uncontrolled clinical studies the drug was noted to cause weight loss *(58)*. A placebo-controlled, double-blind, randomized dose-ranging clinical trial showed a mean percent weight loss from baseline to wk 24 of –2.6% in placebo-treated patients vs –5.0%, –4.8%, –6.3%, and –6.3% in the 64, 96, 192, and 384 mg/d in TPM-treated groups, respectively. Greater percentages of TPM-treated patients lost at least 5 or 10% of body weight compared with placebo. The most frequent adverse events were related to the central or peripheral nervous system, including paresthesia, somnolence, and difficulty with memory, concentration, and attention. Most events were dose-related, occurred early in treatment, and usually resolved spontaneously; only 21% of those receiving TPM withdrew because of adverse events, compared with 11% on placebo. Thus, TPM produced significantly greater weight loss than placebo at all doses and offers a new potential agent for treating obesity *(59)* (Fig. 6).

3.4.2. RIMONABANT

Endocannabinoids may be involved in the leptin pathway that regulates food intake. Rimonabant is a cannabinoid-binding protein agonist that is currently in clinical trials for obesity treatment *(60)*.

3.4.3 ZONISAMIDE

Zonisamide is an antiepileptic drug that blocks sodium and calcium channels as well as affecting the activity of the dopaminergic and serotonergic neurotransmitter systems. It is approved by the FDA as an antiepileptic. In a 16-wk randomized, placebo-controlled trial, 51 of 60 patients completed the 16-wk acute phase. The zonisamide-treated group lost more body weight than the placebo group, 5.9 ± 0.8 kg (6% weight loss) vs 0.9 ± 0.4 kg (1% weight loss). Zonisamide was tolerated well, with few adverse effects. Thus, in

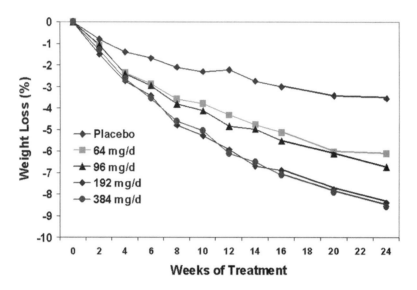

Fig. 6. Weight loss with topiramate *(59)*. In a placebo-controlled, double-blind, randomized dose-ranging clinical trial presented in abstract form, topiramate at doses of 64, 96, 192 and 184 mg/d produced dose-related weight loss, but was also associated with dose-related increases in the number of neurological side effects. (From ref. *59*. Copyright 2002 © American Diabetes Association. Reprinted with permission from Obesity Research.)

one short-term preliminary trial, zonisamide and a hypocaloric diet resulted in more weight loss than placebo and hypocaloric diet in the treatment of obesity *(61)*.

3.4.4. LEPTIN

Leptin is a peptide produced almost exclusively in adipose tissue. Absence of leptin produces massive obesity in mice (ob/ob) and in humans *(62)*, and treatment with this peptide decreases food intake in the ob/ob mouse and the leptin-deficient human *(63)* *(see* Chapter 18). The diabetes mouse (db/db) and the fatty rat, which have genetic defects in the leptin receptor, are also obese but they do not respond to leptin. Leptin levels in the blood are highly correlated with body-fat levels yet obesity persists, suggesting that there may be leptin resistance. In a dose-ranging clinical trial with leptin *(64)*, lean subjects treated for 4 wk and obese subjects treated for 24 wk had modest weight loss with doses ranging from 0.01 mg/kg to 0.3 mg/kg. The side effects of local irritation at the site of injection limit the use of this preparation. A long-acting leptin preparation may provide an improved way to use this drug *(65)*.

3.4.5. AXOKINE

Axokine is a modified form of ciliary neurotrophic factor that acts through the same janus-kinase-signal for the transduction and translation systems that leptin acts through. Axokine will reduce food intake in animals that lack leptin or the leptin receptors *(66)*. It was noted to reduce weight in a clinical trial for amyotrophic lateral sclerosis, and a 3-mo dose-ranging study demonstrated a significantly greater dose-related weight loss in the drug-treated patients *(67)*.

3.5. Peptides That Reduce Food Intake and in Early Stages of Drug Development

3.5.1. NEUROPEPTIDE-Y

NPY is one of the most potent stimulators of food intake and appears to act through NPY Y-5 and/or Y-1 receptors (2). Antagonists to these receptors might block NPY and thus decrease feeding. Several pharmaceutical companies are attempting to identify antagonists to NPY receptors (21).

3.5.2. MELANIN-CONCENTRATING HORMONE

Melanin-concentrating hormone is a cyclic 19 amino acid peptide that is produced in the lateral hypothalamus. When this peptide is injected in the ventricular system of the brain it increases food intake. Genetically engineered animals that overexpress this peptide in the brain become moderately obese, and animals that lack this peptide have a thin phenotype. Thus, antagonists to this peptide have potential therapeutic usefulness (68).

3.5.3. CHOLECYSTOKININ

Cholecystokinin (CCK) reduces food intake in human beings and in experimental animals (2). This effect does not require an intact hypothalamic feeding-control system but does appear to require an intact vagus nerve. Peptide analogs have been developed and tested experimentally but clinical data have not yet been published. A second strategy to modify CCK activity is to reduce the degradation of CCK. This approach is likewise under evaluation.

3.5.4. GLUCAGON AND GLUCAGON-LIKE PEPTIDE-1 (GLP-1)

Pancreatic glucagon produces a dose-related decrease in food intake (2). A fragment of glucagon (amino acids 6-29) called glucagon-like peptide-1 (GLP-1) reduced food intake when given either peripherally (69) or into the brain. Exendin, an analog of GLP-1, has been used in humans because infusion of GLP-1 in humans reduces food intake (70).

3.5.5. PRAMLINTIDE

Pramlintide, an analog of amylin, is in clinical trial for diabetes.

4. DRUGS THAT ALTER ABSORPTION OR METABOLISM

4.1. Drugs Approved by the FDA

4.1.1. ORLISTAT

4.1.1.1. PHARMACOLOGY

Orlistat is a potent selective inhibitor of pancreatic lipase that reduces intestinal digestion of fat. The drug has a dose-dependent effect on fecal fat loss, increasing it to about 30% of ingested fat on a diet that has 30% of energy as fat (71). Orlistat has little effect in subjects eating a low-fat diet, as might be anticipated from the mechanism by which this drug works (71).

Table 6
Effect of Orlistat in Clinical Trials of 1 and 2 Yr in Duration

Year (reference)	No. of subjects P	No. of subjects D	Dose mg/d	Duration of study	Run in (weeks)	Diet	Initial weight loss (kg) P	Initial weight loss (kg) D	Weight loss (kg or %) P	Weight loss (kg or %) D	Comments
1997 (71)	23	23	120 tid	52	4	600 kcal/d deficit	99	100	-2.6 kg	-8.4 kg	Wt. loss at 12 mo
1998 (72)	125			24	4	500 kcal/d deficit	35 [a]		-6.5%		Multicenter Dose-ranging
		122	30 tid					35		-8.5%	
		124	60 tid					34		-8.8%	
		122	120 tid					35		-9.8%	
		120	240 tid					34		-9.3%	
1998 (73)	340	343	120 tid	104	4	600 kcal/d deficit (yr 1) maintenance (yr 2)	99.8	99.1	-6.1 kg / -6.1%	-10.3 kg / -10.2 %	European multicenter Crossover 52-wk data
1998 (79)	159	162	120 tid	52	5	500 kcal/d deficit 30% fat	99.7	99.6	-4.3 kg	-6.2 kg	US diabetic study
1999 (74)	223	657	120 tid	104	4	600 kcal/d deficit (yr 1) maintenance (yr 2) 30% fat	100.6	100.7	-5.8 kg / -5.8%	-8.8 kg / -8.7%	US multicenter Crossover 52-wk data
1999 (75)	188/138			52	24	1000 kcal/d deficit (6 mo); Enrolled if wt loss >8%	90.8		-5.9 kg		Multicenter trial with initial dietary weight loss and test of maintenance of weight loss
	187/140		30 tid					89.3		-5.15 kg	
	173/133		60 tid					92.4		-6.16 kg	
	181/126		120 tid					89.7		-7.24 kg	
2000 (12)	108	110	120 tid	52	4	600 kcal/d deficit	98.4	97.9	-5.4%	-8.5%	British 1 yr
2000 (77)	243/136			104	4	600 kcal/d deficit (yr 1) maintenance (yr 2) 30% fat	97.7		-4.5%		Multicenter European trial
	242/140		60 tid					99.1		-7.0%	
	244/159		120 tid					96.7		-7.8%	
								(2yr data on completers)			
2000 (76)	212/91			104	4	5020 kJ/d if wt <90 kg; or 6275 kJ/d	101.8		-1.5 kg		Multicenter US trial in family practice setting
	213/120		60 tid					100.4		-4.6 kg	
	210/117		120 tid					100.5		-5.2 kg	
2000 (78)	186	190	120 tid	52	2	600 kcal/d deficit; 30% fat	95.9	96.1	-4.3 kg	-5.6 kg	Multicenter trial of individuals with high coronary heart disease risk

P, placebo-treated patients; D, drug-treated patients.
[a] BMI, body mass index.

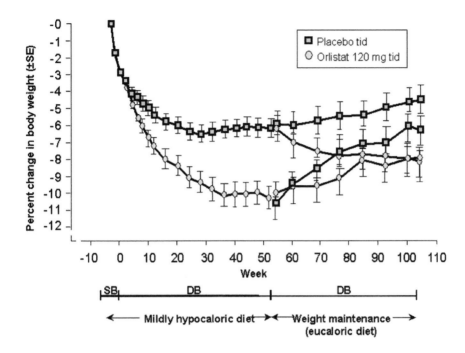

Fig. 7. Effect of orlistat on weight loss during yr 1 and weight maintenance during yr 2 *(72)*. A total of 743 patients were randomized to receive either orlistat (120 mg three times daily) or placebo for the first year and were then re-randomized to the same groups for a second year. Following the 4-wk single-blind (SB) run-in, the first double-blind (DB) period utilized a diet that was calculated to be 600 kcal/d below maintenance, and the second DB period used a diet that was intended to maintain body weight. (From ref. *72*. Reprinted with permission from Elsevier.)

4.1.1.2. EFFICACY

4.1.1.2.1. Effect on Weight

A number of long-term clinical trials with orlistat lasting 6 mo to 2 yr have been published (Table 6) *(12,72–82)*. The results of one 2-yr trial *(74)* are shown in Fig. 7. The trial consisted of two parts. In the first year, patients received a hypocaloric diet calculated to be 500 kcal/d below the patient's requirements. During the second year, the diet was calculated to maintain weight. By the end of yr 1 the placebo-treated patients lost –6.1% of their initial body weight and the drug-treated patients lost –10.2%. The patients were re-randomized at the end of yr 1. Those patients switched from orlistat to placebo gained weight from –10% to –6.0% below baseline. Those switched from placebo to orlistat lost from –6% to –8.1%, which was essentially identical to the –7.9% in the patients treated with orlistat for the full 2 yr. In a second 2-yr study, 892 patients were randomized *(75)*. One group remained on placebo throughout the 2 yr (*n* = 97 completers) and a second group remained on 120 mg three times/d of orlistat for 2 yr (*n* = 109 completers). At the end of 1 yr, two-thirds of the group treated with orlistat for 1 yr were changed to 60 mg of orlistat three times a day (*n* = 102 completers) and the others to placebo (*n* = 95 completers) *(76)*. After 1 yr, the weight change was –8.67 kg in the orlistat-treated group and –5.81 kg in the placebo group (*p* < 0.001). During the second

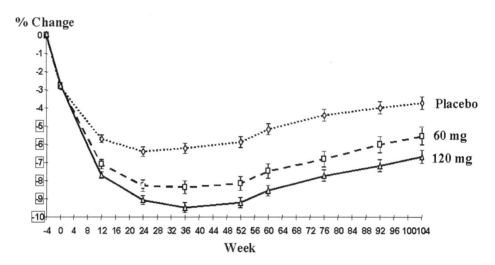

Fig. 8. Hoffman La Roche pooled data *(76)*. The percent change in body weight over 2 yr of orlistat at 60 mg and 120 mg. At the end of 2 yr, the orlistat group receiving 120 mg three times daily were 5.2 kg below their baseline weight compared to –1.5 kg for the group treated with placebo. (Data on file—Hoffmann La Roche—figure provided by J. Hauptman.)

year, those switched to placebo after 1 yr reached the same weight as those treated with placebo for 2 yr (–4.5% in those with placebo for 2 yr and –4.2% in those switched from orlistat to placebo during yr 2). In a third 2-yr study, 783 patients enrolled in a trial where, for 2 yr, they remained in the placebo group or one of two orlistat-treated groups at 60 or 120 mg three times a day *(77)*. After 1 yr with a weight-loss diet, the completers in the placebo group lost –7.0 kg, which was significantly less than the –9.6 kg in the completers treated with 60 mg of orlistat thrice daily or –9.8 kg in the completers treated with 120 mg of orlistat thrice daily. During the second year when the diet was liberalized to a "weight-maintenance" diet, all three groups regained some weight. At the end of 2 yr, the completers in the placebo group were –4.3 kg below baseline, the completers treated with 60 mg of orlistat three times a day was –6.8 kg and the completers treated with 120 mg of orlistat three times daily were –7.6 kg below baseline. Another 2-yr trial that has been published was carried out on 796 subjects in a general practice setting *(77)*. After 1 yr of treatment with orlistat (120 mg/d), completers ($n = 117$) had lost –8.8 kg compared to –4.3 kg in the placebo completers ($n = 91$). During the second year when the diet was liberalized to "maintain body weight" both groups regained some weight. At the end of 2 yr, the orlistat group receiving 120 mg three times daily were 5.2 kg below their baseline weight compared to –1.5 kg for the group treated with placebo (Fig. 8).

Weight maintenance with orlistat was evaluated in a 1-yr study *(76)*. Patients were enrolled who lost more than 8% of their body weight over 6 mo eating a 1000 kcal/d (4180 kJ/d) diet. The 729 patients were one of four groups randomized to receive placebo or 30 mg, 60 mg, or 120 mg of orlistat three times daily for 12 mo. At the end of this time, the placebo-treated patients had regained 56% of their body weight, compared with 32.4% in the group treated with 120 mg of orlistat, three times daily. The other two doses of orlistat were not statistically different from placebo in preventing the regain of weight.

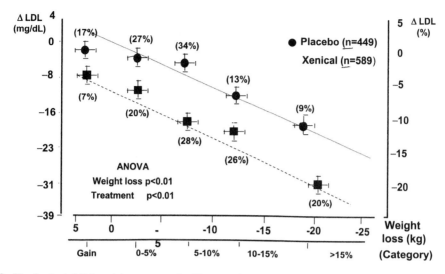

Fig. 9. Xenical: Additional incremental effect on low-density lipoprotein-cholesterol (LDL-C) beyond weight loss. Meta-analysis of the phase III data that showed that improvement in the initial LDL-C was also highly significant. Furthermore, the reduction in LDL-C among Xenical-treated patients was greater than would be expected for the same weight loss with diet alone. The effect of Xenical on LDL-C levels was additional to the effect of weight loss and is probably the result of the inhibition of the absorption of cholesterol (by decreasing solubility and by sequestering cholesterol in an oil phase). *Note.* Xenical significantly improves LDL/HDL ratios. The LDL/HDL ratio, a well-known predictor of cardiovascular risk, was significantly improved after year 1 ($p < 0.001$) and year 2 ($p < 0.001$) in the Xenical group compared with the placebo group.

4.1.1.2.2. Effects on Lipids and Lipoproteins

The modest weight reduction observed with orlistat treatment may have a beneficial effect on lipids and lipoproteins *(23)*. Orlistat seems to have an independent effect on LDL-C. From a meta-analysis *(83)* of the data relating orlistat to lipids, orlistat-treated subjects had almost twice as much reduction in LDL-C as their placebo-treated counterparts for the same weight-loss category reached after 1 yr. This is illustrated in Fig. 9.

One study is representative of the effects of orlistat on weight loss and on cardiovascular risk factors, particularly serum lipids, in obese patients with hypercholesterolemia *(84)*. The main findings were that orlistat promoted clinically significant weight loss and reduced LDL-C in obese patients with elevated cholesterol levels more than could be attributed to weight loss alone.

The ObelHyx study demonstrates an additional 10% LDL-C lowering in obese subjects with baseline-elevated LDL-C levels compared to placebo *(85)*. Table 6 provides mean percentage changes in LDL-C after 24 wk of double-blind treatment in three 2-yr controlled trials, where the majority of patients were normocholesterolemic at baseline. These data indicate that the difference in mean percentage change in LDL-C between orlistat and placebo is roughly 10 to 12% in all studies, whether this difference is computed as change from the start of the single-blind placebo dietary run-in or from the start of double-blind treatment. It is noteworthy that LDL-C levels continued to decline after the start of double-blind treatment in orlistat-treated subjects in all trials, but that LDL-C either remained largely unchanged or increased during double-blind therapy in placebo-treated recipients, despite further weight loss (Table 6). This independent cholesterol-lowering effect probably reflects a reduction in intestinal absorption of cholesterol. Because lipase inhibition by orlistat prevents the absorption of approx 30% of dietary fat, the prescribed diet of 30% of energy from fat becomes in effect a 20 to 24% fat diet when associated with orlistat treatment. It has been hypothesized that inhibition of GI lipase activity may lead to retention of cholesterol in the gut through a reduction in the amount of fatty acids and monoglycerides absorbed from the gut, and/or may lead to sequestration of cholesterol within a more persistent oil phase in the intestine. Partial inhibition of intestinal fat and cholesterol absorption probably leads to decreased hepatic cholesterol and saturated fatty acid concentration, upregulation of hepatic LDL receptors, and decreased LDL-C levels. The decrease in LDL-C observed in the study with hypercholesterolemic subjects *(84)* is comparable to the 14% LDL-C reduction that was previously achieved with a plant stanol ester-containing margarine but is of a lesser magnitude than the LDL-C lowering effects that are commonly observed with fibrate or statin drugs *(86,87)*.

4.1.1.2.3. Effects on Glucose Tolerance and Diabetes

The orlistat-treated subjects in trials lasting for at least 1 yr were analyzed by Heymsfield and coworkers *(88)*, who found that orlistat reduced the conversion of impaired glucose tolerance (IGT) to diabetes from 11% in placebo-treated patients to 6.6% in orlistat-treated patients and the transition from normal glucose tolerance to IGT from 7.6 to 3.0% in subjects treated with orlistat for 1 yr *(88)*. Although these data are based on a retrospective analysis of 1-yr trials in which data on glucose tolerance was available, it shows that modest weight reduction—with pharmacotherapy—may lead to an important risk reduction for the development of type 2 diabetes.

One study *(81)* randomized 550 insulin-treated patients to receive either placebo or 120 mg of orlistat three times a day for 1 yr. Weight loss in the orlistat-treated group was $-3.9 \pm 0.3\%$ compared to $1.3 \pm 0.3\%$ in the placebo-treated group. HbA1c was reduced -0.62% in the orlistat-treated group, but only -0.27% in the placebo group. The required dose of insulin decreased more in the orlistat group, as did plasma cholesterol *(81)*.

Orlistat, in a study in patients with diabetes *(80)*, improved metabolic control with a reduction of up to 0.53 % in HbA1c and a decrease in the concomitant ongoing antidiabetic therapy, despite limited weight loss. Independent effects of orlistat on lipids were also shown in this study *(80)*. Orlistat also has an acute effect on postprandial lipemia in overweight patients with type 2 diabetes *(89)*. By lowering both remnant-like particle cholesterol and free fatty acids in the postprandial period, orlistat may contribute to a reduction in atherogenic risk *(89)*.

The longest clinical trial with orlistat is the Xenical Diabetes Outcome Study *(91)*. In this 4-yr randomized, placebo-controlled clinical trial, 1640 patients were assigned to received 120 mg of orlistat three times daily plus lifestyle and 1637 patients to receive matching placebos plus lifestyle. The study enrolled Swedish patients with a BMI of 30 kg/m^2 or more with normal glucose tolerance or IGT (21%). More than 52% of the orlistat and 34% of the placebo-treated patients continued to adhere to the clinical protocol. The patients receiving orlistat were -6.9 kg below their baseline weight by the end of yr 4 compared to -4.1 kg for the placebo-treated group ($p < 0.001$). Cumulative incidence of diabetes was 9% in the placebo group and 6.2% in the orlistat group, a 37% reduction in relative risk. Thus, it is clear that long-term clinical trials of anti-obesity drugs can be implemented.

In an analysis of orlistat's effect on patients with Syndrome X (*see* Chapter 10 for additional information about Syndrome X), Reaven et al. *(92)* subdivided patients who participated in previously reported studies into those in the highest and lowest quintile for TGs and HDL-C. Those with high TG and low HDL were labeled Syndrome X or metabolic syndrome and those with the lowest TG and highest HDL were in the non-Syndrome X controls. In this analysis, there were almost no males in the non-Syndrome X group compared with an equal gender breakdown in the Syndrome X group. The other differences between these two groups were the slightly higher SBP and DBP in those with Syndrome X and the nearly twofold higher level of fasting insulin. With weight loss, the only difference besides weight between placebo and orlistat-treated patients was the drop in LDL-C. However, the Syndrome X subgroups showed a significantly greater decrease in TG and insulin than those without Syndrome X. HDLC rose more in the Syndrome X subgroup, but LDL-C showed a smaller decrease than in the non-Syndrome X control group.

An analysis of quality of life in patients treated with orlistat showed improvements over the placebo group despite concerns about GI symptoms. In addition, orlistat-treated patients showed a significant decrease in serum cholesterol and LDL-C that is greater than can be explained by the weight loss alone.

4.1.1.3. SAFETY

Orlistat is not absorbed to any significant degree and its side effects are thus related to the blockade of TG digestion in the intestine *(71)*. Fecal fat loss and related GI symptoms are common initially, but subside as patients learn to use the drug *(74,75)*. During treatment, small, but significant, decreases in fat-soluble vitamins can occur, although these almost always remain within normal concentrations *(93)*. However, a few patients may need supplementation with fat-soluble vitamins that can be lost in the stools. Because it is impossible to tell *a priori* which patients need vitamins, we routinely provide a multivitamin with instructions to take it before bedtime. Absorption of other drugs does not seem to be significantly affected by orlistat.

4.1.1.4. COMBINING ORLISTAT AND SIBUTRAMINE

Because orlistat works peripherally to reduce TG digestion in the GI track and sibutramine works on noraderenergic and serotonergic reuptake mechanisms in the brain, their mechanisms do not overlap at all and combining them might provide additive weight loss. To test this possibility, Wadden and his colleagues *(94)* randomly assigned patients to orlistat or placebo following 1 yr of treatment with orlistat. During the additional 4 mo of treatment, there was no further weight loss. This result was a disappointment, but additional studies are obviously needed before firm conclusions can be made about combining therapies (*see* Chapter 17).

4.2. Drugs Approved by the FDA for an Indication Other Than Obesity

4.2.1. ANDROGENS AND ANDROGEN ANTAGONISTS

4.2.1.1. DEHYDROEPIANDROSTERONE

Dehydroepiandrosterone is a weak androgen that induces weight loss in several animal species. Clinical trials in humans have shown no effect *(2)*.

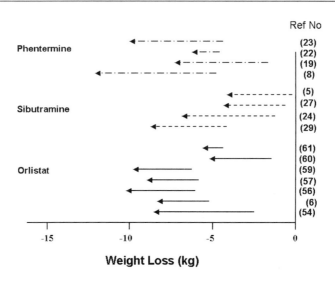

Fig. 10. Effect sizes for three weight loss drugs *(95)*. Each line is a separate study with either phentermine, sibutramine or orlistat. Reference to each study is in parentheses. The right-hand end of the arrow is the weight loss of the placebo-treated group and the tip of the arrow is the weight loss of the drug-treated group (Copyright © 2001 George A. Bray.)

4.2.1.2. TESTOSTERONE

In men, testosterone and the anabolic steroid oxandrolone have been reported to reduce visceral fat. A trial of an anti-androgen and nandrolone in women did not show any effects on visceral fat *(2)*.

5. COMPARISON OF AVAILABLE DRUGS

Of the drugs that we have discussed in this review, three, phentermine, orlistat, and sibutramine, are the most widely used in the United States. The other drugs in the sympathomimetic category, benzphetamine, phendimetrazine, and diethylpropion, are less widely used and they lack sufficient long-term information.

To provide a comparison of the three drugs that are available to the clinician, we have plotted the weight loss of the placebo and drug-treated groups in Fig. 10 *(95)*. All of the trials included in Fig. 10 lasted 6 mo or more. The weight loss of the placebo group is at the beginning of the arrow on the right, and the weight loss of the drug-treated group at the tip of the arrowhead to the left. The length of the arrow is the magnitude of the difference between drug and placebo. In all of the studies plotted, the difference between the two groups was greater than 4 kg, except for one study with phentermine and one study with orlistat. Three trials with phentermine had weight losses exceeding 5 kg, whereas most of the others were around 5 kg.

The effect size, expressed as the difference between the drug-treated and placebo-treated group in each study, is plotted in Fig. 11 *(95)*. The weight loss of the phentermine and orlistat groups was greater than the sibutramine group, but so was the weight loss of the placebo-treated group. When the difference is plotted on the right side of each of the three groups, sibutramine and phentermine produced a similar amount of weight loss that was slightly greater than with orlistat.

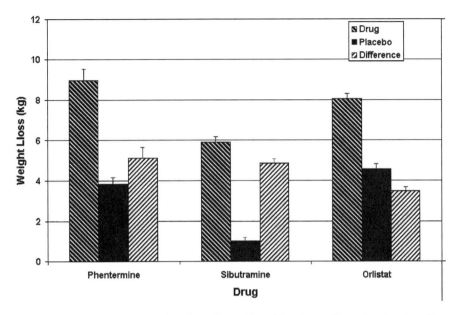

Fig. 11. Effect sizes for three weight loss drugs *(95)*. The drug effect, the placebo effect, and the difference are plotted for the studies (Copyright © 2001 George A. Bray.)

6. DRUGS THAT INCREASE ENERGY EXPENDITURE

6.1. Drugs Approved by the FDA for an Indication Other Than Obesity

6.1.1. EPHEDRINE AND CAFFEINE

6.1.1.1. PHARMACOLOGY

Ephedrine is a derivative of PPA and is used to relax bronchial smooth muscles in patients with asthma. It also stimulates thermogenesis in human subjects *(96,97)*. Caffeine is a xanthine that inhibits adenosine receptors and phosphodiesterase. In experimental animals, the combination of ephedrine and caffeine reduces body weight, probably through stimulation of thermogenesis and a reduction in food intake *(2)*.

6.1.1.2. EFFICACY

One long-term placebo-controlled clinical trial enrolled 180 patients treated with ephedrine, caffeine, or the combination of ephedrine and caffeine *(97)*. Patients treated with the combination of ephedrine and caffeine lost more weight than did patients treated with ephedrine alone, caffeine alone, or placebo (Fig. 12). In a 6-mo open-label extension, subjects who completed the initial trial were offered additional treatment with ephedrine and caffeine. Nearly two-thirds of the group opted for this treatment and were able to maintain their initial weight loss for the next 6 mo. No other long-term data are available using ephedrine and caffeine. During controlled metabolic studies, patients treated with ephedrine and caffeine lost less lean tissue than did those in the placebo-treated group. Using the changes in body composition from these studies, Astrup and his colleagues have estimated the contribution of thermogenesis and food intake to the weight loss *(98)*. They concluded that 60 to 75% of the weight loss was the result of

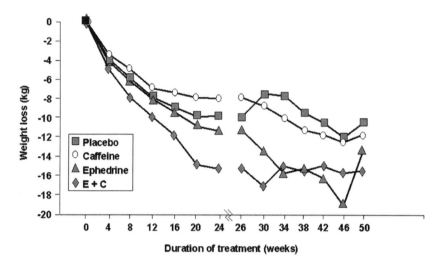

Fig. 12. Effect of ephedrine and caffeine on weight loss and weight maintenance for 1 yr *(98)*. A total of 180 patients were randomly assigned to four groups that were then treated in a double-blind fashion for 6 mo and with an open-label protocol for another 6 mo. The weight losses in the groups receiving placebo, ephedrine alone, and caffeine alone were not significantly different and were smaller than in the group receiving the combination of ephedrine and caffeine. During the 6-mo open-label study when those who wished to received ephedrine and caffeine, weight loss was maintained with no significant difference between groups. (From ref. *98*.)

decreased food intake and 25 to 40% was owing to thermogenic effects of ephedrine and caffeine.

6.1.1.3. SAFETY

Although caffeine and ephedrine have a long record of clinical use separately, neither drug alone nor the combination is approved for treatment of obesity.

6.2. Thyroid Hormone Analogs

Thyroid hormones are known to reduce body weight and body fat in human and animals, but have been limited in use because of the detrimental effects on heart rate and bone mineral metabolism. The thyroid hormone receptor subtype-β is thought to mediate the effects on cholesterol lowering and metabolic rate, whereas the receptor subtype-α mediates the effects of heart rate. An analog of triiodothyronine, which is relatively selective for the β-thyroid receptor, has been shown to increase oxygen consumption with a 10-fold selectivity and to lower cholesterol with a 27-fold selectivity vs heart rate in rodents. Such a drug offers interesting potential for treating human obesity *(99)*.

6.3. β_3-Adrenergic Receptor Agonists in Early Stages of Drug Development

The sympathetic nervous system has a tonic role in maintaining EE and BP. Blockade of the thermogenic part of this system reduces the thermic response to a meal. Norepinephrine, the neurotransmitter of the sympathetic nervous system, may also decrease food intake by acting on β_2- or β_3-adrenergic receptors. Several synthetic β_3-agonists have been developed against rodent β_3-receptors, but the clinical responses have been disappointing *(2)*. After cloning of the human β_3-receptor, new compounds are being developed to evaluate in obese human subjects.

One clinical trial of a third generation β_3 drug has been reported in an abstract; it showed no significant effect on thermogenesis in human subjects when studied in a metabolic chamber after treatment for 28 d *(100)*. Other drugs are being tested.

7. HERBAL PREPARATIONS FOR TREATMENT OF OBESITY

Several different herbal preparations have been recommended for use in treating obesity. These include chromium picolinate, garcinia cambogia as a source of hydroxycitrate, chitosan as a fiber source that is claimed to reduce fat absorption, and ma huang as a source of ephedra alkaloids with or without guarana or kola nut as a source of caffeine. Clinically controlled trials with these preparations are few. Herbal medications usually do not carry the approval of the FDA because the federal law allows them to be sold directly to the consumer through the over-the-counter route.

7.1. Chromium Picolinate

There are no randomized, placebo-controlled clinical trials in human subjects with chromium picolinate as a single agent that would allow us to evaluate of its effectiveness as a treatment for obesity *(2)*.

7.2. Garcinia Cambogia

There is a single published randomized placebo-controlled 3-mo clinical trial with Garcinia cambogia as a source of hydroxycitrate *(101)*. There was no difference in the weight loss between the herbal-treated group and the placebo group.

7.3. Chitosan

Two recent studies have evaluated the effect of chitosan on fecal fat loss and body weight. Using human subjects where fecal fat samples were collected, Guerciolini et al. *(102)* showed that chitosan did not increase fecal fat loss. In a 4-wk dietary study, chitosan or placebo was given randomly to subjects with no dietary advice. At the end of 1 mo there was no difference in weight change between the two groups, suggesting that chitosan has no effect in a short term on body weight *(103)*.

7.4. Ephedra (Ma Huang) and Caffeine (Guarana or Kola Nut)

Owing to concerns about the safety of using this combination of drugs, the FDA removed them from the market in 2004, except for herbal practitioners. Two randomized, placebo-controlled clinical trials have been published using these herbal preparations *(104,105)*. In an 8-wk study with one product (Metabolife 356) *(104)*, the patients treated with the herbal preparation lost more weight and body fat, but the authors commented on the number of side effects and urged caution until longer studies were available. A second *(105)* 6-mo randomized, placebo-controlled trial was of a generic mixture of ephedra alkaloids (30 mg from Ma huang) and caffeine (132 mg from kola nut) given in three divided doses. The patients treated with the ephedra/caffeine combination lost significantly more weight (-5.3 ± 5.0 kg) than the placebo-treated group (-2.6 ± 3.2 kg, $p < 0.001$). In this trial, Holter monitors and ambulatory BP were evaluated at baseline and after 2 and 4 wk of treatment to detect effects on cardiac rhythmicity and BP. Compared to baseline, the only significant changes in any of the cardiac parameters were measured time by group interactions in pulse and percent with bradycardia. Pulse rate increased 4 bpm from baseline in the groups treated with ephedra and guarana. BP fell 1 to 3 mmHg in the placebo group and rose 1 to 2 mmHg in the herbal group.

8. CONCLUSION

Drugs to treat obesity can be divided into three groups: those that reduce food intake; those that alter metabolism; and those that increase thermogenesis. Monoamines acting on noradrenergic receptors, serotonin receptors, dopamine receptors, and histamine receptors can reduce food intake. A number of peptides also modulate food intake. The noradrenergic drugs phentermine, diethylpropion, benzphetamine, and phendi-metrazine are approved only for short-term use. Sibutramine, an NE–serotonin reuptake inhibitor, is approved for long-term use. Also approved for long-term use is orlistat, which inhibits pancreatic lipase and can block hydrolysis of 30% of the dietary TG in subjects eating a 30% fat diet. The thermogenic combination of ephedrine and caffeine has not been approved by regulatory agencies. Several new drugs are under investigation. Medications for obesity treatment should be viewed as useful adjuncts to diet and physical activity prescription and may help selected patients achieve and maintain weight loss. Thus, physicians must be knowledgeable regarding the efficacy and safety profiles of currently available medications.

At present, only two drugs are approved for long-term treatment of obesity. Sibutramine inhibits the re-uptake of serotonin and NE. In clinical trials it produces a dose-dependent 5 to 10% decrease in body weight. Its side effects include dry mouth, insomnia, asthenia, and constipation. In addition, in clinical trials, sibutramine produces a small mean increase in BP and pulse that mandates attention to BP monitoring on follow-up visits. Sibutramine is contraindicated in some individuals with heart disease. Orlistat is the other drug approved for long-term use in the treatment of obesity. It works by blocking pancreatic lipase and thus increasing the fecal loss of TG. One valuable consequence of this mechanism of action is the reduction of serum cholesterol that averages about 5% more than can be accounted for by weight loss alone. In clinical trials, it produces a 5 to 10% loss of weight. Its side effects are entirely the result of undigested fat in the intestine (steatorrhea) that can lead to increased frequency and change in the character of stools. It can also lower fat-soluble vitamins. The ingestion of a vitamin supplement before bedtime is a reasonable treatment strategy when orlistat is prescribed. All medications currently available for obesity management should be used as adjuncts to dietary and physical activity approaches to weight management. Patients who meet prescribing guidelines (BMI $\geq$ 30 kg/m^2 or $\geq$ 27 kg/m^2 with a cormorbid condition) and who are motivated to undertake concurrent lifestyle change may receive health benefits from the additional weight loss that accompanies medication use.

REFERENCES

1. National Institutes of Health, National Heart, Lung, and Blood Institute. Clinical Guidelines on the Identification, Evaluation, and treatment of overweight and obesity in adults—the Evidence report. Obes Res 1998; 6:51S–210S.

2. Bray GA, Greenway FL. Current and potential drugs for treatment of obesity. Endocr Rev 1999; 20: 805–875.

3. Weintraub M, Bray GA. Drug treatment of obesity. Med Clin North Am 1989; 73:237–249.

4. Cole JO, Levin A, Beake B, Kaiser PE, Scheinbaum ML. Sibutramine: a new weight loss agent without evidence of the abuse potential associated with amphetamines. J Clin Psychopharmacol 1998; 18(3): 231–236.

5. Bray GA. Obesity——a time-bomb to be defused. Lancet 1998; 352:160–161.

6. Connolly HM, Crary JL, McGoon MD, et al. Valvular heart disease associated with fenfluramine–phentermine. N Engl J Med 1997; 337:581–588.

7. Ryan DH, Bray GA, Helmcke F, et al. Serial echocardiographic and clinical evaluation of valvular regurgitation before, during, and after treatment with fenfluramine or dexfenfluramine and mazindol or phentermine. Obes Res 1999; 7:313–322.

8. Jick H. Heart valve disorders and appetite-suppressant drugs. JAMA 2000; 283:1738–1740.

9. Hensrud DD, Connolly HM, Grogan M, Miller FA, Bailey KR, Jensen MD. Echocardiographic improvement over time after cessation of use of fenfluramine and phentermine. Mayo Clin Proc 1999; 74: 1191–1197.

10. Mast ST, Jollis JG, Ryan T, Anstrom KJ, Crary JL. The progression of fenfluramine-associated valvular heart disease assessed by echocardiography. Ann Intern Med 2001; 134:261–266.

11. McMahon FG, Fujioka K, Singh, BN, et al. Efficacy and safety of sibutramine in obese white and African-American patients with hypertension. Arch Int Med 2000; 160:2185–2191.

12. Finer N, James WP, Kopelman PG, Lean ME, Williams G. One-year treatment of obesity: a randomized, double-blind, placebo-controlled, multicentre study of orlistat, a gastrointestinal lipase inhibitor. Int J Obes Relat Metab Disord 2000; 24:306–313.

13. Flechtner-Mors M, Ditschuneit HH, Johnson TD, Suchard MA, Adler G. Metabolic and weight loss effects of long-term dietary intervention in obese patients: four-year results. Obes Res 2000; 8:399–402.

14. Munro JF, MacCuish AC, Wilson EM, et al. Comparison of continuous and intermittent anorectic therapy in obesity. Br Med J 1968; 1:352–354.

15. Greenway FL, Ryan Greenway FL, Ryan DH, et al. Pharmaceutical cost savings of treating obesity with weight loss medications. Obes Res 1999; 7:523–531.

16. Astrup A, Breum L, Tourbro S, et al. The effect and satiety of an ephedrine/caffeine compound compared to ephedrine, caffeine and placebo in obese subjects on an energy restricted diet. A double blind trial. Int J Obes 1992; 16:260–277.

17. Sjostrom CD, Lissner L, Wedel H, Sjostrom L. Reduction in incidence of diabetes, hypertension and lipid disturbances after intentional weight loss induced by bariatric surgery: the SOS Intervention Study. Obes Res 1999; 7:477–484.

18. Foster GD, Wadden TA, Vogt RA, et al. What is a reasonable weight loss? Patients expectations and evaluations of obesity treatment outcomes. J Consult Clin Psychol 1997; 65:79–85.

19. Bray GA. Evaluation of drugs for treating obesity. Obes Res 1995; 3:425S–434S.

20. Zhang Y, Proenca R, Maffei M, Barone M, Leopold L, Friedman JM. Positional cloning of the mouse obese gene and its human homologue. Nature 1994; 372:425–432.

21. Bray GA, Tartaglia LA. Medicinal strategies in the treatment of obesity. Nature. 2000; 404:672–677.

22. National on the Task Force Prevention and Treatment of Obesity. Long-term pharmacotherapy in the management of obesity. JAMA 1996; 276:1907–1915.

23. Astrup A, Hansen DL, Lundsgaard C, Toubro S. Sibutramine and energy balance. Int J Obes Relat Metab Disord 1998; 22:S30–S42.

24. Hansen DL, Toubro S, Stock MJ, Macdonald IA, Astrup A. Thermogenic effects of sibutramine in humans. Am J Clin Nutr 1998; 68:1180–1186.

25. Sykas SL, Danforth E Jr, Lien EL. Anorectic drugs which stimulate thermogenesis. Life Sci 1983; 33:1269–1275.

26. Lupien JR, Bray GB. Effect of mazindol, D-amphetamine and diethylpropion on purine nucleotide binding to brown adipose tissue. Pharmacol Biochem Behav 1986; 25:733–738.

27. Scoville B. Review of amphetamine-like drugs by the Food and Drug Administration: Clinical data and value judgments. In: Obesity in Perspective. Pub. No. 75-708. Department of Health, Education, and Welfare, Washington, DC, 1975, pp. 441–443.

28. Silverstone JJ, Solomon T. The long-term management of obesity in general practice. Br J Clin Pract 1965; 19:395–398.

29. McKay RHG. Long-term use of diethylpropion in obesity. Curr Med Res Opin 1973; 1:489–493.

30. Langlois KJ, Forbes JA, Bell GW, Grant GF Jr. A double-blind clinical evaluation of the safety and efficacy of phentermine hydrochloride (Fastin) in the treatment of exogenous obesity. Curr Ther Res 1974; 16:289–296.

31. Gershberg H, Kane R, Hulse M, Pensgen E. Effects of diet and an anorectic drug (phentermine resin) in obese diabetics. Curr Ther Res 1977; 22:814–820.

32. Campbell CJ, Bhalla IP, Steel JM, Duncan LJP. A controlled trial of phentermine in obese diabetic patients. Practitioner 1977; 218:851–855.

33. Williams RA, Foulsham BM. Weight reduction in osteoarthritis using phentermine. Practitioner 1981; 225:231–232.

34. Yanovski SZ, Yanovski JA. Obesity. N Engl J Med 2002; 346:591–602,

35. Bray GA, Ryan DH, Gordon D, Heidingsfelder S, Cerise F, Wilson K. A double-blind randomized placebo-controlled trial of sibutramine. Obes Res 1996; 4:263–270.

36. Bray GA, Blackburn GL, Ferguson JM, et al. Sibutramine produces dose-related weight loss. Obes Res 1999; 7:189–198.

37. Apfelbaum M, Vague P, Ziegler O, Hanotin C, Thomas F, Leutenegger E. Long-term maintenance of weight loss after a very-low-calorie diet: a randomized blinded trial of the efficacy and tolerability of sibutramine. Am J Med 1999; 106:179–184.

38. Fanghanel G, Cortinas L, Sanchez-Reyes L, Berber A. A clinical trial of the use of sibutramine for the treatment of patients suffering essential obesity. Int J Obes 2000; 24:144–150.

39. James WPT, Astrup A, Finer N, et al., for the STORM study group. Effect of sibutramine on weight maintenance after weight loss: a randomized trial. Lancet 2000; 356:2119–2125.

40. Cuellar GEM, Ruiz AM, Monsalve MCR, Berber A. Six-month treatment of obesity with sibutramine 15 mg: a double-blind, placebo-controlled monocenter clinical trial in a Hispanic population. Obes Res 2000; 8:71–82.

41. Smith IG, Goulder MA. Randomized placebo-controlled trial of long-term treatment with sibutramine in mild to moderate obesity. J Fam Pract 2001;50:505–512.

42. Dujovne CA, Zavoral JH, Rowe E, Mendel CM. Effects of sibutramine on body weight and serum lipids: a double-blind, randomized, placebo-controlled study in 322 overweight and obese patients with dyslipidemia. Am Heart J 2001; 142:489–497.

43. Wirth A, Krause J. Long-term weight loss with sibutramine. JAMA 2001; 286:1331–1339.

44. Fujioka K, Seaton TB, Rowe E, et al., and the Sibutramine/Diabetes clinical study group. Weight loss with sibutramine improves glycemic control and other metabolic parameters in obese type 2 diabetes mellitus. Diab Obes Metab 2000; 2:1–13.

45. Gockel A, Karakose H, Ertorer EM, Tanaci N, Tutuncu NB, Guvener N. Effects of sibutramine in obese female subjects with type 2 diabetes and poor blood glucose control. Diabetes Care 2001; 24: 1957–1960.

46. Serrano-Rios M, Melchionda N, Moreno-Carretero E. Role of sibutramine in the treatment of obese Type 2 diabetic patients receiving sulphonylurea therapy. Diabet Med 2002; 19:119–124.

47. McMahon FG, Weinstein SP, Rowe E, Ernst KR, Johnson F, Fujioka K. Sibutramine is safe and effective for weight loss in obese patients whose hypertension is well controlled with angiotensin-converting enzyme inhibitors. J Hum Hypertens 2002; 16:5–11.

48. Weintraub M, Rubio A, Golik A, Byrne L, Scheinbaum ML. Sibutramine in weight control: A dose-ranging, efficacy study. Clin Pharmacol Ther 1991;50:330–337.

49. Finer N, Bloom SR, Frost GS, Banks LM, Griffiths J. Sibutramine is effective for weight loss and diabetic control in obesity with type 2 diabetes: a randomised, double-blind placebo-controlled study. Diab Obes Metab 2000; 2:105–112.

50. Hazenberg BP. Randomized, double-blind, placebo-controlled, multicenter study of sibutramine in obese hypertensive patients. Cardiol 2000; 94:152–158

51. Sramek, JJ, Seiowitz MT, Weinstein SP, et al. Efficacy and safety of sibutramine for weight loss in obese patients with hypertension well controlled by β-adrenergic blocking agents: a placebo-controlled, double-blind, randomized trial. Am J Hyperten 2002; 16:13–19.

52. Berube-Parent S, Prud'homme D, St-Pierre S, Doucet E, Tremblay A. Obesity treatment with a progressive clinical tri-therapy combining sibutramine and a supervised diet-exercise intervention. Int J Obes Relat Metab Disord 2001; 25:1144–1153.

53. Wadden RA, Berkowitz RI, Sarwer DB, Prus-Wisniewski R, Steinberg CM. Benefits of lifestyle modification in the pharmacologic treatment of obesity: a randomized trial. Arch Intern Med 2001; 161:218–227.

54. Van Gaal LF, Wauters M, De Leeuw IH. The beneficial effects of modest weight loss on cardiovascular risk factors. Int J Obes 1997; 21(Suppl 1): S5–S9.

55. Kernan WN, Viscoli CM, Brass LM, et al. Phenylpropanolamine and the risk of hemorrhagic stroke. N Engl J Med 2000; 343:1826–1832.

56. Anderson JW, Greenway FL, Fujioka K, Gadde KM, McKenney J, O'Neil PM. Bupropion SR significantly enhances weight loss: a 24-week double-blind, placebo-controlled trial with placebo group randomized to bupropion SR during 24-week extension. Obes Res 2002; 10:633–641.

57. Haddock CK, Poston WSC, Dill PL, Foreyt JP, Ericsson M. Pharmacotherapy for obesity: a quantitative analysis of four decades of published randomized clinical trials. Int J Obes Relat Metab Disord 2002; 26:262–273.

58. Reife R, Pledger G, Wu S. Topiramate as add-on therapy: pooled analysis of randomized controlled trials in adults. Epilepsia 2000; 41:S66–S71.

59. Bray GA, Hollander P, Klein S, et al. A 6-month randomized, placebo-controlled, dose-ranging trial of topiramate for weight loss in obesity. Obes Res 2003; 11:722–733.

60. DiMarzo V, Goparaju SK, Wang L, et al. Leptin-regulated endocannabinoids are involved in maintaining food intake. Nature 2001; 410:822–825.

61. Gadde KM, Franciscy DM, Wagner HR 2nd, Krishnan KR. Zonisamide for weight loss in obese adults: a randomized controlled trial. JAMA 2003; 289:1820–1825.

62. Montague CT Farooqi IS, Whitehead JP, et al. Congenital leptin deficiency is associated with severe early-onset obesity in humans. Nature 1997; 387:903–908.

63. Farooqi IS, Jebb SA, Langmack G, et al. Effects of recombinant leptin therapy in a child with congenital leptin deficiency. N Engl J Med 1999; 341:879–884.

64. Heymsfield SB, Greenberg AS, Fujioka K, et al. Recombinant leptin for weight loss in obese and lean adults: a randomized, controlled, dose-escalation trial. JAMA 1999; 282:1568–1575.

65. Huckshorn CJ, Saris, WH, Westerterp-Plantenga MS, et al. Weekly subcutaneous pegylated recombinant native human leptin (PEG-OB) administration in obese men. J Clin Endocrinol Metab 2000; 85:4003–4009.

66. Lambert PD, Anderson KD, Sleeman MW, et al. Ciliary neurotrophic factor activates leptin-like pathways and reduces body fat, without cachexia or rebound weight gain, even in leptin-resistant obesity. Proc Nat Acad Sci 2001; 98:4652–4657.

67. Ettinger MP, Littlejohn TW, Schwartz SL, et al. Recombinant variant of ciliary neurotrophic factor for weight loss in obese adults: a randomized, dose-ranging study. JAMA 2003; 289:1826–1832.

68. Ludwig DS, Tritos NA, Mastaitis JW, et al. Melanin-concentrating hormone overexpression in transgenic mice leads to obesity and insulin resistance. J Clin Invest 2001; 107:379–386.

69. Flint A, Raben A, Astrup A, Holst JJ. Glucagon-like peptide 1 promotes satiety and suppresses energy intake in humans. J Clin Invest 1998; 101:515–520.

70. Al-Barazanji KA, Arch JR, Buckingham RE, Tadayyon M. Central exendin-4 infusion reduces body weight without altering plasma leptin in (fa/fa) Zucker rats. Obes Res 2000; 8:317–323.

71. Hauptman J. Orlistat: selective inhibition of caloric absorption can affect long-term body weight. Endocrine 2000; 13:201–206.

72. James WP, Avenell A, Broom J, Whitehead J. A one-year trial to assess the value of orlistat in the management of obesity. Int J Obes Relat Metab Disord 1997; 21(Suppl 3):S24–S30.

73. Van Gaal LF, Broom JI, Enzi G, Toplak H. Efficacy and tolerability of orlistat in the treatment of obesity: a 6-month dose-ranging study. Eur J Clin Pharm 1998; 54:125–132.

74. Sjostrom L, Rissanen A, Andersen T, et al. Randomised placebo-controlled trial of orlistat for weight loss and prevention of weight regain in obese patients. European Multicentre Orlistat Study Group. Lancet 1998; 352:167–172.

75. Davidson MH, Hauptman J, DiGirolamo M, et al. Long-term weight control and risk factor reduction in obese subjects treated with orlistat, a lipase inhibitor. JAMA 1999; 281:235–242.

76. Hill JO, Hauptmann J, Anderson JW, et al. Orlistat, a lipase inhibitor, for weight maintenance after conventional dieting: a 1-y study. Am J Clin Nutr 1999; 69:1108–1116.
77. Hauptmann J, Lucas C, Boldrin MN, Collins H, Segal KR for the Orlistat Primary Care Study Group. Orlistat in the long-term treatment of obesity in primary care settings. Arch Fam Med 2000; 9:160–167.
78. Rossner S, Sjostrom L, Noack R, Meinders AE, Noseda G, on behalf of the European Orlistat Obesity Study Group. Weight loss, weight maintenance, and improved cardiovascular risk factors after 2 years treatment with orlistat for obesity. Obes Res 2000; 8:49–61.
79. Lindgarde F, on behalf of the Orlistat Swedish Multimorbidity study group. The effect of orlistat on body weight and coronary heart disease risk profile in obese patients: the Swedish Multimorbidity study. J Intern Med 2000; 248:245–254.
80. Hollander P, Elbein SC, Hirsch IB, et al. Role of orlistat in the treatment of obese patients with type 2 diabetes. Diab Care 1998; 21:1288–1294.
81. Kelley D, Bray G, Pi-Sunyer FX, et al. Clinical efficacy of orlistat therapy in overweight and obese patients with insulin-treated type 2 diabetes mellitus: a one-year, randomized, controlled trial. Diab Care 2002; 25:1033–1041.
82. Miles JM, Leiter L, Hollander P, et al. Effect of orlistat in overweight and obese patients with type 2 diabetes treated with metformin. Diab Care 2002;25:1123–1128.
83. Zavoral JH. Treatment with orlistat reduces cardiovascular risk in obese patients. J Hypertens 1998; 16: 2013–2017.
84. Muls E, Kolanowski J, Scheen A, Van Gaal LF. The effects of orlistat on weight and on serum lipids in obese patients with hypercholesterolemia: a randomized, double-blind, placebo-controlled, multi-center study. Int J Obes Relat Metab Disord 2001; 25:1713–1721.
85. Tonstad S, Pometta D, Erkelens DW, et al. The effects of gastrointestinal lipase inhibitor, orlistat, on serum lipids and lipoproteins in patients with primary hyperlipidaemia. Eur J Clin Pharmacol 1994; 46: 405–410.
86. Linton MF, Fazio S. Re-emergence of fibrates in the management of dyslipidemia and cardiovascular risk. Curr Atheroscler Rep 2000; 2:29–35.
87. Maron DJ, Fazio S, Linton MF. Current perspectives on statins. Circ 2000; 101:207–213.
88. Heymsfield SB, Segal KR, Hauptman J, et al. Effects of weight loss with orlistat on glucose tolerance and progression to type 2 diabetes in obese adults. Arch Intern Med 2000; 160:1321–1326.
89. Tan MH. Current treatment of insulin resistance in type 2 diabetes mellitus. Int J Clin Pract Suppl 2000; 113:54–62.
90. Ceriello A. The postprandial state and cardiovascular disease: relevance to diabetes mellitus. Diabetes Metabol Res Rev 2000; 16:125–132.
91. Sjostrom L et al. Xendos. Presentation. International Congress on Obesity, Sao Paolo, Brazil, 2002.
92. Reaven G, Segal K, Hauptman J, Boldrin M and Lucas C. Effect of orlistat-assisted weight loss in decreasing coronary heart disease risk in patients with Syndrome X. Am J Cardiol 2001; 87:827–831.
93. Drent ML, van der Veen EA. First clinical studies with orlistat: A short review. Obes Res 1995; 3: S623–S625.
94. Wadden TA, Berkowitz RI, Womble LG, Sarwer DB, Arnold ME, Steinberg CM. Effects of sibutramine plus orlistat in obese women following 1 year of treatment by sibutramine alone: a placebo-controlled trial. Obes Res 2000; 8:431–437.
95. Bray GA. Drug treatment of obesity. Endocr Metab Disor 2001; 2:403–418.
96. Astrup A, Bulow J, Madsen J, Christensen NJ. Contribution of BAT and skeletal muscle to thermogenesis induced by ephedrine in man. Am J Physiol 1985; 248:E507–E515.
97. Astrup A, Breum L, Toubro S. Pharmacological and clinical studies of ephedrine and other thermogenic agonists . Obes Res 1995; 3:537S–540S.
98. Astrup A, Breum L, Toubro S, Hein P, Quaade F. Ephedrine and weight loss. Int J Obes Relat Metab Disord 1992; 16:715.
99. Grover GJ, Mellstrom K, Ye L, et al. Selective thyroid hormone receptor-β activation: a strategy for reduction of weight, cholesterol, and lipoprotein (a) with reduced cardiovascular liability. Proc Natl Acad Sci USA 2003. Electronic publication in advance of print publication.
100. Larsen TM, Toubro S, van Baak MA, et al. No thermogenic effect after 28 days treatment with L-796,568, a novel β-3-adrenoceptor, in obese men. Obes Res 2000; 8(Suppl 1):44S.

101. Heymsfield SB, Allison DB, Vasselli JR, Pietrobelli A, Greenfield D, Nunez C. Garcinia cambogia (hydroxycitric acid) as a potential antiobesity agent: a randomized controlled trial. JAMA 1998; 280:1596–600.
102. Guerciolini R, Radu-Radulescu L, Boldrin M, Moore R. Fecal fat excretion induced by treatment with orlistat or chitosan: a 3-week randomized crossover design study. Obes Res 2000; 8:43S.
103. Pittler MH, Abbot NC, Harkness EF, Ernst E. Randomized, double-blind trial of chitosan for body weight reduction. Eur J Clin Nutr 1999; 53:379–381.
104. Boozer CN, Nasser JA, Heymsfield SB, Wang V, Chen G, Solomon JL. An herbal supplement containing Ma Huang-Guarana for weight loss: a randomized, double-blind trial. Int J Obes Relat Metab Disord 2001; 25:316–324.
105. Boozer CN, Daly PA, Blanchard D, Nasser JA, Solomon JL, Homel P. Herbal ephedra/caffeine for weight loss: A 6-month safety and efficacy trial. Int J Obes Relat Metab Disord 2002; 26:593–604.

17 Combination Therapies for Obesity

Richard L. Atkinson and Gabriel Uwaifo

KEY POINTS

- Obesity is like most chronic diseases, and single treatments are often ineffective.
- Obesity is a complex syndrome that requires complex treatment.
- Most patients will need more than one medication for maximal weight loss, but it may be reasonable to start with only one medication to determine whether the patient is highly sensitive and will do well with only one medication. Additional medications would be added as necessary.
- Long-term, careful follow-up is needed, and because obesity treatment requires a great deal of patient education, it is best done with a team of a physician and at least one allied health professional.

1. INTRODUCTION: OBESITY AS A DISEASE

With the realization that obesity is a disease, not a psychological problem, the horizons of obesity treatment have widened. The concept of drug treatment of obesity has gained more widespread acceptance, and the most recent and exciting developments in obesity treatment have involved the use of drugs as an integral component. Using the concept of obesity as a chronic disease, this chapter discusses the integration of the standard treatments of obesity, including diet, exercise (*see* Chapter 13), and behavior modification (*see* Chapter 14), with single medications or combinations of medications, as potentially more effective regimens for the long-term maintenance of weight loss than without use of medications (Table 1).

Most scientists who study obesity now believe that obesity is the result of environmental factors acting on a genetic predisposition for obesity *(1)*. Currently, it is not possible to manipulate the genes for obesity, but the environment certainly can be manipulated. The genetic contribution to obesity helps explain why medical treatment of obesity, consisting of diet, exercise, and behavior modification, has had a poor long-term success rate. Only a long-term, comprehensive program of lifestyle modification appears to increase the success rate, and few people are able to consistently modify their behavior life long. Although surgical treatment of obesity (*see* Chapter 20) has a good success rate,

From: *The Management of Eating Disorders and Obesity, Second Edition*
Edited by: D. J. Goldstein © Humana Press Inc., Totowa, NJ

Table 1
Overview of Chapter

it is generally reserved for massively obese individuals and therefore is not an option for the average overweight person.

2. NECESSITY FOR LONG-TERM TREATMENT AND EXPERIENCE WITH STANDARD THERAPY

Obesity is a chronic disease *(1,2)*. Chronic diseases require chronic treatments, and when the treatment stops, the disease comes back. Many patients, and even many health care professionals, look for short-term solutions. They do not understand the necessity for lifelong intensive treatment. Massively obese patients who meet the criteria for obesity surgery achieve long-term weight loss in a good percentage of cases because the effects of the surgery are permanent. For the remainder of less obese patients, some form of continuous medical treatment is the only option. Behavioral treatments produce satisfying initial weight loss in the majority of patients, but long-term weight maintenance is much more critical and is more difficult to achieve. Routine medical treatment of obesity consisting of nutrition education, behavior modification, exercise therapy, and activity training was reported to have a failure rate of greater than 95% over 5 to 10 yr when treatment was not continued *(3–6)*. A recent review/meta-analysis was slightly more optimistic, finding that the long-term failure rate is about 85% *(7)*. Even with surgery for obesity, weight is regained if the surgical procedure is reversed. This discouraging information points out the absolute necessity of continual treatment over the lifetime of an obese person with the methods currently available.

3. RATIONALE FOR COMBINING THERAPIES

Unfortunately, obesity is like most chronic diseases, and single treatments are often ineffective. The general lack of success with nonpharmacologic treatment has been noted previously, and the modest results with pharmacological treatment alone are described here. These observations suggest that obesity treatment should mimic treatments of other chronic diseases. If a single intervention is not effective, combinations of therapies should be instituted. The remainder of this chapter addresses the use of medicines, alone or in combination, that may be combined with standard therapy of diet and increased activity. If multiple combinations are evaluated for each individual who seeks therapy, it may be possible to achieve sustained weight loss in many, if not most, obese patients.

4. RATIONALE FOR USE OF OBESITY PHARMACOTHERAPY

Although diet, exercise, and behavior modification of lifestyle can be successful in reducing body weight, the necessity to not eat when hungry and to eat less palatable foods when highly palatable foods are available wears thin with time. Also, dramatic increases in exercise and activity levels are difficult to sustain. The genetic predisposition to obesity mandates that obese people cannot behave as thin people do. To become thin, they have to do more than thin people. The ob/ob mouse and Zucker obese rat are models for obese humans. If these animals are pair fed to lean littermates, they remain obese *(8)*. To weigh the same as their lean littermates, they have to eat half of what their lean littermates eat. Although perhaps not as drastic, similar requirements undoubtedly are present for obese humans. It is extremely difficult to continue such restricted behavior indefinitely with the American environment that is so conducive to eating high-energy–high-fat foods excessively and that is so lacking in necessity for activity. It has been amply shown that few obese people who have sought treatment for obesity continue diet, exercise, and behavior-modification regimens for their entire lifetimes *(3–7)*. Obesity medications are a more passive way of changing the physiology and biochemistry of obesity. By definition, effective pharmacotherapies change the biochemistry of the body. As described here, most of the obesity medications continue to be effective as long as they are taken.

5. INDICATIONS AND CONTRAINDICATIONS FOR OBESITY PHARMACOTHERAPY

As noted earlier, pharmacotherapy of obesity will only be effective if the medications are continued indefinitely. Therefore, obesity medications must be used carefully and only with appropriate indications. Table 2 lists criteria for use of obesity drugs. A panel of experts convened by the North American Association for the Study of Obesity (NAASO) recommended that drugs may be indicated for individuals with a body mass index (BMI) of 27 or above *(9)*. The US Food and Drug Administration (FDA), National Institutes of Health (NIH), and World Health Organization criteria for use of obesity drugs are a BMI of at least 30 (kg/m^2), or a BMI of at least 27 if complications of obesity are present *(10,11)*. Many investigators and clinicians favor these more conservative criteria. Any use of obesity drugs in individuals who weigh less than the FDA/NIH criteria should be very carefully documented and justified in the medical record. The practice of giving obesity drugs to individuals who are not overweight

Table 2
Criteria and Contraindications for Use of Obesity Medications

---

1. Criteria for use
    a. NAASO[a] Criteria
        i. BMI >27 kg/m^2
        ii. BMI >25 kg/m^2, with complications
    b. FDA, NIH, WHO[b] Criteria
        i. BMI $\geq$30 kg/m^2
        ii. BMI $\geq$27 kg/m^2, with complications
2. Contraindications or cautions for use
    a. Pregnancy or lactation
    b. Unstable cardiac disease
    c. Uncontrolled hypertension
    d. Presence of any severe systemic illness (caution)
    e. Severe psychiatric disorder or anorexia (contraindication or caution)
    f. Other drug therapy, if incompatible
    g. Closed angle glaucoma (caution)
    h. Age younger than 18 yr or older than 65 yr (caution)

---

[a] North American Association for the Study of Obesity *(74)*.

[b] Food and Drug Administration, National Institutes of Health *(10)*, World Health Organization *(11)*.

should be deplored. However, there may be a number of mitigating factors that justify use in individuals below the cutoffs. These include complications of obesity such as hypertension, diabetes, and hyperlipidemia. Another is the presence of excess intra-abdominal fat (visceral obesity), a major risk factor for diabetes, heart disease, and strokes *(12)*. Visceral obesity in people with a BMI below 27 can be documented with magnetic resonance imaging or computed tomography scan. Certain racial and ethnic groups, Asians and Hispanics in particular, are prone to depositing visceral fat at much lower BMIs than Caucasians *(13,14)*. There has been significant debate about whether the cutpoints for defining obesity should be based on racial identity *(13,14)*.

Individuals who have a past history of a BMI greater than 27, but less than 30 in the past, but who have been able to maintain weight loss only with great difficulty, also may be considered for treatment with obesity drugs. It makes no sense to have such individuals regain their weight before they become eligible for obesity pharmacotherapy.

Some patients have significant psychological concerns regarding excess body weight. The physician should carefully evaluate such patients before prescribing obesity drugs to determine whether there is any evidence of an eating disorder. In some cases, referral for psychological or psychiatric counseling to deal with these concerns may be a better choice than prescription of obesity medications.

6. CLASSIFICATION OF OBESITY PHARMACOTHERAPIES

Table 3 lists drugs that are used for the treatment of obesity in the United States or elsewhere in the world. The list includes drugs that are approved by the FDA for the treatment of obesity, drugs previously approved but no longer available, drugs that are FDA-approved for marketing for non-obesity indications, and drugs that are still in the research stage and have not yet come on the market. With the exceptions of sibutramine, approved

Table 3
Categories of Weight Loss Medications and Drug Enforcement Agency (DEA) Schedules

1. Adrenergic agonists
   a. Schedule II: Amphetamine,[a] Methamphetamine,[a] Phenmetrazine
   b. Schedule III: Benzphetamine, Chlorphentermine,[a] Chlortermine,[a] Phendimetrazine
   c. Schedule IV: Diethylpropion, Mazindol,[a] Phentermine
   d. OTC: Phenylpropanolamine,[b] Ephedrine and caffeine [b]
2. Monoamine agonists and reuptake inhibitors
   a. Schedule IV serotonin agonists: D,L-Fenfluramine,[b] D-Fenfluramine [b]
   b. Not scheduled serotonin reuptake inhibitors: Fluoxetine,[c] Sertraline,[c] Citalopram [c]
   c. Serotonin, norepinephrine, and dopamine reuptake inhibitor: Sibutramine
3. Drugs affecting absorption
   a. Fat: Orlistat
   b. Carbohydrate: Acarbose [c]
4. Other Mechanisms
   a. Dopamine and serotonin reuptake inhibition: Bupropion
   b. Anticonvulsants: Topiramate,[c] Zonisamide [c]

[a] Not currently marketed for the treatment of obesity in the US.
[b] Withdrawn from market in US.
[c] Marketed for other indications, not FDA approved for the treatment of obesity.
OTC, over-the-counter or nonprescription.

for marketing in early 1998, and of orlistat, approved for marketing in 1999, all of the currently available drugs approved by the FDA for obesity are no longer patent protected. Chapter 16 more fully discusses obesity pharmacotherapies.

6.1. Centrally Acting Obesity Pharmacotherapies

With the exception of orlistat, all obesity pharmacotherapies currently or previously approved in the United States act on the central nervous system as adrenergic, serotonergic, or as a combined adrenergic–serotonergic agonists or reuptake inhibitors.

Adrenergic drugs increase norepinephrine (NE) and/or dopamine activity in specific brain regions including those involved in regulating food intake, satiety, and energy expenditure. All of the adrenergic that are currently indicated as obesity pharmacotherapies are scheduled by the Drug Enforcement Agency (DEA) to indicate abuse potential, despite little or no evidence that they are abused, as indicated in Table 3. Schedule II (e.g., dexamphetamine) pharmacotherapies should not be used for obesity, and there is little reason to use schedule III pharmacotherapies. The adrenergic agonists that are used most frequently by prescription in the United States are phentermine and diethylpropion, both of which are DEA schedule IV. Phentermine was found to be more effective than diethylpropion in one controlled trial (15). Phendimetrazine is in DEA schedule III and has not been shown to be more effective than phentermine in controlled trials (16–18). All of the adrenergic agents were approved by the FDA many years ago and were expected to be used only briefly (12 wk or less) (16–18). Thus, use for more than 12 wk is considered "off label."

Phenylpropanolamine (PPA) once was the most commonly used drug for obesity in the United States because it was present in a large number of over-the-counter (OTC) diet aids. The FDA removed PPA from the market because of a fear that it increased the risk of cerebral vascular accidents (stroke). It remains available in some countries. PPA acts on α-adrenergic receptors in the brain to produce a decrease in appetite and a modest weight loss.

There are no pure serotonin agonists currently on the market. Dexfenfluramine and D,L-fenfluramine, two previously available obesity pharmacotherapies, were removed in 1997 because they produced pulmonary hypertension and damage to the heart valves, particularly the aortic and mitral valves (19–22). Later, more rational evaluation of the degree of the problem of heart valve damage concluded that the prevalences were not as great as initially reported (19), and cardiac valve damage regressed or did not change (20–22). Although they are not approved by the FDA for the treatment of obesity, many physicians have used selective serotonin reuptake inhibitor (SSRI) antidepressant agents including fluoxetine, sertraline, citalopram, and others for weight reduction (23–30) (Table 3).

Sibutramine is a monoamine reuptake inhibitor of both serotonin and NE, so it increases both neurotansmitters (31,32). It is also a dopamine reuptake inhibitor, but has minimal dopamine agonist activity. Although it does not appear to have abuse potential, it has been assigned as a schedule IV drug by the DEA and FDA.

6.2. Non-FDA-Approved, Centrally Acting Pharmacotherapies With Potential for Treating Obesity

In addition to the SSRIs mentioned previously, there are a number of other centrally active agents that potentially may be useful for the treatment of obesity. Some of these agents are already on the market and approved for other indications, but have been shown anecdotally or in clinical trials to produce weight loss. Others have not been fully tested and their roles for obesity therapy are not yet known.

The combination of ephedrine and caffeine, with or without the addition of aspirin, has been extensively used in Europe and is reported to produce weight loss (33,34). Methyl-xanthines (caffeine, theophylline, theobromine, etc.) and/or aspirin potentiate the effects of ephedrine and increase weight loss and metabolic rate by slowing the degradation of norepinephrine (33–36). Ephedrine–caffeine stimulates NE secretion. Caffeine enhances NE activity by inhibiting phosphodiesterase, the enzyme that metabolizes cyclic adenosine monophosphate, through which NE acts. Aspirin enhances NE activity by inhibiting adenosine, which is involved in NE inactivation. The combination may be associated with increases in heart rate, blood pressure (BP), and metabolic rate (33–38). The increases in heart rate and BP associated with ephedrine–caffeine appear to be short-lived, but the effect on thermogenesis persists (34).

Pure ephedrine and caffeine have been used very sparingly in the United States for obesity treatment. However, numerous OTC dietary supplements contain ephedra and a methylxanthine (usually caffeine) as plant extracts. These preparations probably were the most commonly used anti-obesity products used in the United States, dwarfing any of the single obesity prescription medications. The FDA moved to ban ephedra from use in dietary supplements for obesity in December 2003. This ban does not prohibit physicians from prescribing ephedrine, usually in combination with caffeine or other methylxanthine as pure prescription preparations. However, the legal vulnerability, should side effects occur, markedly reduce enthusiasm for its use.

Bupropion is an aminoketone class antidepressant that is chemically related to the phenylethylamines, with a structure similar to diethylpropion. It has adrenergic and serotonergic reuptake inhibitor activity. Anderson et al. *(39)* found that it produced a 1-yr weight loss of about 10% of initial body weight.

Topiramate is an anticonvulsant with an undetermined mechanism of action. Significant weight loss was reported as a side effect of treatment in seizure patients. Bray et al. *(40)* reported a multicenter, 6-mo, randomized trial that found a weight loss of about 6% of initial body weight. Side effects included glaucoma and paresthesias.

Zonisamide is another anti-convulsant with serotonergic and dopaminergic activity in addition to blockade of sodium and calcium channels. Gadde et al. *(41)* reported a 16-wk randomized, blinded trial with a 16-wk open-label extension. Weight loss was about 6% of initial body weight.

Leptin, a peptide made by adipose tissue, signals the brain regarding peripheral fat stores. Clinical trials were disappointing and it is not clear whether this will have a role in obesity treatment with the exception of a tiny number of subjects who were found to have a leptin gene defect.

Rimonabant, octreotide, axokine, and several other agents (*see* Chapters 16 and 18) are in phase II–III clinical trials, but it is too early to determine whether any of these will prove useful for treating obesity. Peptide YY 3-36, glucagon-like peptide-1, enterostatin, ghrelin antagonists, neuropeptide YY antagonists, β-3 adrenergic agents and many others are under evaluation in animals and humans and at least some of these may prove to be useful for obesity.

6.3. Malabsorptive Agents for Obesity

Orlistat is the only obesity drug currently approved by the FDA that is not absorbed into the body. It acts within the gastrointestinal (GI) tract by inhibiting intestinal lipase, thus blocking the digestion and absorption of about one-third of dietary fat that is ingested *(42–48)*. The portion of dietary fat that is not absorbed passes through to the colon and is metabolized and utilized by colonic bacteria or is excreted. Orlistat does not have prolonged activity and must be taken with a meal to be effective. There is an independent effect of orlistat on serum lipids *(44–46)*, but no independent effect on serum glucose *(44–47)*. Orlistat has the distinction of being the only FDA approved anti-obesity medication for use in children and adolescents *(48)*.

Acarbose, an amylase inhibitor that blocks complex carbohydrate absorption *(49)*, is approved for the treatment of diabetes in the United States. Acarbose has been shown to be ineffective in the treatment of obesity when used as a single agent, although anecdotal reports suggest that it occasionally may produce modest additional weight loss when used in combination. Acarbose is a good choice for the obese, non-insulin-dependent diabetic patient because it acts to improve glucose tolerance, decrease insulin resistance, and potentially produces some weight loss.

7. RESULTS OF COMBINATION OF SINGLE MEDICATIONS, DIET, AND EXERCISE FOR OBESITY

A large number of studies have evaluated treatment of obesity with a single drug combined with diet and exercise therapy. The vast majority of these studies were for brief periods of time, most commonly about 12 wk. Scoville *(16)* summarized more than 200 studies of single agents and concluded that obesity drugs were poorly effective, because weekly weight loss was only about one-half pound greater on drug than on placebo. Silverstone *(17)* compared several drugs and noted weight losses that were statistically significant with all of these drugs as compared to placebo. The actual weight losses were modest, but the study times were short. In 1994, Goldstein et al. *(18)* evaluated all of the studies in the literature to that date that had lasted longer than 6 mo. The 1-yr average weight losses ranged from 2.3 kg to 14.2 kg. Losses with mazindol were greatest at 14.2 and 12.0 kg. Fluoxetine produced weight losses of 2.3 to 13.9 kg. Losses with fenfluramine and dexfenfluramine varied from 5.2 to 9.8 kg.

Phentermine, sibutramine, and orlistat are the three drugs used most often in the United States, and all produce a weight loss of about 6 to 13%. The longest reported use of phentermine was 36 mo, in two studies from Monroe's laboratory *(50,51)*. Both of these studies reported weight losses of 13% of initial body weight. In neither of these trials was there a strong diet and exercise component to the weight-loss program.

The initial reports on effectiveness of sibutramine demonstrated a weight loss of about 6 to 8% of initial body weight *(31)*. The Sibutramine Trial of Obesity Reduction and Maintenance trial, which included intensive lifestyle intervention plus sibutramine, reported an average weight loss of about 13% at 1 yr *(52)*, and Wadden et al. *(53)* reported an average loss of 11.6% at 1 yr. However, Padwal et al. *(54)* performed a Cochrane review of all published studies of obesity drugs with at least 1 yr of follow-up. Five sibutramine trials were included and the average weight loss was 4.3 kg or 4.6% more than in the placebo group in these studies. All of these studies included a diet and exercise component.

Initial reports of the effectiveness of orlistat demonstrated a weight loss of about 5 to 12% of baseline body weight at 1 to 2 yr *(42–48)*. The Cochrane review by Padwal et al. *(54)* evaluated 11 orlistat studies. Average weight loss was 2.7 kg or 2.9% greater than placebo.

Almost all of the studies noted here were not a pure test of drug vs placebo because they included at least some dietary and behavioral therapy. The large variability of weight losses between studies may have been influenced by the success of subjects at different sites combining diet, exercise, and behavior modification with the drug treatment. Also, investigators placed greater emphasis on diet and exercise at some sites compared with others.

Another potential explanation for variability in weight loss is the observation that some people are more sensitive to obesity drugs, and could be classified as "responders." Sayler et al. *(55)* attempted to identify factors that would predict success of treatment with fluoxetine and found a series of variables that gave significant results. However, the variation was large and the variables were nonspecific, so that the formula has little clinical usefulness. Additional studies are indicated to determine whether clinically useful predictors can be identified.

8. COMBINATION PHARMACOTHERAPY OF OBESITY

Pharmacologics are therapies of choice for most chronic diseases. For chronic medical conditions like hypertension, diabetes, dyslipidemia and asthma, if one medication does not completely alleviate the problem, a second, third, or more are added. However, the use of combinations of medications for obesity has been surprisingly sparse. Combinations of medications that have been used for obesity include ephedrine–methylxanthines–aspirin, phenylpropanolamine–benzocaine, fenfluramine–phentermine, fluoxetine–phentermine, dexfenfluramine–fluoxetine, and sibutramine–orlistat *(23,28–30,33–34,53,56–63)*. Data from a sampling of these studies are described next.

8.1. Ephedrine Combinations

The combination of ephedrine with caffeine and/or aspirin results in fat loss with preservation of lean body mass *(33–38,64)*. Toubro et al. *(34)* compared placebo, ephedrine alone (60 mg/d), caffeine alone (600 mg/d), and the combination of ephedrine and caffeine over a period of 24 wk in 180 subjects. None of the substances caused weight loss alone, compared with placebo, but the combination produced a mean weight loss of 16 kg. A 26-wk open-label extension revealed that the 16 kg weight loss persisted for 50 wk in the 99 of 180 subjects who completed the protocol. Molnar et al. *(64)* treated adolescents with ephedrine–caffeine for 20 wk and found a weight loss of 14.4vs 2.2% for placebo treatment. Side effects were not different than placebo and there were no withdrawal effects. Boozer et al. *(37,38)* performed randomized, double-blind studies of dietary supplements containing ephedra and caffeine. This group noted significant weight loss vs placebo, with only modest side effects in their carefully selected subjects. They evaluated cardiac status by 24hr Holter monitoring and noted no differences in arrhythmias compared to placebo *(38)*. Kalman et al. *(65)* evaluated the cardiac effects of a dietary supplement over a 14 d period and found no meaningful differences from the placebo group.

Physicians in the United States rarely prescribe this combination of drugs, but before removal from the market, large amounts were bought by consumers as "dietary supplements" in health food stores and other commercial distributors. A very large number of adverse events were reported to the FDA in users of ephedra or ephedra–caffeine combinations including myocardial infarctions, cerebrovascular accidents, and sudden death. These were anecdotal reports rather than scientific data, so the FDA commissioned the Rand Corporation to prepare a report. After reviewing the literature and the anecdotal reports of adverse events that were sent to the FDA, the authors of this report noted the large number of adverse events and concluded that the combination was associated with some potentially concerning side effects *(66)*. They stated that there was insufficient evidence to conclude that ephedrine/ephedra and caffeine was responsible for the morbidity and mortality seen anecdotally, but that the evidence warranted controlled studies. Reviews of the literature by Greenway *(67)* and by Shekelle et al. *(68)* came to the same conclusions. However, the FDA decided that the potential risks of dietary supplements containing ephedrine/ephedra outweighed the potential benefits and in December 2003, banned the use of ephedra in dietary supplements for weight loss in the United States *(69)*.

8.2. Phenylpropanolamine–Benzocaine

Benzocaine, a local anesthetic agent reputed to "numb the taste buds," is in some OTC weight reduction aids. Greenway and colleagues *(56,57)* found that the combination of PPA and benzocaine was no more effective than placebo, so this combination cannot be recommended for clinical use.

8.3. Phentermine–Fenfluramine Combination

Although fenfluramine and dexfenfluramine are no longer on the market, the results of the seminal studies of Weintraub et al. *(58,59)* using this combination for obesity are instructive. Weintraub et al. *(59)* kept 121 subjects on the combination of phentermine resin and fenfluramine for up to 3.5 yr. All subjects were treated with diet, exercise, and behavior modification. At 60 wk, patients on continuous treatment had lost 15.8 kg. This was the first long-term study of drug-combination therapy for obesity, and demonstrated that significant weight loss persisted as long as the drugs were given. When subjects discontinued medications at the end of the study, weight gain back toward baseline levels was rapid. Atkinson et al. *(60)* reported weight loss of about 16.5% of initial body weight (17 kg) at 1 yr and about 8% at 3 yr in patients on fenfluramine and phentermine hydrochloride (HCL). Dramatic reductions were noted in systolic and diastolic BP in hypertensive patients (28 mmHg and 17 mmHg, respectively) and in serum cholesterol and triglycerides (27 mg/dL and 79 mg/dL, respectively) in hyperlipidemic patients *(60)*. Hartley et al. *(61)* found a 17% weight loss on phentermine–fenfluramine. However, as noted previously, fenfluramine and dexfenfluramine were reported to cause cardiac valve lesions, and were removed from the market in 1997 *(19–22)*.

8.4. Fenfluramine–Fluoxetine Combination

Pedrinola et al. *(62)* carried out a randomized, double-blind trial of fluoxetine–fenfluramine vs fluoxetine–placebo in 33 women for 8 mo. The fluoxetine–fenfluramine group lost 13.4 kg vs 6.2 kg for fluoxetine–placebo. Unfortunately, a fenfluramine–placebo treatment group was not included.

8.5. Phentermine–Fluoxetine Combination

Dhurandhar et al. *(23)* reported in abstract form that the combination of fluoxetine (20–60 mg/d) and phentermine HCL (18.75–37.5 mg/d) produced significant weight losses that were similar to those produced by the combination of fenfluramine (20–60 mg/d) and phentermine HCL (18.75–37.5 mg/d). In two letters to the editor and a book for the lay audience, Anchors *(28–30)* reported that fluoxetine–phentermine in doses of 10 to 20 mg/d and 30 mg/d, respectively, produced long-term weight losses approaching 15% of initial body weight. Devlin et al. *(63)* treated overweight females with binge-eating disorder with fluoxetine–phentermine in an open-label trial and noted significant weight loss that persisted at 18 mo in subjects who continued medication.

8.6. Sibutramine and Orlistat

Wadden and colleagues *(53)* added orlistat to the regimen of 34 obese female subjects who had lost about 11% of initial body weight after 1 yr on sibutramine and lifestyle modification. There was no additional weight loss during a 16-wk extension on the drug combination.

The data presented here on combinations of drugs to treat obesity suggest that some combinations produce weight loss that is greater than can be attained with single drug treatment. The most effective was phentermine–fenfluramine, which is no longer available since fenfluramine was removed from the market. Phentermine–fluoxetine holds some promise, but the studies of this combination are not adequate and more work is needed before this can be accepted as a standard therapy. Anecdotal, nonpublished reports indicate that some private physicians use combinations including phentermine and topiramate, phentermine and zonisamide, fluoxetine and bupropion, fluoxetine and topiramate, and metformin with either phentermine or sibutramine. Until controlled studies are performed with these combinations, physicians should use them only with great caution and only after obtaining written, informed consent regarding the off-label status of such combinations.

9. PRACTICAL ASPECTS OF OBESITY PHARMACOTHERAPY

9.1. Side Effects and Adverse Events

Obesity medications, although generally quite safe, may be associated with side effects that require careful follow-up. Most side effects of the adrenergic agents and sibutramine occur early in the course of treatment and improve or resolve within the first month. Dry mouth is common and often persists, as does fatigue or asthenia. Sleep disturbances, such as insomnia, drowsiness, and vivid dreams tend to resolve. GI disturbances occur (e.g., diarrhea with serotonin agonists and constipation with adrenergic agonists). It is important for patients to drink large amounts of water to help constipation and because sweating is another side effect that may contribute to dehydration. Because patients may not be hungry, they also may neglect to drink adequate fluids.

Sibutramine is associated with slight pulse rate increases and BP increases in normotensive subjects, but most hypertensive subjects have reductions in BP *(31,32,52)*. A small percentage of patients report a paradoxical increase in hunger with sibutramine.

Severe side effects including abnormalities of cardiac valves and primary pulmonary hypertension occurred with fenfluramine and dexfenfluramine *(19–22,70–73)*, but there is no evidence to suggest that adrenergic agents or sibutramine produce either of these.

Because orlistat reduces fat absorption, it is associated with GI complaints of loose stools, diarrhea, and in a small percentage of patients, incontinence *(42–49)*. The GI complaints are self-limited and may be easily controlled by stopping the drug or reducing the amount of fat in the diet. Most physicians and patients consider the increased GI symptoms a good behavioral stimulus to control dietary fat intake. Rarely are the GI symptoms sufficiently severe to require discontinuing the medication.

9.2. Medication Regimens and Administration

There are few data to guide physicians as to the optimal medication regimen for a given patient. It is very clear that different people respond differently to the combination of obesity drugs, diet, and exercise. It also is clear that dosage sensitivity of drugs varies widely. In their study on the combination of diet, exercise, phentermine, and fenfluramine, Weintraub et al. *(58,59)* showed that most subjects lost weight with low doses of phentermine and fenfluramine. In subjects who did not lose well initially, increasing the dosage to full levels did not cause additional weight loss. A practical philosophy for use of obesity drugs is summarized in Table 4 (*see also* Chapter 16). Because obesity pharmacotherapies may have adverse effects, it is important to use them only when indicated and to use the lowest dose that will give maximum weight loss with tolerable side effects. By starting at a low dose, some of the side effects may be avoided. Most patients will need more than one medication for maximal weight loss, but it may be reasonable to start with only one medication to determine whether the patient is highly sensitive and will do well with only one medication. Additional medications would be added as necessary. If an increase in dosage does not cause additional weight loss, the dosage should be reduced.

Table 4
Philosophy for Use of Obesity Pharmacotherapy

1. Start at a low to very low dose.
2. Increase the dosage when a plateau is reached.
3. Reduce the dose to previous level if an increase does not cause more weight loss.
4. Discontinue if a drug does not appear effective.
5. Use the lowest maintenance dose possible.
6. Add additional drugs as needed.
7. Use clinical judgment to determine if side effects require cessation.

If a new medication does not contribute to reducing weight or complications, it should be discontinued. The physician must use clinical judgment to determine whether a given patient should discontinue one medication or all pharmacotherapy. Often patients are reluctant to discontinue medication, even in the face of significant side effects, because the pharmacotherapy is effective and weight regain is highly likely with cessation of pharmacotherapy. Physicians need to inquire about side effects and unilaterally intervene if the necessity arises.

10. CONCLUSION

Obesity is a complex syndrome that requires complex treatment. Obesity rarely may be treated with only one form of therapy. All patients need the underlying basic treatments of diet, exercise, and behavior modification for a healthy lifestyle. Obesity drugs may make it much easier for patients to follow such lifestyle modifications. Single drug therapy or low-dose combination drug therapy has been very helpful in producing sustained weight loss, but if the drugs are effective, it is likely that they will be needed life long. Cessation of treatment almost invariably results in weight regain. Although generally safe, there may be significant side effects with obesity drugs, so ineffective agents should be discontinued. Almost never is there an indication for temporary treatment or treatment of non-obese patients with obesity drugs. Long-term, careful follow-up is needed, and because obesity treatment requires a great deal of patient education, it is best done with a team of a physician and at least one allied health professional (*see* Chapter 22). Appropriate team members may include a dietitian, nurse, exercise physiologist, psychologist, social worker, or other educator. The optimal regimen for each patient will differ, and until additional research is done, choosing a regimen is a matter of trial and error.

REFERENCES

1. Friedman JM. A war on obesity, not the obese. Science 2003; 299:856–858.
2. Bray GA. Risks of obesity. Prim Care 2003; 30:281–299, v–vi.
3. Andersen T, Stokholm KH, Backer OG, Quaade F. Long-term (5-year) results after either horizontal gastroplasty or very-low calorie diet for morbid obesity. Int J Obesity 1988; 12:277–284.
4. Wadden TA, Sternberg JA, Letizia KA, Stunkard AJ, Foster GD. Treatment of obesity by very low calorie diet, behavior therapy, and their combination: a five year perspective. Int J Obesity 1989; 13: 39–46.

5. Wilson GT. Behavioral treatment of obesity: thirty years and counting. Adv Behav Res Ther 1993; 16:31–75.
6. Perri MG. Improving maintenance of weight loss following treatment by diet and lifestyle modification. In: Wadden TA, VanItallie TB, eds. Treatment of the seriously obese patient. New York, NY: Guilford, 1992, pp. 456–477
7. Ayyad C, Andersen T. Long-term efficacy of dietary treatment of obesity: a systematic review of studies published between 1931 and 1999. Obes Rev 2000; 1:113–119.
8. Coleman DL. Obese and diabetes: two mutant genes causing diabetes-obesity in mice. Diabetologia 1979; 14:141–148.
9. Pi-Sunyer X.Guidelines for the approval and use of obesity drugs. Obes Res 1995; 3:473–478.
10. Clinical Guidelines on the Identification, Evaluation, and Treatment of Overweight and Obesity in Adults—The Evidence Report. Obes Res 1998;6:51S–209S.
11. WHO Consultation. Preventing and managing the global epidemic of obesity: report of a WHO Consultation on Obesity. Geneva, 3–5 June, 1997. Geneva, Switzerland: WHO/NUT/NCD98.1, 1998.
12. Kissebach AH, Vydelingum N, Murray R, et al. Relation of body fat distribution to metabolic complications of obesity. J Clin Endocrinol Metab 1982; 54:254–260.
13. Misra A. Revisions of cutoffs of body mass index to define overweight and obesity are needed for the Asian-ethnic groups. Int J Obes Relat Metab Disord 2003; 27:1294–1296.
14. Stevens J. Ethnic-specific revisions of body mass index cutoffs to define overweight and obesity in Asians are not warranted. Int J Obes Relat Metab Disord 2003; 27:1297–1299.
15. Valle-Jones JC, Brodie NH, O'Hara H, O'Hara J, McGhie RL. A comparative study of phentermine and diethylpropion in the treatment of obese patients in general practice. Pharmatherapeut 1983; 3: 300–304.
16. Scoville BA. Review of amphetamine-like drugs by the Food and Drug Administration. In: Bray GA, ed. Obesity in perspective. Fogarty International Center for Advanced Studies in the Health Sciences, Series on Preventive Medicine, Vol. II. Washington, DC: US Government Printing Office, 1976, pp. 441–443.
17. Silverstone T. Appetite suppressants: a review. Drugs 1992; 43:820–836.
18. Goldstein DJ, Potvin JH. Long-term weight loss: the effect of pharmacologic agents. Am J Clin Nutr 1994; 60:647–657.
19. Connolly HM, Crary JL, McGoon MD, et al. Valvular heart disease associated with fenfluramine–phentermine. N Engl J Med 1997; 337:581–588.
20. Gardin JM, Schumacher D, Constantine G, Davis KD, Leung C, Reid CL. Valvular abnormalities and cardiovascular status following exposure to dexfenfluramine or phentermine/fenfluramine. JAMA 2000; 283:1703–1709.
21. Weissman NJ. Appetite suppressants and valvular heart disease. Am J Med Sci 2001; 321:285–291.
22. Tellier P. Fenfluramines, idiopathic pulmonary primary hypertension and cardiac valve disorders: facts and artifacts. Ann Med Interne (Paris) 2001; 152:429–436.
23. Dhurandhar NV, Atkinson RL. Comparison of serotonin agonists in combination with phentermine for treatment of obesity. FASEB J 1996; 10:A561.
24. Goldstein DJ, Rampey AH Jr, Dornseif BE, Levine LR, Potvin JH, Fludzinski LA. Fluoxetine: a randomized clinical trial in the maintenance of weight loss. Obes Res 1993; 1:92–98.
25. Goldstein DJ, Rampey AH Jr, Roback PJ, et al. Efficacy and safety of long-term fluoxetine treatment of obesity–maximizing success. Obes Res 1995; 3:481S–490S.
26. Wadden TA, Bartlett SJ, Foster GD, et al. Sertraline and relapse prevention training following treatment by very low-calorie diet: a controlled clinical trial. Obes Res 1995; 3:549–557.
27. Ricca V, Mannucci E, Di Bernardo M, Rizzello SM, Cabras PL, Rotella CM. Sertraline enhances the effects of cognitive–behavioral treatment on weight reduction of obese patients. J Endocrinol Invest 1996; 19:727–733.
28. Griffen L, Anchors M. The "phen–pro" diet drug combination is not associated with valvular heart disease. Arch Intern Med 1998; 158:1278–1279.
29. Anchors M. Safer than phen–fen. Rocklin, CA: Prima Publishing, 1997.
30. Anchors M. Fluoxetine is a safer alternative to fenfluramine in the medical treatment of obesity. Arch Intern Med 1997; 157:1270.

31. Ryan DH, Kaiser P, Bray GA. Sibutramine: a novel new agent for obesity treatment. Obes Res 1995; 3:553S–559S.
32. Heal DJ, Aspley S, Prow MR, Jackson HC, Martin KF, Cheetham SC. Sibutramine: a novel anti-obesity drug. A review of the pharmacological evidence to differentiate it from D-amphetamine and D-fenfluramine. Int J Obes 1998; 22:S18–28.
33. Daly PA, Krieger DR, Dulloo AG, Young JB, Landsberg L. Ephedrine, caffeine and aspirin: safety and efficacy for treatment of human obesity. Int J Obes 1993; 17:S73–78.
34. Toubro S, Astrup AV, Breum L, Quaade F. Safety and efficacy of long-term treatment with ephedrine, caffeine, and an ephedrine/caffeine mixture. Int J Obes 1993; 17:S69–S72.
35. Dulloo AG. Ephedrine, xanthines and prostaglandin-inhibitors: actions and interactions in the stimulation of thermogenesis. Int J Obes 1993; 17:S35–S40.
36. Arner P. Adenosine, prostaglandins and phosphodiesterase as targeted for obesity pharmacotherapy. Int J Obes 1993; 17(Suppl 1):S57–S59.
37. Boozer CN, Nasser JA, Heymsfield SB, Wang V, Chen G, Solomon JL. An herbal supplement containing Ma Huang–Guarana for weight loss: a randomized, double-blind trial. Int J Obes Relat Metab Disord 2001;25:316–324.
38. Boozer CN, Daly PA, Homel P, et al. Herbal ephedra/caffeine for weight loss: a 6-month randomized safety and efficacy trial. Int J Obes Relat Metab Disord 2002; 26:593–604.
39. Anderson JW, Greenway FL, Fujioka K, Gadde KM, McKenney J, O'Neil PM. Bupropion SR enhances weight loss: a 48-week double-blind, placebo- controlled trial. Obes Res 2002; 10:633–641.
40. Bray GA, Hollander P, Klein S, Kushner R, Levy B, Fitchet M, Perry BH. A 6-month randomized, placebo-controlled, dose-ranging trial of topiramate for weight loss in obesity. Obes Res 2003; 11: 722–733.
41. Gadde KM, Franciscy DM, Wagner HR 2nd, Krishnan KR. Zonisamide for weight loss in obese adults: a randomized controlled trial. JAMA 2003; 289:1820–1825.
42. Drent ML, van der Veen EA. First clinical studies with orlistat: a short review. Obes Res 1995; 3: 623S–625S.
43. James WP, Avenell A, Broom J, Whitehead J. A one year trial to assess the value of orlistat in the management of obesity. Int J Obesity 1997; 21:S24–S30.
44. Sjostrom L, Rissanen A, Andersen T, et al. Randomised placebo-controlled trial of orlistat for weight loss and prevention of weight regain in obese patients. European Multicentre Orlistat Study Group. Lancet 1998; 352:167–172.
45. Tonstad S, Pometta D, Erkelens DW, et al. The effect of the gastrointestinal lipase inhibitor, orlistat, on serum lipids and lipoproteins in patients with primary hyperlipidaemia. Eur J Clin Pharmacol 1994; 46:405–410.
46. Lucas CP, Boldrin MN, Reaven GM. Effect of orlistat added to diet (30% of calories from fat) on plasma lipids, glucose, and insulin in obese patients with hypercholesterolemia. Am J Cardiol 2003; 91:961–964.
47. Hollander PA, Elbein SC, Hirsch IB, et al. Role of orlistat in the treatment of obese patients with type 2 diabetes. A 1-year randomized double-blind study. Diab Care 1998; 21:1288–1294.
48. McDuffie JR, Calis KA, Uwaifo GI, et al. Three-month tolerability of orlistat in adolescents with obesity-related comorbid conditions. Obes Res 2002; 10:642–650.
49. Berger M. Pharmacological treatment of obesity: digestion and absorption inhibitors-clinical perspective. Am J Clin Nutr 1992; 55:318S–319S.
50. Munro JF, MacCuish AC, Wilson EM, Duncan LPJ. Comparison of continuous and intermittent anorectic therapy in obesity. Br Med J 1968; 1:352–354.
51. Steel JM, Munro JF, Duncan LJ. A comparative trial of different regimens of fenfluramine and phentermine in obesity. Practitioner 1973; 211:232–236.
52. James WP, Astrup A, Finer N, et al. Effect of sibutramine on weight maintenance after weight loss: a randomised trial. STORM Study Group. Sibutramine Trial of Obesity Reduction and Maintenance. Lancet 2000; 356:2119–2125.
53. Wadden TA, Berkowitz RI, Womble LG, Sarwer DB, Arnold ME, Steinberg CM. Effects of sibutramine plus orlistat in obese women following 1 year of treatment by sibutramine alone: a placebo-controlled trial. Obes Res 2000; 8:431–437.

54. Padwal R, Li S, Lau D. Long-term pharmacotherapy for obesity and overweight. Cochrane Database Syst Rev 2003; 4:CD004094.

55. Sayler ME, Goldstein DJ, Roback PJ, Atkinson RL. Evaluating success of weight loss programs, with an application to fluoxetine weight reduction clinical trial data. Int J Obes Relat Metab Disord 1994; 18:742–751.

56. Greenway FL. Clinical studies with phenylpropanolamine: a metaanalysis. Am J Clin Nutr 1992, 55: 203S–205S.

57. Greenway F, Herber D, Raum W, Herber D, Morales S. Double-blind, randomized, placebo controlled clinical trials with non-prescription medications for the treatment of obesity. Obes Res 1999; 7:370–378.

58. Weintraub M, Hasday JD, Mushlin AI, Lockwood DH. A double blind clinical trial in weight control: use of fenfluramine and phentermine alone and in combination. Arch Intern Med 1984; 144: 1143–1148.

59. Weintraub M. Long-term weight control: the National Heart, Lung, and Blood Institute funded multimodal intervention study. Clin Pharmacol Ther 1992; 51:581–646.

60. Atkinson RL, Blank RC, Schumacher D, Dhurandhar NV, Ritch DL. Long-term drug treatment of obesity in a private practice setting. Obesity Research 1997; 5:578–586.

61. Hartley GG, Nicol S, Halstenson C, Khan M, Pheley A. Phentermine, fenfluramine, diet, behavior modification, and exercise for treatment of obesity. Obes Res 1995; 3:340s.

62. Pedrinola F, Sztejnsznajd C, Lima N, Halpern A, Medeiros-Neto G. The addition of dexfenfluramine to fluoxetine in the treatment of obesity: a randomized clinical trial. Obes Res 1996; 4:549–554.

63. Devlin MJ, Goldfein JA, Carino JS, Wolk SL. Open treatment of overweight binge eaters with phentermine and fluoxetine as an adjunct to cognitive–behavioral therapy. Int J Eat Disord 2000; 28: 325–332.

64. Molnar D, Torok K, Erhardt E, Jeges S. Safety and efficacy of treatment with an ephedrine/caffeine mixture. The first double-blind placebo-controlled pilot study in adolescents. Int J Obes Relat Metab Disord 2000; 24:1573–1578.

65. Kalman D, Incledon T, Gaunaurd I, Schwartz H, Krieger D. An acute clinical trial evaluating the cardiovascular effects of an herbal ephedra–caffeine weight loss product in healthy overweight adults. Int J Obes Relat Metab Disord 2002; 26:1363–1366.

66. Paul Shekelle, Hardy M, Morton SC, et al. Ephedra and Ephedrine for Weight Loss and Athletic Performance Enhancement: Clinical Efficacy and Side Effects. Rand Corporation, AHRQ Publication No. 03-E022, Contract No. 290-97-0001, Task Order No. 9, February 2003.

67. Greenway FL. The safety and efficacy of pharmaceutical and herbal caffeine and ephedrine use as a weight loss agent. Obes Rev 2001; 2:199–211.

68. Shekelle PG, Hardy ML, Morton SC, et al. Efficacy and safety of ephedra and ephedrine for weight loss and athletic performance: a meta-analysis. JAMA 2003; 289:1537–1545.

69. FDA Press Release. FDA Announces Plans to Prohibit Sales of Dietary Supplements Containing Ephedra. Website: (http://www.fda.gov/oc/initiatives/ephedra/december2003).

70. Brenot F, Herve P, Petitpretz P, Parent F, Duroux P, Simonneau G. Primary pulmonary hypertension and fenfluramine use. Br Heart J 1993; 70:537–541.

71. Abenhaim L, Moride Y, Brenot F, et al. Appetite-suppressant drugs and the risk of primary pulmonary hypertension. N Engl J Med 1996; 335:609–616.

72. Manson JE, Faich GA. Pharmacotherapy for obesity–do the benefits outweigh the risks? N Engl J Med 1996; 335:659–660.

73. Dhurandhar NV, Atkinson RL. Appetite-suppressant drugs and primary pulmonary hypertension. N Engl J Med 1997; 336:511.

74. Pi-Sunyer X. The NAASO position paper on approval and use of drugs to treat obesity. Obes Res 1995; 3:471–472.

18 Genetics and Potential Treatments of Obesity

José R. Fernández and David J. Goldstein

KEY POINTS

- The current "epidemic" of obesity is the result of increasing disruption between the balance of energy intake and energy expenditure related to the action and interaction of biological and nonbiological causes.
- Animal models are extremely useful in identifying the contributions of genes because they can be subjected to genetic manipulation.
- Studies with monozygotic and dizygotic twins have estimated that body mass index (BMI = kg/m^2) is about 70% heritable.
- Use of genetic tools has been beneficial in increasing our understanding of the neurohumoral controls of energy balance.
- Recent advances have begun uncovering many of the genetic–environment interactions that result in obesity.

1. INTRODUCTION

The incidence of obesity and other comorbidities in the US population has increased dramatically during the past two decades. According to the Center for Disease Control, the number of states in the United States that have obesity prevalence rates greater than 15% has increased from none in 1985 and 1990 to 25 states in 1995 and 49 states in 2000 (Fig. 1).

This increase in the prevalence of obesity is the result of increasing disruption between the balance of energy intake and energy expenditure related to the action and interaction of biological and nonbiological causes (1). The regulation of body weight and food intake is a highly complex and redundant homeostatic system set to ensure positive energy balance (2). Its main purpose, prevention of starvation, provides an evolutionary advantage under circumstances of uncertain food supply to assuage the effects of prolonged starvation (3). As a consequence, in an environment of plentiful food, many individuals gain excessive weight (4). Body weight is regulated by interactions of both peripheral and central nervous system mechanisms including drives for palatability and variety and neurohormonal stimulation of centers in the dorso-medial hypothalamus, arcuate nucleus, and nucleus tractus solitarius (5,6).

From: *The Management of Eating Disorders and Obesity, Second Edition*
Edited by: D. J. Goldstein © Humana Press Inc., Totowa, NJ

Table 1
Chapter Overview

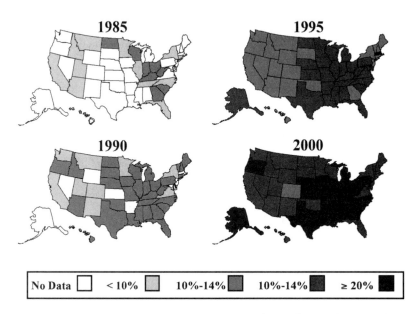

Fig. 1. Obesity trend in the adult population of the United States from 1985 to 2000 (From the US Center for Disease Control, Website: www.cdc.gov.)

To understand these aspects, scientists have investigated the role that genetic and environmental factors play in the etiology of this condition. Advances in molecular biology, the development of animal models for genetic manipulation, and the enterprise of the human genome project have greatly contributed to the identification of

DNA sequences that may play pivotal roles in the development of obesity. As of this time the scientific literature identifies approx 236 DNA sequences across the mouse and human genomes *(7)* with some type of influence on various measures related to excessive body fat.

The field of obesity genetics has grown dramatically during the past decade. This chapter, outlined in Table 1, describes general findings that support the influence of genes on obesity, as well as the results of genetic associations identified to influence aspects of energy intake, energy expenditure, and nutrient partitioning in both rodents and humans. The relationship of recent genetic findings to future obesity therapies is reviewed.

2. ANIMAL AND HUMAN MODELS OF OBESITY

The ultimate goal of obesity research is to develop strategies to prevent excessive fat accumulation after identifying those factors that cause this condition in individuals. As a complex trait, obesity results from the influence of genetic and environmental factors and their interaction. Both animal and human models have been used to investigate the role of genes in obesity-related research.

In mammals, genetic information occurs in pairs. Each individual receives one copy of genetic information, from the mother and the other copy from the father (a condition referred to as diploid). For any piece of DNA, the two copies, constituting a pair, can be identical (homozygous) or different (heterozygous). To investigate the function of DNA fragments, this material is separated or cut into pieces containing sequences of bases. Some of those pieces are not necessarily functional (i.e., do not have all the necessary information for the coding of a protein) and are often referred to as "markers." Some other pieces have been previously studied and the protein coded by the sequence is known. Those sequences are traditionally referred as "genes." Variants of markers and genes (called "alleles") occur in the population, creating genotypic variation, known as "polymorphism." These variants can be the result of differences in length, number of base repeats, or single nucleotide substitutions that alter the protein product by the substitution of one amino acid for another. Obesity-related gene-mapping techniques are used to identify the allele(s) that have an effect on different measurable traits (phenotypes) related to obesity.

2.1. Animal Studies

Animal models are extremely useful in identifying the contributions of genes because they can be subjected to genetic manipulation. Breeding experiments in which specific inbred strains are mated to produce a genetically controlled progeny have been utilized to explore environmental and genetic sources of variation. Genetic manipulation has allowed the addition or deletions of specific genes in animals of identical genetic background, generating meaningful insights into the understanding of the role of various genes and its products in mechanisms related to obesity. Also, the use of animal models permits control of energy intake, energy expenditure, and other environmental stressors that markedly reduce environmental variability. Many of the most important breakthroughs in the obesity field have resulted from experiments involving animal physiological manipulations. For example, the identification of the feeding-inhibiting hormone leptin and the leptin receptor occurred as a result of parabiosis experiments in which two rodents were surgically attached by suturing their skin together after making an incision through the skin of both rodents. This permitted transfer of small molecular-weight substances for one rodent to the other. If both animals lacked the ability to make leptin, they both became obese. If both animals lacked a receptor to recognize leptin, they both became fat. If the one that lacked the ability to produce leptin is joined to the one that lacked the receptor, the receptor-deficient animal overproduced the hormone, suppressing the appetite of the hormone-deficient animal. Consequently, adiposity was reduced in both animals.

2.2. Human Studies

Various human models are used to answer specific questions regarding obesity in the population. Twin, adoption, and family studies have supported the presence of genetic influences. Family pedigrees have also provided information regarding the linkage of genetic sequences with obesity phenotypes. Cross-sectional studies have been used for many genotype–phenotype associations, experiments regarding energy intake and expenditure, intervention strategies, and evaluation of racial differences in obesity.

2.2.1. EARLY EVIDENCE OF THE GENETIC BASIS OF OBESITY

Early evidence for a genetic component of obesity came from twin and adoption studies and was based on the determination of heritability. Heritability refers to the portion of the phenotypic variation that is owing to genetic variation. Studies with monozygotic and dizygotic twins have estimated that BMI is about 70% heritable (8–10). On the other hand, an estimate of 20 to 60% has been obtained from adoption studies considering biological/adoptive siblings (12).

2.2.2. MONOGENETIC MUTATIONS

The study of mutant alleles of individual genes has contributed to the understanding of certain molecular mechanisms of obesity, particularly those studies where the presence of mutant genes creates obesity phenotypes in animals and/or humans. Table 2 summarizes information about "traditional" rodent genetic models of obesity. Although the interaction of these monogenic forms is not completely understood, it has been proposed that in humans, the hypothalamic binding of leptin with leptin receptor stimulated a signaling cascade (see Fig. 2) in which neuropeptide Y (NPY) is inhibited, and α-melanocyte-stimulating hormone (α-MSH) is stimulated to act on the melanocortin-4-receptor (MC4R) (13). The hypothalamus also signals MSH (a precursor of pro-opiomelanocortin [POMC]) for a decrease in appetite and possibly signals for increased energy expenditure (14). Some of these monogenic mutants are described here.

2.2.2.1. LEPTIN

Parabiosis experiments in the 1950s (summarized in Subheading 2.1.) demonstrated that obesity on the mouse strain ob/ob was owing to a missing substance that regulated body weight. This substance was identified as leptin (15), the product of the ob gene, which was sequenced and cloned in the 1990s (16). Mice that are homozygous ob/ob do not produce leptin and develop obesity and type 2 diabetes (17). Leptin, one of several adipocytokines, is a protein produced primarily in adipocytes and antagonizes the action of NPY. Mutations in the leptin gene and the leptin receptor cause obesity, hyperphagia,

Table 2
Clinical Appearance (Phenotype), Mode of Inheritance, and Molecular Defects Owing to Monogenic Lesions (Genotypes) in Obese Rodents

Molecular defect	Species	Genotype	Mode of inheritance	Phenotype	Reference
Absent leptin activity	Mouse	ob	AR	Severe obesity; hypoglycemia	16
Mutation in leptin receptor	Mouse	db	AR	Severe obesity; hyperglycemia	78,79
	Rat	fa	AR	Severe obesity; hyperglycemia	
Leptin receptor nul	Koletsky ("corpulent") obese rat	fak	AR	Hyperphagia, obesity, hyperlipidemic	80
Mutation in carboxypep-tidase E which processes neuropeptides such as NPY		fat	AR	Gradual obesity; hyperglycemia	81
Overexpression of melano-cortin antagonist, agouti protein		Agouti	AD	Yellow coat; gradual obesity	82
Sulfonylurea receptor defect		Tubby	AR	Mild obesity; hyperinsulinemia	83–85
Obese Zucker	Rat		Rat	hyperphagic	
Absent CCK(A) receptors	OLETF Rat			Mild obesity, NIDDM	46,86
Overexpression of agouti protein (MC4R antagonist)	Obese viable yellow mouse	AgRP gene	Avy/a	Increased food intake, increased body weight	87
Attractin affects balance between agonist and antagonist on melanocytes	Mahogony mouse				88
	WDF			Higher body weight, higher fasting blood glucose, insulin, triglyceride	89
	Mouse	NZO	polygenic		
	Mouse	KK	polygenic		
Syndrome X	WOK W rat			Syndrome X: obesity, coronary heart disease, hypertension, dyslipidemia, impaired glucose tolerance	90

AR, autosomal recessive; AD, autosomal dominant; NZO, New Zealand Obese; OLETF, Otsuka Long Evans Tokushima Fatty; WDF, Obese diabetic Wistar rat.

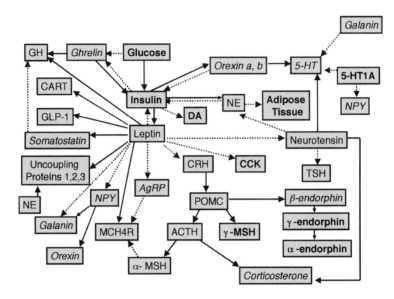

Fig. 2. Neuroendocrine pathways involved in energy balance. Solid lines indicate agonist effects. Broken lines indicate antagonist effects. Non-bolded *italic* font represents orexigenic hormones, non-bolded normal font represents anorexigenic hormones.

and reduced energy expenditure in both humans and rodents *(17–20)*. Despite expectations that individuals with higher plasma concentrations of leptin would have reduced food intake and increased energy expenditure, that is not the case with the vast majority of obese humans who have high plasma leptin concentration relatively proportionate to their fat mass *(13)*. Although exogenous administration of leptin induces dose-related mean weight loss, exogenous administration of leptin in non-leptin *nul* obese individuals produces modest mean weight reduction consistent with leptin insensitivity *(21)*. The primary effect of leptin may be to regulate food intake to prevent starvation rather than to limit body weight. Despite the limited effect of leptin in reducing obesity in humans, the characterization of leptin was pivotal in elucidating many of the neuroendocrine hormones that regulate energy intake and expenditure.

2.2.2.2. Melanocortin Receptor 4

The MC4R is expressed in the hypothalamus and has been associated with obesity *(24)*. Several investigations have provided support for the relationship between MC4R and obesity. Mice that are homozygous for a MC4R mutant allele have shown late-onset obesity with increased food intake. Chagnon and colleagues *(25)* reported an association between MC4R and percent body fat, and mutations on this receptor have been correlated with obesity *(28)*, suggesting that mutations in MC4R contribute to hyperphagia and hyperinsulinemia in obese individuals. Branson and colleagues *(29)* have also supported a role of MC4R in binge-eating disorders (*see* Chapter 11).

2.2.2.3. Neuropeptide Y

Studies have demonstrated that leptin binds the NPY receptor to block NPY activity, reducing energy intake and expenditure *(2,30)*. When NPY is administered to mice, an increase in food intake is observed *(31)*. However, NPY knockout mice have normal body weight with only slight responses to food deprivation *(2)*, suggesting a role of NPY in body-weight homeostasis. It has been proposed that the action of NPY is through the production of agouti-related peptide that promotes energy intake and decreases energy expenditure by antagonizing α-MSH through MC4R *(32)*.

2.2.2.4. PRO-OPIOMELANOCORTIN

POMC has also been associated with obesity, particularly because a loss of POMC function results in obesity in mice *(33)* and humans *(34)*. Quantitative trait loci (QTL) have been identified for obesity-related traits in chromosome 2, which encompasses the POMC gene *(35–38)*. An amino acid missense substitution in the POMC gene, R236G, produces an aberrant fusion protein that can interfere with signaling through MC4R *(39)*. The binding of this protein to the MC4R receptor acts as an agonist, reducing the normal antagonist effect of α-MSH, thereby leading to a predisposition to obesity through hyperphagia.

2.2.3. ASSOCIATION STUDIES

A great deal of information regarding genetics of obesity comes from studies that identify DNA sequences across the genome that are statistically associated with an obesity phenotype. Approaches for the identification of DNA markers influencing a phenotype include the QTL and candidate gene approach. In the QTL approach, various DNA sequences contribute a small portion to a measured quantitative trait. In the candidate-gene approach, an association is sought with known genes located across the genome. A great amount of different association results have been related to different aspects of obesity. For BMI alone, associations have been identified in regions of chromosomes 1–8, 10–13, 16, and 18–20 of the human genome. Chagnon et al. *(7)* provides a comprehensive review of genetic associations with various obesity-related phenotypes.

The identification of genotype–phenotype associations traditionally results from the statistical consideration of the phenotype of interest with only one genetic marker. Consequently, when many markers of interest are considered in a study, multiple statistical tests are required, and statistical adjustments are necessary to reduce false-positive rates. Although sophisticated approaches have been recently developed to understand the role of more than one gene on a complex trait *(40)*, very few studies count with the large sample size required for the exploration of interaction of multiple genes in a complex trait. To overcome this limitation, molecular geneticists have developed techniques such as the microarray technology, in which thousands of strands of DNA sequences of interest are arrayed on a physical surface, where they serve as a matching template to identify the presence or absence of DNA material on individuals in a sample. Although recent applications of the microarray technology include genotyping, this technique was originated to identify DNA expression, particularly the expression occurring in specific tissues as a consequence of an experimental condition or environmental influence. Microarrays provide unique and vital information about the role of multiple genes in a phenotype of interest, the effect of environmental factors in such, and the interaction of genes and environment in a phenotypic outcome.

The following sections summarize the most relevant associations supporting a role of genetics in energy intake, energy expenditure, and nutrient partitioning.

2.2.3.1. ENERGY INTAKE

The extent to which individuals consume food responds mainly to appetite, taste perceptions, and satiety (see Chapter 19). Examples of mediators of these effects include TAS1R genes, and cholecystokinin (CCK).

Inbred strains of mice have been used to identify genetic influences in sweet taste. In testing for the sensitivity to saccharin, researchers identified Sac, a locus on mouse chromosome 4 (41). Within 20,000 base pairs of Sac, the gene Tas1r3, expressed in taste receptor cells, was identified (42). The TAS1r3 product, T1r3 protein, is a member of the family of G protein-coupled receptors. The human TAS1R3 gene has been mapped. It is expressed in taste receptor cells and is believed to be a sweet-ligand taste receptor (43). Two other T1r genes, T1r1 and T1r2, which code for receptors, T1R1 and T1R2, may be responsible for variation in sweet taste within a single taste bud (44). Regarding food intake, evidence from twin studies have supported a heritability estimate of 23% of the variance in before-meal palatability ratings (45), suggesting that energy intake might be mediated by genes influencing predisposition to highly palatable foods. Experiments with rats have proposed a role of the peptide CKK in food satiety (46).

2.2.3.2. ENERGY EXPENDITURE

Recent investigations have proposed a genetic predisposition to physical activity (see Chapter 13). Genetic differences in muscle fiber types can be the predisposing factor for people to engage in physical activity (47). Lean individuals have more slow-twitch muscle fibers, obese individuals have a much greater proportion of fast-twitch muscle fibers (48,49).

Two genetic associations support a genetic role in physical activity. Angiotensin I-converting enzyme (ACE) has been proposed as a candidate gene for exercise-related phenotypes (50), based on the observation that individuals with one or two insertion alleles in the ACE gene had a greater duration in repetitive arm flexion time after exercise training (51). Another candidate gene is the uncoupling protein 3, a gene involved in the disposal of excess energy within the skeletal muscle (52,53), that is believed to influence resting metabolic rate in individuals (54).

2.2.3.3. NUTRIENT PARTITIONING

Nutrient partitioning is an important component to obesity. If the nutrients obtained from energy intake were distributed throughout the body in fat-free components, there would be no risk for obesity. In understanding this nutrient partitioning, investigators have paid attention into the identification of genes influencing fat accumulation and distribution.

Studies have suggested that adrenoreceptors have a role in fat accumulation. Dionne and colleagues (55) reported that individuals carrying one or two copies of the allele that causes a substitution of the amino acid Arg instead of Gly (Gly389Arg polymorphism) in the human β_1-adrenoceptor gene had greater body weight and BMI. They argued that this association attributable to greater fat mass as measured by dual x-ray absorptometry. Similarly, greater fat mass has been observed on individuals homozygotes for the Gln27Glu polymorphism of the β_2-adrenoceptor (56). In addition, a mutation on the Trp64Arg polymorphism of the β_3-adrenoceptor (57–60), has been associated with excess body fat and low energy expenditure.

Another interesting association regarding nutrient partitioning is peroxisome proliferator-activated receptor γ 2 (PPAR-γ2), a transcription factor that is believed to play a role in adipocyte differentiation. Ristow *(61)* reported that 4 out of 121 obese subjects had a missense mutation in the gene for PPAR-γ2, whereas none of 237 normal-weight subjects had this mutation, suggesting that this mutation may accelerate adipocyte differentiation resulting in an obese phenotype.

2.2.4. GENETICS IN THE POPULATION

One of the challenges of investigating genetic influences in obesity-related traits in humans is the identification and decomposition of genetic and environmental sources of variation. To control for environmental factors, many studies are designed to consider groups of individuals that live in specific locations, that share a particular cultural background, or that identify themselves as members of a specific group. The study of different populations is of epidemiological importance, particularly when considering that, in addition to the increasing prevalence of obesity in the general population, certain groups have higher levels of obesity and other related traits than others.

Research findings have demonstrated that genetic and non-genetic factors influence fat accumulation in different ways in different populations. For example, whereas Euro-American (EA) females of higher socioeconomic status (SES) tend to have lower prevalence of obesity, African-American (AA) females of higher SES have higher overweight prevalence *(62)*. In addition, AA females have higher prevalence of obesity even after controlling for SES *(63)*, lower levels of energy expenditure *(64–67)*, and higher bone mineral density *(68,69)* than EA females, suggesting the role of genetic influences underlying these differences.

Genetic associations within members of specific groups have been reported in the literature *(7)*. Most recently, the genetic components accounting for these differences have also been explored by considering the genetic ancestral background of admixed populations. This genetic admixture approach relies in the assumption that common cultural and social backgrounds provide environmental control and that by modeling the ancestral background of individuals in a population, insightful information can be obtained about the role of genes, environment, and their interaction in obesity. Recent investigations have used genetic admixture to account for racial differences in obesity-related traits *(70,71)*, reporting associations for BMI in chromosomes 1, 11, and 12 of the human genome.

3. POTENTIAL TREATMENTS

Prior to 1990, treatments for obesity were serendipitous or extensions of serendipity (*see* Chapter 16). At this time, however, many of the treatments being explored are based on recent discoveries related to the genetic basis of obesity and its role in understanding the neuroendocrine pathways involved in energy balance (Fig. 2). As noted earlier, additional explorations of interactions between environment and genetics using novel technology and statistical methodologies that permit screening of extremely large numbers of individuals, such as use of microarrays of DNA chips, are being used to identify genes that might be associated with low or high adiposity *(72,73)*. Unfortunately, these findings are nascent and unlikely to be translated to available pharmacotherapies during this decade.

3.1. Therapies Based on Genetic Discoveries

As noted in Subheading 2.2.2.1., human studies have indicated that leptin will be unsatisfactory as a therapy for obesity, except in rare leptin-deficient individuals. Based on newer understandings of the genetics of obesity, another cytokine, genetically engineered ciliary neurotrophic factor (CNF), has recently been studied in man and has demonstrated some efficacy. Genetically engineered CNF (*see* [Website: http://www.regeneron.com/investor/press_detail.asp?v_c_id=169] Regeneron, Tarrytown, NY, *[74]*), injected subcutaneously in obese patients, produced dose-related weight loss in shorter trials and last-observation-carried-forward mean weight loss of 2.8 kg vs 2.0 kg for placebo treatment at 1 yr. About 30% of patients developed antibodies to CNF, but the consequences and limitations related to this are not clear. Although these cytokines may not be commercially viable, they have demonstrated that our early understanding of the genetics of obesity can lead to further uncovering of the mechanisms involved and new opportunities.

Another compound, the canabinoid-1 antagonist SR141716, rimonabant, has been studied in obesity and genetic tools have been used to uncover its mode of action *(77)*. Rimonabant reduces food intake and body weight in rodents. One of its actions is to increase Acrp30 mRNA expression. Acrp30 is an adipose tissue-derived plasma protein that induces free fatty acid oxidation, decreases hyperglycemia and hyperinsulinemia, and reduces body weight *(75)*. A 16-wk human study has been completed and longer term studies are underway.

Another compound, L-796568, a selective β_3-agonist, increased energy expenditure 8% and lipolysis, as assessed by increased plasma glycerol and free fatty acid concentrations, after a single 1000-mg dose without apparent cardiovascular adverse effects *(76)*. It can be anticipated that genetic studies may help in designing newer selective β_3-agonists that could prove useful in man and avoid difficulties of earlier compounds.

Some treatments designed from genetic discoveries are showing some promise in animal studies. Although lead compounds may demonstrate the difficulties of translation from animals to man, it can be expected that genetic methods will uncover reasons for these limitations and help in the design of future refinements.

4. CONCLUSION

Use of genetic tools has been beneficial in increasing our understanding of the neurohumoral controls of energy balance. Recent advances have begun uncovering many of the genetic-environment interactions that result in obesity. Eventually, treatments designed from this information will be forthcoming, but are not expected in the near term.

Future experimental designs will need to include environmental measures that may influence the development of obesity in individuals. This will require use of large sample sizes and sophisticated statistical models. The technology is advancing so that such endeavors are becoming practical and cost efficient. The understanding and identification of genetic influences in obesity will impact on the development of public health initiatives to reduce and prevent obesity.

REFERENCES

1. Comuzzie AG, Allison DB. The search for human obesity genes. Science 1998; 280:1374–1377.
2. Wilding JP. Neuropeptides and appetite control. Diabet Med 2002; 19:619–627.

3. Kahn RC. The role of obesity in diabetes mellitus. Curr Opin Endocrinol Diabet 1996;3:1–2.
4. Kaplan LM. Genetics of obesity and body weight regulation. Curr Opin Endocrinol Diabet 2000; 7: 218–224.
5. Hillebrand JJ, de Wied D, Adan RA. Neuropeptides, food intake and body weight regulation: a hypo-thalamic focus. Peptides 2002; 23:2283–2306.
6. Sainsbury A, Cooney GJ, Herzog H. Hypothalamic regulation of energy homeostasis. Best Pract Res Clin Endocrinol Metab 2002; 16:623–637.
7. Chagnon YC, Rankinen T, Snyder EE, Weisnagel SJ, Perusse L, Bouchard C. The human obesity gene map: the 2002 update. Obes Res 2003; 11:313–367.
8. Segal NL, Allison DB. Twins and virtual twins: bases of relative body weight revisited. Int J Obes Relat Metab Disord 2002; 26:437–441.
9. Allison DB, Kaprio J, Korkeila M, Koskenvuo M, Neale MC, Hayakawa K. The heritability of body mass index among an international sample of monozygotic twins reared apart. Int J Obes Relat Metab Disord 1996; 20:501–506.
10. Barsh GS, Farooqi IS, O'Rahilly S. Genetics of body-weight regulation. Nature 2000; 404:644–651.
11. Maes HH, Neale MC, Eaves LJ. Genetic and environmental factors in relative body weight and human adiposity. Behav Genet 1997; 27:325–351.
12. Allison DB, Pietrobelli A, Faith MS, Fontaine KR, Gropp E, Fernández JR. Genetic Influences on Obesity 2003.
13. Jequier E. Leptin signaling, adiposity, and energy balance. Ann N Y Acad Sci 2002; 967:379–388.
14. Michaud JL. The developmental program of the hypothalamus and its disorders. Clin Genet 2001; 60: 255–263.
15. Halaas JL, Gajiwala KS, Maffei, M, et al. Weight-reducing effects of the plasma protein encoded by the obese gene. Science 1995; 269:543–546.
16. Zhang Y, Proenca R, Maffei M, Barone M, Leopold L, Friedman JM. Positional cloning of the mouse obese gene and its human homologue. Nature 1994;372:425–432.
17. Ingalls AM, Dickie MM, Snell GD. Obese, a new mutation in the house mouse. Obes Res 1996; 4:101.
18. Montague CT, Farooqi IS, Whitehead JP, et al. Congenital leptin deficiency is associated with severe early-onset obesity in humans. Nature 1997; 387:903–908.
19. Chua SC, Jr., Chung WK, Wu-Peng XS, et al. Phenotypes of mouse diabetes and rat fatty due to mutations in the OB (leptin) receptor. Science 1996; 271:994–996.
20. Clement K, Vaisse C, Lahlou N, et al. A mutation in the human leptin receptor gene causes obesity and pituitary dysfunction. Nature 1998; 392:398–401.
21. Heymsfield SB, Greenberg AS, Fujioka K, et al. Recombinant leptin for weight loss in obese and lean adults: a randomized, controlled, dose-escalation trial. JAMA 1999; 282:1568–1575.
22. Mergen M, Mergen H, Ozata M, Oner R, Oner C. A novel melanocortin 4 receptor (MC4R) gene mutation associated with morbid obesity. J Clin Endocrinol Metab 2001; 86:3448.
23. Fan W, Boston BA, Kesterson RA, Hruby VJ, Cone RD. Role of melanocortinergic neurons in feeding and the agouti obesity syndrome. Nature 1997; 385:165–168.
24. Huszar D, Lynch CA, Fairchild-Huntress V, et al. Targeted disruption of the melanocortin-4 receptor results in obesity in mice. Cell 1997; 88:131–141.
25. Chagnon YC, Chen WJ, Perusse L, et al. Linkage and association studies between the melanocortin receptors 4 and 5 genes and obesity-related phenotypes in the Quebec Family Study. Mol Med 1997; 3:663–673.
26. Farooqi IS, Yeo GS, Keogh JM, et al. Dominant and recessive inheritance of morbid obesity associated with melanocortin 4 receptor deficiency. J Clin Invest 2000; 106:271–279.
27. Dubern B, Clement K, Pelloux V, et al. Mutational analysis of melanocortin-4 receptor, agouti-related protein, and a-melanocyte-stimulating hormone genes in severely obese children. J Pediatr 2001; 139: 204–209.
28. Farooqi IS, Keogh JM, Yeo GS, Lank EJ, Cheetham T, O'Rahilly S. Clinical spectrum of obesity and mutations in the melanocortin 4 receptor gene. N Engl J Med 2003; 348:1085–1095.
29. Branson R, Potoczna N, Kral JG, Lentes KU, Hoehe MR, Horber FF. Binge eating as a major phenotype of melanocortin 4 receptor gene mutations. N Engl J Med 2003; 348:1096–1103.
30. Schwartz MW, Seeley RJ, Campfield LA, Burn P, Baskin DG. Identification of targets of leptin action in rat hypothalamus. J Clin Invest 1996; 98:1101–1106.

31. Stanley BG, Kyrkouli SE, Lampert S, Leibowitz SF. Neuropeptide Y chronically injected into the hypothalamus: a powerful neurochemical inducer of hyperphagia and obesity. Peptides 1986; 7:1189–1192.

32. Marsh DJ, Hollopeter G, Huszar D, et al. Response of melanocortin-4 receptor-deficient mice to anorectic and orexigenic peptides. Nat Genet 1999; 21:119–122.

33. Yaswen L, Diehl N, Brennan MB, Hochgeschwender U. Obesity in the mouse model of pro-opiomelanocortin deficiency responds to peripheral melanocortin. Nat Med 1999; 5:1066–1070.

34. Krude H, Biebermann H, Luck W, Horn R, Brabant G, Gruters A. Severe early-onset obesity, adrenal insufficiency and red hair pigmentation caused by POMC mutations in humans. Nat Genet 1998; 19: 155–157.

35. Comuzzie AG, Hixson JE, Almasy L, et al. A major quantitative trait locus determining serum leptin levels and fat mass is located on human chromosome 2. Nat Genet 1997; 15:273–276.

36. Hager J, Dina C, Francke S, et al. A genome-wide scan for human obesity genes reveals a major susceptibility locus on chromosome 10. Nat Genet 1998; 20:304–308.

37. Rotimi CN, Comuzzie AG, Lowe WL, Luke A, Blangero J, Cooper RS. The quantitative trait locus on chromosome 2 for serum leptin levels is confirmed in African-Americans. Diabetes 1999; 48:643–644.

38. Hixson JE, Almasy L, Cole S, et al. Normal variation in leptin levels in associated with polymorphisms in the proopiomelanocortin gene, POMC. J Clin Endocrinol Metab 1999; 84:3187–191.

39. Challis BG, Pritchard LE, Creemers JW, et al. A missense mutation disrupting a dibasic prohormone processing site in pro-opiomelanocortin (POMC) increases susceptibility to early-onset obesity through a novel molecular mechanism. Hum Mol Genet 2002; 11:1997–2004.

40. Fernandez JR, Tarantino LM, Hofer SM, Vogler GP, McClearn GE. Epistatic quantitative trait loci for alcohol preference in mice. Behav Genet 2000; 30:431–437.

41. Capeless CG, Whitney G. The genetic basis of preference for sweet substances among inbred strains of mice: preference ratio phenotypes and the alleles of the Sac and dpa loci. Chem Senses 1995; 20: 291–298.

42. Li X, Inoue M, Reed DR, et al. High-resolution genetic mapping of the saccharin preference locus (Sac) and the putative sweet taste receptor (T1R1) gene (Gpr70) to mouse distal chromosome 4. Mamm Genome 2001; 12:13–16.

43. Max M, Shanker YG, Huang L, et al. Tas1r3, encoding a new candidate taste receptor, is allelic to the sweet responsiveness locus Sac. Nat Genet 2001; 28:58–63.

44. Lewcock JW, Reed RR. Sweet successes. Neuron 2001; 31:515–517.

45. de Castro JM, Plunkett SS. How genes control real world intake: palatability—intake relationships. Nutr 2001; 17:266–268.

46. Moran TH. Cholecystokinin and satiety: current perspectives. Nutr 2000; 16:858–865.

47. Weinsier RL, Hunter GR, Heini AF, Goran MI, Sell SM. The etiology of obesity: relative contribution of metabolic factors, diet, and physical activity. Am J Med 1998; 105:145–150.

48. Howard BV, Bogardus C, Ravussin E, et al. Studies of the etiology of obesity in Pima Indians. Am J Clin Nutr 1991; 53:1577S–85S.

49. Wade AJ, Marbut MM, Round JM. Muscle fibre type and aetiology of obesity. Lancet 1990; 335:805–808.

50. Bray MS. Genomics, genes, and environmental interaction: the role of exercise. J Appl Physiol 2000; 88:788–792.

51. Montgomery HE, Marshall R, Hemingway H, et al. Human gene for physical performance. Nature 1998; 393:221–222.

52. Vidal-Puig A, Solanes G, Grujic D, Flier JS, Lowell BB. UCP3: an uncoupling protein homologue expressed preferentially and abundantly in skeletal muscle and brown adipose tissue. Biochem Biophys Res Commun 1997; 235:79–82.

53. Boss O, Samec S, Kuhne F, et al. Uncoupling protein-3 expression in rodent skeletal muscle is modulated by food intake but not by changes in environmental temperature. J Biol Chem 1998; 273:5–8.

54. Rolfe DF, Newman JM, Buckingham JA, Clark MG, Brand MD. Contribution of mitochondrial proton leak to respiration rate in working skeletal muscle and liver and to SMR. Am J Physiol 1999; 276:C692–C699.

55. Dionne IJ, Garant MJ, Nolan AA, et al. Association between obesity and a polymorphism in the B(1)-adrenoceptor gene (Gly389Arg ADRB1) in Caucasian women. Int J Obes Relat Metab Disord 2002; 26:633–639.

56. Large V, Hellstrom L, Reynisdottir S, et al. Human B-2 adrenoceptor gene polymorphisms are highly frequent in obesity and associate with altered adipocyte B-2 adrenoceptor function. J Clin Invest 1997; 100:3005–3013.

57. Widen E, Lehto M, Kanninen T, Walston J, Shuldiner AR, Groop LC. Association of a polymorphism in the B 3-adrenergic-receptor gene with features of the insulin resistance syndrome in Finns. N Engl J Med 1995; 333:348–351.

58. Garcia-Rubi E, Starling RD, Tchernof A, et al. Trp64Arg variant of the B3-adrenoceptor and insulin resistance in obese postmenopausal women. J Clin Endocrinol Metab 1998; 83:4002–4005.

59. Walston J, Silver K, Bogardus C, et al. Time of onset of non-insulin-dependent diabetes mellitus and genetic variation in the B 3-adrenergic-receptor gene. N Engl J Med 1995; 333:343–347.

60. Shuldiner AR, Silver K, Roth J, Walston J. Beta 3-adrenoceptor gene variant in obesity and insulin resistance. Lancet 1996; 348:1584–1585.

61. Ristow M, Muller-Wieland D, Pfeiffer A, Krone W, Kahn CR. Obesity associated with a mutation in a genetic regulator of adipocyte differentiation. N Engl J Med 1998; 339:953–959.

62. Gordon-Larsen P, Adair LS, Popkin BM. The relationship of ethnicity, socioeconomic factors, and overweight in US adolescents. Obes Res 2003;11:121–129.

63. Allison DB, Edlen-Nezin L, Clay-Williams G. Obesity among African American women: prevalence, consequences, causes, and developing research. Womens Health 1997; 3:243–274.

64. Gallagher D, Heymsfield SB, Heo M, Jebb SA, Murgatroyd PR, Sakamoto Y. Healthy percentage body fat ranges: an approach for developing guidelines based on body mass index. Am J Clin Nutr 2000; 72:694–701.

65. Nicklas BJ, Berman DM, Davis DC, Dobrovolny CL, Dennis KE. Racial differences in metabolic predictors of obesity among postmenopausal women. Obes Res 1999; 7:463–468.

66. Hunter GR, Weinsier RL, Darnell BE, Zuckerman PA, Goran MI. Racial differences in energy expenditure and aerobic fitness in premenopausal women. Am J Clin Nutr 2000; 71:500–506.

67. Lovejoy JC, Champagne CM, Smith SR, de Jonge L, Xie H. Ethnic differences in dietary intakes, physical activity, and energy expenditure in middle-aged, premenopausal women: the Healthy Transitions Study. Am J Clin Nutr 2001; 74:90–95.

68. Wright NM, Papadea N, Veldhuis JD, Bell NH. Growth hormone secretion and bone mineral density in prepubertal black and white boys. Calcif Tissue Int 2002; 70:146–152.

69. Wagner DR, Heyward VH. Measures of body composition in blacks and whites: a comparative review. Am J Clin Nutr 2000; 71:1392–1402.

70. Williams RC, Long JC, Hanson RL, Sievers ML, Knowler WC. Individual estimates of European genetic admixture associated with lower body-mass index, plasma glucose, and prevalence of type 2 diabetes in Pima Indians. Am J Hum Genet 2000; 66:527–538.

71. Fernandez JR, Shriver MD, Beasley TM, et al. Association of African Genetic Admixture with Resting Metabolic Rate and Obesity Among Women. Obes Res 2003; 11:904–911.

72. Schadt EE, Monks SA, Drake TA, et al. Genetics of gene expression surveyed in maize, mouse and man. Nature 2003; 422:297–302.

73. Glazier AM, Nadeau JH, Aitman TJ. Finding genes that underlie complex traits. Science 2002; 298: 2345–2349.

74. Ettinger MP, Littlejohn TW, Schwartz SL, et al. Recombinant variant of ciliary neurotrophic factor for weight loss in obese adults: a randomized, dose-ranging study. JAMA 2003; 289:1826–1832.

75. Bensaid M, Gary-Bobo M, Esclangon A, et al. The cannabinoid CB1 receptor antagonist SR141716 increases Acrp30 mRNA expression in adipose tissue of obese fa/fa rats and in cultured adipocyte cells. Mol Pharmacol 2003; 63:908–914.

76. van Baak MA, Hul GB, Toubro S, et al. Acute effect of L-796568, a novel B 3-adrenergic receptor agonist, on energy expenditure in obese men. Clin Pharmacol Ther 2002; 71:272–279.

77. Fernández JR, Allison DB. Rimonabant Sanofi-Synthelabo. Curr Opin Investig Drugs 2004; 5: 430–435.

78. Chen H, Charlat O, Tartaglia LA, et al. Evidence that the diabetes gene encodes the leptin receptor: identification of a mutation in the leptin receptor gene in db/db mice. Cell 1996; 84:491–495.

79. Tartaglia LA, Dembski M, Weng X, et al. Identification and expression cloning of a leptin receptor, OB-R. Cell 1995; 83:1263–1271.

80. Kahle EB, Butz KG, Chua SC, et al. The rat corpulent (cp) mutation maps to the same interval on (Pgm1-Glut1) rat chromosome 5 as the fatty (fa) mutation. Obes Res 1997; 5(2):142–145.

81. Naggert JK, Fricker LD, Varlamov O, et al. Hyperproinsulinaemia in obese fat/fat mice associated with a carboxypeptidase E mutation which reduces enzyme activity. Nat Genet 1995; 10:135–142.

82. Wilson BD, Ollmann MM, Kang L, Stoffel M, Bell GI, Barsh GS. Structure and function of ASP, the human homolog of the mouse agouti gene. Hum Mol Genet 1995; 4:223–230.

83. Kapeller R, Moriarty A, Strauss A, et al. Tyrosine phosphorylation of tub and its association with Src homology 2 domain-containing proteins implicate tub in intracellular signaling by insulin. J Biol Chem 1999; 274:24,980–24,986.

84. Kleyn PW, Fan W, Kovats SG, et al. Identification and characterization of the mouse obesity gene tubby: a member of a novel gene family. Cell 1996; 85:281–290.

85. Noben-Trauth K, Naggert JK, North MA, Nishina PM. A candidate gene for the mouse mutation tubby. Nature 1996; 380:534–538.

86. Moralejo DH, Wei S, Wei K, et al. Identification of quantitative trait loci for non-insulin-dependent diabetes mellitus that interact with body weight in the Otsuka Long-Evans Tokushima Fatty rat. Proc Assoc Am Physicians 1998; 110(6):545–558.

87. Adan RA, Vink T. Drug target discovery by pharmacogenetics: mutations in the melanocortin system and eating disorders. Eur Neuropsychopharmacol 2001; 11(6):483–490.

88. Jackson IJ. The mahogany mouse mutation: further links between pigmentation, obesity and the immune system. Trends Genet 1999; 15(11):429–431.

89. Carrascosa JM, Molero JC, Fermin Y, Martinez C, Andres A, Satrustegui J. Effects of chronic treatment with acarbose on glucose and lipid metabolism in obese diabetic Wistar rats. Diabetes Obes Metab 2001; 3(4):240–248.

90. Kovacs P, van den Brandt J, Kloting I, et al. Genetic dissection of the syndrome X in the rat. Biochem Biophys Res Commun 2000; 269(3):660–665.

19 The Role of Hunger and Satiety in Weight Management

Michael Penn and David J. Goldstein

KEY POINTS

- Studies of specific dietary constituents and preloads fail to identify any particular food type that results in decreased intake.
- Higher fiber foods and large quantities of noncaloric beverages might serve to reduce overall intake.
- Low-caloric density foods may help to reduce overall intake.
- Effective dietary interventions need to include ways to control emotional eating and novelty eating.
- Low-carbohydrate diets are easy to follow for the short term because it is easier to avoid certain foods than to limit the amounts. It may be particularly effective in the snacking patient because it markedly reduces snacking. This diet tends to be monotonous and eventually the patients break it. Furthermore, because new low-carbohydrate foods are now commercially available, it is more likely that snacking is again possible reducing the initial weight-loss effect.

1. INTRODUCTION

Hunger is a craving, desire, or urgent need for food, an uneasy sensation occasioned normally by the lack of food and resulting directly from stimulation of the sensory nerves of the stomach by the contraction and churning movement of the empty stomach, metabolic, nutrient, environmental (orosensory and social), and psychological factors. Hunger leads to initiation of eating. Eating activates inhibitory signals producing satiety. Satiety is the quality or state of being fed or gratified to or beyond capacity mediated in the short term by mechanical factors related to swallowing and gastric distention, chemical factors related to taste and smell, and psychological factors (sensory-specific satiety) and in the long term by chemoreception of nutrients and gastrointestinal (GI) peptides and neuroendocrine and neuronal factors and is a major motivation for terminating eating (1).

Numerous investigations have attempted to identify mechanical factors, nutrients or food components, or neuroendocrine hormones that could modify hunger or satiety. Many of these studies involve giving defined meals (preload) after an overnight fast,

From: *The Management of Eating Disorders and Obesity, Second Edition*
Edited by: D. J. Goldstein © Humana Press Inc., Totowa, NJ

Table 1
Chapter Overview

assessing the satiety that results at periodic intervals, and assessing food choices and overall calories eaten in a subsequent "cafeteria"(or buffet)-type meal from which the patient can select. The cafeteria diet selection consists of a variety of premeasured items of various foods such that the calories from protein, fat, and carbohydrate can readily be assessed and the patients can choose which foods and how much they choose to eat. As these studies have become more sophisticated, "shakes" (liquid test meals) of defined composition and taste are given to blind the patients as to the composition of their preload. Sometimes, the preload is given by gavage to avoid orosensory effects, such as smell, taste, consistency, and son on, that might influence the patient. Additionally, the time that the patient takes to eat the meal is also assessed.

Limitations of most of these studies is that they test acute effects and there might be longer term effects of dietary manipulations that might either enhance or obscure short-term effects. There is also the potential for bias. For example, a brownie and a scoop of macaroni and cheese may have identical protein, fat, and carbohydrate composition and total calories, but the attraction for the patient might be entirely different, particularly if the macaroni does not look appealing. Thus, the selection of items in the "cafeteria" might influence the result.

In this chapter, we describe the factors influencing hunger and appetite, relate this to the low-carbohydrate diet developed by Atkins *(2)*, and hypothesize about the role of hunger and satiety in weight reduction (Table 1).

2. MECHANICAL AND LOCAL FACTORS

2.1. Gastric Capacity

One hypothesis about obese patients was that they had a larger gastric capacity or more rapid gastric emptying leading them to eat more to achieve satiety. As a consequence, surgical techniques were developed to reduce gastric capacity. Studies have not confirmed these ideas, suggesting that intrinsic differences in gastric capacity do not cause obesity; however, there were unexpected findings regarding the production of gastric-derived ghrehlin *(3)*.

Studies of gastric size and time for gastric emptying do not demonstrate an intrinsic difference between obese and lean individuals. Geliebter and Hashim *(4)* evaluated gastric capacity in 10 bulimics, 6 obese binge eaters, and 5 obese non-binge eaters, and 10 non-obese non-bulimic controls. The bulimics and the binge-eating obese subjects had larger gastric capacity than the controls and non-binge-eating obese subjects who did not differ from each other. They concluded that binge eating influenced the size of the stomach and that obesity did not. Similarly, Kim et al. *(5)* evaluated gastric volume and satiety while fasting and postprandial by photon emission computed tomography (PET). No differences were noted between the 13 obese or 19 non-obese subjects for either fasting or postprandial gastric volumes or the ratio of the volumes, the amount ingested to maximum tolerability or satiety. Chilkoiro et al. *(6)* evaluated gastric emptying in normal and obese children by ultrasound. They noted a significant correlation between fasted gastric antral area 3.9 cm^2 for the very obese and 3.6 cm^2 for the obese, and 3.5 cm^2 in normal children and body mass index (BMI). No difference was noted in gastric emptying time.

Nevertheless, within an individual, it seems that after surgery, gastric size does influence subsequent weight. Forsell *(7)* demonstrated a correlation between the size of the gastric pouch and the amount of weight lost after adjustable gastric banding. It may be that functional alteration in gastric size within an individual may have an effect on weight, however, this has not been demonstrated. Recent evidence suggests that decreased stomach-derived ghrelin plays an additional role in the weight loss associated with gastric bypass surgery *(3)* (*see* Subheading 5.).

2.2. Fiber and Volume

Fiber has been hypothesized to increase satiety and to reduce hunger by filling the stomach with noncaloric material and by slowing gastric emptying. The data from studies of these hypotheses is mixed, suggesting that fiber has little significant effect on hunger or satiety. Many of the studies evaluating the effect of fiber are summarized here.

Kromhout et al. *(8)* evaluated the relationship of various factors on body fat. They noted that on a population level, the job-related physical activity and dietary fiber intake predicted the level of body fat as indicated by subscapular skinfold thickness.

Howarth et al. *(9)* reviewed the relationship of dietary fiber and weight reduction. The specific results varied depending on whether the diet was restricted and whether the subject was overweight or lean; however, overall, fiber intake reduces hunger, increases satiety, and reduces energy intake. Overweight individuals demonstrate a greater effect than lean individuals. The effect is independent of type of fiber. The absolute weight effect of adding fiber to diet is relatively modest, a weight loss of about 2 kg. Some of the studies evaluating the effect of supplementing diet with fiber are summarized here.

Rolls and Roe *(10)* administered treatments (no gastric tube inserted and no preload, gastric tube inserted but preload covertly diverted, 200 kcal in 200 mL, 200 kcal in 400 mL, 400 kcal in 400 mL) as preloads administered over 15 min intragastrically beginning 30 min prior to lunch to 25 lean and 29 obese women on 5 separate days.

They noted that increased volume, but not increased calories, reduced subsequent energy intake when orosensory cues are bypassed.

Kaplan and Greenwood *(11)* examined the effects of equal caloric amounts of high-carbohydrate (potato and glucose drink) and low-carbohydrate (barley) with placebo on hunger, satiety, and subsequent lunch intake in 10 men and 10 women, ages 60 to 82, on four mornings, after fasting overnight. Potatoes produced greater satiety than barley, which produced more satiety than glucose and placebo. There was less hunger with potatoes than with barley, glucose, or placebo. The subjects reported greater fullness with potatoes and barley than with glucose and placebo. The subsequent lunch intake was decreased more for potatoes and barley than for glucose and placebo. The differences in plasma glucose among the groups did not predict these results. Thus, it suggests that greater bulk, as a result of increased fiber, results in greater satiety.

Landstrom et al. *(12)* evaluated the wakefulness and satiety effects of food alternatives with differing energy content and bulk (100, 500, and 1000 kcal and low bulk, 100 kcal in 10 food- and sleep-deprived subjects. There were no differences in wakefulness, but subjects were more satiated after higher energy and higher bulk.

Birketvedt et al. *(13)* evaluated the effect of fiber on weight control in 53 moderately obese women who were on a daily 1200 kcal diet for 24 wk. The patients were randomly allocated to fiber, initially 6 g/d, then 4 g/d maintenance, supplementation, or placebo. The fiber supplementation resulted in 8 kg vs 5.8 kg weight loss.

Mattes and Rothacker *(14)* attempted to evaluate the effects of viscosity using 220 kcal shakes that were matched on weight, volume (325 mL), temperature, energy, macronutrient content, and energy density in 84 adults in a crossover design by assessing reduction in hunger, size and time to first meal as well as 24-hr intake. Reductions in hunger were observed with a thicker shake, no significant differences occurred in the size or time to the first meal or 24-hr intake.

Pasman et al. *(15)* evaluated the effect of a 1-wk fiber supplementation vs no supplementation in obese women who had lost weight. In 17 subjects who were not on a restricted diet, mean energy intake decreased significantly after fiber supplementation without changing hunger or satiety. In 14 patients with fixed energy intake (6 MJ/d or 4 MJ/d) hunger scores were less with fiber supplementation with the more restricted diet but not different with the 6 MJ diet.

Pasman et al. *(16)* evaluated the effects of supplementation with 20 g/d of fiber vs placebo for 14 mo after an energy-restricted diet (very low-calorie diet) in 31 females. The fiber group ($n = 20$) who were at least 80% compliant and the control group ($n = 11$) showed the same weight regain, whereas the noncompliant fiber-supplemented group regained more weight. Thus, there did not seem to be an effect of dietary fiber intake on longer term weight maintenance. Rather, this suggests that compliance to the fiber diet may be a marker for better weight maintenance.

Burton-Freeman et al. *(17)* evaluated the effect of fiber on glucose, insulin, and cholecystokinin (CCK) and the subjects assessed their hunger, desire to eat, fullness, and prospective consumption via visual analog scales. Fasted males ($n = 7$) and females ($n = 8$) completed a crossover study evaluating the effects of isoenergetic low-fat/low-fiber, high-fat/low-fiber and low-fat/high-fiber breakfasts. The high-fiber/low-fat diet suppressed peak glucose and insulin concentrations compared with the low-fiber/low-fat breakfasts. In women, higher fat and higher fiber meals resulted in greater feelings of satiety and higher plasma concentrations of CCK. In males, the levels of CCK did not correlate to changes in the amount of fat or fiber in the meals. In females, the high-fiber/high-fat diets produced higher CCK concentrations than the low-fat/low-fiber diet. This study suggests that fiber induces CCK, similar to fat and thus increases satiety (*see* Subheading 3.3.). The apparent difference in gender in this study may not be artifact.

Del Parigi et al. *(18)* evaluated regional cerebral blood flow using PET to evaluate gender differences in human neuroanatomical response to hunger and satiation. After fasting and thus during hunger, males had greater activation of the frontotemporal and paralimbic areas. After satiation, women had greater activation in occipital and parietal sensory association areas and dorsolateral prefrontal cortex. Men had greater activation of ventro-medial prefrontal cortex. They suggested that this reflected possible gender differences in cognitive and emotional processing of hunger and satiation.

2.3. Gastric Acid, Use of Histamine-2 Receptor (H$_2$) Antagonists

It was also proposed that the production of gastric acid was one of the cures for hunger and that inhibition of the effects of gastric acid would reduce hunger, and possibly increase satiety. One strategy for blocking the effects of gastric acid was the use of H$_2$ antagonists.

Stoa-Birketvedt *(19)* evaluated the weight loss effect of cimetidine (200 mg tid before meals) vs placebo in 60 overweight to obese patients who were taking a 5 MJ/d diet supplemented with 9 g/d fiber over 8 wk. The cimetidine-treated patients lost 7.3 kg more than placebo-treated patients. In a similar study, Rasmussen et al. *(20)* evaluated the weight loss effect of cimetidine suspension 200 mg/10 mL vs placebo in 60 moderately obese patients taking a 5 MJ/d diet supplemented with 9 g/d of dietary fiber. There was no difference between the groups after 8 wk. Stoa-Birketvedt et al. *(21)* used a higher dose of cimetidine (400 mg tid) over 12 wk in 43 overweight patients in a parallel, randomized, double-blind, placebo-controlled study. The cimetidine-treated patients lost 5 kg vs 1.3 kg for placebo and had significant reductions in appetite and body fat. Birketve et al. *(22)* subsequently evaluated long-term use of cimetidine for 8 wk twice a year with a dietary restriction and exercise vs nonintervention for 42 wk. The cimetidine and behavior-modification group had a 15.1% weight loss compared with a weight gain of 8.6% in the nonintervention group. Overall, cimetidine appears to improve compliance with a weight-reduction diet when given at a sufficient dose. Whether this is related to blockade of the effects of gastric acid is not known. In addition, the ideal timing of use of cimetidine is not known.

3. NUTRIENT EFFECTS ON SUBSEQUENT INTAKE

Some researchers hypothesized that eating certain foods prior to a meal would induce changes in later appetite such that the subsequent meal would be smaller than normal and that the total caloric intake would be reduced. The results of some studies testing this hypothesis are summarized here.

3.1. Carbohydrate

Preloads of sucrose, fructose, and citrate have been evaluated to determine whether they would reduce the caloric intake of the subsequent meal. Although differences in the amounts ingested in a subsequent meal occur depending on the preload, the overall caloric intake was not reduced compared with a placebo preload. Many of the studies are summarized here.

Woodend and Anderson *(23)* noted that a preload of sucrose at 0, 418, 836, and 1254 kJ in the same volume suppressed average appetite more than nonsucrose control. The sucrose preload dose dependently decreases food intake of the subsequent meal by nearly the amount of calories of the sucrose given. Several studies investigated the effects of glycemic carbohydrates on subsequent satiety or food intake. In evaluating the effects of sugar-containing beverages *(24)*, the highest glycemic response was greatest with glucose followed by polycose, sucrose, amylopectin, a fructose–glucose mixture, and amylose, respectively. This was confirmed by another study *(25)*. High-glycemic carbohydrate reduced satiety at about 1 hr and lower-glycemic carbohydrates reduced satiety at 2 and 3 hr. This effect was unrelated to plasma glucose. Food intake at 1 hr was inversely related to that of plasma glucose concentration.

Van de Ven et al. *(26)* evaluated the effect of four different 250 mL preloads (2% fructose with 2% fiber, 10% fructose with 2% fiber, 10% fructose with 4% fiber, artificial sweeteners) on lunch ingestion 60 min later in 24 healthy women. There was no significant overall effect in that any reduction in lunch eaten was less than the caloric intake of the preload and there was no effect on overall 24-hr ingestion.

Kovacs and Westerterp-Plantenga et al. *(27)* treated 14 normal to moderately obese women with placebo, hydoxycitric acid (HCA) and HCA with medium-chain triglyceride in a crossover design to assess effects on satiety and energy intake. After 2 wk of each treatment, all treatments were associated with weight loss, but there was no difference in satiety or reduced 24-hr caloric intake among treatments.

Westerterp-Plantenga and Kovacs *(28)* administered 300 mg HCA in tomato juice vs plain tomato juice three times daily for 2 wk to 12 overweight males and 12 overweight females to evaluate its effects on satiety and energy intake. The 24-hr food intake decreased by 15 to 30% compared with placebo, despite no significant change in appetite profile, dietary restraint, taste perception, or hedonics.

3.2. Protein

Protein has been proposed as being more satiating than carbohydrate and this forms a part of the argument supporting the Atkins low-carbohydrate diet (*see* Subheading 6.). Several studies have tried to address this question, but most have limitations that make an absolute conclusion elusive. It has also been hypothesized that proteins are digested into peptides that trigger satiety signals from the gut via CCK-A and opioid receptors *(29)* contributing to satiating properties of protein intake.

Barkeling et al. *(30)* reviewed studies that used meals with various proportions of protein and carbohydrate and evaluated post-meal fullness. They found mixed results, with three studies indicating that a high-protein meal will reduce subsequent cravings, and two showing no difference between high-protein and high-carbohydrate meals in subsequent feelings of fullness or the calories consumed in the subsequent meal. Barkeling et al. performed a study using 20 healthy normal BMI women who were given meals with equal calories, fat, and fiber and a glass of water. They were randomly allocated to eat either a high-protein meal (meat and whole-meal spaghetti) or a high-carbohydrate meal (vegetables and ordinary spaghetti). Subjects were to consume the entire meal and water.

They then fasted until the standard dinner meal, which was provided in excessive quantity. They were instructed to eat until pleasantly full. Subjects who had eaten the high-protein meal consumed 12% less calories at dinner. This short-term effect was somewhat artificial because of the balance of fiber provided in the test meal that would not generally occur in a low-carbohydrate meal outside the investigative setting.

In a review of 11 studies that addressed the issue of high- vs low-calorie diets *(31)*, 8 of the 11 indicated that a low-carbohydrate, high-protein diet reduced subsequent hunger. It was uncertain whether the subjects might have been biased by being able to identify the foods they ate. To address this question, they did a study that incorporated three similar-appearing liquid test meals (high-protein, high-carbohydrate, and mixed 50/50) as a 450-cal lunch in a crossover design in 12 female college students. They were told to consume as much of a cafeteria-style dinner as they wished. They consumed less after the protein meals than the carbohydrate meals.

Gendall et al. *(32)* evaluated the effects on subsequent food cravings, binge eating, nutrient intake, and mood of high-protein, high-carbohydrate, and mixed meals on 3 separate days in nine women who had food cravings at least once a week over the 2 mo prior to beginning the study. After the high-protein meal, the patients craved more sweet carbohydrate-rich foods than they did after the other meals.

Rosen et al. *(33)* evaluated obese subjects who were given 2 wk of low-carbohydrate diet followed by high-carbohydrate diet or visa versa in a crossover study. There was a decrease in appetite and elevation in psychological reactions to dieting after 2 wk of dieting that did not differ between the type of diet.

3.3. Fat

The effect of fat in diets is important because of the recommendation to reduce the amount and types of fat in diets. Additionally, in the low-carbohydrate diet (*see* Subheading 6.), because carbohydrate intake is severely restricted, the amount of fat in the diet tends to be high as many high-protein, low-carbohydrate foods also have high-fat content.

The effect of an equal calorie and density high-protein, high-carbohydrate, high-fat, or mixed breakfast on the amount eaten at lunch was evaluated in 16 normal-weight men *(34)*. Hunger was significantly less after the high-protein and the mixed breakfasts. They consumed more calories at lunch after the high-fat breakfast.

Orosco et al. *(35)* tested the effects of different fats on 5-HT concentrations. Lard and high-saturated fat-enriched margarines caused a reduction in 5-HT concentration and increased sucrose consumption. Sunflower oil- and olive oil-enriched margarines did not significantly alter 5-HT concentrations.

Rissanen et al. *(36)* evaluated dietary preference for fat by evaluating responses by monozygotic twins who were discordant for obesity as evidenced by at least a 3 BMI difference. The obese twins reported a current preference for fatty foods three times more frequently than their non-obese co-twins. In addition, when recalling taste preferences at the time they left their parental home, the twins reported that the obese twin had a greater preference for fatty foods.

Woodend and Anderson *(23)* noted that a preload of safflower oil at 0, 418, 836, and 1254 kJ suppressed average appetite more than non-safflower control. The highest safflower preload dose decreased food intake of the subsequent meal by about half the calories of the safflower given. Furthermore, safflower oil suppressed the food intake of the subsequent meal less than a sucrose preload with comparable calories.

St. Onge and Jones *(37)*, after a review of the literature, concluded that medium-chain triglycerides might result in faster satiety, and increased energy expenditure compared with long-chain triglycerides through hypothesized actions on CCK, peptide YY, gastric inhibitory peptide, neurotensin, and pancreatic polypeptide.

CCK is released after fat intake (*see* Subheadings 2.2 and 5). In addition, recent evidence suggests that high-fiber meals also increase CCK concentrations *(17)* examined CCK-associated satiety in seven males and eight females, who had been fasted, when they received differing amounts of fat in three isoenergetic breakfast meals (low-fiber and low-fat; high-fiber and low-fat; low-fiber and high-fat) in a randomized crossover design. Plasma samples were analyzed for CCK, insulin, glucose, and triacylglycerols.

4. ENVIRONMENTAL FACTORS

4.1. Effect of Exercise

Long et al. *(38)* evaluated lean males, of whom 14 were regular exercisers and 9 were nonexercisers, to determine whether exercise improved accuracy of regulation of food intake in compensation for prior energy intake. The subjects were given liquid preloads that were blinded as to content (2513 kJ high energy, 1008 kJ low energy) followed by a buffet lunch 1 hr later. They found that the nonexercisers did not significantly alter their intake based on the preload, whereas the exercisers reduced their lunch intake after the high-energy intake. There were no differences in hunger or satiety ratings following the preloads for either group. Although this supports the benefits of exercise on short-term regulation of food intake, because this evaluation was not randomized, this finding could be an intrinsic difference in exercisers and nonexercisers rather than a consequence of exercise.

4.2. Oro-Sensory Component

Food consistency makes a difference with thicker consistency enhancing satiety. Mattes and Rothasker *(14)* tested shakes with different consistencies. The thicker the consistency, the more hunger was reduced. However, there was no difference in the total intake of the subsequent 24 hr.

Appearance affects eating behavior. Linne et al. *(39)* evaluated the amount of food eaten by nine blind and nine matched normal subjects with and without blindfolding. The eating behavior of the normal and blind subjects did not differ. The subjects ate 22% less food and ate more quickly when blindfolded than when they could see.

Taste can influence the perception of satiety. The effects of lemon-flavored sucrose (2160 kJ in 575 mL), maltose (67 kJ, 575 mL), and water drinks taken orally were compared in six normal males to evaluate the potential effects on appetite and gastric emptying *(40)*. The sucrose and maltose solutions slowed gastric emptying compared with water, but maltose delayed gastric emptying more than sucrose. Sucrose was more effective in increasing fullness and in reducing intake during the subsequent 3 hr. In a second study using another six volunteers, the sucrose and maltose were given by gavage. The effect on gastric emptying remained, but there were no differences in hunger, fullness, or consumption. This suggests that the sweet taste of the sucrose was responsible for the perception of increased fullness and decreased subsequent consumption.

The effects of sucrose (sucrose-containing 251kJ pastilles chewed over 10 min, sucrose jelly 251 kJ consumed over 5 min, sucrose drink 251kJ consumed within 2 min, and water consumed within 2 min) on subsequent suppression of appetite was evaluated in 10 male and 10 female subjects *(41)*. There was no difference in hunger and fullness among the treatments, but after chewing the pastilles, the lunch intake was reduced, compared with the sucrose solution and the water. This suggested that the orosensory component resulted in suppression of subsequent intake.

Zandstra et al. *(42)* evaluated food intake after a mid-morning yogurt snack consisting of 67 kcal or 273 kcal/200 mL, each with a specific flavor, given on alternating days for 40 d to evaluate whether the subject's lunch food intake compensated for the differing snack intakes. Lunch intake was reduced after both yogurt snacks compared to lunch without a snack. This effect did not change after repeated exposures. When the flavors were switched after 40 d, subjects increased their intake after eating the high-calorie yogurt with the low-calorie taste, but did not reduce their calorie intake after eating the low-calorie yogurt with the high-calorie taste.

4.3. Novelty and Palatability

Frequent and repeated exposure to a particular food results in satiation or monotony. This effect has neuroanatomical basis. Rolls et al. *(43)* tested sensory-specific satiety by measuring neuronal response to repeated stimulation in the caudofrontal cortex taste area. When monkeys were fed to satiety with a specific taste, neurons in their caudolateral orbitofrontal cortex decreased in their response to that particular taste. When subjects were allocated to no chocolate except during test days (*n* = 15), 67 g chocolate per day (*n* = 20), or increasing amounts of chocolate from 57 g/d to 86 g/d (*n* = 18) over a 15-d period, the desire for and pleasantness of chocolate declined over time for the chocolate-eating subjects. However, there was no reduction in chocolate intake.

Consistent with this study, McCrory et al. *(44)* noted that dietary energy intake was related to palatability and that dietary variety was an important predictor of body fatness. Looking at this from the opposite perspective, Bell et al. *(45)* showed that the volume of food rather than its energy density determined the perception of that food's palatability and as a consequence larger food volume results in earlier termination of eating.

Gosnell et al. *(46)* concluded that the amount and number of different foods presented significantly influenced how much food was consumed. Ten male and female subjects (ages 18 to 65), 5 with binge-eating disorder (*see* Chapter 11) and 5 without, were tested in a feeding laboratory setting. They were examined with either one or two binge foods in either twice to four times their self-reported binge-eating episode amounts. Energy intake, hunger, fullness, anxiety, and depression were measured. Results showed that the amount and selection of foods did significantly affect the amount of food consumed irrespective of the binge-eating disorder. This suggests that patients are more likely or capable of over-eating because of the variety and palatability of foods.

5. NEUROENDOCRINE HORMONES

With societal obsession with obesity and weight loss, many media stories and scientific publications have focused on a physiological mechanism for obesity. Chapter 18 presents the molecular evidence related to neurohormones affecting ingestion and body weight. The effects of many of the neuroendocrine hormones involved in body weight are summarized briefly here.

Although many have attributed obesity to psychological issues including lack of self-control, emotional problems, research does not fully support this. For example, Pearcey et al. *(47)* examined the energy balance (diet and activity diaries) and influencing factors of subjects who had been gaining weight during the prior 6 mo (*n* = 19) compared to subjects who were weight stable (*n* = 19) in an attempt to determine whether there were differences between the two groups. In addition to their intake and activity, each subject recorded the environmental, social, and psychological factors associated with each meal in a 7-d diary. Weight gain was associated with increased caloric intake, but none of the other assessed factors. Thus, determination of the causes of increased ingestion, would be valuable in controlling weight gain.

Neuroendocrine hormones have been suggested a physiological factor causing obesity and weight gain. The neuroendocrine hormones that regulate feeding behaviors are discussed in Chapters 9 and 18. Those neuroendocrine hormones that regulate eating through effects on hunger or satiety are discussed here. These hormones, usually produced peripherally, act as satiety signals and do little to regulate body fat stores. Many of these satiety signals act through the serotonergic system *(48)*. The GI tract releases CCK, ghrelin, glucagon-like peptide (GLP)-1, and GLP-2. These peptides cause gastric relaxation through gastric sensory, direct central nervous system, and indirect vagal effects. Fat stimulates CCK release that, acting through CCK-A receptors, transmits via the vagal nerve to the nucleus tractus solitaris and then to the lateral parabrachial nucleus, amygadala, and other sites. Heini et al. *(49)* evaluated the effects of fiber supplementation in a 5-wk randomized, double-blind, crossover study in 25 obese females on an 800 kcal/d (3.3 MJ) diet. They noted that 2-hr postprandial CCK concentrations were increased after a fiber-supplemented meal but not after a meal without fiber supplementation.

As glucose is released from food, pancreas β-cells co-secrete insulin and islet amyloid polypeptide (amylin) *(50)*. Insulin acts to increase hunger, whereas, amylin acts to decrease hunger. Amylin also inhibits postprandial glucagon secretion and delays gastric emptying. Both of these effects result in a blunted hyperglycemia. Both amylin and insulin act in concert in the area postrema of the hindbrain to reduce food intake *(51,52)*.

The human analogue of bombesin, gastrin inhibitory peptide, reduces food intake *(53)*. A double-blind, placebo-controlled study evaluated the effects of a 165-min infusion of bombesin on satiety and food intake in seven obese and seven lean women, with a preload of banana slices at 60 min. Bombesin reduced food eaten more than saline infusion by lean individuals, but not by the obese women, indicating that obese women are less sensitive to the effects of bombesin *(54)*.

Enterostatin, a petapeptide, is produced in enterochromaffin cells in the antrum and duodenum and in the exocrine pancreas as pancreatic procolipase *(55)*. It is released in response to dietary fat and reduces fat intake *(56)*. It has been shown by microdialysis to increase serotonin and dopamine in the lateral hypothalamus *(57)*.

Ghrelin derived from the stomach and in the hypothalamus, stimulates food intake by acting in the arcuate nucleus and other brain locations *(58,59)*. Ghrelin augments neuropeptide Y (NPY) gene expression and blocks leptin-induced feeding reductions *(59)*. Ghrelin plasma concentrations rise before meals and drop after meals. The concentrations increase during a weight-reduction diet and markedly decrease after gastric bypass surgery *(3)*. At present, ghrelin antagonism is being proposed as a potential pharmaceutical target *(60)*.

Hellstrom and Naslund *(61)* note that after food intake, CCK, GLP-1, and GLP-2 are released from the GI tract to mediate satiety. CCK and GLP-1 mediate satiety in both lean and obese humans. These peptides may act centrally, via the vagus nerve, or through gastric sensory mechanisms. In the brain, GLP-1is synthesized in the arcuate nucleus and acts in the area postrema, caudal nucleus of the solitary tract, lateral parabrachial nucleus, hypothalamic paraventricular nucleus, bed of the nucleus stria terminalis, and central nucleus of the amygdala *(62)*. GLP-2 is synthesized in the nucleus of the solitary tract.

Adiposity signals circulate in proportion to body adiposity and influence body weight by modifying the action of meal-generated satiety signals. Insulin and leptin, two such neuroendocrine hormones, are transported into the brain to modulate expression of hypothalamic neuropeptides. Leptin suppresses appetite and insulin increases appetite. NPY, β-endorphin, orexin (hypcretin), galanin, and melanin-concentrating hormone increase food intake. Corticotrophin-releasing hormone/urocortin (CRH), leptin, cocaine amphetamine-regulated transcript, and α-melanocyte-stimulating hormone (α-MSH) reduce food intake. CRH, α-MSN, and β-endorphin are cleavage products of pro-propriomelanocortin, which is released from other arcuate neurons after leptin stimulation.

NPY, orexin, and melanocortin-4 receptor (MC4R)-containing neurons are located in the hypothalamus. Leptin and insulin inhibit the NPY neurons in the arcuate nucleus, the paraventricular nucleus, and the lateral hypothalamus suppressing NPY release, but in periods of undernutrition or when genetic mutations result in inactive or reduced leptin, they are overactive as a result of release of this inhibitory control *(63)*. Additionally, recent studies in rats may suggest that NPY neurons develop resistance to the satiety actions of leptin in the hypothalamus *(64)*. This may explain the failure of leptin in weight-loss trials. Neurons expressing prepro-orexin, the precursor of orexin A and orexin B, are located in the lateral hypothalamus and are stimulated by hypoglycemia and are inhibited by food ingestion. The orexins transiently increase feeding *(65)*.

Activation of α-MSH neurons in the arcuate nucleus occurs coincident with meal termination, indicating that it is a satiety mediator *(66)*. α-MSH activates MC4R to inhibit feeding probably by blocking the action of agouti gene-related peptide, which is co-expressed with NPY in arcuate neurons. This may reduce overeating of palatable foods.

Galanine, β-endorphin, and other opioids, particularly μ-selective agonists, induce potent increases in food intake, sucrose, salt, saccharine, and ethanol. Based on studies using macronutrient selection, regional specificity, role of output structures, c-Fos mapping, analysis of motivational state, and enkelphalin gene expression, Kelley et al. concluded that opioid receptors in the ventral striatal medium spiny neurons mediate the affective hedonic response to food (liking or food pleasure).

5.1. Medications

Because diets tend to fail for most individuals, particularly over the long term, attempts have been made to identify herbals or medications that could be used to reduce weight. Most such agents, such as sibutramine, phentermine, fluoxetine, dexfenfluramine, fenfluramine, phenylpropanolamine, and ephedra (ma huang), act by increasing satiety. This permits patients to better adhere to a behavior modification weight-loss program (*see* Chapter 14). The amount of weight loss for such agents has proven to be minimal and tends to decrease over time *(67)*. Many of the neuroendocrine hormones noted earlier, as well as other strategies, such as efforts to increase metabolic rate (e.g. α_2-adrenergic agonists), may prove more effective; however, it is also possible that the complex regulation of energy intake, designed to prevent starvation and thus tilted toward accumulation of energy stores to permit survival when food supplies are tenuous, may require intervention with multiple concurrent mechanisms.

6. LOW-CARBOHYDRATE (ATKINS) DIET

The low-carbohydrate diet has been extremely popular *(2)*. For the initiation (induction) period, the amount of carbohydrate is severely restricted. During the later phases (ongoing weight loss, premaintenance stage, maintenance stage), more carbohydrate is added to the diet, but it is still significantly restricted with white flour, milk, refined sugar-containing foods, white bread, or white rice being permanently excluded from the diet. As a consequence, the dietary protein and fat intake increases. Proponents claim that this diet suppresses appetite, increases metabolic rate, decreases metabolic efficiency, and shunts nutrients away from storage *(68)*. Because restriction of carbohydrates prevents stimulation of insulin secretion, the effect is an insulin surge such as that which occurs after ingestion of simple sugars or refined carbohydrates. Because the carbohydrates in the diet are restricted, the body converts protein to sugar and burns fat for energy needs. Part of the popularity of the diet is the large, rapid initial weight loss seen by many users. Although some of the weight loss is the result of reduction in fat and lean body mass, much is owing to diuresis that occurs as a consequence of this diet as the body rids itself of the byproducts of fat and protein metabolism. The proponents additionally claim that the low-carbohydrate diet is practical because it is easily adhered to (*see* Table 2).

Proponents of this diet claim that it results in marked improvement of cardiovascular risk, as evidenced by reduction in cholesterol and triglyceride concentrations *(68)*. These risk factors have been noted to decrease as a consequence of weight loss, but they have not shown that this effect is specific to the low-carbohydrate diet. The adversaries, who will be called proponents of a "balanced" diet, argue that eating large amounts of fats used during the low-carbohydrate diet is potentially risky and that although the cholesterol and triglycerides drop, no long-term data on improvement in the risk for cardiovascular disease exists. These balanced diet proponents believe that there is a longer term risk that has not yet been identified. Until the long-term effects are studied, the diet should be avoided.

Balanced-diet proponents further argue that by substituting complex carbohydrates found in whole grains and vegetables, the insulin surge is also avoided. In this way, the diet would be better balanced because fruits, vegetables, and whole grains would compose the majority of the diet. Proponents of the low-carbohydrate diet counter that this has been proposed for years and that the majority of people have shown that they are incapable of maintaining such a diet. So, they add, theory is nice, but practicality supports the low-carbohydrate diet because it appears to be easy to follow.

There are additional arguments claiming that the low-carbohydrate diet is potentially unsafe. The low-carbohydrate diet should not be used by individuals who have increased risk for liver or kidney damage because of the high protein load and the fat metabolites. Low-carbohydrate diet proponents agree that these individuals should not use this diet.

Table 2
Arguments Related to the Benefits of the Low-Carbohydrate Diet [a]

Issues	Claims for low-carbohydrate diet	Counter claims
Satiety	Greater satiety after fat and protein; carbohydrate stimulates appetite through insulin surge	Reduction of high-caloric density foods with reduction in refined sugar and carbohydrates and increased fruits and vegetables provides a more healthful, better balanced diet with the benefits of natural ingredients (e.g., flavinoids and carotinoids) that have independent health benefits
Cardiovascular risk	Reduction in cholesterol and triglyceride reducing cardiovascular complications	The amount of improvement is related to the weight loss and not specific to the low carbohydrate diet
Hepatic and renal risk		High-protein and high-fat diet can be dangerous if there is an underlying organ compromise
Patient acceptance and compliance	This diet can be followed by patients more easily than the balanced low-fat diet because it tends to be more compatible with the American "meat and potatoes diet"	Requires that patients restrict highly palatable foods and replace them with whole grains and vegetables that they may not find desirable
Adverse effects	Improvement in various symptoms: sleep, concentration	Evidence suggest worsening of many of these symptoms

[a] For references, see text.

High-protein diets are associated with higher excretion of calcium, which might predispose the individual to osteoporosis and kidney stones. Balanced-diet proponents further argue that the low-carbohydrate diet lacks fiber and other nutrients, such as flavinoids and other photonutrients found in fruits, vegetables, and whole grains, that are important for protecting against cancer, particularly colon cancer, and heart disease and that high fat intake is associated with breast and prostate cancer. They note that if the amount of carbohydrate is insufficient, there will be insufficient glycogen stores for long-term exercise. The antagonists also note that if ketosis occurs, the dieter will have ketotic breath, bad body odor, and foul-smelling stools. Finally, they express concerns that the metabolism of medications might be altered by the diet and ensuing diuresis and that the diet-induced diuresis might result in dehydration and loss of potassium. They would like to see long-term studies evaluating the long-term medical effects such as frequencies of malignancies, and so on.

Interestingly, little scientifically has been published on the low-carbohydrate diet. For example, which patients are most likely to benefit? What proportion of patients fail and why? Our hypothesis is that one advantage of the low-carbohydrate diet is the reduction of snacking. Mormonier et al. *(69)* showed that snacking contributes to overweight. They assessed both behavioral and metabolic results from high-carbohydrate and high-protein snacking and concluded that between-meal snacking, irrespective of composition, has poor satiating efficiency and, as a result, contributes to obesity. When one considers the most common snacks—chips, popcorn, crackers, pretzels, candy, cookies, cake, and ice cream—these would be excluded in the low-carbohydrate diet because of their high-carbohydrate load. What would constitute a low-carbohydrate snack? Chicken or turkey leg, bacon, hamburger patty, egg salad. None are likely candidates for snacking. Thus, individuals who eat between meals would be those most likely to benefit from the low-carbohydrate diet because an absolute prohibition is easier to follow than restricted amounts ("Bet you can't eat just one!"). Furthermore, as noted in Subheading 4.2., larger portions of a single food or a more monotonous diet may lead to reduced intake as a result of decreased perception of palatability *(45)*.

Westman et al. *(70)* described an uncontrolled, 6-mo low-carbohydrate diet with no restriction on caloric intake in 51 overweight or obese volunteers who were given a nutritional supplement and exercise recommendations. The mean weight decrease was 10.3 ± 5.9% from baseline with a 2.9 ± 3.2% fat mass reduction for completers. Ten patients did not complete the program. Although the patients had reduction in cholesterol and triglycerides and reasonable weight loss, it is interesting that the majority of weight loss was of nonfat mass. Given these findings, Foster et al. *(71)* did a controlled trial to evaluate the low-carbohydrate diet. They found that the mean weight loss on the low-carbohydrate diet was greater than that of the conventional diet group initially, but the difference decreased over time and was not significant at the 12-mo endpoint. BP and glucose control showed similar effects to weight. Triglycerides had a significant mean decrease for the low-carbohydrate diet compared with no change for the conventional group. The conventional diet group had greater decreases in mean cholesterol (total and low-density lipoprotein) and less mean increase in high-density lipoprotein cholesterol. Although this was a relatively small study, it suggests that the claims supporting the low-carbohydrate diet do not hold up to scrutiny and add weight to the need to define the subset of patients who have a better outcome.

Proponents of low-carbohydrate diets claim that the diet will relieve fatigue, depression, irritability, headaches, and joint and muscle aches. They also claim that it will improve sleep by reducing the diurnal cortisol surge that occurs in response to the insulin surge produced by the release of sugars in the normal carbohydrate diet. Interestingly, the proponents of a balanced diet claim that the low-carbohydrate diet can cause fatigue, dull headaches, abdominal pain, nausea and vomiting, many of the same complaints that low-carbohydrate proponents claim are improved. Such claims should be relatively easy to resolve using a randomized trial and food supplied by the study.

Thus, further evaluation of the low-carbohydrate diet are needed to dissect the profile of the patients who benefit the most and those who benefit little. Furthermore, the reasons for such success or failure need to be elucidated. Finally, the long-term effects of this diet need to be defined. It may be that there are points of intersection of this and more standard diets that would help individuals find a practical, safe, and effective diet. It is likely that we could achieve similar benefits by incorporating the best points of the low-carbohydrate and low fat diets, such as increasing the fruits and vegetables and whole grains in our diets and restricting saturated fats, refined sugar, white rice, and white flour. At present, the industry produces low-fat foods with increased sugar or salt to increase palatability and foods that are low in carbohydrate are being introduced. Will these new low-carbohydrate formulations have substituted fat and salt for carbohydrate? Because consumers seem to like the convenience and taste of such foods, and in response to low-fat claims, seem to increase their overall intake in the misguided belief that low-fat somehow translates to "eat all you want," it will be helpful if the food industry could devise more nutritious foods as snacks instead of the high-fat, high-sugar, high-salt, starch foods that are primarily marketed. It will remain incumbent on medical practitioners to educate patients that such foods still need to be eaten in moderation.

7. CONCLUSION

Physiological processes defend the body from starvation. As a consequence, there is a tendency for overconsumption (72) and weight gain. The onset and termination of eating episodes are subject to facilitating and inhibitory processes that are controlled by environmental circumstances such as food availability, food type and variety, and environmental (habitual) routines.

Although numerous studies have been performed in an effort to understand factors that influence taste, consistency, hunger, and satiety, these have not been well integrated to give a conclusive overall picture of effective ways that can benefit the patient to lose weight. In addition, most of the individual interventions that show a statistically significant effect in well-designed and controlled studies demonstrate minor effects that tend to dwindle over time. Use of various foods as preloads that could reduce intake during a subsequent meal do not reduce the total intake over the longer term.

Unfortunately much of the ingestion by individuals is not primarily owing to hunger, but rather to emotional eating and to the novelty of foods (73). We can see this effect of palatability and novelty in house pets, particularly canines, which tend to gain weight when given table scraps or other palatable foods in addition to, or instead of, their formulated chow. In humans, we see this at a buffet when individuals eat a second dessert despite having been full prior to the first. As a consequence, effective interventions need to include ways to control emotional and novelty eating (see Table 3).

Table 3
Possible Strategies for Reducing Hunger and Enhancing Satiety to Assist in Weight Reduction

	Do	Avoid
Between meals	• Drink lots of noncaloric liquids • Snacks of high-fiber, low-caloric dense foods	• High-calorie drinks • Snacks of high-fat and high-sugar foods
During meals	• Drink lots of noncaloric liquids • Eat high-fiber foods (e.g., vegetables) • Eat low-caloric density foods	• High-calorie drinks • Eating until "stuffed" • Rushing through the meal • High-caloric dense foods • All-you-can-eat buffets • Large portion size
Food selection	• Replace high-caloric density foods with low-caloric density • Limit refined sugars and grains • Prepare smaller portions	• High-caloric dense foods • Foods that do not require preparation

Methods that reduce hunger and increase satiety can enhance dietary restriction to improve weight loss. For example, enhancing satiety by increasing mechanical effects by filling the stomach with water and fiber during a meal, and with water and fiber or low energy-dense foods between meals can result in an overall decrease in total energy input. Substitution of high-density foods with low-density foods and of refined foods with natural grains and vegetables can also be used to enhance satiety and reduce the postprandial surge in insulin and enhance weight reduction. Although such strategies can help patients lose weight while they are restricting intake, the ready availability of a wide variety of highly palatable food and the natural tendency to seek novelty in eating can undercut efforts to restrict intake. Other strategies discussed in this book, including behavioral therapy (*see* Chapter 14) and physical activity and exercise (*see* Chapter 13) need to be utilized as parts of a complete weight loss program. Finally future drug therapies may be helpful in adhering to a weight loss program.

REFERENCES

1. Plata-Salaman CR. Regulation of hunger and satiety in man. Dig Dis 1991; 9:253–268.
2. Atkins RC. Dr. Atkins' new diet revolution. New York, NY: Simon and Schuster, 1998.
3. Cummings DE, Weigle DS, Frayo RS, et al. Plasma ghrelin levels after diet-induced weight loss or gastric bypass surgery. N Engl J Med 2002; 346:1623–1630.
4. Geliebter A, Hashim SA. Gastric capacity in normal, obese, and bulimic women. Physiol Behav 2001; 74:743–746.
5. Kim DY, Camilleri M, Murray JA, Stephens DA, Levine JA, Burton DD. Is there a role for gastric accommodation and satiety in asymptomatic obese people. Obes Res 2001; 9:655–661.
6. Chilkoiro M, Caroli M, Gurra V, Lodadea Piepoli A, Riezzo G. Gastric emptying in normal weight and obese children—an ultrasound study. Int J Obes Relat Metab Disord 1999; 23:1303–1306.
7. Forsell P. Pouch volume, stoma diameter and weight loss in Swedish adjustable gastric banding (SAGB). Obes Surg 1996; 6:468–473.
8. Kromhout D, Bloemberg B, Seidell JC, Nissinen A, Menotti A. Physical activity and dietary fiber determine population body fat levels: the Seven Countries Study. Int J Obes Relat Metab Disord 2001; 25:301–306.

 9. Howarth NC, Saltzman E, Roberts SB. Dietary fiber and weight regulation. Nutr Rev 2001; 59:129–139.
10. Rolls BJ, Roe LS. Effect of the volume of liquid food infused intragastrically on satiety in women. Physiol Behav 2002; 76:623–631.
11. Kaplan RJ, Greenwood CE. Influence of dietary carbohydrates and glycaemic response on subjective appetite and food intake in healthy elderly persons. Int J Food Sci Nutr 2002; 53:305–316.
12. Landstrom U, Knutsson A, Lennernas M, Stenudd A. Onset of drowsiness and satiation after meals with different energy contents. Nutr Health 2001; 15:87–95.
13. Birketvedt GS, Aaseth J, Florholmen JR, Ryttig K. Long-term effect of fibre supplement and reduced energy intake on body weight and blood lipids in overweight subjects. Acta Medica (HradecKralove) 2000; 43:129–132.
14. Mattes RD, Rothacker D. Beverage viscosity is inversely related to postprandial hunger in humans. Physiol Behav 2001; 74:551–557.
15. Pasman WJ, Saris WH, Wauters MA, Westerterp-Plantenga MS. Effect of one week of fibre supplementation on hunger and satiety ratings and energy intake. Appetite 1997; 29:77–78.
16. Pasman WJ, Westerterp-Plantenga MS, Muls E, Vansant G, van Ree J, Saris WH. The effectiveness of long-term fibre supplementation on weight maintenance in weight-reduced women. Int J Obes Relat metab Disord 1997; 21:548–555.
17. Burton-Freeman B, Davis PA, Schneeman BO. Plasma cholecystokinin is associated with subjective measures of satiety in women. Am J Clin Nutr 2002; 76:659–667.
18. Del Parigi A, Chen K, Gaitier JF, et al. Sex differences in the human brain's response to hunger and satiation. Am J Clin Nutr 2002; 75:1017–1022.
19. Stoa-Birketvedt G. Effect of cimetidine suspension on appetite and weight in overweight subjects. BMJ 1993; 306:1091–1093.
20. Rasmussen MH, Andersen T, Breum L, Gotzsche PC, Hilsted J. Cimetidine suspension as adjuvant to energy restricted diet in treating obesity. BMJ 1993; 306:1093–1096.
21. Stoa-Birketvedt G, Paus PN, Ganss R, Ingebretsen OC, Florholmen J. Cimetidine reduces weight and improves metabolic control in overweight patients with type 2 diabetes. Int J Obes Metab Disord 1998; 22:1041–5.
22. Birketvedt GS, Thom E, Bernersen B, Florholmen J. Combination of diet, exercise and intermittent treatment of cimetidine on body weight and maintenance of weight loss: a 42 months follow-up study. Med Sci Monit 2000; 6:699–703.
23. Woodend DM, Anderson GH. Effect of sucrose and safflower oil preloads on short term appetite and food intake of young men. Appetite 2001; 37:185–195.
24. Anderson GH, Catherine NL, Woodend DM, Wolever TM. Inverse association between the effect of carbohydrates on blood glucose and subsequent short-term food intake in young men. Am.J Clin Nutr 2002; 76:1023–1030.
25. Anderson GH, Woodend D. Effect of glycemic carbohydrates on short-term satiety and food intake. Nutr Rev 2003; 61:S17–26.
26. Van de Ven ML, Westerterp-Plantenga MS, Wouters L, Saris WH. Effects of liquid preloads with different fructose/fibre concentrations on subsequent food intake and ratings of hunger in women. Appetite 1994; 23:139–146.
27. Kovacs EM, Westerterp-Plantenga MS, de Vries M, Brouns F, Saris WH. Effects of 2-week ingestion of (–)-hydroxycitrate ands (–)-hydroxycitrate combined with medium-chain triglycerides on satiety and food intake. Physiol Behav 2001; 74:543–549.
28. Westerterp-Plantenga MS, Kovacs EM. The effect of (–)-hydroxycitrate on energy intake and satiety in overweight humans. Int J Obes Relat Metab Disord 2002;26:870–872.
29. Pupovac J, Anderson GH. Dietary peptides induce satiety via cholecystokinin-A and peripheral opiod receptors in rats. J Nutr 2002; 132:2775–2780.
30. Barkeling B, Rossner S, Bjorvell H. Effects of a high-protein meal (meat) and a high-carbohydrate meal (vegetarian) on satiety measured by automated computerized monitoring of subsequent food intake, motivation to eat and food preferences. Int J Obes 1990; 14:743–751.
31. Latner JD, Schwartz M. The effects of a high-carbohydrate, high-protein or balanced lunch upon later food intake and hunger ratings. Appetite 1999; 33:119–128.
32. Gendall KA, Joyce PR, Abbott RM. The effects of meal composition on subsequent craving and binge eating. Addict Behav 1999; 24:305–315.

33. Rosen JC, Gross J, Loew D, Sims EA. Mood and appetite during minimal-carbohydrate and carbohy-drate-supplemented hypocaloric diets. Am J Clin Nutr 1985; 42:371–379.

34. Stubbs RJ, O'Reilly LM, Johnstone AM, et al. Description and evaluation of an experimental model to examine changes in selection between high-protein, high-carbohydrate and high-fat foods in humans. Eur J Clin Nutr 1999; 53:13–21.

35. Orosco M, Rouch C, Dauge V. Behavioral response to ingestion of different sources of fat. Involvement of serotonin? Behav Brain Res 2002; 132:103–109.

36. Rissanen A, Hakala P, Lissner L, Mattlar CE, Koskenvuo M, Ronnemaa T. Acquired preference espe-cially for dietary fat and obesity: a study of weight-discordant monozygotic twin pairs. Int J Obes Relat Metab Disord 2002; 26:93–97.

37. Woodend DM, Anderson GH. Effect of sucrose and safflower oil preloads on short term appetite and food intake of young men. Appetite 2001; 37:185–195.

38. St-Onge MP, Jones PJ. Physiological effects of medium-chain triglycerides: potential agents in the prevention of obesity. J Nutr 2002; 132:329–332.

39. Long SJ, Hart K, Morgan LM. The ability of habitual exercise to influence appetite and food intake in response to high- and low-energy preloads in man. Br J Nutr 2002; 87:517–523.

40. Linne Y, Barkeling B, Rossner S, Rooth P. Vision and eating behavior. Obes Res 2002; 10:92–95.

41. Lavin JH, French SJ, Read NW. Comparison of oral and gastric administration of sucrose and maltose on gastric emptying and appetite. Int J Obes Metab Disord 2002; 26:80–86.

42. Lavin JH, French SJ, Ruxton CH, Read NW. An investigation of the role of oro-sensory stimulation in sugar satiety? Int J Obes Relat Metab Disord 2002;26:384–388.

43. Zandstra EH, Stubenitsky K, De Graaf C, Mela DJ. Effects of learned flavour cues on short-term regulation of food intake in a realistic setting. Physiol Behav 2002;75:83–90.

44. Rolls ET, Sienkiewicz ZJ, Yaxley S. Hunger modulates the responses to gustatory stimuli of single neurons in the caudolateral orbitofrontal cortex of the macaque monkey. Eur J Neurosci 1989; 1:53–60.

45. McCrory MA, Fuss PJ, Saltzman E, Roberts SB. Dietary determinants of energy intake and weight regulation in healthy adults. J Nutr 2000; 130:276S–279S.

46. Bell EA, Roe LS, Rolls BJ. Sensory-specific satiety is affected more by volume than by energy content of a liquid food. Physiol Behav 2003; 78:593–600.

47. Gosnell BA, Mitchell JE, Lancaster KL, Burgard MA, Wonderlich SA, Crosby RD. Food presentation and energy intake in a feeding laboratory study of subjects with binge eating disorder. Int J Eat Disord 2001; 30:441–446.

48. Pearcey SM, de Castro JM. Food intake and meal patterns of weight-stable and weight-gaining persons. Am J Clin Nutr 2002; 76:107–112.

49. Halford JC, Blundell JE. Separate systems for serotonin and leptin in appetite control. Ann Med 2000; 32:222–232.

50. Arnelo U, Blevins JE, Larsson J, et al. Effects of acute and chronic infusion of islet amyloid polypeptide on food intake in rats. Scand J Gastroenterol 1996; 31:83–89.

51. Riediger T, Schmidt HA, Lutz TA, Simon E. Amylin and glucose co-activate area postrema neurons of the rat. Neurosci Lett 2002; 328:121–124.

52. Rushing PA, Lutz TA, Seeley RJ, Woods SC. Amylin and Insulin interact to reduce food intake in rats. Horm Metab Res 2000; 32:62–65.

53. Hampton LL, Ladenheim EE, Akeson M, et al. Loss of bombesin-induced feeding suppression in gastrin-releasing peptide receptor-deficient mice. Proc Natl Acad Sci USA 1998; 95:3188–3192.

54. Lieverse RJ, Masclee AA, Jansen JB, Lam WF, Lamers CB. Obese women are less sensitive for the satiety effects of bombesin than lean women. Eur J Clin Nutr 1998; 52:207–212.

55. Sorhede M, Erlanson-Albertsson C, Mei J, Nevalainen T, Aho A, Sundler F. Enterostatin in gut endo-crine cells—immunocytochemical evidence. Peptides 1996; 17:609–614.

56. Koizumi M, Sato H, Seguro K, Ide H, Morinaga Y, Kimura S. Effects of enterostatin (Val–Pro–Asp–Pro–Arg) on fat intake and blood levels of glucose and insulin in rats. Methods Find Exp Clin Pharmacol 2001; 23:235–239.

57. Koizumi M, Kimura S. Enterostatin increases extracellular serotonin and dopamine in the lateral hypo-thalamic area in rats measured by in vivo microdialysis. Neurosci Lett 2002; 320:96–98.

58. Wren AM, Small CJ, Abott CR, et al. Ghrelin causes hyperphagia and obesity in rats. Diabetes 2001; 50:2540–2547.

59. Nakazato M, Murakami N, Date Y, et al. A role for ghrelin in the central regulation of feeding. Nature 2001; 409:194–198.
60. Flier JS, Maratos-Flier E. The stomach speaks–ghrelin and weight regulation. NEJM 2002; 346: 1662–1663.
61. Hellstrom PM, Naslund E. Interactions between gastric emptying and satiety, with special reference to glucagon-like peptide-1. Physiol Behav 2001; 74:735–741.
62. Rowland NE, Crews EC, Gentry RM. Comparison of Fos induced in rat brain by GLP-1 and amylin. Regul Pept 1997; 71:171–174.
63. Williams G, Bing C, Cai XJ, Harold JA, King PJ, Liu XH. The hypothalamus and the control of energy homeostasis: different circuits, different purposes. Physiol Behav 2001; 74:683–701.
64. Sahu A. Resistance to the satiety action of leptin following chronic central leptin infusion is associated with the development of leptin resistance in neuropeptide Y neurones. J Neuroendocrinol 2002; 14: 796–804.
65. Cai XJ, Liu XH, Evans M, Clapham JC, Wilson S, Arch JR, Morris R, Williams G. Orexins and feeding: special occasions or everyday occurrence? Regul Pept 2002; 104:1–9.
66. Olszewski PK, Wirth MM, Shaw TJ, et al. Role of α-MSH in the regulation of consummatory behavior: immunohistochemical evidence. Am J Physiol Regul Integr Comp Physiol 2001; 281:R673–680.
67. Goldstein DJ, Potvin J. Long-term weight loss: effect of pharmacological agents. Amer J Clin Nutr 1994; 60:647–657.
68. Volek JS, Westman EC. Very-low-carbohydrate weight-loss diets revisited. Cleveland Clinic J Med 2002; 68:849–862.
69. Marmonier C, Chapelot D, Fantino M, Louis-Sylvestre J. Snacks consumed in a nonhungry state have poor satiating efficiency: influence of snack composition on substrate utilization and hunger. Am J Clin Nutr 2002; 76:518–528.
70. Westman EC, Yancy WS, Edman JS, Tomlin KF, Perkins CE. Effect of 6-month adherence to a very low carbohydrate diet program. Am J Med 2002; 113:30–36.
71. Foster GD, Wyatt HR, Hill JO, et al. A randomized trial of a low-carbohydrate diet for obesity. N Engl J Med 2003; 34:2082–2090.
72. Koleva M, Kadiiska A, Markovska V, Nacheva A, Boev M. Nutrition, nutritional behavior, and obesity. Cent Eur J Public Health 2000; 8:10–3.
73. Raynor HA, Epstein LH. Dietary variety, energy regulation, and obesity. Psychol Bull 2001; 127: 325–341.

20

Surgical Interventions
for the Management of Obesity

Scott A. Shikora, David Smith, and Julie J. Kim

KEY POINTS

- For the extremely obese, nonsurgical treatment strategies consistently fail to achieve and/or sustain meaningful weight loss. As a consequence, surgical solutions have been gaining popularity as an alternative therapy.
- Surgical procedures have become safer with the introduction of laparascopic techniques and more effective in either limiting nutrient absorption or reducing food intake, but no one procedure is uniformly accepted as "the gold standard."
- Bariatric operations that result in nutrient partitioning include intestinal bypassing, biliopancreatic diversion, and biliopancreatic diversion with duodenal switch.
- Bariatric operations that result in nutrient restriction include bariatric bypass, gastric bypass, and gastric banding.
- Careful patient selection and comprehensive long-term follow up are the cornerstones to long-lasting success.
- When significant surgically induced weight-loss results, obesity-associated conditions improve or resolve.
- Surgery is best utilized in the setting of a multidisciplinary treatment model.

1. INTRODUCTION

The prevalence of obesity is increasing at an alarming rate worldwide. In the United States, it is estimated that 64% of all adults are overweight or obese *(1)*. Furthermore, 4.7% are extremely (morbidly) obese, defined as a body mass index (BMI) greater than or equal to 40 kg/m². This means that the number of extremely obese adults in the United States has reached a staggering 14 to 16 million people. The impact of obesity is not limited to the United States but is spreading worldwide. Globally, the prevalence of overweight/obesity was recently estimated at 1.7 billion people *(2)*. This accounts for more than 2.5 million deaths per year *(3)*. This high prevalence is not limited to adults, as there is a growing epidemic of overweight adolescents.

From: *The Management of Eating Disorders and Obesity, Second Edition*
Edited by: D. J. Goldstein © Humana Press Inc., Totowa, NJ

Table 1
Chapter Overview

This chapter reviews the various surgical procedures, patient selection process, operative complications, and postoperative outcomes (Table 1).

Obesity is more than just a cosmetic problem (*see* Chapter 10). Obese individuals suffer from a wide range of comorbidities and comprise the second largest group of preventable deaths after smoking (>300,000 per year) *(4)*. Comorbid conditions are many and can cause early death or disruption of the quality of life in the severely obese (Table 2). Inability to perform activities of daily living, immobility, psychosocial and economic problems, and disability are common accompaniments. Furthermore, the cost of treating the obese is staggering, and is estimated at approx $70 billion per year *(5)*.

For the extremely obese, nonsurgical treatment strategies consistently fail to achieve and/or sustain meaningful weight loss. Since its introduction in the 1950s, surgery has slowly evolved into a safe and effective treatment option for the extremely obese. In addition to the technical advances, including the adoption of minimally invasive technology, the decrease in operative risk and increase in long-term success can be attributed to improvements in patient selection, preparation, and, postoperative care. The resultant weight loss has been demonstrated to improve the health and quality of life for the majority of these patients. As society becomes more aware of these facts (with the aid of the recent success of high-profile celebrities), bariatric surgery, as it is called, has become one of the fastest growing fields in all of medicine. It has been estimated, that approx 30,000 procedures were performed in the United States last year. Projections indicate that 50,000 surgeries will be performed in 2004, 75,000 in 2005, and more than 100,000 in 2006.

Table 2
Obesity-Associated Medical Conditions

Cardiovascular	Endocrine	Hepatobiliary/Gastrointestinal
• Cardiomyopathy	• Amenorrhea	• Hepatic steatosis
• Cerebrovascular disease	• Diabetes mellitus	• Gallstones
• Coronary artery disease	• Hirsutism	• Gastroesophageal reflux
• Dyslipidemia	• Infertility	• Steatohepatitis
• Hypertension		
• Sudden death	Musculoskeletal/skin	Psychological
	• Accident proneness	• Depression
Miscellaneous	• Chronic back pain	• Low self esteem
• Chronic fatigue	• Degenerative joint disease	• Poor quality of life
• Malignancies	• Diaphoresis	• Poor relationships
• Pseudotumor cerebri	• Hernia	• Suicide
• Urinary stress incontinence	• Immobility	
	• Infections	Venous disease
Pulmonary/respiratory	• Intertrigenous dermatitis	• Deep vein thrombosis
• Dyspnea		• Lower limb edema
• Obesity hypoventilation		• Pulmonary embolus
• Obstructive sleep apnea		• Venous stasis
		• Venous stasis ulcers

Table 3
Current Surgical Procedures

Purely restrictive	Malabsorptive < restrictive
• Gastric balloons [a]	• Biliopancreatic diversion (BPD)
• Vertical banded gastroplasty	• BPD with duodenal switch
• Gastric adjustable banding	• Very long limb Roux en-Y gastric
Restrictive > malabsorptive	Purely malabsorptive
• Short limb or proximal Roux en-Y gastric bypass	• Jejunal-ileal bypass [b]
• Long limb or distal Roux en-Y gastric bypass	• Jejunal-colonic bypass [b]

[a] Not approved for use in the United States.
[b] No longer considered a safe surgical option

2. OVERVIEW OF SURGICAL WEIGHT-LOSS STRATEGIES

At present, several operations are being performed worldwide. All of these procedures can be viewed by their mechanism of action (Table 3). They are designed to either limit nutrient absorption or to reduce food intake. Some procedures rely on a combination of both mechanisms. It would be fair to state that currently no one procedure would be uniformly accepted as "the gold standard." Each has favorable and unfavorable attributes. There is no consensus as to which procedure is superior and the answer will vary from surgeon to surgeon and location to location. For example, in the United States, nutrient intake-restrictive procedures with or without some degree of malabsorption (Roux en-Y gastric bypasses) are currently considered the operations of choice for most patients. In Europe, Australia, and other countries, purely restrictive procedures (laparoscopic adjustable gastric bands) are overwhelmingly more common. In addition, the popularity of these procedures is likely to change with time.

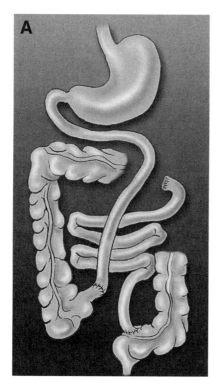 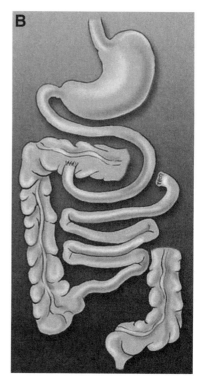

Fig. 1. Intestinal bypasses. (A) Jejuno-ileal bypass where the proximal jejunum is anastomosed to the terminal ileum. (B) Jejuno-colic bypass where the proximal jejunum is anastomosed to the transverse colon. (Reprinted with permission from the American Society for Bariatric Surgery.)

3. BARIATRIC OPERATIONS: NUTRIENT PARTITIONING

3.1. Intestinal Bypassing

Intestinal bypassing was the first type of operative procedure developed to induce significant weight loss (6). First reported in the early 1950s, these procedures were based on the common knowledge that after major small bowel resection or failure, most patients lost weight because of inadequate nutrient absorption surface area. Intestinal bypassing involves connecting the very proximal jejunum to the very distal ileum (or even the colon). Typically, only 10% of the small bowel was kept in the circuit and exposed to the luminal nutrients (Fig. 1). Patients could eat without restriction, but most complained of frequent foul-smelling bowel movements.

Intestinal bypasses were relatively low-risk procedures in otherwise high-risk patients. Operative mortality was reported to be less than 3%. Although perioperative complications were frequent (about 30%), most were minor in severity. This led to a rapid increase in popularity. During the 1960s and 1970s tens of thousands of patients had intestinal bypasses. Unfortunately, many patients experienced a number of late complications (Table 4), some very serious in nature (7). Approximately 25% of patients required hospitalization within the first 2 yr for control of severe diarrhea, dehydration, electrolyte abnormalities, abdominal pain, and vomiting. More serious complications included liver dysfunction, protein malnutrition, renal disease, and stone formation. Bacterial over-

Table 4
Late Complications of Jejuno-Ileal Bypass

• Liver disease	• Nephrolithiasis	• Cholelithiasis
• Arthropathies	• Vitamin deficiencies	• Chronic diarrhea
• Protein malnutrition	• Dermatitis	• Bone demineralization
• Electrolyte deficiencies	• Mineral deficiencies	• Intussusception

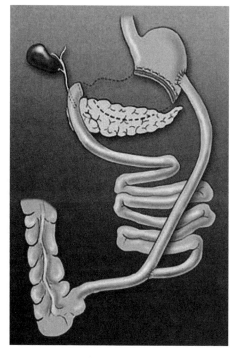

Fig. 2. Biliopancreatic diversion. After a partial gastrectomy, the ileum is anastomosed to the stomach remnant. The intestinal limb that drains the bile and pancreatic juices is anastomosed to the terminal ileum. (Reprinted with permission from the American Society for Bariatric Surgery.)

growth in the bypassed segment of intestine was considered to be the etiology of the complications that could not be directly attributed to malabsorption.

Hepatic disease, the most potentially life-threatening problem, was reported in about 29% of patients followed long term. This would progress to cirrhosis in about 7%. The fatty deposition and fibrosis was described to be quite similar to alcoholic liver changes. Some patients have since required liver transplantation for intestinal bypass-related cirrhosis (8). For these reasons, intestinal bypasses are no longer recommended. Patients who underwent intestinal bypass operations may need reversal if they develop any of the sequelae.

3.2. Biliopancreatic Diversion

The biliopancreatic diversion (BPD) is a modified intestinal bypass (Fig. 2). First developed by Scopinaro et al. in 1976, it was intended to cause nutrient malabsorption, yet minimize the potential complications associated with the intestinal bypasses (9).

Although the BPD seems similar to the intestinal bypass, there is no blind limb so the consequences of bacterial overgrowth are thought to be eliminated. The operation involves a partial gastrectomy with the gastric remnant anastomosed to the distal ileum. The proximal ileum is then anastomosed to the terminal ileum to create a "common channel" approx 50 to 100 cm from the ileocecal valve. Although the mechanism of action for weight loss is predominantly nutrient malabsorption, the partial gastrectomy is thought to initiate the weight loss by nutrient restriction. The intestinal bypassing is thought to maintain weight loss long term while allowing patients to eat "normally." Scopinaro has published results reporting 72% excess weight loss in patients followed for up to 18 yr *(10)*.

The weight loss achieved by the BPD is considered superior to that achieved by nutrient-restrictive procedures; however, this is accomplished at greater risk. The severity of complications is greater. The most serious potential complications include protein malnutrition and severe vitamin deficiency leading to bone demineralization that has been reported to occur in up to 15% *(10)*. Some of these complications have been reduced by lengthening the common channel from 50–100 cm to 150–200 cm. Ulceration of the ileum at the gastric connection is also a common complication. With the high incidence of complications, it is unlikely that the BPD or its variants will ever replace the gastric bypass as the most popular procedure in the United States. However, there may be a potential application for BPD in those patients who fall into the super superobese category (BMI >70 kg/m^2, where the weight loss from nutrient-restrictive procedures may not be sufficient to reverse weight-associated morbidity.

3.3. BPD With Duodenal Switch

In 1992, Marceau et al. described the BPD with duodenal switch. This updated variant of the BPD involves a sleeve gastrectomy of the greater curvature of the stomach instead of the removal of the distal fundus and antrum (Fig. 3). The antrum, pylorus, and first portion of the duodenum remain in continuity with the alimentary stream, thereby reducing the incidence of stomal ulceration of the ileum and dumping syndrome *(11)*. This procedure is growing in popularity in the United States.

4. BARIATRIC OPERATIONS: NUTRIENT RESTRICTION

4.1. Gastric Bypass (Fig. 4)

The failure of the original intestinal bypassing to provide safe weight loss led to the development of operative procedures based on nutrient-intake restriction. Gastric partitioning, commonly referred to as "gastric stapling," was conceptualized from the longstanding experience of gastrointestinal (GI) surgeons with subtotal gastric resections. Most patients, after partial gastrectomy, lost weight and were not capable of eating large (or even average-sized) meals. Based on these observations, Mason et al. performed the first gastric bypasses (GBP) for weight loss in 1967 *(12)*.

There is some recently published work regarding *ghrelin*, a peptide hormone that is secreted by the stomach in response to substrate, which is thought to promote appetite (*see* Chapter 18). Levels of this hormone increase in patients subjected to dieting and weight loss. This increase in ghrelin stimulates appetite, which causes weight gain *(14)*. Interestingly, ghrelin levels were found to be nonexistent in a small cohort of patients who had undergone GBP *(14)*. This may be another explanation for sustained weight loss after GBP.

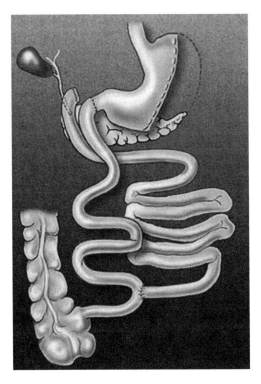

Fig. 3. Biliopancreatic diversion with duodenal switch. Similar to the biliopancreatic diversion except that a sleeve gastrctomy is done and the ileum is anastomosed to the duodenum. (Reprinted with permission from the American Society for Bariatric Surgery.)

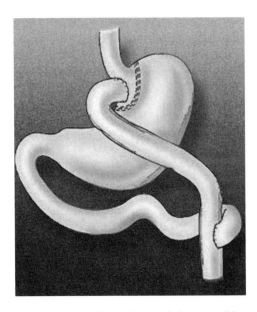

Fig. 4. Roux-en-Y gastric bypass. A small gastric pouch is created by staple partition (as in this picture) or staple transection of the stomach. The pouch is anastomosed to the jejunum. (Reprinted with permission from the American Society for Bariatric Surgery.)

Table 5
Long-Term Considerations of Gastric Bypass Surgery

Nutritional issues

- Anemia
- Dehydration

- Dumping syndrome
- Malnutrition

- Vitamin and mineral deficiencies
- Weight loss failure

Gastrointestinal issues

- Abdominal pain
- Constipation
- Diarrhea
- Gallstones

- Gastritis
- Incisional hernias
- Internal hernias
- Intestinal obstructions

- Marginal ulcers
- Nausea
- Vomiting

With more than 20 yr of experience, the GBP is currently the most common operative procedure performed in the United States for the treatment of morbid obesity. It is the method against which all others are judged. The operative mortality has been reported to range from 0.3 to 1.6% *(15,16)*. Perioperative complications occur in about 10% of patients. Fortunately, serious complications are rare. Long-term complications are more common but are usually easily managed (Table 5). These include anemia, vitamin and mineral deficiencies, dehydration, persistent vomiting, and dumping syndrome. With the appropriate patient selection, education, and after-care, 75 to 80% of patients will lose more than 50% of their excess weight *(15,17)*.

4.2. Gastroplasty

The original versions of the GBP were technically difficult and the complication rates were significant *(18)*. In the mid-1970s, a simplified version of gastric restriction, called *gastroplasty* was introduced. These procedures maintained the small pouch, yet eliminated the need for an intestinal connection. The small gastric pouch was constructed by staple partitioning of the stomach. The pouch drained into the main body of the stomach through a small gastric channel. The narrow channel functions similarly to the anastomosis of the GBP, delaying pouch emptying, thereby causing satiety after consuming a small meal.

Unfortunately, some of the earlier varieties were prone to fail from dilatation of the gastric pouch or from disruption of the staple line partition. However, one procedure seemed to perform more successfully. The vertical-banded gastroplasty (VBG), also first described by Mason et al. in 1982 *(19)*, utilizes a vertically oriented 30-cc pouch that drains through a narrow gastric channel into the gastric fundus (Fig. 5). The pouch outlet is 1 cm in diameter and reinforced by a polypropylene band, which prevents it from stretching. The VBG has a lower perioperative complication rate than the GBP, and because there is no malabsorption, cases of vitamin deficiency and anemia are almost never occur.

It was initially thought that the VBG would be an acceptable alternative to the GBP, possibly even a replacement. The VBG, however, has been shown to be inferior to the GBP in many aspects. Studies comparing the efficacy of the VBG to the GBP have found that the GBP produces better weight loss *(20,21)*. This may be because after VBG,

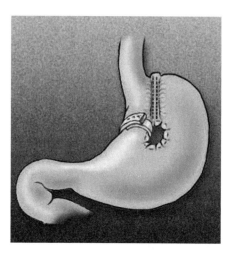

Fig. 5. Vertical banded gastroplasty. A small gastric pouch is created by staple partition (as in this picture) or staple transection of the stomach. A band is placed around the outlet to slow food movement. (Reprinted with permission from the American Society for Bariatric Surgery.)

patients can still tolerate sweets and high-calorie liquids, whereas after GBP, patients experience dumping syndrome with those same foods. Dumping syndrome seen after GBP functions as a built-in deterrent to eating foods high in sugar and fat. To study this, Sugerman et al. *(22)* segregated patients to GBP or VBG based on preoperative dietary habits. Those noted to be "sweet-eaters" were selected for GBP and those not considered "sweet-eaters" were offered VBG. By not performing VBG on patients with sweet-eating tendencies, he hoped to improve the results of the VBG. Surprisingly, despite this selection process, patients having VBG still lost less weight. In addition, the VBG has proven over time to be inferior in other aspects as well. There is a greater incidence of staple-line breakdown and risk of band erosion. In addition, a significant number of patients, after VBG, experience various degrees of food intolerance and vomiting.

4.3. Gastric Banding

In the 1970s, gastric banding was offered as an alternative to gastric stapling. These procedures place tight plastic bands around the upper stomach, creating small proximal pouches. The initial material used to create the band was similar to that of vascular grafts. Gastric-banding procedures function very similarly to the VBG in that the resultant weight loss is solely owing to intake restriction. Gastric banding is considered to have less operative risk and a shorter recovery period than GBP. However, the initial experience with banding was poor with significant complications related to the band. These included band migration, band erosion, or pouch dilatation. Migration and erosion led to significant vomiting. Pouch dilatation or dietary noncompliance led to weight-loss failure. In the late 1980s, gastric banding was rejuvenated with the introduction of adjustability. Kuzmak et al. developed the adjustable silicone gastric band, implanted via laparotomy *(23)*. The design was a hollow expandable band connected to a saline reservoir by a thin tube. The reservoir was placed below the skin on the abdominal wall. The band could be "tightened" by injecting saline into the reservoir and "loosened" by withdrawing saline.

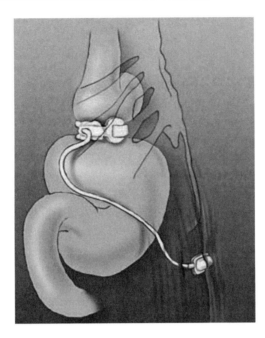

Fig. 6. Laparoscopic adjustable gastric band. An adjustable band is placed around the top of the stomach. Its diameter can be adjusted by inserting or removing saline from the reservoir. (Reprinted with permission from the American Society for Bariatric Surgery.)

The next big advance in gastric banding came in 1993 when the gastric band was modified for laparoscopic insertion (Fig. 6). First reported by Belachew et al. *(24)*, the device, the laparoscopic adjustable gastric band (LAGB), has become popular in Europe, Australia, the Middle East, Mexico, and other areas outside of the United States. Like its predecessor, the LAGB is positioned around the upper stomach, just below the gastroesophageal junction, where it acts to limit food intake by constricting the stomach to a shape similar to an hourglass. The upper chamber is a small 15–20 cc gastric pouch. Like the VBG, the LAGB is a purely restrictive operation with no malabsorptive component. This eliminates any concern for anemia, vitamin deficiencies, or dumping; but like the VBG, LAGB mandates greater compliance from the patient to be successful. It differs from the VBG in that it does not require stapling, is adjustable, and reversible. Because it is adjustable, vomiting is less of a problem than with VBG. Although there is a still a learning curve associated with laparoscopic band placement, it is technically easier than the laparoscopic GBP.

More than 100,000 LAGB have been implanted worldwide, confirming its safety, with weight-loss results similar to that seen with the VBG *(25,26)*. However, until June 2001, LAGB was not available in the United States. Based on the results of a multicenter trial with 300 American patients, the US Food and Drug Administration (FDA) approved the use of one version of the LAGB called the Lap-Band®. However, several European and Australian series seem to show consistently better weight-loss results when compared to the US trial. The reason for this is not known, but may reflect cultural influences affecting dietary behavior as well as the learning curve with the device.

Complications with the LAGB include band slippage, band erosion, pouch dilatation, reservoir infection, and tube leakage. The incidence of these seems to have decreased as certain technical modifications to the procedure have been made. Pouch dilatation with or without esophageal dilatation, may be related to overfilling of the band. Better results with the LAGB in American patients have recently been reported by Rubenstein *(27)*. In a 3-yr study of his personal series of 63 patients, he reported results more similar to the European experience than the FDA trial. This lends support to the argument that a learning curve was the reason for the poor results of the FDA trial.

The LAGB is an appealing addition to the armamentarium of the bariatric surgeon primarily because it is less invasive and adjustable. Only prospective, randomized trials and long-term follow up, however, will confirm whether this procedure is truly efficacious.

5. LAPAROSCOPIC BARIATRIC SURGERY

As with other areas in surgery, minimally invasive technologies such as laparoscopy have become quite popular. The difference between the traditional open procedure and its laparoscopic counterpart is the access to the organs. The procedures are still similar internally and have similar risks and outcomes. There are clear benefits to laparoscopic surgery especially in this patient population. Major benefits are related to the wound(s). With laparoscopy, the risk of wound complications, such as hernia or wound infection, is reduced from almost 30% with open, to less than 1% with laparoscopic, techniques *(28,29)*. The other well-described perioperative benefits of laparoscopic surgery (i.e., less pain, shorter hospitalization, better wound healing, improved cosmesis, and more rapid convalescence) are particularly beneficial to this patient population. In addition, Nguyen et al. found that extremely obese patients undergoing laparoscopic GBP surgery demonstrated improved pulmonary function compared to patients having open GBP surgery *(30)*. Decreased cytokine release has also been reported, suggesting that laparoscopy may produce less metabolic stress.

Currently, all of the bariatric procedures can be performed laparoscopically and estimates are that 30% of all bariatric procedures are now performed laparoscopically. However, the learning curve is quite steep, as many of these procedures are technically very difficult. Not surprisingly, because of this need for developing experience, complication rates are initially higher with laparoscopic surgery. Table 6 lists our complication rates of the first 100 and second 100 laparoscopic GBPs. The complication rate was decreased by 60%. Consistent with our experience, many centers specializing in laparoscopic bariatric surgery now report outcomes similar to that seen with open techniques *(29–33)*. As a consequence, the proportion of procedures done laparoscopically should dramatically increase in the near future as many surgeons are obtaining the necessary training.

6. ELECTRICAL GASTRIC STIMULATION: A LOOK INTO THE FUTURE?

In the future, one would anticipate the continued development of less-invasive and risky procedures. The currently performed operations for weight loss all involve some degree of altering the anatomy and function of the GI tract. In addition, they do so at the cost of both significant operative risk and long-term consequences. Electrical gastric stimulation with a pacemaker-like device, offers an exciting and novel alternative.

Table 6
Reduction in Perioperative Complications With the Laparoscopic
Roux-en-Y Gastric Bypass at Tufts-New England Medical Center

	Perioperative complications	
Complication	First 100 cases	Second 100 cases
Wound infection	9 (9%)	1 (1%)
Intraabdominal bleed	3 (3%)	0
Intraluminal bleed	1 (1%)	3 (3%)
Anastomotic leak	1 (1%)	0
Staple line leak	2 (2%)	0
Gastric remnant necrosis	1 (1%)	0
Ischemic Roux limb	1 (1%)	0
Incomplete gastric division	1 (1%)	0
Internal hernia	1 (1%)	2 (2%)
Enteroenterostomy Obstruction	3 (3%)	2 (2%)
Death	1 (1%)	0
Total	24 (24%)	8 (8%)

The stomach, like the heart, has a native pacemaker that is located along the greater curvature. The concept of "pacing" or altering the intrinsic pacesetter activity originated in the 1960s and 1970s. The application in humans to affect appetite was first proposed by Cigaina et al. in Italy *(34)*. They found that long-term antral pacing could reduce feed intake in young growing swine *(34)*. Since that time, an implantable gastric stimulator (IGS), analogous to a cardiac pacemaker, has been created and is currently being investigated both in Europe and the United States. The IGS has already been shown through clinical trials to be safe. However, the degree of success for inducing weight loss is still under investigation *(35)*. Further research is also being performed to better elucidate the precise mechanism of action, which is still unclear. The device consists of bipolar leads, which can be implanted laparoscopically within a sero-muscular tunnel along the less curvature of the stomach. The leads are connected to an electrical pulse generator that is positioned subcutaneously on the abdominal wall. At our institution, we are currently involved in the second phase of US clinical trials and have seen encouraging preliminary results. Because of the relatively high safety profile, gastric pacing is an exciting modality that warrants further investigation regarding its long-term efficacy.

7. QUALIFICATION FOR SURGERY

7.1. Indications for Surgery

Even with the tremendous advances in minimally invasive techniques, as well as improvements in perioperative care, surgery still remains an invasive and potentially life-threatening option, and should be reserved for only a small subset of patients seeking treatment. Surgery should be offered only to well-informed patients in whom the potential benefits clearly outweigh the operative risks. Currently, few studies have evaluated the cost-effectiveness of surgical vs nonoperative therapies. One study, by Martin and colleagues, found that surgery was a less costly treatment option for patients with extreme obesity and had a significantly greater success rate *(36)*.

According to guidelines set by the National Institutes of Health consensus panel, patients must first meet strict weight criteria *(37)*. Potential surgical patients must weigh more than 200% of their ideal body weight (BMI >40 kg/m^2) or have a BMI >35 kg/m^2 and suffer from obesity-associated comorbidities such as diabetes, hypertension, or sleep apnea, that should improve with weight loss. In addition, all potential candidates should have demonstrated repeated failure to control weight by medical means, including supervised dietary programs.

Traditionally, bariatric surgery was limited to patients who were older than 18 and younger than 50 yr of age *(38)*. This was based on some earlier studies that demonstrated higher operative morbidity and mortality in older patients. Better perioperative patient management as well as advancements in minimally invasive techniques has enabled many surgeons to offer surgery to older patients *(39)*. In our practice, we have safely operated on patients who were in their seventh decade of life. Currently, most bariatric programs will consider patients who are in their sixth decade of life, assuming they are otherwise acceptable candidates. The other end of the age spectrum is still controversial. Extremely obese adolescent patients will usually be physically healthy and pose minimal operative risk. However, they may not have yet reached the level of emotional maturity required to cope with the drastic life changes associated with surgery that are paramount to its success. In that setting, a good surgical outcome may not translate into a good long-term result. As the prevalence of adolescent obesity continues to grow, younger patients are increasingly being considered for surgery, particularly if they possess the appropriate behavioral support structures required. Many have demonstrated excellent weight loss with vast improvements in quality of life *(40)*.

7.2. Initial Screening

Careful patient selection and comprehensive long-term follow up are the cornerstones to long-lasting success. Dietary indiscretion and maladaptive eating behavior can result in complications and/or weight-loss failure despite an excellent surgical result. Therefore, patient screening needs to be performed to identify patients unlikely to comply. The selection process is quite comprehensive and should rely on a multidisciplinary group of clinicians in addition to the surgeons. Team members may include bariatric internists, psychologist/psychiatrists, and dietitians. After determining that a potential candidate meets the standard weight criteria, the screening process is then initiated. This process is designed to prevent undesirable candidates from undergoing surgery.

7.2.1. Comorbidities

A thorough medical evaluation is performed to affirm known comorbidities and uncover those that are often overlooked by non-bariatric physicians, such as sleep apnea. Medical conditions, such as diabetes and hypertension, must be optimally controlled prior to surgery and the degree of perioperative cardiopulmonary monitoring that will be required must be determined. Despite the complexity of the surgery and the general acknowledgment that obesity represents a high-risk condition, medical comorbidity will only disqualify patients for surgery if the medical conditions are prohibitive and the predictive operative mortality is significant enough to pose an unacceptable risk.

7.2.2. PSYCHOLOGICAL EVALUATION

Although most medical conditions do not disqualify patients from surgical consideration, behavioral issues might. Because behavior modification is necessary for long-term success following surgery, patients with significant active psychiatric disorders or mental retardation should rarely if ever be considered. In addition, a strong history of substance abuse or self-destructive behavior, including eating disorders, may preclude patients from consideration. A thorough psychological evaluation is also performed. The current living conditions, life stresses, family relationships, and childhood histories are obtained. As previously mentioned, histories of substance abuse or maladaptive behavior would preclude patients from consideration. An unstable living environment may also negatively impact results. A thorough dietary and eating history is also obtained. Patients considered for surgery must not display evidence of eating patterns (i.e., active bulimia, binge eating) that will preclude compliance with the postoperative dietary restrictions. However, patients initially rejected from surgical consideration because of behavioral issues may be reevaluated for surgery at a later time if they respond favorably to psychiatric or psychological therapy.

8. PREOPERATIVE ASSESSMENT AND PREPARATION

After clearing patients for surgery, a thorough preoperative evaluation is necessary to identify significant comorbidity. This work up should include standard surgical laboratory and radiographic studies as well as gallbladder ultrasonography, cardiac evaluation, pulmonary function tests, and upper GI fluoroscopy when indicated. Specialty consults, such as cardiology, endocrinology, and pulmonary, may also be required prior to surgery. Although comorbidities rarely exclude patients from consideration for surgery, they may alter the surgical and anesthetic management of the patient in the perioperative period. A difficult airway and chronic pain with narcotic dependence are some examples. We generally require patients to lose approx 10% of their body weight prior to surgery in hope of decreasing intra-abdominal adiposity and hepatic steatosis. This may decrease operative complications.

Patient education is also an important component of the preoperative preparatory process. During this preoperative period, extensive teaching, counseling, and supervised dietary instructions are provided. A good understanding of the operative changes to gastric capacity and function, dietary restrictions, and potential long-term nutritional concerns is critical to a good outcome. Patients unable to grasp these issues may not make good operative candidates. Patients should also have a full understanding of the potential operative complications.

9. PERIOPERATIVE AND POSTOPERATIVE MANAGEMENT

Perioperative management should focus on minimizing postoperative complications. This involves consideration of standard postoperative issues as well as those that are more unique to the obese patient. Venous access and fluid management must be addressed prior to surgery. Although most patients are extubated and removed from mechanical ventilation at the conclusion of surgery, pulmonary toilet and gas exchange must be carefully monitored, particularly for those patients with sleep apnea. We encourage patients with diagnosed sleep apnea who are on home continuous positive airway pressure devices

(CPAP) to continue using CPAP until the time surgery and we restart CPAP on the first postoperative day.

Patient-controlled analgesia has improved early postoperative pain management and pulmonary toilet. In our program, because the majority of procedures are performed laparoscopically, epidurals are rarely used. However, they may be of great benefit for open surgeries. Most surgeons will utilize compression sleeves and/or low-dose heparin to decrease the likelihood of venous thrombosis. Some studies have advocated the use of low-molecular-weight heparins, but dosing in the obese is not currently known *(41)*. Early ambulation is also critical. Patients are encouraged to ambulate on the evening after surgery. A nasogastric tube, traditionally used after many GI procedures, is rarely left in place after surgery. Patients start oral intake with small volumes of water usually on the first postoperative day and progress through a defined dietary protocol. Most patients are discharged from the hospital by the second or third day after surgery on a nutritious liquid diet. They are then transitioned to solids as outpatients over the next 5 wk.

Because obesity is a high-risk condition, clinicians must be alert to signs of a potential postoperative complication, since early recognition and treatment are often critical. Respiratory insufficiency may be seen with pneumonia, atelectasis, pulmonary embolus, and even congestive heart failure. Leg swelling or pain may indicate deep vein thrombosis. The most severe complication that may be seen in the early postoperative period is GI leak and the rapid development of severe peritonitis. Obese patients with peritonitis rapidly manifest severe shock and multiple organ dysfunction and therefore the diagnosis and treatment must be done quickly. Fever, tachycardia, tachypnea, severe abdominal or back pain, excessive fluid requirements, anxiety, or the "feeling of doom" are some of the signs and symptoms. A gastrograffin swallow radiograph or computed tomography scan should be obtained to detect a leak. However, if the patient appears to be deteriorating or if the index of suspicion of a leak is high despite no evidence of leak on x-ray, an emergent reoperation is justified.

10. LONG-TERM CONSIDERATIONS

A good surgical result does not ensure a successful long-term outcome. The degree of weight loss and the ability to keep it off long-term appears to be as much behavioral as surgical. Bothe et al. described the process as containing three priorities; cue control and food-avoidance behavior change, establishment of increased activity patterns, and weight-reducing surgery *(13)*. Despite our ability to surgically reduce gastric storage capacity, patients must modify their eating behaviors and increase their physical activities. Guidelines and diet plans are often necessary to prevent the tendency to resume inappropriate eating. One such set of eating guidelines dictates that patients consume three small solid meals daily. These meals are eaten very slowly with approx 1 min between each bite. No liquids are allowed with meals, and the meal should cease when the sensation of restriction occurs.

In our experience, patient compliance and outcome are directly related to the number of follow-up office visits. Follow-up visits should address psychological issues, ongoing nutritional concerns, as well as screen for signs of potential failure. Patients given access to seminars, tutorial sessions, and group meetings develop the sense of partnership in their weight-loss program and are more eager to participate. Patients who do not participate or those rarely seen in follow-up, tend to do less well or ultimately fail. Again, the vast resources of a multidisciplinary team are quite useful.

Despite the excellent weight-loss results after surgery, patients after GBP may present with various problems. These can be divided into nutritional and GI categories (see Table 5). Nutritional concerns include malnutrition, dehydration, vitamin deficiencies, and weight-loss failure. The GI issues are those related directly to the abdominal viscera.

Most problems after surgery can be easily diagnosed and treated. Vitamin deficiencies are prevalent after GBP and BPD (42–45). Serum iron, folate and B_{12} are the most common deficiencies. Other vitamin and mineral deficiencies include vitamin A deficiency, noted in 10% of patients, hypokalemia in 56%, and hypomagnesemia in 34% (43). Our program also screens for vitamin D deficiency, but the incidence is low. Most patients will require lifelong supplementation. The VBG and LAGB generally cause few nutritional deficiencies (46). However, deficiencies may develop in patients with intractable vomiting or deficient intake. For all patients, serum vitamin levels need to be checked yearly and deficiencies promptly corrected.

Dehydration is commonly seen after most bariatric procedures. Patients often have difficulty drinking adequate fluids. It typically occurs in the first few months following surgery and during the summer months. Furthermore, vomiting and diarrhea may exacerbate fluid derangements. Once dehydrated, these patients have great difficulty "catching up" because they cannot drink fluid quickly. For patients not vomiting, fluid status can be managed by encouraging patients to travel with a fluid source (i.e., sports bottle) and drink throughout the day one swallow at a time until the symptoms of dehydration are relieved. For those patients with vomiting, intravenous fluid may be necessary to restore lost intravascular volume.

Weight-loss failures occur in approx 20 to 25% of patients (17). Few failures can be traced to technical errors. In most cases, dietary noncompliance or behavioral changes are to blame. In these cases, patients chronically overeat and/or abuse calorie-dense foods, candies, or sweets. Patients may present with chronic vomiting, increasing appetite, increasing meal capacity, and gradual weight gain. Most will also have abandoned exercise.

GI problems can occur even in patients who are doing well after their surgery. Nausea, vomiting, abdominal pain, and constipation are common complaints that require evaluation. Persistent nausea can be found in some patients in the first few months after surgery. It can be caused by a number of factors including eating habits and medications. If it is not associated with vomiting, it can usually be treated conservatively, occasionally with the aid of anti-emetics. Vomiting poses more of a potential problem. Vomiting has been described to occur in up to one-third of patients postoperatively (18). It is usually the result of overeating or incomplete chewing. The incidence of vomiting can be minimized with the appropriate use of the dietary and behavioral support structures both before and after surgery. However, vomiting may also have anatomic causes and may need further evaluation. Outlet stenosis, marginal ulcerations, internal hernias, partial small bowel obstructions, medications, gallstones, and even constipation can cause vomiting. Other less common causes (pregnancy, gastroenteritis, food poisoning, etc.) that may cause vomiting in people who have not had gastric restrictive surgery should also be considered. As with vomiting, abdominal pain can be encountered anytime after surgery and can be the result of causes both related and unrelated to the operation.

Table 7
Expected Long-Term Outcomes After Gastric Restrictive Surgery

Comorbidity	Improved or resolved
Diabetes	100%
Coronary artery disease	100%
Hypercholesterolemia	96%
Gastroesophageal reflux disease	96%
Obstructive sleep apnea	93%
Hypertension	88%
Osteoarthritis	88%
Hypertriglyceridemia	86%
Depression	55%

Adapted from ref. *42*.

Generally speaking, the workup should be the same as for any patient presenting with abdominal pain after an abdominal procedure.

Internal herniation is an uncommon complication after GBP. It is caused by the migration of bowel into abnormal spaces created at time of surgery. The bowel may kink or obstruct. The diagnosis is often difficult to make as radiographic studies are usually negative. The diagnosis should be considered in any patient with unexplained pain. This pain is typically episodic, recurrent, sudden, severe, and without any logical patterns. Exploration is necessary and often done laparoscopically even when the original surgery was an open procedure.

11. SURGICAL RESULTS

All of the current procedures for weight loss can achieve approx 40 to 60% of excess weight loss. Weight loss after GBP is reported to be about 60% of excess weight within the first 2 yr and remains stable over time *(15,20)*. The very long limb gastric bypass and biliopancreatic bypass often exceed this amount. More significant than the amount of weight loss is the ability to sustain the loss over time. As previously stated, long-term success requires more than a good procedure. It also requires a programmatic effort to provide ongoing aftercare that includes both medical and behavioral follow-up. Obesity programs that can provide these services succeed at maintaining excellent long-term results. For example, Pories and coworkers *(15)* reported sustained weight loss 14 yr after GBP (49% of excess weight). Similar results have been reported by Scopinaro and associates for the BPD *(10,47)*.

Although excellent weight loss and its resultant cosmetic benefits are not insignificant, the primary goal of the surgery is to induce sufficient weight loss to ameliorate associated medical problems such as diabetes, heart disease, and respiratory abnormalities. Although it is currently not known what magnitude of weight loss is necessary to improve the health of the severely obese patient, it appears that the obesity-associated medical conditions improve or resolve at more modest weight loss than that achieved with surgery (*see* Chapter 10). Currently, a number of reports have demonstrated improvement and even resolution of these morbid obesity-associated diseases with surgically induced weight loss (Table 7).

Diabetes and glucose intolerance improve greatly after bariatric surgery. Herbst and coworkers *(48)* first reported improvement in blood sugar control in 23 morbidly obese patients with adult-onset diabetes mellitus 6 wk after surgery. Fourteen of their patients no longer required insulin and another seven patients were able to reduce their insulin requirements by 72%. Weight loss in this group averaged only 30 kg. Pories et al. *(15)* more recently reported similar results with a significantly larger patient population. In more than 500 patients, they found that 82.9% of patients with preoperative non-insulin-dependent diabetes and 98.7% of patients with glucose impairment maintained normal levels of plasma glucose, glycosylated hemoglobin, and insulin postoperatively.

The beneficial effects of weight loss on cardiovascular disease have also been described. Gleysteen et al. *(49)* reported decreased serum triglyceride levels and improved lipid profiles in 42 morbidly obese patients 1 yr after surgery. The group had a mean weight loss of 61% of excess weight. They also noted maintenance of the improved lipid profiles 5 to 7 yr postoperatively despite a 12% weight regain. Alpert and coworkers *(50)* studied ventricular function using echocardiography in morbidly obese patients both pre-operatively and after weight loss. They reported significant improvements in left ventricular ejection fraction and lesser improvements in chamber size and ventricular wall thickness. They also noted improvement in blood pressure. Successful treatment of hypertension was also reported by Foley et al. *(51)*.

Pulmonary manifestations of morbid obesity include the obesity-hypoventilation syndrome and the sleep apnea syndrome. Both problems are life-threatening and can occur together (Pickwickian Syndrome). Sugerman and coworkers *(52)* found an incidence of at least one of these disorders in 14% of their patients. After GBP (mean loss of 45% of excess weight), they found improvement or cure in most of their patients. Improvements in arterial blood oxygenation, carbon dioxide retention, lung volumes, frequency of episodes of sleep apnea, and resolution of polycythemia vera were also described.

A number of other obesity-associated medical problems have also been shown to improve or resolve after surgically induced weight loss. These include infertility, arthritis, chronic back pain, skin conditions, gastroesophageal reflux, pseudotumor cerebri, venous stasis disease, chronic lower extremity edema, dyspnea on exertion, and depression.

12. CONCLUSION

The incidence of extreme obesity is increasing worldwide. The consequences and the cost to society are significant. There is still no cure. Nonsurgical treatments are still inadequate for achieving significant and/or sustained weight loss. Surgical approaches have evolved into safe and effective options. Laparoscopic techniques continue to advance the field and may prove to become the new "gold standard" of the future. For appropriately selected and carefully prepared patients, surgery can achieve the weight loss necessary to improve or prevent the development of significant medical conditions and improve quality of life. However, it is best utilized in the setting of a multidisciplinary treatment model. Until science finds a cure to the underlying biologic derangements that cause obesity, surgery will continue to be the most cost-effective and successful treatment option available.

REFERENCES

1. Flegal KM, Carroll MD, Ogden CL, et al. Prevalence and trends in obesity among US adults, 1999–2000. JAMA 2002; 288:1723–1727.

2. Professor Philip James, Chair of the London-based International Obesity Task Force, Monte Carlo, March 17, 2003. Website: (www.iotf.org/media).
3. World Health Report 2002. Website: (www.iotf.org).
4. Mokdad AH, Ford ES, Bowman BA, et al. Prevalence of obesity, diabetes, and obesity-related health risk factors, 2001. JAMA 2003; 289:76–79.
5. Colditz GA. Economic costs of obesity and inactivity. Medicine Sports 1999; 31:S663–S667.
6. Kremen AJ, Linner JH, Nelson CH. An experimental evaluation of the nutritional importance of proximal and distal small intestine. Ann Surg 1954; 140:439–448.
7. Halverson JD, Scheff RJ, Gentry K, et al. Jejunoileal bypass. Late metabolic sequelae and weight gain. Am J Surg 1980; 140:347–350.
8. Lowell JA, Shenoy S, Ghalib R, et al. Liver transplantation after jejunoileal bypass for morbid obesity. J Am Coll Surg 1997; 185:123–127.
9. Scopinaro N, Gianetta E, Civalleri D, et al. Bilio-pancreatic bypass for obesity. II. Initial experience in man. Br J Surg 1979; 66:618–620.
10. Scopinaro N, Gianetta E, Adami GF, et al. Biliopancreatic diversion for obesity at eighteen years. Surgery 1996; 119:261–268.
11. Marceau P, Hould FS, Simard S, et al. Biliopancreatic diversion with duodenal switch. World J Surg 1998; 22:947–954.
12. Mason EE, Ito C. Gastric bypass in obesity. Surg Clin North Am 1967; 47:1345–1352.
13. Bothe A, Bistrian BR, Greenberg I. Energy regulation in morbid obesity by multidisciplinary therapy. Surg Clin North Am 1979; 59:1017–1031.
14. Cummings DE, Wiegle DS, Fray RS, et al. Plasma ghrelin levels after diet induced weight loss or gastric bypass surgery. NEJM 2002; 346:1623–1630.
15. Pories WJ, Swanson MS, MacDonald KG, et al. Who would have thought it? An operation proves to be the most effective therapy for adult-onset diabetes mellitus. Ann Surg 1995; 222:339–352.
16. Benotti, PN, Forse, RA. The role of gastric surgery in the multidisciplinary management of severe obesity. Am J Surg 1995; 169:361–367.
17. MacLean LD, Rhode BM, Sampalis J, et al. Results of the surgical treatment of obesity. Am J Surg 1993; 165:155–159.
18. Halverson JD. Metabolic risk of obesity surgery and long-term follow-up. Am J Clin Nutr 1992; 55: 602s–605s.
19. Mason EE. Vertical banded gastroplasty for obesity. Arch Surg 1982; 117:701–706.
20. Capella, JF, Capella RF. The weight reduction operation of choice: vertical banded gastroplasty or gastric bypass? Am J Surg 1996; 171:74–74.
21. Brolin RE, Robertson LB, Kenler HA, et al. Weight loss and dietary intake after vertical banded gastroplasty and roux-en- bypass. Ann Surg 1994; 220:782–790.
22. Sugerman HJ, Londrey GL, Kellum JM, et al. Weight loss with vertical banded gastroplasty and Roux-Y gastric bypass for morbid obesity with selective versus random assignment. Am J Surg 1989; 157: 93–102.
23. Kuzmak L. Silicone gastric banding: a simple and effective operation for morbid obesity. Contemp Surgery 1986; 28:13–18.
24. Belachew M, Legrand M, Defechereux T, et al. Laparoscopic adjustable silicone gastric banding in the treatment of morbid obesity: a preliminary report. Surg Endosc 1994; 8:1354–1356,.
25. Cadiere GB, Himpens J, Vertruyen M, et al. Laparoscopic gastroplasty (adjustable silicone gastric banding). Semin Laparosc Surg 2000; 7:55–65.
26. O'Brien PE, Brown WA, Smith A, et al. Prospective study of a laparoscopically placed, adjustable gastric band in the treatment of morbid obesity. Br J Surg 1999; 86:113–118.
27. Rubenstein RB. Laparoscopic adjustable gastric banding at a U.S. center with up to 3-year follow-up. Obes Surg 2002; 12:380–384.
28. Sugerman HJ, Kellum JM, Reines HD, et al. Greater risk of incisional hernia with morbidly obese than steroid-dependent patients and low recurrence with prefascial polypropylene mesh. Am J Surg 1996; 171:80–84,.
29. Wittgrove AC, Clark GW. Laparoscopic gastric bypass, Roux-en-Y- 500 patients: technique and results, with 3–60 month follow-up. Obesity Surg 2000; 10:233–239.

30. Nguyen NT, Lee SL, Goldman C, et al. Comparison of pulmonary function and postoperative pain after laparoscopic versus open gastric bypass: a randomized trial. J Am Coll Surg 2001; 192:469–476.
31. Higa KD, Boone KB, Ho T. Complications of the laparoscopic roux-en-Y gastric bypass: 1040 patients—what have we learned? Obes Surg 2000; 10:509–513.
32. Schauer PR, Ikramuddin S, Gourash W, et al. Outcomes after laparoscopic roux-en-Y gastric bypass for morbid obesity. Ann Surg 2000; 232:515–529.
33. Nguyen NT, Ho HS, Palmer Ls, et al. A Comparison study of laparoscopic versus open gastric bypass for morbid obesity. J Am Coll Surg 2000; 191:149–157.
34. Cigaina VV, Saggioro A, Rigo VV, et al. Long-term effects of gastric pacing to reduce feed intake in swine. Obes Surg 1996; 6:250–253.
35. Cigaina V. Gastric pacing as therapy for morbid obesity: preliminary results. Obes Surg 2002; 12:12S–16S.
36. Martin LF, Tan T-L, Horn JR, et al. Comparison of the costs associated with medical and surgical treatment of obesity. Surgery 1995; 118:599–607.
37. Gastrointestinal surgery for severe obesity. National Institutes of Health Consensus Development Conference Statement. Am J Clin Nutr 1992; 55:615s–619s.
38. Printen KJ, Mason EE. Gastric bypass for morbid obesity for patients more than 50 years of age. Surg Gynecol Obstet 1977; 144:192–194.
39. MacGregor AMC, Rand CS. Gastric surgery in morbid obesity: outcome in patients aged 55 and older. Arch Surg 1993; 128:1153–1157.
40. Strauss RS, Bradley LJ, Brolin RE. Gastric bypass surgery in adolescents with morbid obesity. J Pediatr 2001; 138:499–504.
41. Kalfarentzos F, Stavropoulou F, Yarmenitis S, et al. Prophylaxis of venous thromboembolism using two different doses of low-molecular-weight heparin (nadroparin) in bariatric surgery: a prospective randomized trial. Obesity Surgery 2001; 11:670–676.
42. Avinoah E, Ovnat A, Charuzi I. Nutritional status seven years after Roux-en-Y gastric bypass surgery. Surgery 1992; 111:137–142.
43. Halverson JD. Micronutrient deficiencies after gastric bypass for morbid obesity. Am Surg 1986; 52: 594–598.
44. Amaral JF, Thompson WR, Caldwell MD, et al. Prospective hematologic evaluation of gastric exclusion surgery for morbid obesity. Ann Surg 1985; 201:186–192.
45. Rhode BM, Arseneau P, Cooper BA, et al. Vitamin B-12 deficiency after gastric bypass surgery for obesity. Am J Clin Nutr 1996; 63:103–109.
46. Printen KJ, Halverson JD. Hemic micronutrients following vertical banded gastroplasty. Am Surg 1988; 54:267–268.
47. Scopinaro N, Adami GF, Marinari GM, et al. Biliopancreatic diversion. World J Surg 1998; 22:936–946.
48. Herbst CA, Hughes TA, Gwynne JT, et al. Gastric bariatric operation in insulin-treated adults. Surgery 1984; 95:209–214.
49. Gleysteen JJ, Barboriak JJ, Sasse EA. Sustained coronary-risk-factor reduction after gastric bypass for morbid obesity. Am J Clin Nutr 1990; 51:774–778.
50. Alpert MA, Singh A, Terry BE, et al. Effect of exercise on left ventricular systolic function and reserve in morbid obesity. Am J Card 1989; 63:1478–1482.
51. Foley EF, Benotti PN, Borlase BC, et al. Impact of gastric restrictive surgery on hypertension in the morbidly obese. Am J Surg 1992; 186:294–297.
52. Sugerman HJ, Fairman RP, Baron PL, et al. Gastric surgery for respiratory insufficiency of obesity. Chest 1986; 90:81–86.

21 Clinical Experience in a Comprehensive Weight-Management Center

Judy Loper and Richard A. Lutes

KEY POINTS

- Obesity treatment requires a multifaceted approach that can be optimally delivered in a comprehensive weight-management program.
- Lifestyle modification and education remain the cornerstone of obesity treatment.
- Obesity treatment requires long-term commitment and follow-up.

1. INTRODUCTION

The treatment of obesity is very rewarding and challenging. We have enjoyed nearly 26 yr of providing a comprehensive weight-management program to our community. Our program began in one small room and now fills four large office suites throughout Columbus, Ohio. What follows is a description of a comprehensive weight-management program that has proven successful through many years. Along with this is a description of the experience of a typical patient, Mary S., who participated in all phases of our program. The chapter is outlined in Table 1.

2. PROGRAM DESCRIPTION

Our program is divided into seven phases. Phase 1 is the free orientation visit and phase 2 includes the nutritional assessment by the dietitian. Phase 3 is the doctor's physical examination and evaluation for the very low-calorie diet (VLCD) treatment. Phase 4 is the active weight-loss phase and can be time-limited or open-ended. If this phase is time-limited, then the patient may choose to follow the VLCD for 12 or 16 wk and then begin transition. If a patient chooses an open-ended program, he or she may follow the regimen until the desirable or healthy weight is reached. Phase 5 is refeeding or transition back to a regular low-calorie maintenance diet. In this phase, the patient can choose to enter a research protocol utilizing combination anti-obesity medications, which would continue throughout the final phase of the program. Phase 6 is lifestyle

From: *The Management of Eating Disorders and Obesity, Second Edition*
Edited by: D. J. Goldstein © Humana Press Inc., Totowa, NJ

Table 1
Chapter Overview

1. Introduction
2. Program Description
    2.1. Phase 1: Patient Orientation
    2.2. Phase 2: Nutritional Assessment
    2.3. Phase 3: Physician Evaluation
    2.4. Phase 4: Active Weight Loss
    2.5. Phase 5. Refeeding
    2.6. Phase 6: Behavior Modification and Maintenance
    2.7. Phase 7: Long-Term Intervention
3. Caveats
4. Conclusion

Table 2
Program Description

Phase 1:	Orientation visit
	Explanation of program, staff, options, risks, and costs
Phase 2:	Nutritional assessment by dietitian
	Develop personalized plan
	Rapport-building
Phase 3:	Physician evaluation
Phase 4:	Active weight loss
Phase 5:	Refeeding, transition to maintenance
Phase 6:	Lifestyle modification and maintenance
Phase 7:	Long-term intervention
Caveats:	Empathy
	Staff selection
	Marketing

modification and maintenance. This phase can be either an individual appointment with the dietitian or in a group setting with other maintenance patients. The final phase (Phase 7) is long-term intervention that can continue for many years according to the needs of the patient (*see* Table 2).

2.1. Phase 1: Orientation Visit

Mary S. was approved to participate in our comprehensive weight-management program. She came to the center for an evening orientation accompanied by her husband, and she listened attentively to the presentation by the dietitian. She completed a questionnaire about her weight history. There are seven patients attending this orientation and they ask questions about the different weight-management options. After the information session is completed, Mary met with the office manager to discuss insurance concerns and with the dietitian to discuss her diet options. The medical assistant obtained her baseline height, weight, and blood pressure. She was interested in the VLCD option and scheduled an appointment for the initial evaluation.

Our philosophy of the treatment of obesity is presented at the free group orientation session. We treat obesity as a chronic disease and we tell the participants that we offer them lifelong support. The dietitian, knowledgeable about all aspects of the center, leads the group presentation. Participants are asked about their individual weight histories and how they heard about our comprehensive weight-management program. The professional qualifications of our staff along with a description of the various treatment options are presented.

Among the treatment options are VLCDs, low-calorie diets, special diets, and various combinations of these (*see* Chapter 16). The VLCD provides 70 to 100 g of high-quality protein per day either in a powdered formulation that must be mixed with water, or a low calorie fluid, or in the form of lean meat, fish, or fowl. The VLCD of lean meats generally contains 1.2 g of protein per kilogram of desirable body weight as described by Bistrian *(1)*. Small amounts of carbohydrate are also contained in the regimen. High-fiber bars are used by some patients with the VLCD. Another option for patients is part formula and part food. This option is individualized for each patient. This individualization would be based on the patient's medical history, lifestyle, and personal preferences. A brief discussion of the history of the VLCD development, indications for use, and common side effects, risks, and benefits of the VLCD are presented. Finally, the treatment results of our program are shared with the group.

2.2. Phase 2: Nutritional Assessment

Mary met with the dietitian for her initial nutritional assessment. She completed a lifestyle inventory, depression inventory, health history form, and read the informed consent. She is 68 in tall, weighed 310 lb, and had a calculated body mass index (BMI) of 47.1. Her percentage of body fat was 43%. She had a chest circumference of 50 in, waist circumference of 48 in, and hip circumference of 44 in. She met with the dietitian to discuss the diet plan, nutritional assessment results, and informed consent. Mary chose the formula VLCD. The dietitian reviewed her plan and together they made out a feeding schedule. The medical assistant took some photographs of Mary. Blood was drawn for laboratory work and an electrocardiogram I(EKG) was performed.

In Phase 2, the dietitian reviews a lifestyle inventory that includes a 1-d dietary recall, family history of obesity, previous weight-management attempts, family support, and body image. The dietitian also addresses patient motivation to lose weight and the patient's expectations. Body composition is determined by bioelectrical impedance. Resting metabolic rate is determined by the BodyGem™, a handheld instrument that determines metabolic rate. The medical assistant measures height, weight, chest circumference, waist circumference, hip circumference, and blood pressure. BMI (weight in kilograms divided by height in meters squared) and the waist-to-hip ratio are calculated by the dietitian. The body composition results include the percentage of body fat, body fat in pounds, the percentage of lean body mass, the lean body mass in pounds, the percentage of body water, and an optimal weight based on these findings.

The dietitian uses the above calculated information and the patient's weight history to discuss a target or healthy weight with the patient. Photographs—side and frontal view—are taken for identification purposes and to provide a visual form of motivation for the patient.

The diet plan that is determined to be most appropriate by a review of all the patient's information and the patient's personal preferences is reviewed in detail by the dietitian. Recipes, dietary exclusions, techniques for enhancing compliance, and permitted medications, while on the VLCD plan, are discussed. If the patient chooses the lean meat VLCD, then supplementation with calcium, potassium chloride, and other vitamins and minerals are given. If the patient chooses the formula VLCD, the dietitian reviews formula preparation, recipes, spacing of formula individualized for lifestyle, and calorie-free beverage consumption. Some patients choose a mixture of formula and food. A typical plan may be four supplements plus one meal per day. The meal may consist of four ounces of lean meat and some vegetables in limited quantities. Commercial low-calorie frozen entrees are sometimes used in place of self-prepared food, allowing for ease of preparation, clean-up, and stimuli-narrowing. We find this popular for people who are working and for people who want to eat a meal with their family.

Next, the dietitian reviews the informed consent in detail with the patient. Any questions are answered or referred to the physician, who gives final approval for the chosen diet plan based on the patient's medical history.

This thorough orientation, including the informed consent process, helps build the rapport that is important for long-term success. The patient also is given a notebook that contains program information, including office hours, medical bureau telephone numbers, emergency food lists, and techniques for compliance. The notebook also contains information for other family members in how they may encourage, enhance, and support the dieter throughout the entire program. Family and friends can be a great deal of support if they are well informed and understand the treatment modality and goals of the patient.

2.3. Phase 3: Physician Evaluation

At her physical examination, Mary's weight was 310 lb and her blood pressure (BP) was 150/100. The doctor reviewed her medical history. Her physical examination was remarkable for hyperpigmentation of her neck folds and axillary folds. She had no discernible retinopathy. She had mild inspiratory rales on lung exam and distant heart sounds. Jugular venous distention to 4 cm above the clavicle was seen at 30 degrees. Mild pitting edema was seen in her legs. Review of lab work obtained was remarkable for a fasting blood sugar of 200 mg/dL, high-density lipoprotein of 20 mg/dL, triglycerides of 300 mg/dL,, total cholesterol of 320 mg/dL, and calculated low-density lipoprotein cholesterol of 240 mg/dL. Hepatic tests were mildly elevated. Her EKG was unremarkable except for left-anterior hemiblock. The doctor reviewed the informed consent for a VLCD regimen with her. Modifications of her medications were discussed. A letter to her primary care physician about her VLCD regimen was completed. Mary was asked to change her insulin dosage and to measure home blood glucose at least twice daily. She was given information on how to contact the doctor if she had problems or questions.

The doctor of the comprehensive weight-management program needs to be familiar with fasting physiology. Diuretics are usually discontinued. As the patient loses weight on the VLCD, sodium accompanies the diuresis. The patient may be at risk for hypertension. Diabetic patients often benefit significantly as glucotoxicity is rapidly reversed.

As blood sugars often decline rapidly with the VLCD, insulin and other hypoglycemic therapy need to be adjusted at the initial physical examination visit. Metformin is theoretically not problematic as it decreases hepatic glucose production and is not a hypoglycemic agent. The comprehensive weight-management program doctor assumes the responsibility of monitoring diet-related medical problems that might arise during treatment. Patients referred by their primary care physicians to our dietitians for low-calorie diet options are managed in conjunction with the primary care physician.

2.4. Phase 4: Active Weight Loss

At her first office visit, Mary attended a group lecture on stress management. She lost 10 lb the first wk and her insulin requirements dropped from 160 U/d to 20 U/d. She had experienced no hypoglycemic episodes. Her home glucose values ranged from 90 to 200. She was breathing better and reported having more energy. Her hunger was diminished. The dietitian complimented her on her 100% compliance. She was encouraged to keep up the good work.

Patients on the VLCD regimen attend weekly office visits. Group classes last 30 to 40 min and are led by the dietitian, psychologist, or exercise psychologist. The format of the group sessions varies from wk to wk with lecture, discussion, and lots of group participation. Twenty-six topics including behavior modification, nutrition education, stress management, the psychological aspects of weight management and exercise are rotated on a weekly basis. One popular topic is a presentation by successful weight maintainers. Many of our patients are very dedicated and contribute to the group interaction. These group sessions are strongly encouraged and occur at the beginning of the office visit session. The patient is then seen individually by the doctor and dietitian. The dietitian reviews compliance and answers any questions related to the diet. Motivation and expectations continue to be discussed with the patient. Each week, the patient is asked about his or her activity level, and moderate exercise is encouraged. We feel the dietitian–patient relationship is important for long-term success with weight maintenance. Continuity of care with the same dietitian and doctor is extremely important. At each visit, the doctor reviews medically related problems of the VLCD and addresses common complaints such as constipation or dizziness. Adjustments in medications are made by the doctor at the weekly office visits. We adhere to standard laboratory monitoring protocols for VLCDs.

2.5. Phase 5: Refeeding

After 16 wk on the VLCD, Mary had lost 60 lb and had adhered to the VLCD remarkably well. She was off insulin and had normal blood sugar. Her energy level had increased and her husband reported less snoring at night. Her BP was normal and her lipids were much improved. She was ready to transition and added food gradually back into her diet. Repeat nutritional assessment by bioelectrical impedance revealed a 10% decrease in body fat. Her BMI was 38. The dietitian discussed transitional feeding with her.

The transition to food is determined in conjunction with the doctor, dietitian, and patient. We find it useful to repeat a nutritional assessment at this time to help determine the time to transition to food. During the VLCD, we provide flexibility of meal plans based on the patient's preferences, lifestyle, and issues such as vacations, meetings, and social events. The frequent office visits make it helpful to problem-solve with the patient. The transition from the VLCD is gradual and structured. Patients are most comfortable with this approach because they have become used to a structured plan on the VLCD. Transitional feeding is sometimes a time of anxiety for these patients. They have been very successful on the VLCD and now have to deal with food and restraint. Some researchers believe that the VLCD is successful with many patients because of stimuli-narrowing *(2)*. Stimuli-narrowing is the concept of having a structured food plan without much choice and variety. We try to maintain some stimuli-narrowing throughout the transitional feeding and long-term maintenance. Throughout transition, specific dietary instruction adding small amounts of food each week is given by the dietitian. This minimizes refeeding edema commonly seen with rapid refeeding. Most medical comorbidities have been eliminated or greatly reduced by this time. We ask patients who desire to continue the VLCD after 16 wk to reread and sign a new informed consent form. Transitional refeeding usually lasts 4 to 6 wk depending on amount of weight lost and compliance.

2.6. Phase 6: Lifestyle Modification and Maintenance

Mary decided to participate in a research protocol studying combination anti-obesity medications and their effect on long-term weight maintenance. The medication used for Mary was phentermine. Mary was on the lowest dose of this medication after the research informed consent form was signed and discussed with her. Common side effects of this medication were reviewed by the comprehensive weight-management program doctor. Mary was now ready for the lifestyle modification phase of the program.

During the lifestyle modification phase of the comprehensive weight-management program, the patient has the option of coming every week to the office. The patient participates in a new group session geared toward people who are back on regular food and eating a low-fat diet. The group session is led by the dietitian with the psychologist and exercise psychologist as occasional leaders. During this phase, the patient learns how to stabilize his or her weight. Exercise habits are strongly emphasized, as well as support from family and friends. Those patients on anti-obesity medications continue to see the doctor every 2 wk for any adjustment in medications. Patients also may see the dietitian individually if they are finishing up the refeeding phase of the program. Maintenance diets can consist of all regular food or commercial frozen low-calorie entrees. Often, a patient may choose to keep some of the formula in the maintenance plan. For example, a patient may continue to take one or two packets of the supplements for breakfast and eat regular meals at lunch and dinner. For patients who prefer to have more choice in their diet, the exchange list system by the American Diabetic and Dietetic Associations can be used *(3)*. Some patients prefer to count calories and some prefer to count fat grams. Maintenance diets are very individualized, and flexibility is the key to long-term success.

2.7. Phase 7: Long-Term Intervention

Mary tolerated the combination anti-obesity medication regimen with only minor side effects. She had dry mouth initially. She lost 20 lb over 6 mo and has maintained that weight loss. She is adhering well to a 1000-cal diet and her blood sugars are normal without diabetic medication. She struggles a bit with weekly family events but has remained in control. She regularly attends the twice-monthly maintenance group sessions for reinforcement of lifestyle modification principles.

The long-term intervention phase of the comprehensive weight-management program involves group sessions and individual appointments with the doctor as needed. In these group sessions, the patient is asked to keep food and activity records. The material presented in these sessions is innovative and is prepared individually by the dietitian. Often, a discussion leads to a presentation the following week. Nutrition information disseminated in the media is often discussed in these groups. The dietitian's responsibility is not just education but motivation as well. The long-term support given by the health professional and the other patients provide the necessary reinforcement to help the patient during high-risk situations (e.g., job changes, vacations, illnesses, family events, and problems with interpersonal relationships). These group sessions have been ongoing for many years, and it is emphasized to the patients frequently that obesity is a chronic disease and requires long-term follow up. Many patients get to know each other well and provide each other with a good deal of support. Diet intake of the maintenance patient is assessed periodically for nutritional adequacy and compliance to his or her plan. Changes are made if necessary on an individual basis.

Mary is continuing in the long-term intervention phase and continues to see the doctor every 2 wk per the research protocol. Mary is maintaining her weight loss and enjoys the group experience. She compliments the staff on their caring attitude and attentiveness. Her primary care physician is happy with the control of her medical conditions. She realizes she has come a long way but needs to stay focused on her healthy habits. Mary is now walking 45 min a day, five times a week. Her husband continues to be supportive and accompanies her occasionally to some office visits.

3. CAVEATS

Our comprehensive weight-management program has treated obese patients for nearly 25 yr. We have changed some philosophies over the years, but have remained consistent with our basic tenets. We approach the treatment of this chronic disease with much empathy.

Staff selection is one of the most important qualities of a successful comprehensive weight-management program. In selecting staff, we choose individuals who will relate to all the different personalities of patients. Staff must have compassion, empathy, common sense, and a caring attitude for the obese patient. Technical skills alone, although important, are not enough to make a successful employee. A caring, compassionate attitude must be present by the receptionist who answers the phone, as well as all other health professionals. The office environment should be friendly and appealing.

In marketing a comprehensive weight-management program, the most effective tool is a happy patient. Most of our patient referrals have been generated by the success of our patients. We have tried various advertising techniques and have found the most effective to be newspaper advertisements. In addition, we prepare and send our own newsletter three times a year to current and past patients, referring physicians, and insurance companies. We also keep local physicians informed about our center and our treatment of obesity.

The biggest criticism of weight-loss programs, in general, is the experience of patients being unable to maintain their weight loss. Some large clinical trials have elucidated results of the VLCD. In one study, of the patients who completed treatment, successful weight maintenance (defined as maintaining 60% or more of the lost excess weight at 18 mo) was achieved in 46% of the patients at the 18-mo follow up *(4)*. In another study, patients had kept off, on average, two-thirds of the weight that was lost during treatment on follow-up after 85 wk *(5)*. In a more recent study, for those patients who completed treatment, 59% maintained a weight loss of 10 kg or more after 1 yr *(6)*. We feel strongly there should be a universal standard to evaluate the success of a program. We decided to study the anti-obesity medications long term to see if we could improve long-term maintenance results at our center. Some of our patients have been on the regimen for 5 yr. Most patients have experienced very few side effects. Although a plateau occurred in weight loss after about 6 mo on the medications, weight regain was very small *(7)*.

4. CONCLUSION

Obesity is a chronic incurable disease that is challenging to treat. Obesity treatment requires a multifaceted approach that can be optimally delivered in a comprehensive weight-management program. Our model of dietitians and physicians working closely together facilitates medical nutritional therapy. The combination of group teaching and individualized counseling optimize resources and allows for affordable treatment. Obesity treatment requires long-term commitment and follow-up. An empathetic staff is critical for success. Obesity treatment requires people skills, expertise in dietary management, patient education skills, and savvy business management skills. Lifestyle modification and education remain the cornerstone of obesity treatment. As obesity has reached epidemic proportions in our country, we need to continue to strive for more effective and efficient treatments.

REFERENCES

1. Bistrian BR, et al. Protein requirements for net anabolism with hypocaloric diet. Clin Res 1975; 23:315A.
2. Wadden T, Kuehnel R. Very-low-calorie diet: reappraisal and recommendations. Weight Control Digest 1993.
3. American Diabetes Association and American Dietetic Association. Exchange lists for weight management. 1995.
4. Hovell MF, Koch A, Hofstelter CR, et al. Long-term weight loss maintenance: assessment of a behavioral and supplemented fasting program regimen. Am J Pub Health 1988; 78:663–666.
5. Kanders BS, Blackburn GL, Lavin P, Norten D. Weight loss outcome and health benefits associated with the Optifast program in the treatment of obesity. Int J Obes 1989; 13:131–134.
6. Wadden TA, Foster GD, Letizia KA, Stunkard AJ. A multicenter evaluation of a proprietary weight reduction program for the treatment of marked obesity. Arch Intern Med 1992; 152:961–966.
7. Lutes RA, JF Loper, EJ Baltes, RK May, JT Broyles. VLCD followed by use of phentermine for weight maintenance. Obes Res 2000; 8:72S.

22 The Multidisciplinary Team in the Management of Obesity

Patrick Mahlen O'Neil and Sherry Rieder

KEY POINTS

- In the most advantageous situation, a full- or part-time team of professionals from the different disciplines should provide a full frontal attack on weight loss and weight maintenance.
- Members of the multidisciplinary team include the registered dietitian (RD), exercise specialist, behavioral/mental health professional, physician, nurse, "lifestyle counselors," and administrative and support staff.
- When obesity treatment sites cannot staff a full-time multidisciplinary team, practitioners should attempt to acquire a cadre of consulting professionals, even if on a part-time basis.

1. INTRODUCTION

This chapter describes the qualifications and functions of each of the members of a multidisciplinary team, suggests ways to organize the functioning of such a team, and discusses ways to capture many of the strengths of the multidisciplinary team in settings where such an on-site team is not feasible (Table 1). Examples of specific situations are provided to demonstrate how the complexities of obesity therapy can require a broad range of expertise. A treatment team comprising representatives of different disciplines can provide such a scope of knowledge and skills.

Obesity is recognized widely as a multifaceted disorder with etiologies and effects spanning levels from the gene to the environment. The study of obesity proceeds in fields as diverse as molecular biology, psychology, medicine, physiology, nutrition, and epidemiology.

Because of the complex nature of obesity and the absence of a common remediable biological defect (i.e., it is a near certainty that the final outcome of obesity results from numerous combinations of causal factors), interventions for obesity are varied and represent management or palliative treatment rather than cure. Approaches to the management of obesity include not only treatments conducted upon the patient (e.g., pharmacotherapy, surgery), but also efforts to direct and motivate cognitive and behavioral changes to be implemented by the patient, especially in the areas of diet and exercise.

From: *The Management of Eating Disorders and Obesity, Second Edition*
Edited by: D. J. Goldstein © Humana Press Inc., Totowa, NJ

Table 1
Chapter Overview

Multipronged treatment requires experience and expertise in numerous areas. That is why professionally directed centers for the management of obesity typically feature a multidisciplinary staff that may include a registered dietitian, exercise physiologist, physician, nurse, and behavioral/mental health specialist, such as psychologist or clinical social worker.

1.1. Illustrative Case Histories

Near the end of a busy evening clinic, an impromptu conclave is underway around the office copier in the staff space. In attendance are a dietitian, a psychologist group leader, a physician, and an exercise physiologist. The topic is patient P.T. During several weeks on a very low-calorie diet (VLCD), P.T. has lost weight at an impressive, some think alarming, rate. He reported to the group leader and dietitian that he was consuming all necessary nutrients, but his rapid loss prompted rough body composition appraisals last week and this week by the exercise physiologist. Both tests suggest excess loss of lean body mass, even when considering the patient's avoidance of exercise. All parties in contact with P.T. report on the data they have that bear on the question. The physician orders extra lab work to ascertain whether P.T. is losing excess protein. When the lab work confirms these suspicions, the patient is referred immediately to the dietitian for a higher calorie diet.

The next wk, a dietitian is informed that another patient, C.H., confessed to the group leader that she had, for several weeks, substituted skim milk for the required VLCD supplement, which she hates. The physician had also received this report from the patient with no alarm, but the group leader consulted the dietitian. The dietitian calls C.H. and corroborates these reports. The dietitian performs some quick computations of the nutritional adequacy of this ad hoc diet, and immediately calls the physician and group leader to urge that C.H. enter the next dietary phase of the program, in which she will move to a food-based plan providing better dietary balance with less reliance on the detested supplement.

Later that wk, the physician is consulted by the group leader because most members of another group of patients had requested a weight-loss medication. The physician confers with the group leader and the dietitian. After the group leader explains that several of these patients are doing extremely well without medication and a few others have recently experienced unusual life stressors, and the dietitian reports on her plans for changes in their food plans, the physician suggests that the three of them meet with the group to explain the pros and cons of a trial of medication at this point. During this meeting, the patient group is somewhat resistant to any deferral of medication, but more than half of the original medication-seekers decide to wait.

2. MEMBERS OF THE MULTIDISCIPLINARY TEAM

2.1. Registered Dietitian

2.1.1. QUALIFICATIONS

Nutrition professionals who meet specific knowledge and educational requirements of the American Dietetic Association (ADA) may obtain registration through that group. Only those who obtain registration are authorized to use the title "registered dietitian." A bachelor's degree, including approved didactic curriculum in dietetics, and an approved practicum or internship are the minimum training level required of RDs. Successful completion of a national examination is also required. The ADA also offers a certificate in training in adult weight management requiring completion of a self-study module, a live workshop, and a posttest. Some states have their own additional licensing procedures for dietetic practitioners. The title "nutritionist" denotes no specialized training or experiences in nutrition in many states where the title can be self-conferred.

2.1.2. FUNCTIONS

The RD can conduct nutritional analyses of patients' dietary intake based on a variety of means including 24-hr recall interviews and patient self-monitoring data. These analyses can be informal, based on within-session review of eating records, or quite detailed using any of a number of existing computer software packages or internet resources. Based in part on the assessment data, the RD (a) provides the dietary prescription for each patient; (b) confers with the patient to provide modifications to the dietary prescription based on weight loss, adherence, changes in health parameters, and changes in the patient's lifestyle; and (c) instructs the patient on important nutritional issues so that the patient has the knowledge to make more healthful food choices.

The counsel of an RD is particularly important for patients who suffer obesity comorbidities, such as type 2 diabetes, hypercholesterolemia, hypertriglyceridemia, and hypertension. These conditions may affect the composition of the recommended diet regardless of caloric level. Furthermore, the RD's ongoing monitoring of the patient's eating patterns can reveal nutritional inadequacies in the weight-loss diet as actually followed, such as vitamin deficiencies, insufficient protein intake, or excessively low caloric intake.

Many RDs learn to employ behavior-modification techniques to enhance the patient's dietary adherence. They also often are familiar with behavioral procedures that can be applied to other aspects of the patient's weight-control plan. Of the nonmedical team members, the RD is often the one with the most medical knowledge and experience.

2.2. Exercise Specialist

2.2.1. QUALIFICATIONS

The generic, unregulated title, "exercise physiologist" can describe people with various, although overlapping, academic backgrounds, including physical education, exercise physiology, exercise science, and others. Exercise physiologists should be expected to have at least a bachelor's degree in one of these or related areas.

The American College of Sports Medicine (ACSM) offers certification in several exercise specialties after the applicant demonstrates the requisite knowledge and skills via combinations of written and practical exams (1). ACSM offers certification in two tracks:

1. Clinical track certifications: These are appropriate for personnel in clinical exercise programs for individuals with cardiovascular, pulmonary, and metabolic disease. The majority of individuals with ACSM clinical certifications are found in cardiac rehabilitation programs. Because of the increased risk status of many obese persons, this may be the more relevant group of certifications for members of the multidisciplinary obesity treatment team. The two certifications within this clinical track are Registered Clinical Exercise Physiologist® and ACSM Exercise Specialist®. The more rigorous Registered Clinical Exercise Physiologist® certification requires a graduate-level degree in exercise science, exercise physiology, or physiology, as well as a specified amount and breadth of clinical experiences. The ACSM Exercise Specialist® certification requires a bachelor's degree in an allied health field and the completion of a prescribed number of hours of practical experience.

2. Health and fitness track certification: The ACSM Health/Fitness Instructor(SM) certification is targeted for exercise personnel who work with apparently healthy individuals who have no history of disease or who have controlled disease. ACSM health/fitness-certified personnel can be found in corporate fitness centers, fitness clubs, wellness programs, and the like.

Another fitness-related organization, the American Council on Exercise, offers certifications for group fitness instructors and for personal trainers based on written examinations. These certifications are found primarily among fitness professionals working with members of the general population rather than with clinical groups.

Finally, although the title is certainly not approved by any exercise group, patients in our center take delight when we refer to our exercise specialists as "exercisers."

Regardless of certification status, any exercise specialist considered for participation on the multidisciplinary team should be knowledgeable about the impact of obesity and associated comorbidities on exercise capacity and should be sympathetic about the often unhappy exercise experiences of many members of this patient population (see Chapter 13).

2.2.2. Functions

The exercise specialist reviews the patient's medical background and confers with the physician to determine the patient's risk level for exercise and the need for additional testing (e.g., stress electrocardiogram [EKG]) prior to beginning self-directed exercise. ACSM guidelines *(1)* provide a useful basis for this decision.

The exercise specialist assesses the patient's baseline fitness level. In the ideal case, this fitness test would include measures of body composition, aerobic capacity, flexibility, and muscular strength. Time, equipment, and funding requirements may limit the extent of this assessment.

The exercise specialist, in collaboration with the patient and, when needed, the physician, then develops a beginning exercise prescription. The patient's progress should be monitored on a regular basis and the exercise plan modified according to progress and changes in the patient's life situation. The exercise specialist also educates the patient about important aspects of fitness, exercise, and how they relate to weight control and obesity. Perhaps most important, he or she is the main source of support, acceptance and problem solving to the patient in the frequently discouraging effort to install exercise as a permanent fixture in the patient's life.

2.3. Behavioral/Mental Health Professional

2.3.1. Qualifications

The person occupying this role on the team will usually be a psychologist or social worker, or less often, a graduate trained nurse or licensed professional counselor.

All states control the use of the "psychologist" title by licensing or certification, and, in all but a very few, the minimal education requirement for independent (unsupervised) practice is the doctoral degree. Usually a PhD Licensure in psychology also requires passing a nationally standardized written exam and, usually, a state-administered oral and/or written exam. Not all licensed psychologists are necessarily qualified to assess patients for the presence of mental disorders and/or to offer counseling or psychotherapy because some will have been trained in other areas of psychology, such as industrial psychology. In many states, licensed psychologists qualified for clinical work may carry an additional designation such as "health service provider."

The minimal educational level that should be expected of a social worker in this position on the team is the master's of social work (MSW). Some, but not all, states limit by licensure the individuals who can call themselves social workers, and it should be noted that some categories of licensure are available to persons without the MSW degree. The National Association of Social Workers offers the Academy of Certified Social Workers certificate to those who meet requirements of education (minimum of MSW), knowledge, and supervised experience.

The advanced practice registered nurse (APRN) is educated at the graduate level (master's of science in nursing education or doctoral), and should be certified nationally in a relevant specialty area, such as psychiatric mental health nursing. APRNs include clinical nurse specialists (independent practitioners) and nurse practitioners.

Counselors with other educational backgrounds are licensed by more than 40 states. The minimum requirements are a master's degree and successful completion of a written examination. Licensed counselors may specialize in mental health practice or in other areas, such as vocational counseling.

2.3.2. FUNCTIONS

The functions of the mental health specialist include, in the most general terms: pretreatment assessment, provision of cognitive–behavioral counseling and education to accomplish weight-control goals, and management of psychological/psychiatric problems whether or not associated with weight.

Initial patient assessment should include appraisal of behavioral and psychosocial factors related to eating and weight control (e.g., situational and emotional antecedents of overeating, self-efficacy regarding weight control), and issues of expectations regarding the magnitude and ease of weight loss and the impact of that weight loss on other areas of life. It is also important in some clinical settings to conduct a pretreatment screening for psychiatric disorders, especially eating disorders and mood disorders like depression and anxiety that have a high base rate in the general population.

Nearly all comprehensive weight-control programs incorporate behavior-modification principles and elements of cognitive–behavioral therapy (*see* Chapter 14). In most well-designed programs, these aspects will be woven throughout the program and integrated into all areas of desired change whether related to diet, exercise or other. In addition, it is useful to teach patients some of the fundamentals of behavioral change (e.g., proper use of goals and rewards, cognitive restructuring) so that they will have knowledge to apply later in unanticipated situations. The behavioral/mental health specialist should participate in designing these elements of the program if they are not present. Although the RD or exercise specialist will be the logical presenter of topics in their domains, even if they contain the application of behavioral principles, the behavioral/mental health specialist is the logical teacher of "Behavior Modification 101," although other team members with adequate training and experience could certainly do so.

In programs using a group-based approach to patient education and counseling, the behavioral specialist is probably most often the group leader. He or she should have knowledge and training in management of such groups. However, many effective groups, when conducted in a "psychoeducational" rather than "group-therapy" format, are led effectively by properly trained team members of other disciplines.

Regarding the third general set of functions of the behavioral specialist, it should be remembered that obesity is neither a psychiatric diagnosis nor a sign of underlying psychological turmoil. However, it is also the case that obesity confers no special protection against prevalent psychiatric disorders, and there is evidence that unlike the obese in the general population, obese people presenting for treatment may have higher rates of psychopathology than rates seen in the general population *(2–4)*. Therefore, a significant minority of obese patients in long-term treatment will at some point be in need of mental health treatment. The behavioral specialist serves screening and referral functions for such patients, and may also take on selected patients in individual treatment aimed at the psychiatric condition.

Although there are scant data supporting the contention that dieting is an expected cause of psychological distress *(4–6)*, clinical experience shows that, as is the case with any significant change in behavioral patterns, the occasional patient will require supportive individual counseling to help deal with specific obstacles. Furthermore, for a very few patients, arrival at a lower weight can entail psychologically stressful consequences, for example, anxiety-provoking sexual attention and loss of body size as the perceived cause of most unhappiness. In these varied situations, the behavioral/mental health specialist again may refer the patient or provide directly the necessary psychotherapy.

It should be noted that the mental health specialist should review carefully his or her other programmatic relations with the patient before agreeing to add a psychotherapeutic relationship to the mix. Some of the demands of the latter relationship may conflict with requirements of other contacts (e.g., behavioral education) concerned with the overall weight-control program, and vice versa. At the least, the specialist should discuss this matter clearly with the patient before taking him or her on as a therapy patient.

2.4. Physician

2.4.1. QUALIFICATIONS

A license to practice medicine is obviously required. No particular specialization is necessary, but knowledge and experience in general internal medicine, family medicine, or endocrinology are particularly useful with this population. "Bariatric physicians" designate themselves as such to indicate a practice concentration in obesity and weight control. However, "bariatric medicine" is not a medical specialty recognized by the American Board of Medical Specialties (ABMS), the umbrella organization for the 24 approved medical specialty boards in the United States that certify specialists in such areas as endocrinology, pediatrics, and the like. As with other members of the team, understanding of the chronic nature of obesity and tolerance of imperfect patient efforts are essential. Physicians without prior experience in obesity may obtain online information and continuing medical education programs at websites such as that of the North American Association for the Study of Obesity (www.naaso.org; *see* Chapter 23).

2.4.2. FUNCTIONS

The physician oversees the entry medical assessment, ordering necessary tests and conducting or supervising the history and physical. He or she also interprets the results of this assessment to the patient and to the team.

The physician informs the RD about special dietary requirements and the exercise specialist about risk status for unsupervised exercise. For diets such as VLCDs that require medical monitoring, the physician provides this oversight with patient visits and appropriate lab work. Improvement in associated risk factors, such as blood lipids and blood glucose, is assessed by tests ordered by the physician.

Although the physician is, of course, responsible for deciding the appropriateness of the individual patient for a trial of medication, in a team setting, the decision to prescribe should be made only after input from other team members about germane patient factors.

2.5. Nurse

2.5.1. QUALIFICATIONS

Professional nurses are registered in each state by the successful completion of a recognized nursing program and a national examination. Registered professional nurses can be educated at the diploma (3 yr), associate (2 yr), or bachelor's degree level as the entry to nursing practice. As previously noted, nurses with graduate degrees may be certified for specialist practice in designated fields.

2.5.2. FUNCTIONS

The nurse may occupy a variety of roles on the team. Besides traditional functions, such as monitoring of vital signs and taking the medical history, many nurses assume other important roles, such as patient education, interviewing about ongoing medical status, and patient counseling regarding program adherence. In most states, APRNs may qualify for limited prescriptive privileges.

2.6. Certified "Lifestyle Counselors"

2.6.1. QUALIFICATIONS

This represents a new group of persons credentialed by one of two groups to provide certain weight control and other wellness counseling services. The designation is intended for people who work within programs directed by traditional health care professionals and/or work more or less independently with individuals whose weight is in the "nonclinical" range, within programs that do not entail services of an intensity that necessitates specialist intervention.

The American Association of LifeStyle Counselors designates as "certified lifestyle counselors in weight control" those persons who have completed a training workshop and passed a qualifying examination. The American Council on Exercise designates individuals as "lifestyle and weight management consultants" who have successfully completed a qualifying examination. Both of these certifications require some knowledge regarding nutritional, behavioral, and exercise aspects of weight control. Some people receiving these new designations have training and, sometimes, credentials in dietetics or exercise, and others do not.

2.6.2. FUNCTIONS

This is a new group of providers, and their role in a professional team is yet to be delineated. As mentioned previously, the intents of their credentialing organizations seem to be to designate persons who can provide the more frequent contact with obese patients as part of a professionally directed team and who can work independently with clients whose weight problems are not yet clinically significant. Their scope of practice within the multidisciplinary team should be defined on a case-by-case basis.

2.7. Administrative and Support Staff

2.7.1. QUALIFICATIONS

Specific employment criteria for the program administrator and support staff are set by the practice or institution, but a few specific factors are worth noting. All administrative staff must be able to interact appropriately and productively with patients who may at times displace their frustration onto program staff. As with clinical staff, no one should be hired for an administrative position who displays any signs of intolerance of obese people (*see* Chapters 23 and 24).

2.7.2. FUNCTIONS

In addition to their expected organizational and business functions, administrative staff can be a rich source of extra information for clinical staff. Patients may confide in front-desk personnel, or inadvertently reveal to them, clinically relevant information that they will not volunteer or admit to clinical staff. Furthermore, support staff with patient contact frequently find themselves in the position of being additional sources of informal support for patients. When a person with a clinical role has programmatic administrative responsibilities, special care must be taken to clarify to patients when he or she is acting in the administrative capacity.

3. ORGANIZATION AND FUNCTION OF THE MULTIDISCIPLINARY TEAM

It should be obvious, from examination of the preliminary examples and the descriptions of team member functions, that use of a multidisciplinary team in addressing clinically the multifaceted problem of obesity can offer advantages over a solo practitioner model. Participation by members of different disciplines offers the patient the benefit of a treatment plan that covers all necessary areas. The presence of more than one clinical professional provides a clinical milieu that communicates to the patient that he or she has a group of supporters and that management of obesity requires efforts in several different domains. It is more difficult for a patient to dismiss difficulties as simply the result of a nonempathetic or disagreeable professional if several team members are allied in their efforts to help the patient.

At the same time, it is possible that without clear guidelines, too many cooks can indeed spoil the broth. Patients may, unwittingly or not, "triangulate" team members by instigating disagreements among them. Team members may inadvertently contribute to this by conveying contradictory messages to patients. Members may also openly have different beliefs and philosophies about the treatment of obesity. Finally, and unfortunately, there always exists the possibility that team members may transfer disagreements among themselves, unintentionally, to their patient interactions.

Clear team guidelines can greatly help to enhance the advantages of a team approach while minimizing its disadvantages. The way that the team is constituted and operates will depend on its mission and its organizational context. In some settings, there may be a nonclinical administrator overseeing the organizational matters with a group of clinicians in a generally flat structure. In a private medical practice, it will be expected that the physician is at the top of an organizational pyramid. Elsewhere, there will be a clinical director from any of several disciplines, with other professionals fulfilling their important roles in accord with their areas of expertise.

Regardless of the organizational milieu, certain operational guidelines (summarized in Table 2) should be in place:

1. The team should collaboratively construct, and unanimously agree to, a coherent approach and philosophy to the management of obesity.
2. Each team member should know in which areas, if any, he or she has decision-making autonomy.
3. Areas in which different team members have overlapping responsibility should likewise be designated.
4. A method of decision making in areas of overlapping responsibility should be specified.
5. An individual should be designated with overall clinical responsibility for ensuring that decisions are made according to specified guidelines.
6. Each team member should communicate freely with all other affected members.
7. All members should take pains to present themselves to patients as a team. This includes explicitly avoiding any agreements to keep any patient information from other team members.

Table 2
Organization Guidelines for the Multidisciplinary Team

- Establish a coherent approach and philosophy
- Define each member's decision-making autonomy
- Note overlapping responsibilities
- Specify decision making when responsibilities overlap
- Designate individual with overall clinical responsibility
- Communicate freely
- Present team image to patients and avoid intra-team secrets
- Establish primary contact for patients
- Design and implement methods of meeting individual needs of patients

Table 3
Creating a "Virtual" Multidisciplinary Team

- Collaborate with the patient's existing health care providers, including mental health professionals
- Develop and use a network of providers in other disciplines
- Learn the basics of other disciplines as they apply to weight control and obesity
- Use patient education materials
- Recognize your limitations

8. Each patient should be given clear guidance as to whom his or her primary clinical contact is. In some situations, a "case manager" model may be useful.
9. Most important, the team's overall approach to obesity management should provide ample mechanisms for tailoring the treatment plan to the individual patient's unique needs.

4. WHEN AN ON-SITE TEAM IS NOT FEASIBLE

Often, obesity treatment sites cannot staff a full-time multidisciplinary team as described here. In practice, most programs use part-time consulting team members in most or all positions. Practitioners should attempt to acquire a cadre of consulting professionals, even if on a part-time basis.

Many health care professionals working with obese patients, however, will operate in solo conditions, or nearly so, because their population of obese patients does not justify even a part-time on-site consulting staff. Here are some suggestions for constructing a "virtual" multidisciplinary team (summarized in Table 3):

1. Collaborate with the patient's existing health care providers. Nonphysicians should always consult with the patient's primary care physician before, and during, direction of any weight-loss effort. If the patient has no physician, he or she should be urged to obtain one before embarking on weight loss. Physicians or nurses in a primary care setting should ascertain whether the patient is currently under the care of a mental health professional, and consult accordingly.
2. Develop a network of providers from other disciplines who can be referred to as needed. Refer, and communicate, frequently. The referral relationships may become reciprocal.

3. Learn the rudiments of disciplines whose practitioners are unavailable. This does not mean that an endocrinologist should try to front as an exercise physiologist, or that a psychologist should attempt to be a dietitian. However, acquiring the basic knowledge of all aspects of weight management can allow the practitioner of any discipline to provide the rudimentary guidance needed by most patients.

4. Use patient education materials (books, videos, computer software, Internet) to enhance communication of information in all topic areas

5. Know your limitations, and make contingency plans. Even if there is no member of a needed discipline available nearby, acquire other resources. For example, a physician in a small rural community without a dietitian may develop a relationship with a dietitian in a larger city within driving distance that will allow the physician to obtain telephone consults or to refer selected patients for infrequent consultations.

5. CONCLUSION

In summary, obesity is a condition with multiple causes, multiple effects, and multiple necessary intervention components. In the most advantageous situations, it may be possible to construct a full- or part-time team of professionals from the different disciplines necessary to provide a full frontal attack on the problem. In the more numerous other cases, the practitioner should attempt, insofar as is feasible, to simulate the same effect by whatever means are available.

REFERENCES

1. American College of Sports Medicine. ACSM's Guidelines for Exercise Testing and Prescription, 6th Ed. Baltimore, MD: Lippincott, Williams & Wilkins, 2000.
2. Brownell KD, O'Neil PM. Obesity. In: x Barlow DH, ed. Clinical Handbook of Psychological Disorders: a Step-By-Step Treatment Manual, 2nd Ed. New York, NY: Guilford, 1993.
3. Friedman MA, Brownell KD. Psychological correlates of obesity: Moving to the next research generation. Psych Bull 1995; 117:3–20.
4. O'Neil PM, Jarrell MP. Psychological aspects of obesity and dieting. In: Wadden TA, VanItallie TB, eds. Treatment of the Seriously Obese Patient. New York, NY: Guilford, 1992.
5. Stunkard AJ, Rush J. Dieting and depression reexamined: a Critical review of reports ofuntoward responses during weight reduction for obesity. Ann Intern Med 1974; 81: 526–533.
6. Williamson DA, O'Neil PM. Behavioral and psychological correlates of obesity. In: Bray G, Bouchard C, James WPT, eds. Handbook of Obesity. New York, NY: Marcel Dekker, 1998.

23

The Internet and Obesity Treatment

David J. Goldstein

KEY POINTS

- Obesity treatment is best performed by a multidisciplinary team, however, the appropriate consultants may not always be available. The Internet can provide access to areas of additional expertise.
- Numerous sites are available for dissemination of educational material on weight loss.
- Methods are being developed to enhance obesity therapy in a cost-effective and efficient manner.
- Various organizations are attempting to develop and evaluate therapeutics on the Internet.

1. INTRODUCTION

Internet resources can be beneficial additions for health care professionals and patients and have the potential to reduce health care costs. For professionals, the Internet can be a source of information and can be used as supplements for patients to augment the benefits provided during office visits. This can be of benefit in both the integrated weight-loss clinic and the smaller practice that has a limited support system.

Patients should be informed of these resources and guided to avoid strictly commercial and fad websites. This chapter summarizes available online information sources, the patient perspective obtained from message boards, and support groups. Table 1 outlines the chapter.

2. THE INTERNET AS SOURCE OF INFORMATION

If one enters "obesity" into an Internet search engine, one will obtain approx 2.5 million hits. "Weight loss" yields 5.15 million hits; and "diet" yields 16.8 million hits. Thus, although there is a substantial amount of information available on the Internet, accessing this information via search engines is not efficient *(1)* and the priority of hits does not reflect a factual or noncommercial priority. In addition, although much of the available medical information tends to be good, it is generally at an academic reading level that is beyond most patients *(1)*. Further information on weight-loss diets tends to be commercial and often lacks a scientific basis *(2)*.

From: *The Management of Eating Disorders and Obesity, Second Edition*
Edited by: D. J. Goldstein © Humana Press Inc., Totowa, NJ

Table 1
Chapter Overview

As a consequence, patients need to be educated about nutrition and cautioned to consult with the physician of health care team on the scientific basis of weight-loss information obtained on the Internet before implementing new behaviors or taking dietary supplements. They can be provided with several reputable websites that are noncommercial or that separate commercial content from information sharing such as those provided here. This list is not exhaustive and organizations and Internet addresses may change. A description of the provided information or services is included for most of the listed websites. Some of the listed organizations provide handouts for patients and some may provide information that might assist a practitioner caring for patients with obesity or help in identifying referral services.

2.1. Disease Information: Obesity

There are several reputable websites and organizations that are noncommercial or that separate commercial content from information-sharing. Several are listed here with a description of the information they provide.

The American Dietetic Association (ADA) (www.eatright.org) media is a professional society for dietitians. Its goals are to promote the science of dietetics and nutrition and to educate the public and professionals in these areas. ADA activities and services include continuing education programs, nutritional research, scholarships, consumer publications, educational publications for professionals, public awareness campaigns, and promulgation of educational standards. The address is 216 West Jackson Boulevard, Suite 800, Chicago, IL 60606-6995; Phone: 800-366-1655, 312-899-0040, 900-CALL-AN-RD; media@eatright.org.

The American Heart Association (AHA) (www.americanheart.org) is a nonprofit, voluntary health agency funded by private contributions which is dedicated to the reduction of death and disability from cardiovascular diseases, including heart diseases and stroke. The address of the AHA is 7272 Greenville Avenue, Dallas, TX 75231-4596; Phone: 800-242-8721, 214-706-1552; Fax: 214-706-2139.

The American Obesity Association (www.obesity.org) is a nonprofit organization dedicated to promoting education, research, and community action. The goals of the organization are improving the quality of life for people with obesity through public education about obesity and its role in causing illness and unnecessary deaths, assisting professionals in caring for people with obesity, supporting efforts to prevent obesity especially in children, and supporting research. The address is 1250 24th St., N.W, Suite 300, Washington, DC 20037; Phone: 800-986-2373, 202-776-7711; Fax: 202-776-7712; pr@obesity.org.

The American Society of Bariatric Physicians (www.asbp.org) is a national medical specialty society of physicians who offer comprehensive programs in the medical treatment of overweight, obesity, and associated conditions. The address is 5453 East Evans Place, Denver, CO 80222-5234; Phone: 303-770-2526, 303-779-4833; Fax: 303-779-4834; info@asbp.org.

The Calorie Control Council (www.caloriecontrol.org) is an international association representing the low-calorie and diet food and beverage industry seeks to provide an effective channel of communication among its members, the public, and government officials, and to assure that scientific, medical, and other pertinent research and information is developed and made available to all interested parties. The Council has sponsored numerous studies on low-calorie sweeteners, foods, and beverages. It supports the availability of aspartame, saccharin, sucralose, and acesulfame K and the approvals of neofame and alitame and reapproval of cyclamate. The Council also supports the continued availability of current fat substitutes and caloric dietary sweeteners. The address is 5775 Peachtree-Dunwoody Road, Suite 500-G, Atlanta, GA 30342; Phone: 404-252-3663; Fax: 404-252-0774; webmaster@caloriecontrol.org.

The Food and Nutrition Information Center, US Department of Agriculture (www. nal.usda.gov/fnic/) provides information on food, human nutrition, and food safety to consumers and professionals. The address is National Agricultural Library, 10301 Baltimore Avenue, Room 105, Beltsville, MD 20705-2351; Phone: 301-504-5719; Fax: 301-504-6409.

The website http://hin.nhlbi.nih.gov/atpiii/calculator.asp has a tool that determines the heart-attack risk during the next 10 yr for a given gender, age, gender, total and high-density lipoprotein cholesterol, blood pressure, and smoking status.

My.webmd.com provides information on food and nutrition, sports and fitness, and health e-tools. Food and nutrition contains articles on diet, exercise, nutrition, including interviews with experts and bulletin boards that permit individuals to ask for advice from these experts. This website also includes some recipes. Sports and fitness contains calculators for target heart rate and calories expended with different exercise regimes. Health e-tools has a diet and exercise log including dessert wizard, which permits one to calculate the amount of exercise required to offset the calories of a specific dessert; target heart rate calculator; and calorie calculator.

The North American Association for the Study of Obesity (NAASO) (www.naaso.org) is a nonprofit scientific organization composed of scientists and clinicians who conduct research or have a scientific interest in the field of obesity. The goal of NAASO is to advance knowledge in the field of obesity and facilitate communication among professionals whose work is relevant to obesity. The address is 8630 Fenton St., Suite 918, Silver Spring, MD 20910; Phone: 301-563-6526; Fax: 301-563-6595.

The President's Council on Physical Fitness and Sports (www.fitness.gov) promotes, encourages, and motivates the development of physical fitness and sport participation for Americans of all ages through its work with partners in government and the private sector.

They provide recognition and incentive programs for individuals and organizations and materials on fitness and physical activity. The address is 200 Independence Avenue, SW, Room 738-H, Washington, DC 20201; Phone: 202-690-9000; Fax: 202-690-5211.

Shape up America! (www.shapeup.org) is a nonprofit national initiative. Its goals are to raise awareness of the importance of healthy eating and increased physical activity for weight management and disease prevention, to promote a new understanding by Americans of the health importance of achieving and maintaining a healthy weight and increasing physical activity, to provide science-based information on the assessment and treatment of obesity, and to increase cooperation among national and community organizations committed to advancing healthy weight and increased physical activity as major public health priorities. The address is 4500 Connecticut Ave., N.W., Suite 414 Washington, DC 20008; Fax: 202-244-3560; suainfo@shapeup.org.

The website www.webhealthcentre.com provides health calculators for determination of body mass index (BMI) and energy utilization. The BMI calculator permits the determination of BMI and interpretation related to level of appropriateness of weight (i.e., underweight, normal, normal, overweight, obese, morbid obesity). It also provides the lower and upper range of normal for that individual assuming normal range of musculature. The energy calculator permits the determination of the minimal (basal) and ambulatory caloric utilization for an individual of a given gender, age, height, and weight.

Weight-Control Information Network, National Institute of Diabetes and Digestive and Kidney Diseases (www.niddk.nih.gov/health/nutrit/win.htm) provides effective treatment for eating disorder patients and their families, specialized training for professionals who treat people with eating disorders, and information. The address is 6101 Executive Boulevard, Suite 300, Rockville, MD 20852; Phone: 877-946-4627, 202-828-1025; Fax: 202-828-1028; win@info.niddk.nih.gov.

2.2. Patient Perspective

In the first edition of *The Management of Eating Disorders and Obesity*, Ron Rogers gave a patient perspective gained in part from patients who replied to the question "If you could teach doctors anything about treating obese patients, what would you teach them?" placed on Internet websites devoted to obesity-related support groups *(4)*. Table 2 provides suggestions for practitioners who see obese patients in their practice based on patients' comments.

3. THE INTERNET AS A MEDIUM FOR THERAPY

The Internet is being studied as a medium for delivering behavioral programs for the induction *(5,6)*, maintenance of weight loss *(7,8)*, and prevention of obesity. Although the results to date are modest, use of the Internet has improved weight loss. The results for weight maintenance are less promising so far. Regardless, it can be anticipated that use of the Internet will expand and the ways of using the Internet will be refined.

3.1. Weight Loss

Tate and colleagues *(5,6)* conducted two randomized, controlled trials of Internet-based weight-loss interventions. In the first study *(5)*, 91 hospital employees received an in-person weight-loss counseling session at which they were instructed in behavioral

Table 2
Practical Suggestions for Improving Obesity Treatment

1. Treat health first and obesity second.
   - Consider the patient's wishes and seek feedback. An obese patient may not wish to lose weight.
   - Provide sufficient information and clarify expectations of treatment for obesity.
   - Help patients identify weight-loss goals.
   - Don't ignore treating obesity, if indicated, just because treatment might fail.
   - Keep up with the latest developments in obesity and its treatment.

2. Treat the patient with respect.
   - Don't treat the obese patient differently from other non-obese patients.
   - Provide truthful, unambiguous and balanced information. Let the patient make decisions about their treatment.
   - Do not make the patient feel guilty. Negative comments and criticism don't help.
   - Provide a complete program. Don't just tell patients to go on a diet and provide a pamphlet.
   - Remember that obesity is not a character flaw or weakness.
   - Listen actively and empathetically.
   - Monitor therapy and modify the treatment and goals accordingly.
   - Treat the patient as an individual.

3. Equip the waiting area appropriately.
   - Provide chairs in the waiting room to accommodate large-size individuals.
   - If reading material is provided, make sure it is appropriate

4. Equip the office appropriately.
   - Have scales that can accommodate sufficient weight.
   - Have adequate access to scales and other equipment.
   - Place scales in a private location.
   - Have adequate-sized hospital gowns
   - Have large blood pressure cuffs.
   - Provide chairs that can accommodate large-size individuals.

weight-control methods and encouraged to self-monitor their eating and exercise behaviors. At the end of that session, participants were randomly allocated to 6-mo trial of Internet-based education or Internet-based behavioral therapy program. All participants received instructions for logging in to a website that directed them to various Internet resources on diet, exercise, self-monitoring, and other elements of lifestyle modification. The behavioral therapy group was instructed to submit weekly records of weight, calorie and fat intake, and physical activity, along with any questions. A therapist sent participants weekly feedback and behavioral therapy lessons via e-mail. Finally, those in the behavioral therapy group had access to an electronic bulletin board, through which they could contact other participants. The Internet-based behavior therapy completers ($n = 33$) had significantly greater mean weight loss (4.1 kg) than the education program completers ($n = 32$) (1.7 kg) at 6 mo. Weight loss was correlated to login frequency.

In the second study *(6)*, after one in-person session, patients at risk for type 2 diabetes mellitus were randomly allocated to either an Internet weight-loss program alone ($n = 46$)

or with the addition of behavioral counseling via e-mail ($n = 46$) for 1 yr. Thus, this study was of longer duration and the Internet intervention was more comprehensive than the previous study (5). The Internet weight-loss program consisted of the recommendation to self-monitor; access to a message board and a website with weight-loss tutorials and links that were updated weekly, and weekly reminders to submit weights. The behavioral counseling by e-mail consisted of weekly submission of self-monitoring records, questions or comments for a therapist, and e-mail responses from a therapist. After 12 mo of treatment, the basic Internet with behavioral e-counseling group lost significantly ($p = 0.04$) more weight (4.4 kg) than the Internet control group (2.0 kg) by intent-to-treat analysis. Other measures such as percent weight loss, BMI, and weight circumference showed similar effects.

Although both these studies (5,6) showed about half the weight loss of in-person lifestyle modification, the more intensive interaction resulted in greater weight loss. It is likely that the interpersonal relationship and improved compliance in the traditional setting result in better weight loss. Consistent with the latter hypothesis, on average, the patients who had greater completion of food records lost more weight than those who were less compliant. Alternatively, it cannot be ruled out that patients who seek Internet therapy differ in some important way from those who seek in-person counseling. The effect of integrating in-person and Internet counseling to increase therapist and patient contact frequency requires study.

Formal online counseling is available at the www.nutrisessions.com website which provides a 30-min counseling session (with a coach) for $39.

3.2. Weight Maintenance

Harvey-Berino and colleagues (7,8) compared on-site and Internet-based weight maintenance programs. In the pilot study (7), after a 15-wk weight-loss program, patients were randomly assigned to (a) therapist-led in-person counseling, (b) therapist-led Internet counseling, or (c) a control group. The therapist-led interventions met every 2 wk. At the end of the 22 wk of the study, there was no significant difference between the two therapist-led interventions for attrition or number of peer-support contacts made. There was also no significant difference in the amount of weight lost. However, patients preferred the in-face intervention.

In the follow-up study (8), all participants received 6 mo of in-person weight-loss behavioral treatment. They were then given a 12-mo maintenance program. They were randomly assigned to (a) frequent in-person support (i.e., twice-monthly group meetings for 52 wk), (b) minimal in-person support (i.e., monthly group meetings for 26 wk, followed by 26 wk of no meetings), or (c) Internet support (i.e., twice-monthly "chat" sessions with other participants and a therapist for 52 wk). The weight loss at the time of randomization did not differ significantly across groups at the end of the 6-mo weight-loss program (9.8, 11.0, and 8.0 kg, for frequent, minimal, and Internet groups respectively). At the end of the first 6 mo of weight-maintenance therapy, the Internet group gained more weight (2.2 kg) than the frequent therapy group (0 kg, $p < 0.05$). The attendance at meetings was significantly greater for the frequent-therapy group compared with the Internet group. At the end of the 12-mo maintenance period, participants in the Internet support group maintained a significantly smaller weight loss (5.7 kg) than participants in the minimal or frequent in-person support groups (10.4 kg for both), but the amount of weight regained was not as different (–0.6, 0.6, and 2.3 kg for the frequent, minimal and Internet groups respectively). This suggests that exclusive Internet-based support does not substitute for in-person support. Further study should evaluate Internet-based support as an adjunct to in-person support.

3.3. Weight-Loss Groups and Organizations

3.3.1. SELF-HELP GROUPS

As noted previously, Internet tools, such as online food journals and message boards, augment weight loss (5,6). Individuals who used these online aids lost three times as much weight as those who did not use these aids. Patients who use online programs with e-mail consultations with a dietitian lost twice as much weight as those who did not utilize this consultative support. Thus, it appears that increased contact achieves greater weight loss. This requires study, but physicians may want to supplement their therapy with these aids.

Many patients use the message boards of diet support groups as a group counseling tool. The cost is generally less than that of office visits or Weight Watchers visits. Examples of Internet sites that offer tools include www.ediets.com ($15/wk for access), www.ivillage.com (free message board), and www.weightwatchers.com ($59.95 sign up and initial fees with $15.95/mo standard fee, discounted for Weight Watchers members). Diet boards are sometimes tailored to the individual needs of the patient. The edsiets.com website has programs for men and for women, recipes, success stories for motivation, and different diet boards for each type of diet. The ivillage.com site is for women and has diet boards based on the both type of diet and stage of dieting.

3.3.2. WEIGHT-LOSS ORGANIZATIONS

The following are some of the weight-loss organizations that can be found online.

TOPS Club, Inc. (Take Off Pounds Sensibly) (www.tops.org) is a nonprofit, noncommercial weight-control support group with approx 10,370 chapters. The TOPS program focuses on weight reduction through sensible dieting, regular exercise, and group support. Members adhere to individual medically prescribed food and exercise plans and participate in mutual support activities such as educational and motivational programs, discussions, an ongoing walking program, lectures, visits, social activities, retreats, and weight-loss competitions and awards. The address is 4575 South Fifth Street, Milwaukee, WI 53207-0360; Phone: 800-932-8677, 414-482-4620.

Overeaters Anonymous (www.overeatersanonymous.org) has as its goal aiding individuals who compulsively overeat to overcome that problem through a 12-step program of recovery modeled on Alcoholics Anonymous. There are no dues or fees. The address is PO Box 44020, Rio Rancho, NM 87174-4020; Phone: 505-891-2664; Fax: 505-891-4320.

Weight Watchers International, Inc (www.weightwatchers.com) is a commercial weight-loss organization that has local chapters that implement weight-loss programs that include group meetings. The website provides information, recipes, chat rooms, information about meetings, and so on.

3.4. Prevention of Obesity

Bartanowski and colleagues reported on the results of the Baylor Girls Health Enrichment Multisite Studies (GEMS) Fun, Food, and Fitness Project (FFFP) pilot study (9).

This study evaluated the effects of two randomly assigned interventions in 35 African-American girls. Both groups attended 4 wk of summer camp followed by 8 wk of Internet intervention, but the treatment group had GEMS–FFFP enhancements, whereas the control group did not. Less than half of the treatment group logged onto the Internet website following camp attendance. The sample size was small and there were no significant differences between the groups, although there were trends for more physical activity and increased fruit and vegetable intake by the treatment group. If such interventions are to be effective, compliance will need to be improved. Whether such interventions, even with good compliance, will prove effective is still unknown because there are many additional barriers to improved food choice or increased exercise than lack of education.

4. CONCLUSION

The potential for the Internet as a resource for information and an adjunct to behavioral therapy is just being explored. Early studies have indicated that there is some potential for this medium, but the effects have been modest. It should be expected that use of the Internet as an adjunct to improve the induction and maintenance of weight loss will expand and become more effective as future research discovers new ways to use the Internet to improve the effects of office-based therapies. It can be expected that use of Internet-based behavioral therapy should provide cost-effective weight-reducing treatments that will reduce the social and economic costs of obesity-related health complications.

REFERENCES

1. Berland GK, Elliott MN, Morales LS, et al. Health information on the Internet: accessibility, quality, and readability in English and Spanish. JAMA 2001; 285:2612–2621.
2. Miles J, Petrie C, Steel M. Slimming on the Internet. J R Soc Med 2000; 93:254–257.
3. Frenn M, Malin S, Sanal N, et al. Addressing health disparities in middle school students' nutrition and exercise. J Community Health Nurs 2003; 20:1–14.
4. Goldstein DJ, Rogers, RS, Lutes RA, Blank RC. Treating obesity in the physician's office. In: Goldstein DJ, ed. The Management of Eating Disorders and Obesity. Totowa, NJ: Humana Press, 1999, pp. 285–312.
5. Tate DF, Wing RR, Winett RA. Using Internet technology to deliver a ehavioral weight loss program. JAMA 2001;285:1172–1177.
6. Tate DF, Jackvony EH, Wing RR. Effects of Internet behavioral counseling on weight loss in adults at risk for type 2 diabetes: a randomized trial. JAMA 2003; 14:1833–1836.
7. Harvey-Berino J, Pintauro SJ, Gold EC. The feasibility of using Internet support for the maintenance of weight loss. Behav Modif 2002; 26:103–116.
8. Harvey-Berino J, Pintauro S, Buzzell P, et al. Does using the Internet facilitate the maintenance of weight loss? Int J Obes Relat Metab Disord 2002; 26:1254–1260.
9. Baranowski T, Baranowski JC, Cullen KW, et al. The Fun, Food, and Fitness Project (FFFP): the Baylor GEMS pilot study. Ethn Dis 2003; 13:S30–S39.

24 Barriers to Treatment

Arthur Frank

KEY POINTS

- The individual health care provider, professional or otherwise, who offers care for the obese patient is obligated to understand barriers to obesity therapy and to develop sophisticated and sustaining ways of coping with them, managing them, or circumventing them.
- The barriers include societal and cultural, patient, familial, provider, and financial issues.
- Each of the barriers impacts significantly on the nature, the format, the cost, and the effectiveness of the care provided.

1. INTRODUCTION

The treatment of obesity is unlike the medical management of any other disease. It is a chronic, alarmingly common, and incurable disease that is remarkably easy to diagnose with appalling associated disabilities. Nevertheless, for almost all overweight people, the traditional medical care system is irrelevant for the management of their problem *(1);* and its treatment, therefore, has traditionally followed a format outside the typical care patterns of other chronic diseases.

A series of barriers interfere with the treatment of obesity. At every level of care, these barriers distort the management of the disease for overweight people who are trying to assess their problem, to obtain care, and to develop skills for sustaining control, preventing obese patients from receiving adequate or appropriate care. An assessment of the nature of these barriers should be helpful for health care professionals and patients in understanding the issues and in managing the problem of obesity with enhanced sophistication and effectiveness.

The medical care that is needed for the management of obesity is distinctly different from the care that is routinely provided for the management of other chronic medical problems. Primary care medicine, insofar as it exists at all for the care of obesity, typically has limited ability to provide counseling in the lifestyle intervention skills that are considered to be a necessary part of careful management *(2).* Although as many as 40 to 50% of American women and 25 to 33% of American men are dieting at any given time *(3–5),* almost all of these dieters (87% of women and 95% of men who are on a diet) manage the problem themselves without an organized program and without professional or other

From: *The Management of Eating Disorders and Obesity, Second Edition*
Edited by: D. J. Goldstein © Humana Press Inc., Totowa, NJ

Table 1
Chapter Overview

1. Introduction
2. Societal and Cultural Barriers
    2.1. False Beliefs That Obesity is a Curable Disease
    2.2. Uncertainties About the Need for Medical Care in the Management of Obesity
    2.3. Blaming the Victim: The Belief That Obesity is the Result of Bad Habits
    2.4. Inflexible Culturally Imposed Eating Rules Complicating Treatment
    2.5. The Belief That Treatment is Futile
    2.6. The Effect of Advertising on Behavior
    2.7. Severe Appearance Standards
    2.8. The Treatment of Obese People As Outcasts
    2.9. Commercial Overstatements and the Lack of Reliable Consumer Information
    2.10. Fad Diets With Simplistic Solutions and Nutritional Misinformation
3. Patient Barriers
    3.1. Food and Fat Dependence
    3.2. The Complexity of Evaluating Self-Treatment
    3.3. Perfectionism and Bias About the Lack of Personal Control
    3.4. Cultural and Language Barriers
    3.5. Neglect of Children and Adolescents
    3.6. Lack of Understanding About the Implications of Obesity
    3.7. Health Benefits Are Remote
    3.8. Inconsistent Patient Behavior in Response to Physician Advice
    3.9. Underutilization of Exercise
    3.10. Unrealistic Patient Expectations
4. Familial Issues
    4.1. Lack of Spousal Commitment
    4.2. Lack of Parental Commitment
5. Provider Issues
    5.1. Skills of Health Care Providers
    5.2. Shortage of Training Programs
    5.3. The Need for Multidisciplinary Programs
    5.4. The Image of Sleaze and Quackery
    5.5   Limited Medical Treatment Options and the Value of Nonmedical Providers
    5.6. Inconsistent Assessment of the Maintenance of Reduced Weight
    5.7. The History of Medication Misuse
    5.8. Inappropriate Expectations of Medications
    5.9. Lack of Prevention and Preventive Services
    5.10. Duration of Treatment
    5.11. Physicians Frequently Fail to Provide Obesity-Related Services
    5.12. Physicians Often Ignore Obesity As a Medical Problem
    5.13. Support Services and Appropriate Teaching Materials Are Often Unavailable
    5.14. Limitations of Obese Health Care Personnel
6. Financial Issues
    6.1. Lack of Reimbursement by Health Insurance Companies
    6.2. Administrative Categorization of Costs in Multidisciplinary Programs
    6.3. The Dilemma of Health Insurance and Managed Care
    6.4. High Costs of Long-Term Treatment

(Continued)

Table 1 *(Continued)*
Chapter Overview

---

assistance *(6,7)*. A relatively small fraction of overweight people depend on an array of commercial, nonprofessional resources for the management of obesity. A smaller fraction still depend on nonphysician professionals such as dietitians, counselors, social workers, and psychologists.

The frequency of the disease and the frequency with which patients manage it themselves have created substantial contradictions for those involved in the care of obesity. Although almost all overweight people choose to lose weight themselves, the frequency of medical complications of obesity is very high *(8)* and it is clear that many should be receiving some professional care. Obese people do not necessarily need medical care for their weight management. Nutritional and dietary education and advice, counseling in the skills of situational management, and exercise programs may be sufficient for many overweight and obese individuals. We have, nevertheless, created no standards for judging which obese individuals should be treated or the degree or intensity of care that should be used *(1)*.

Similarly, although professional involvement is often minimal, there is increasing recognition of the physiological basis and the medical nature of the disease of obesity. Although we have a more sophisticated understanding of the nature of the dysfunctional regulating systems in the control of eating and body weight, this understanding has not created new models for medical management. As we create more medications for the treatment of obesity, we have not developed any way to reorganize the health care system to provide these medications and the support services that should accompany them *(2,9)*. If even a small fraction of the 60 to 80 million obese Americans and 50 million more who are overweight were to seek professional care for their disease, particularly for the use of obesity medications, the cost would be enormous and would overwhelm the personnel and financial resources of the health care system.

The problem is further complicated when we recognize that patients have limited ability to determine the degree of care that they need, to assess the nature of the services provided, and to select from among service providers those who are most likely to be able to meet their needs *(1)*. Ordinary mechanisms for the care of any other medical problem are not applicable for the disease of obesity. At every level of care; for the consumer, the customer, the client, or the patient, and even for the provider of care, a series of barriers exists that impede the identification, the selection, and the provision of services. Since the publication of the first edition of this book (1999), the barriers have increased in number and intensity. Many have been clarified and more thoughtfully examined. None has been eliminated.

It is apparent that a pattern has evolved in which obesity has been shunted aside and is left to be perceived as a social, rather than as a medical problem. Resources for managing it as a medical problem exist in a very limited way and the neglect, apathy and indifference which surround its proper care are pervasive throughout the health care community.

The barriers have been arbitrarily sorted into groups; those that are related to (a) our society or culture, (b) patient and consumer issues, (c) familial issues, (d) providers (or potential providers) of services, (e) financial or cost issues, and (f) government or regulatory agencies (Table 1). Many barriers are universal; some are not. It should be noted that many of these issues are uniquely related to the specific circumstances of the United States. Issues such as public (government) policy, education of professionals, availability of support services, and so on, are not necessarily applicable to health care in other countries. The reader's indulgence in tolerating this parochial approach is appreciated.

2. SOCIETAL AND CULTURAL BARRIERS

2.1. False Beliefs That Obesity is a Curable Disease

Despite the increasing scientific understanding of the abnormal physiology of obesity and the accompanying inability to repair the abnormality, all parts of our society, including health care professionals, have an expectation that the manifestations of obesity can (or should) be resolved with weight loss. This misconception has contributed substantially to the difficulties that many patients have in sustaining the continuing management of their lost weight. The expectation of a cure, along with fear of abuse and addiction to obesity medications *(10)* also have been barriers to the development of medications and their use in long-term management of obesity (*see* Chapter 16). Although a variety of interventions (including medications) *(11)* have been helpful for patients in their efforts to lose weight, care has not usually been organized with any attention to long-term management of a chronic disease. Many patients and health care professionals continue to structure management with the belief that an intervention has been a therapeutic failure if a patient regains weight after that intervention has been discontinued.

2.2. Uncertainties About the Need for Medical Care in the Management of Obesity

Many aspects of obesity can (and should) be managed by nonphysician personnel. Commercial programs can be helpful for many of their clients and many people successfully use self-help and do-it-yourself programs, particularly when they have small amounts of weight to lose. Nevertheless, there is uncertainty because there are no established guidelines to clarify which of these individuals should receive medical care. It is tempting to suggest that medical care be reserved only for patients with associated medical problems or those using medication or surgery. This may be a simplistic model, however, because a very large fraction of obese patients have at least one obesity-associated medical problem. Medical involvement may depend on the severity of the problem or on the likelihood that weight change will have an impact on its management. Patients (and physicians) continue to be troubled by the problems of overuse, misuse, and under use of medical resources *(12)* and uncertainty of what medical resources are applicable for the care of which individuals.

2.3. Blaming the Victim: The Belief That Obesity is the Result of Bad Habits

There are only a few diseases in which the system for the provision of care systematically diminishes its responsibility with the culturally convenient mechanism of blaming the victim. Acquired immunodeficiency syndrome, alcoholism, and sexually transmitted diseases are examples of our social pattern of indifference to people who suffer not only the consequences of their disease, but the opprobrium of others for the "sin" of having developed the disease. Obesity is another example, despite the overwhelming evidence that little about the *cause* of obesity is related to the behavior of the victim. Traditionally, obesity is thought to be caused by a failure of willpower; willful misconduct. This conviction that the disease is *caused* by the patient's behavior creates a substantial burden for health care practitioners and their patients in their efforts to manage it. Patients often perceive that physicians or other health care professionals are indifferent, lack concern, or have a negative attitude about their problem *(13–17)*.

The scientific basis for the regulation of body weight and of eating behavior (*see* Chapter 18) has not yet been sufficiently communicated to the American public or to health professionals. The conviction that obesity and its management are solely related to patient behaviors represents a significant barrier to its appropriate management.

2.4. Inflexible, Culturally Imposed Eating Rules Complicating Treatment

Meal-time patterns in most parts of the world are culturally imposed rather than biologically driven. Food customs and rituals are a product of the society in which they exist. Eating patterns that could be helpful for an individual patient (e.g., shifting meal times, the use of nonmeal-time eating, or the selection of specific nontypical foods at a particular meal) are often difficult to implement in the context of the cultural expectations of family, friends, and colleagues. These rules restrict opportunities for overweight people to select, modify, or manage their eating patterns and thus represent a powerful barrier to flexibility in adapting or adjusting personal eating patterns to manage obesity.

2.5. The Belief That Treatment is Futile

The experience of decades of unsuccessful weight management, particularly unsuccessful weight maintenance, has convinced most obese people that they are unlikely to succeed in any future attempts at managing their weight. The common slogan, "diets don't work," is an unfortunate misunderstanding of the distinction between diets (i.e., losing weight), which are often successful, and maintenance programs, which often are not. Patients and health care professionals struggle with a culturally imposed sense of futility and fatalism. The sense of hopelessness, with no expectation of success, is a substantial barrier to the appropriate management of obesity *(18,19)*.

2.6. The Effect of Advertising on Behavior

Many of the factors that affect behavior in our society are driven by the substantial resources of the food industry including the use of advertising. In no other place and in no other time has universally plentiful and affordable food been such a dominant factor in inducing people, who are otherwise not biologically hungry, to eat for non-nutritional reasons. In the United States in 2001 more than $5.8 billion was spent on advertising food, confections, and beverages. This was the fourth largest category exceeded only by automobiles, retail stores, and motion pictures. Restaurants (primarily "fast-food" franchises) spent $3.5 billion in 2001 in the promotion of their products; in most cases promoting abundant portions of high-calorie foods *(23–25)*. As an example, the 18th largest US advertiser in 2001 was McDonald's, which spent $1.2 billion in promotional advertising

(26). The intense message of food as pleasure and comfort is reinforced by our daily exposure to food marketing campaigns *(20,21)*. This is a particularly powerful message for children because food is the most frequently advertised product on children's television and children are particularly susceptible to the impact of these promotions *(20–22)*. Remarkably, the same message, that you can eat what you want and still lose weight, represents a significant part of the commercial promotion of the weight-loss industry. Food-promoting messages overwhelm the senses of even the most insensitive and appear to have a substantial impact on behavior and consumer choices.

2.7. Severe Appearance Standards

Cultural and societal standards of appearance and idealized weight are overwhelming for both men and women. They are typically more demanding than goals that are based on data or clinical judgments of health, morbidity, or mortality. The standards are more severe for women. Complex expectations of women's appearance are often not realistically practical in achievement or in maintenance. Nevertheless, the negative perception of the appearance of moderate or even mildly overweight women is suffused with discrimination and social penalties; in education, employment, income, and social status. It is particularly regrettable that these standards are profoundly influenced by the commercial exploitation of the fashion and entertainment industries. Attempts to achieve impractical goals create a pattern of despair, failure, frustration, and a sense of futility, all of which complicate more modest expectations of weight-loss efforts and achievement *(27,28)*.

2.8. The Treatment of Obese People As Outcasts

In some cultures, obesity is viewed as a sign of affluence, social distinction, fertility, and leisure *(29,30)*. Historically, in a culture with the likelihood of a shortage of food and starvation, obesity provided security as a survival mechanism during an anticipated famine. In the developed world, obesity no longer has survival value, and obese people are viewed in strongly negative terms. As a consequence, there is discrimination against overweight people in employment, education, income, and social status *(13,14, 17,24,31)* and in the health care provided by physicians *(15,28)* and dietitians *(16,17)*. The provision of professional services is often compromised by negative stereotyping by professional service providers *(28)*. Discrimination represents a strong motivator for losing weight and maintaining weight loss. However, discrimination socially isolates overweight people, increasing their despair and often reinforcing the patients' defiant and hostile view of the harsh world in which they live.

2.9. Commercial Overstatements
and the Lack of Reliable Consumer Information

Many consumers of obesity services have experience in contracting for weight-management services that were misrepresented and that failed to fulfill their promises. There is no system that provides consistent characterization of the services provided, identifies the type and qualifications of the service providers *(1)*, accreditation of obesity-related services, or regulation or certification that services are appropriately promoted *(32,33)*. Consumers of obesity services are often unsure about what services they need and they lack reliable sources of information about how to select appropriate services *(1)*.

Commercial obesity programs in the United States often exaggerate their skills and successes and oversell their products and services. They often inappropriately assume the care of patients who require greater skills than they can offer and have usurped the role that physicians and professional personnel have relinquished owing to their limited skills and reluctance to care for obesity. Such commercial misrepresentation of program characteristics and successes produces negative consumer experience and reinforces skepticism and uncertainty. Consumers are reluctant, therefore, to trust other service providers and their own judgment in selecting alternate providers of care.

2.10. Fad Diets With Simplistic Solutions and Nutritional Misinformation

Closely related to the problem of commercial overstatements is the abundance of obesity therapies including fad diets with the attendant misinformation and simplistic solutions. There is no shortage of miracle cures, ancient remedies, and potent natural products, all typically characterized as newly discovered. A walk down the aisle of a health food store can be an impressive experience for a naive and vulnerable patient who is exposed to a copious supply of treatments for obesity along with those for curing cancer and arthritis. Late-night television infomercials can be very tempting for someone who is desperate. Novelty diets (and diet books) are likely to create short-term success; however, the more unusual they are, the more likely they are to produce transient weight loss. The ultimate failure of these commercial fad therapies creates a public cynicism about all providers of obesity management, including those who are skilled and competent, and it reinforces skepticism and confusion in patients who do not know what to do, where to get help, or which sources to trust.

3. PATIENT BARRIERS

3.1. Food and Fat Dependence

Many people use food and eating as a way of managing stress—the "food-dependent" pattern. For these patients, eating is a particularly effective way of calming the complexity and turbulence of their everyday existence. In addition, a smaller number of people also use the state of being overweight—the "fat-dependent" pattern—to enable them to cope with aspects of their lives *(13)*.* Patients can use their obese state as a mechanism for avoiding their resolution of potential problem issues, such as responsibility, achievement, sexuality, or personal relationships. In both cases, but more so with fat dependence, efforts involved in losing weight and in maintaining lost weight increases stress by affecting the availability and the use of these coping mechanisms. Such patients are unlikely to lose weight or to maintain their weight loss unless the issues that are related to these coping mechanisms are addressed and resolved. New and difficult issues are created for individual patients as they lose weight. Failure to recognize the importance of these patterns and to modify or manage them frequently accentuates the difficulty of weight management and creates substantial obstacles for patients and the providers of the care they receive.

---

*I am indebted to my colleague, William Picon, PhD, for discussions and his formulation of the model and terminology of food and fat dependence.

3.2. The Complexity of Evaluating Self-Treatment

Most people who lose weight depend entirely on their own effort *(6)*, generally using a "do-it-yourself" program, a personally formulated diet, or instructions from a variety of sources including books and magazine articles *(1)*. Programs for the personal management of obesity are insufficiently studied because the subjects are not part of an organized system of care *(34–36)*. The randomness of these individual efforts and their separation from structured analysis makes it difficult to assess the patterns, techniques, and effectiveness of self-care. As a consequence, because so little is known about these do-it-yourself weight-loss programs, we are unable to incorporate the beneficial aspects of these programs into more structured obesity care.

3.3. Perfectionism and Bias About the Lack of Personal Control

People expect, and like to believe, that they can control their lives. It is not clear, however, whether patients can perform a specific behavior merely because they are told, and believe, (a) that it will have a positive effect, (b) that other people think they can perform this behavior, and (c) that it is actually under their control *(37)*. Obese and overweight women actually reported a lower sense of self-efficacy in exercise and eating than their nonoverweight peers *(37)*. Because individuals are unlikely successfully to impose permanent or sustained control on a biologically driven, dysfunctional weight-regulating system, the unrealistic expectation of this control, particularly for people with substantial obesity, has a devastating impact on patient morale. This expectation of perfectionism in the management of obesity creates a sense of helplessness and hopelessness that compounds the existing difficulty in obesity management.

3.4. Cultural and Language Barriers

Because many minority groups are particularly susceptible to obesity, large numbers of obese people have a cultural heritage and a primary language that is different from the American mainstream *(38–41)*. Some of these cultures may have a genetic susceptibility to obesity; others have a traditional social preference for obesity, particularly in women *(24,42)*. Because most services for these groups are not provided by people of similar culture or with similar language skills, the opportunities for minority groups to obtain adequate care, and the availability of culture specific options and strategies are severely limited *(43)*. This is particularly important when attempting to devise culturally relevant strategies for dietary and behavioral counseling. Moreover, because many of these groups have a more limited income, cost barriers (see Section 6) are an even larger issue.

3.5. Neglect of Children and Adolescents

Obese children, their parents, and health care professionals responsible for their care often do not know what to do or how adequately to manage the problem. Pediatricians inconsistently refer patients to obesity consultants *(19,44)*. Weight-management services for obese children and adolescents are seldom available and comprehensive programs are almost nonexistent. Although studies on the treatment of obesity in children and adolescents suggest that the entire family unit needs to be treated to enhance the possibility of success for the patient *(45)*, no effective system for its implementation exists. Any systematic public health approach to the management of obesity that depends on early intervention will face the barrier of the lack of effective services for this segment of the obese population.

3.6. Lack of Understanding About the Implications of Obesity

In the United Sates, the incidence of obesity-associated complications and medical comorbidities is significantly increased in people with low income and less education *(1)*. These at-risk people are least likely to be informed of the effect of obesity on their health, its impact on their survival, and the value of its management. In addition, many patients and physicians neglect the aggressive management of obesity that is otherwise linked to other specific comorbidities because the patient is feeling otherwise well *(46)*.

3.7. Health Benefits Are Remote

Although the advantages of weight loss in health, comfort, and appearance are immediate and often gratifying, the long-term benefits of sustaining maintenance of this weight loss are remote and intangible and often more difficult for many people to value. The understanding that losing weight improves health competes with the complexity of the short-term needs of the daily existence of many patients. Lowering the barrier of the obscurity of remote benefits will only be achieved by a continuing, effective, long-term public education campaign to develop greater appreciation of the value of delayed gratification and long-term rewards.

3.8. Inconsistent Patient Behavior in Response to Physician Advice

Patients do not always follow medical advice, nor are they necessarily able to do what both the patient and doctor (or other health professionals) may judge to be appropriate. Patients may choose to ignore advice, or they may not be motivated or interested or prepared to make changes at specific times in their lives *(47)*. They may not understand or agree with the counseling, have no confidence in the physician, or have conflicts with their work or family. They may be currently untroubled by their excess weight, may be unable to afford the costs of what is asked of them, or may need repeated advice or more effective education than they had previously received *(46,48–52)*. There is often a delicate balance between the physician's repeated effort to have the patient lose weight and the patient's perception that this is bothersome or annoying when the patient is unwilling or unable to make the necessary changes.

3.9. Underutilization of Exercise

Although there is a universal recognition that exercise plays an important role in good health generally, and with weight loss more specifically, it is also understood that relatively few patients exercise enough (frequency, duration, intensity, and sufficiently sustained effort) for adequate weight control (*see* Chapter 13). Moreover, many patients who exercise in a specifically structured part of their day do not necessarily extend the pattern of increased activity sufficiently to the remaining part of the day, during which many patients may sustain a pattern of profound sedentary behavior.

The problem of the implementation of exercise as part of ordinary activity is intensified with the conveniences of ordinary life in America. The car, television set, and computer have complicated the problem.Eighty-four percent of trips in the United States, and 75% of trips of less than 1 mile, are taken by car. Only one-fourth of high school students participate in daily physical activity or education at school *(56)*. About 40% of Americans are not regularly active and 25% are entirely inactive *(53)*. One report noted that 22.6% of obese adults thought of themselves as too fat to exercise *(54)* and overweight and obese women were less confident than normal weight women in their ability to exercise *(37)*. Many obese patients are embarrassed about exercise. As a consequence, it has been noted that successful exercise programs require intensive and repeated counseling *(55)*

3.10. Unrealistic Patient Expectations

Patients often think of successful weight management based on the expectation that they will lose all of their excess weight and maintain all of that weight loss indefinitely thereafter *(57)*. Although a smaller amount of weight loss has a beneficial effect on a number of measures of health, patients are often disappointed with lesser amounts of weight loss. It is often difficult to convince patients of the advantages of losing 10 to 15% of their initial weight, or of the usefulness of losing weight in stages with consistently smaller interventions spread over a longer time. The urgency that patients feel in their need to complete the task immediately is a measure of how desperate they are to resolve the problem.

4. FAMILIAL ISSUES
4.1. Lack of Spousal Commitment

Although it is generally assumed that families are supportive of the patient's effort to lose weight, this is not invariably true. Family members may have conflicting feelings about the patient's weight loss and are not always willing or able to devote the time, support, and energy to the management of this disease, which the patient may be willing and obliged to commit. Many patients find that spouses have a vested interest in maintaining the status quo. For example, a husband might wish to maintain his wife's dependency on him and feel threatened by the attention she attracts after she loses weight. The opposite pattern, "lose weight or else," may be equally destructive to a patient's efforts by adding intolerable stress to the weight-loss effort. In either case, the treatment of obesity, particularly because it involves a large financial and time commitment and a continuing, lifelong effort, necessarily involves the patient's family *(58,59)*. The resolution of all the obstacles involved in these familial relationships is important for the successful treatment of obesity *(60)*.

4.2. Lack of Parental Commitment

No treatment program for children or adolescents is likely to be effective in the absence of significant and supportive parental involvement *(51)*. Parental involvement is not always available or helpful. The treatment of childhood or adolescent obesity requires a sustaining effort for the parents, as well as for the child *(45)*.

5. PROVIDER ISSUES
5.1. Skills of Health Care Providers

A major barrier to the treatment of obesity, at any level of care, relates to the insufficient number of skilled health care providers and an inadequate knowledge base among providers of care. Physicians typically are not trained extensively in nutrition and certainly not often in the treatment of obesity, including the management of low-calorie physiology and dietary therapy *(61–63)*. They often do not consider obesity as a disease and usually do not incorporate the model of its chronic care into its management *(64,65)*. Counselors, such as psychologists and social workers, often lack skills and training in the complex issues surrounding eating behavior. Exercise therapists, including those who have participated in formal training programs, are usually insufficiently trained in the general principles of nutrition or diet therapy. Even dietitians who might well be able to manage diet therapy are often incompletely trained in techniques of behavior therapy and about the metabolic basis of obesity. Many providers who recognize their insufficient training lack confidence in their skills, avoid dealing with the problems of obesity and avoid any role in its management *(48,49)*.

5.2. Shortage of Training Programs

The problem of insufficient provider skills is compounded by the absence of training programs in nutrition, obesity, low-calorie physiology, and psychological issues in weight management. Although primary care physicians *(48)*, pediatricians, pediatric nurse practitioners, and dietitians all expressed high interest in obtaining additional training in obesity management, training opportunities are limited or unavailable *(51)*. Thus, even highly motivated providers have difficulty acquiring the skills necessary for the management of obesity.

5.3. The Need for Multidisciplinary Programs

Patients with substantial excess weight, those with complicated associated medical problems, and those for whom weight loss has been particularly intractable are likely to be more rigorously managed in a multidisciplinary program; those with physicians, psychologists, behavior and exercise therapists, and dietitians *(see* Chapter 22). Surveyed practitioners note, however, the lack of available support services *(51)*. Establishing these programs requires a significant commitment of staff and investment of capital *(9)*. However, these commitments are often not made because of concerns that a multidisciplinary program will not be financially sustainable unless a "critical mass" of patients can be drawn to the program to enable it to maintain its financial solvency. As a consequence, this effort is typically beyond the means of an individual provider and depends on a hospital or some alternate institutional base and a reliance on expectations of long-term financial stability.

5.4. The Image of Sleaze and Quackery

A basic principle in the provision of medical care is that when no adequate treatment programs are available for a disabling condition, quacks and charlatans will fill the vacuum. For decades, this has been the case with obesity. In the effort to treat obesity, we have seen a rogue's gallery of rascals and snake-oil-salesmen, a library of junk science and nutritional gibberish, and a catalogue of nonsense cures and commercial hustle. Rightfully, the public has become skeptical and distrusting of those involved in treating obesity. The barrier of this image will be sustaining until ethical therapists and treatment programs exist in sufficient quantity to discourage the efforts of commercial opportunists *(18,32,33)*. Paradoxically, the pattern had recurred in a somewhat different format (with a minor variation on the theme) with the renewed interest in the rational use of medications for the extended management of obesity. The emergence of "phen-fen" practitioners from 1992 to 1997 who dispensed pills or prescriptions indiscriminately with no associated medical care, counseling, or weight-management support services was a new variation on an old theme and an example of the sad history of therapeutic abuse in the management of obesity *(66)*.

5.5. Limited Medical Treatment Options and the Value of Nonmedical Providers

Physicians and others who might be inclined to undertake the management of obesity are often thwarted in their efforts by their inability to offer the patient much assistance. They recognize that some services needed for obesity management are best provided by nonphysician personnel, that physician counseling alone is often insufficient, and that the variety of skills needed are typically not conveniently organized in therapeutic units. Unfortunately, many of the specialists with needed skills are not readily available in every community. Barriers to integrated medical management will only be resolved by improving access to an array of available skills and services *(9)*.

5.6. Inconsistent Assessment of the Maintenance of Reduced Weight

There is a general misunderstanding of the role of weight-loss programs and their relation to weight maintenance. The public, and many health professionals, have a long tradition of assuming that a weight-loss program should enable a patient to sustain that lost weight based, in part, on the naïve assumption that once weight is lost, the patient should be cured. However, most weight-loss programs, regardless of their success at weight loss, have relatively little impact on weight maintenance; and as a consequence there is a continuing dismissal of the success of any weight-loss program with the declaration that "the patients all regain their weight."

Although many programs are reasonably successful at weight loss, very few maintenance programs have been established and even fewer have shown any evidence of continuing, long-term success. This is partly related to the absence of a consistent, quantitative system for measuring and comparing the effects of weight-maintenance programs *(67–70)*. Thus, although weight-loss programs are being asked to provide information on their weight-maintenance success rates *(1)*, these data are not generally available. The failure to recognize the distinction between weight loss and maintenance, with the attendant dismissal of weight loss alone, contributes to the difficulty in developing successful weight-loss and weight-maintenance programs.

5.7. The History of Medication Misuse

The misuse of medications (e.g., dinitrophenol, digitalis preparations, thyroid, chorionic gonadotropin, chromium picolinate) for weight management, the overuse and misuse of anorectic medications (e.g., amphetamines, phendimetrazine), the largely unforeseen complications of a medication that appeared otherwise to have been useful (fenfluramine), and the careless promotion of unregulated and potentially dangerous over-the-counter preparations of unpredictable potency (e.g., ephedra *[71,72]*) has clouded the treatment of obesity for decades *(10)*. These examples have created a generation of overweight people who are fearful of using medications to manage their illness

(73) and have led to consideration that those physicians who prescribed these medications were exceeding the limits of mainstream health care *(18)*. The historical barrier created by misuse of medications will continue to be an obstacle for many overweight people until convincing evidence about the safety and effectiveness of the pharmacological approach is made available to the public.

5.8. Inappropriate Expectations of Medications

There is no expectation that insulin can be discontinued in the treatment of type 1 diabetes or that medications should be discontinued in the treatment of hypertension, schizophrenia, hypercholesterolemia, or other chronic diseases. Nevertheless, patients, physicians, and regulatory authorities are typically skeptical about sustaining use of drugs for the treatment of obesity. Long-term management of obesity with medications has, until recently, not been an option in the United States because regulations limited the duration of use of obesity drugs. For decades, the value of medications for the treatment of obesity was trivialized because patients typically regained their weight when medications were discontinued. This reflects the complexity and the slow evolution of the understanding of the physiology of the disease, the recognition of its chronic nature, and the adjustments needed by medical personnel in their use of continuing medications. It has created a devastating double standard for obesity medications because they are held to a higher standard of success (i.e., a cure) than is expected of medications for the treatment of other chronic medical problems.

5.9. Lack of Prevention and Preventive Services

Although the value of preventive services is widely endorsed by the public, health care providers, government agencies, and the health insurance and managed care systems, there is almost no funding of such services. Although there is a general agreement that much might be accomplished by programs to prevent obesity or to intervene early in its treatment, there is no practical way of doing this and certainly no payment mechanism to support such an effort *(1,7,74)*. Many obesity-treatment programs specifically exclude patients with small amounts of excess weight, or those normal-weight patients who, with an ominous family history or with a history of successful maintenance of weight loss, are at high risk for gaining or regaining excess weight. This exclusion, however justified by the limitation of existing management techniques, is inconsistent with the development of preventive services and effectively eliminates the possibility of prevention or early intervention in the management of this disease. This is true despite a number of studies that suggest that more intensive treatment programs will produce greater effects *(75,76)*. Because of cost and the need for a greater commitment of time and effort, few patients select this approach without public funding. Thus, the anticipated expense and effort vs perceived value are limiting factors in any program.

5.10. Duration of Treatment

Obesity is a chronic disease with no expectation of a cure in the foreseeable future. Any program for the treatment of obesity must establish mechanisms for lifelong treatment. Because of the difficulty in treating obesity, as for any chronic disease that requires the patient to sustain changes in the complex social and cultural patterns of food selection and eating formats, all treatments must necessarily be intense and continuing.

Treatment programs of this nature, that involve sustaining and chronic care, generally do not exist and successful treatment models, including the long-term use of medications for long-term control, have not been tested or established.

5.11. Physicians Frequently Fail to Provide Obesity-Related Services

Many services for the management of obesity can be provided by nonphysician professionals or, in many cases, by nonprofessional (commercial) programs. The participation of physicians is surely important, however, for many patients, particularly those with severe obesity, complicating medical problems, or those who need the reinforcement that can be provided by a skillful physician. Patients are more likely to undertake a behavior if they are told by others, particularly by those who are perceived as authorities, that they should perform it or that it will have a beneficial effect *(37)*.

Physicians, even those involved in primary care, often choose not to be involved in the management of obesity *(48)*. One survey noted that only 42% of obese patients were advised to lose weight by health care professionals. Many factors are cited for this lack of involvement. Obesity services are time consuming and health insurance benefits are not paid for the treatment of obesity. Physicians do not want to raise the issue for fear of embarrassing a reluctant patient. Furthermore, they may be concerned that, if they raise the issue, they are then obligated to assist the patient in its management and they often feel that there is little that they can offer to help the patient succeed *(48,51)*.

5.12. Physicians Often Ignore Obesity As a Medical Problem

Obesity has some of the neglect patterns that have been reported for hypertension *(46)*. Many physicians see weight gain as an inevitable part of increasing age and do not view it as a medical condition requiring treatment. As a consequence, weight is inconsistently documented in medical records. In one study, less than 30% of residents in a family practice training program documented patients' weight or body mass index (BMI) *(77)*. A pervasive sense of futility appears to have a negative impact on professional behavior and the professional obligation to gather information and intervene *(18)*.

5.13. Support Services and Appropriate Teaching Materials Are Often Unavailable

Many aspects of obesity management require the skills and services of nonphysician personnel (e.g., dietitians, counselors). Health care professionals frequently note difficulty in identifying appropriate support services for these aspects of care. Even when professional service providers are available, they are often insufficiently trained in obesity management.

Patients struggle with current fad diets, best-selling books offering erroneous weight-management advice, and a culture of quick-fix solutions. Appropriate teaching materials for professionals or teaching materials for patients cannot keep current with the deluge of styles in popular culture. As a result, little material is available to enable the professional or the patient to analyze or cope with the current dietary fads *(48)*.

5.14. Limitations of Obese Health Care Personnel

Although it is possible that the problem of obesity is less common among health care personnel than the general public, it is likely that a substantial fraction of these professionals, including those who would otherwise be responsible for the management of obese patients, are themselves overweight or obese. Patients report, however, that they are less receptive to weight-management advice from obese physicians *(78)*, rendering this group of health care providers less effective in their efforts to manage their patients' obesity because of their own difficulty with weight control. The prevalence of the problem, and the ease that patients have in identifying if their physician is obese, decreases the potential effectiveness of a significant group of providers who might otherwise be skilled in the professional management of obesity.

6. FINANCIAL ISSUES

6.1. Lack of Reimbursement by Health Insurance Companies

Probably the major barrier to the treatment of obesity from the patient's perspective is the failure of health insurance companies (in the United States) to reimburse patients for the costs associated with the treatment of obesity *(79,80)*. Almost no health insurance programs reimburse patients for nutritional services or for the medical treatment of obesity. Health insurance payments, if any, are likely to be related to the treatment of obesity comorbidities. Thus, otherwise healthy obese patients do not receive obesity-related insurance payments until they have medical complications of their obesity. One report *(81)* noted that only 11% of pediatrician treatment of obesity was reimbursed by health insurance. That treatment is difficult, or that success of treatment is infrequent, seems an unconvincing rationale for this policy; the same argument can be made for cancer or substance abuse. That the problem cannot be resolved, or that no effective form of therapy exists, is equally unconvincing; the same argument can be made for senility or mental retardation. That the disease is "self-inflicted" is also unconvincing; the same argument can be made for tobacco-induced lung cancer or motorcycle accidents.

Multiple arguments for the denial of insurance benefits can be dismissed *(79)* and it appears then that the reason for insurance denial of benefits is entirely related to questions of anticipated costs or the cost-effectiveness of treatment. This argument is also unconvincing; it would be difficult to establish the cost effectiveness of treating Alzheimer's disease or many forms of cancer.

The avoidance of responsibility by the health insurance and managed care systems has created a complex series of alternate management mechanisms used by physicians who care for obese patients. These physicians often complete health insurance claims based on alternate or comorbid diagnoses. Physicians in managed care, particularly those who are using medications for obesity treatment, are often forced into a "therapeutic underground" with their patients. They use a nonspecific characterization of the nature of their patient encounter. This pattern of miscoded patient records has the unfortunate effect of making it difficult for anyone to collect accurate data on obesity treatment. It may have the effect of sustaining treatment by the physician without appropriate support services with the result that incomplete services are thus provided by the most expensive personnel, rather than by less-expensive and more effective nonphysician staff. It appears unlikely that any rational treatment program for obesity can be developed unless a systematic financing mechanism can be developed.

6.2. Administrative Categorization of Costs in Multidisciplinary Programs

Traditional health insurance programs reimburse patients for the costs of specific services. In multidisciplinary program models (such as pain clinics, cancer programs, diabetes treatment and, of course, obesity programs) it is often not possible to separate (i.e., unbundle) a package of services provided by many individuals on a treatment team. This typically makes it impossible to meet the specific administrative requirements of health insurance companies. The barrier of unbundling the diverse services of a multidisciplinary team will have to be modified as part of the rationalization of health insurance payment.

6.3. The Dilemma of Health Insurance and Managed Care

If health insurance and managed care programs are going to be enlightened about establishing programs for the treatment of obesity, they will have to be convinced that such treatment programs will be cost-effective *(80,82)*. A simple analysis of costs will not be complete because, although it may be expensive to treat obesity, it is also very costly not to treat it. It is estimated that obese patients with a BMI of 30 cost about 25% more than non-obese patients in a managed care program and those with a BMI of 35 cost about 44% more *(83)*. Health care for type 2 diabetics, 85% of whom are obese, costs substantially more than the care of non-diabetics; it seems likely that even marginally effective weight-control treatment for obese diabetics would be cost effective *(84)*, particularly if it can reduce or delay obesity-related medical complications.

Can any obesity treatment program decrease the total costs of a managed care program, number and duration of hospitalizations, frequency of laboratory tests, or number of medications? Although convincing arguments can be made for the effectiveness of treating an individual in an individual program, it is likely that managed care plans will need definitive evidence that the cost of providing effective obesity treatment (lifesaving as it may be) does not exceed the cost of doing nothing. It is, of course, possible for patients to choose obesity coverage in selecting plans but, in the reality of the market, this option is never offered.

Regardless of any economic analysis, there should be a recognition that no other decisions on insurance benefit payments are made on the basis of cost effectiveness. Nevertheless, the unique obligation to establish a financial benefit for the treatment of obese patients is inconsistent with any other aspect of health insurance and is morally and ethically indefensible. There is little evidence to suggest that insurance plans will offer to provide obesity services unless compelled to do so by regulatory or statutory obligations.

6.4. High Costs of Long-Term Treatment

The cost of any effective long-term treatment program, particularly obesity treatment which is lifelong and intense, will be substantial and beyond the financial means of most individuals. Regardless of any reimbursement mechanisms, the reality of total cost is invariably a substantial barrier to the treatment of obesity.

7. GOVERNMENT AND REGULATORY ISSUES

7.1. Inconsistent Rules About Medications

It is likely that the role of medications in the management of obesity will increase as the underlying physiological mechanisms that control eating are more clearly understood (*see* Chapter 18). Many aspects of the use of medications are, however, distorted by confusion, ambivalence, and the legacy of years of inappropriate use and misunderstanding.

First, obesity is clearly a chronic disease. If medications might control eating behavior it seems likely that they will be needed as permanent pharmacotherapy; much as they would be used for diabetes, hypertension, or hypercholesterolemia. Because of the obligations of the drug manufacturers to establish the safety and efficacy of long-term use, the expense of doing these studies, and evolving requirements by the US Food and Drug Administration (FDA), medications have a variety of duration specifications in the labels. Some medications (e.g., phentermine or phendimetrazine) are authorized for "short-term (a few weeks)" use. Phenylpropanolamine, when it was available, had a labeled authorization for use of not more than 3 mo. Some medications have a label that specifies that "safety and efficacy have not been studied in long term use" (e.g., sibutramine and orlistat are not studied beyond 2 yr). This limitation on long-term use constrains the concept of the continuous use of medications for the chronic disease of obesity. Because of these inconsistencies, and the sustaining public focus on weight loss rather than on maintenance, many physicians have a persistent reluctance to use these medications chronically.

Second, the problem of physician prescription is further complicated by a tangled variety of state and local regulations that limit the duration of use of specific drugs, obligate the frequent rewriting of prescriptions, or selectively limit the use of specific medications. Many state and local governments, cautious about amphetamine analogues and the history of the abuse of diet drugs, have imposed rules that exceed federal regulatory obstacles. There is no current systematic effort to modify the suffocating requirements of some state and local regulatory authorities that threaten physicians with a variety of penalties including the possibility of withdrawal of their license to practice. It is clear that this obstacle will need modification if pharmaceutical treatment of obesity is to be made widely available *(73,85,86)*.

Third, health insurance plans do not typically pay benefits for the treatment of obesity and do not, therefore, pay for the cost of obesity medications. In one survey of 375 employers representing almost 12 million beneficiaries, more than 80% specifically excluded appetite-suppression products in the health insurance plan *(87)*. Only nine states cover anti-obesity pharmaceutical products as a benefit in their Medicaid program *(88)*. Medicare has no current benefits for any medications but proposals under consideration (in 2003) typically used the same exclusionary language as Medicaid, excluding benefits for weight-loss drugs *(88)*.

Fourth, widely promoted over-the-counter and herbal preparations are typically sold without specifying the duration of use. Weight-loss products sold as dietary supplements have included potent ingredients, such as ephedrine, that are sold without thorough evaluation of safety and efficacy. Preparations are not certified as to purity and potency. Manufacturing procedures are not monitored and labeling specifications are often found to be inconsistent with content. Reported adverse reactions, including deaths, have elicited editorial pleas for increased regulations *(71,72)*.

7.2. Inconsistent Federal Government Policies on Obesity

All US government agencies that have reviewed the issue of obesity characterize it as a serious chronic disease with substantial public health implications. In one form or another, a statement of this character has been presented by all health or health-related agencies.* Despite this, three institutions that have a specific responsibility to pay benefits for health services, Medicare, Medicaid, and the Federal Employee Health Benefit Program, have consistently declined to pay benefits for obesity treatment. This is particularly regrettable because these agencies often set policies for health insurance coverage that tend to become standards in the health insurance and managed care industries. The federal government has, in effect, recognized the importance of the problem but has declined to pay for its care.

7.3. Lack of Research Funding

It is likely that current treatment programs, based entirely on behavioral and nutritional changes, when optimally administered, are close to maximizing their effectiveness. No manipulation of the existing patterns, however subtle or bold, is likely to have a significant additional impact on the short or long term treatment of obesity. Funding for innovative research, and a clearer understanding of the neurochemical, molecular, and genetic basis for eating and body weight regulation, seem to be necessary for the development of treatment programs, with or without new medications.

Despite the recognition of the seriousness of obesity less than 0.7% of the NIH budget in 1999 was allocated to obesity-related research *(89)*. Public health education related to obesity is similarly underfunded. Although $9.3 billion was spent in 2001 for advertising and promotion of foods, confections, beverages, and restaurants *(23,26)*, only $100 million (about 1% of what was spent on the promotion of eating) was spent in 2003 on public and private advertising to educate the public or to prevent diabetes, asthma, and obesity *(90)*. Only a fraction of this 1% will be spent on obesity.

7.4. Absence of Accreditation and Certification

Anyone, professional or otherwise, can provide treatment for obesity in almost any jurisdiction. There is no scrutiny, at any governmental level, of the character or quality of any treatment programs. No systematic effort has been made to sort treatment programs or to develop any rational system to match specific programs to specific patients *(1)*. No effort has been made to verify the quality, the successes, the staffing, or the honesty of any commercial or professional program. Governmental agencies have been generous in their criticism of the existing system *(91)* but have been unable to develop any legislative or regulatory solutions. It may be helpful to develop an accreditation system *(32,33)* to protect the consumer and to avoid the burden of government overregulation.

8. CONCLUSION

The catalogue of barriers seems formidable. Indeed, it is. So too is the treatment of obesity. The individual health care provider, professional or otherwise, who offers care

---

* This includes, *inter alia*, the National Institutes of Health (NIH) and various agencies of the NIH, the Centers for Disease Control, the Public Health Service, the Department of Health and Human Services, the FDA, the Federal Trade Commission, the Social Security Administration, the Surgeon General, the Department of Agriculture and a number of government related or international agencies including the Institute of Medicine of the National Academy of Sciences, the World Health Organization, and the International Classification of Diseases.

for the obese patient, is obligated to understand these barriers and to develop sophisticated and sustaining ways of coping with them, managing them, or circumventing them.

For the individual provider, the difficulties in coping with the barriers is characterized perhaps most clearly by the example of the mixed or contradictory messages of comprehensive care *(79)*. The first message is that the provider is encouraged to undertake the careful and thoughtful care of obese patients; failure to do so is neglect of professional responsibility. Second, the patient may express relative passivity and may be eager to use medication or surgery, often with unrealistic expectations of the simplicity and benefits of these interventions. These patients shift the responsibility for managing this disease to drugs or surgery and hope that these interventions will solve the problem. These same patients then tend to assume that there is no need for a deliberate effort to modify diet, behavior, or exercise patterns. A third message is that the care of obesity should be provided in a comprehensive manner with medical, dietetic, behavioral, psychological, and exercise personnel. Implied in the latter is the assumption that anything less is inadequate. Yet most providers, however willing they might be to treat obese patients, do not have access to these services in their professional offices, and are not organized as part of a multidisciplinary team. The eagerness of an individual to provide services is diluted by the recognition that the team does not necessarily exist and cannot easily be created. A final message is the complicated recognition that, regardless of how the other obstacles are resolved, there is no consistent mechanism for paying for any of it.

Understanding the barriers is a first step toward resolution of these impediments to successful treatment. Eventually, new therapies and improved understanding of the molecular basis of obesity will help to break down these barriers. Until that time, health care providers who have an understanding of the barriers will have an enhanced ability to care for their patients, and they will be able to offer them the option of managing this disease in a more sophisticated manner.

Each of the barriers impacts significantly on the nature, the format, the cost, and the effectiveness of the care provided. Still, as with the management of any patient with any disease, care has to be given one patient at a time. Global issues surrounding the management of obese patients impinge on the relationship and affect whether or not the relationship will be successfully established or sustained. The barriers, which have added substantially to the difficulty, complexity, cost, availability, and effectiveness of treatment, substantially increase the burden of obesity. No other disease has as many obstacles to its effective management as does obesity. It seems regrettable that this disease, so difficult to treat in ideal circumstances, should be additionally burdened by these barriers.

REFERENCES

1. Thomas PR, ed. Weighing the Options: Criteria for Evaluating Weight Management Programs. Prepared by the Committee to Develop Criteria for Evaluating the Outcomes of Approaches to Prevention and Treatment of Obesity. Food and Nutrition Board, Institute of Medicine, Washington, DC: National Academy Press, 1995.
2. US Dept of Health and Human Services. The Practical Guide: Identification, Evaluation and Treatment of Overweight and Obesity in Adults. NIH Publication No. 00-4084. October, 2000.
3. National Research Council. Diet and Health: Implications for Reducing Chronic Disease Risk. Prepared by the Committee on Diet and Health, Food and Nutrition Board and Committee on Life Sciences, Washington, DC: National Academy Press, 1989.
4. Horn J, Anderson K. Who in America is trying to lose weight? Ann Int Med 1993; 119:672–676.

5. Williamson DF, Serdula MK, Andra RF, Levy A, Byers T. Weight loss attempts in adults: goals, duration and rate of weight loss. Am J Public Health 1992; 82:1251–1257.

6. Levy AS, Heaton AW. Weight control practices of US adults trying to lose weight. Ann Int Med 1993; 119:661–666.

7. Heaton AW, Levy AS. Information sources of US adults trying to lose weight. J Nutr Educ1995; 27: 182–190.

8. Pi-Sunyer FX. Medical hazards of obesity. Ann Int Med 1993; 119:655–660.

9. Frank A. A multidisciplinary approach to weight management: the physician's role and team care alternatives. J Am Diet Assoc 1998; 98: S44–S48.

10. Cerulli J, Shafer A. ASHP therapeutic position statement on the safe use of pharmacotherapy for obesity management in adults. Am J Health-Syst Pharm 2001; 58:1645–1655.

11. Weintraub, M. Long term weight control: The National Heart, Lung and Blood Institute funded multimodal intervention study. Clin Pharm Ther 1992; 51:581–646.

12. McNeil BJ. Shattuck lecture—hidden barriers to improvement in the quality of care. N Engl J Med 2001; 345:1612–1619.

13. Sarlio-Lahteenkorva S, Stunkard A, Rissanen A. Psychological factors and quality of life in obesity. Int J Obes 1995; 19:s1–s5.

14. Kral JG, Sjostrom LV, Sullivan MB. Assessment of quality of life before and after surgery for severe obesity. Am J Clin Nutr 1992; 55:611S–614S.

15. Kaminsky J, Gadaleta D. A study of discrimination within the medical community as viewed by obese patients. Obes Surg 2002; 12:14–18.

16. Harvey EL, Summerbell CD, Kirk SFL, Hill AJ. Dietitians' views of overweight and obese people and reported management practices. J Hum Nut Diet 2002; 15:331–347.

17. McArthur LH, Ross JK. Attitudes of registered dietitians toward personal overweight and overweight clients. J Am Diet Assoc 1997; 97:63–66.

18. Frank A. Futility and avoidance: medical professionals in the treatment of obesity. JAMA 1993; 269: 2132–2133.

19. Grizzard T. Undertreatment of obesity. JAMA 2002; 288:2177.

20. Taras HL, Gage M. Advertising foods on children's television. Arch Ped Adolesc Med 1995; 149: 649–652.

21. Coon KA, Tucker KL. Television and children's consumption patterns. A review of the literature. Minerva Pediatr 2002; 54:423–436.

22. Borzekowski DL, Robinson TN. The 30-second effect: an experiment revealing the impact of television commercials on food preferences of preschoolers. J Am Diet Assoc 2001; 101:42–46.

23. Domestic advertising spending by category: ranked by measured U.S. expenditures in 2001. AdAge. com. Crain Communications. (Accessed February 18, 2003). Website: (http://www.adage.com/page).

24. Prentice AM. Overeating: the health risks. Obes Res 2001; 9:234S–238S.

25. Welch G. Spending in the U.S. on advertising for fast food, sodas and automobiles. Food for thought regarding the type 2 diabetes epidemic. Diabetes Care 2003; 26:546–547.

26. 100 leading national advertisers: ranked by total U.S. advertising spending in 2001. AdAge.com. Crain Communications. (Accessed February 18, 2003). Website: (http://www.adage.com/page).

27. Bordo S. Unbearable weight: feminism, western culture and the body. Berkeley, CA: University of California Press, 1993.

28. Thompson RL, Thomas DE. A cross-sectional survey of the opinions on weight loss treatments of adult obese patients attending a dietetic clinic. Int J Obes 2000; 24:164–170.

29. Sobal J. Obesity and socioeconomic status: a framework for examining relationships between physical and social variables. Med Anthropol 1991; 13:231–247.

30. Wilson H. Egyptian food and drink. Bucks, UK: Shire Publications Ltd. 1988.

31. Wadden TA, Stunkard AJ. Social and psychological consequences of obesity. Ann Int Med 1985; 103:1062–1067.

32. Frank A. Accreditation and certification: the rationalization of obesity management services. Am J Clin Nutr 1995; 62:439–440.

33. Frank A. It's time to regulate the diet industry. Med Econ 1993; 70:23–30.

34. Schachter S. Recidivism and self cure of smoking and obesity. Am Psychologist 1982; 37:436–444.

35. Rzewnicki R, Forgays DG. Recidivism and self-cure of smoking and obesity: an attempt to replicate. Am Psychologist 1987; 42:97–100.
36. Klem M, Wing R, McGuire M, Seagle H, Hill J. A descriptive study of individuals successful at long term maintenance of substantial weight loss. Am J Clin Nutr 1997; 66:239–246.
37. Pinto BM, Maruyama NC, Clark MM, Cruess DG, Park E, Roberts M. Motivation to modify lifestyle risk behaviors in women treated for breast cancer. Mayo Clin Proc 2002; 77:122–129.
38. Kuczmarski RJ, Fegal KM, Campbell ST, and Johnson CL. Increasing prevalence of overweight among US adults: the National Health and Nutrition Examination Surveys, 1990 to 1996. J Am Med Assoc 1994; 272:205–211.
39. Uba L. Cultural barriers to health care for southeast Asian refugees. Pub Health Reports 1992; 107: 544–548.
40. Valdez RB, Giachello A, Rodriguez-Trias H, Gomez P, de la Rocha C. Improving access to care in Latino communities. Pub Health Reports 1993; 108:534–539.
41. Woloshin S, Bicknell NA, Schwartz LM, Gany F, Welch HG. Language barriers in medicine in the US. JAMA 1995; 273:724–728.
42. van der Sande A, Bailey R, Faal H, et al. Nationwide prevalence study of hypertension and related non-communicable diseases in The Gambia. Trop Med Int Health 1997; 2:1039–1048.
43. Ashton CM, Haidet P, Paterniti DA, et al. Racial and ethnic barriers in the use of health services. J Gen Int Med 2003; 18:146–152.
44. Miller LA, Grunwald GK, Johnson SL, Krebs NF. Disease severity at time of referral for pediatric failure to thrive and obesity: time for a paradigm shift? J Pediatr 2002; 141:6–7.
45. Uzark KC, Becker MH, Dielman TE, Rocchini AP, Katch V. Perceptions held by obese children and their parents: implications for weight control intervention. Health Education Q 1988; 15:185–198.
46. Gupta K, Gupta S. Undertreatment of hypertension: a dozen reasons. Arch Int Med 2002; 162: 2246–2247.
47. Rossi SR, Rossi JS, Rossi-DelPrete LM, Prochaska JO, Banspach SW, Carleton RA. A processes of change model for weight control for participants in community-based weight loss programs. Int J Addict 1994; 29:161–177.
48. Kushner RF. Barriers to providing nutrition counseling by physicians: a survey of primary care practitioners. Prev Med 1995; 24:546–552.
49. Bowerman S, Bellman M, Saltsman P, et al. Implementation of a primary care physician network obesity management program. Obes Res 2001; 9:321s–325s.
50. Oliveria SA, Lapuerta P, McCarthy BD, L'Italien GJ, Berlowitz DR, Asch SM. Physician-related barriers to the effective management of hypertension. Arch Int Med 2002; 162:413–420.
51. Story MT, Neumark-Stzainer DR, Sherwood NE, et al. Management of child and adolescent obesity: attitudes, barrier skills, and training needs among health care professionals. Pediatr 2002; 110:210–214.
52. Ling BS, Moskowitz MA, Wachs D, Pearson B, Schroy PC. Attitudes toward colorectal cancer screening tests. J Gen Intern Med 2001; 16:822–830.
53. American Obesity Association. Physical activity for adult weight control. Healthy Weight 2010. Objective #2.7. Washington, DC: American Obesity Association (AOA), January 20, 2000.
54. Ball K, Crawford D, Owen N. Too fat to exercise? Obesity as a barrier to physical activity. Aust N Z J Public Health 2000; 24:331–333.
55. Chakravarthy MV, Joyner MJ, Booth FW. An obligation for primary care physicians to prescribe physical activity to sedentary patients to reduce the risk of chronic health conditions. Mayo Clin Proc 2002; 77:165–173.
56. American Obesity Association. A pound of prevention for a healthier tomorrow. American Obesity Association (AOA) Report 1999; 3.
57. Foster GD, Wadden TA, Phelan S, Sarwer DB, Sanderson RS. Obese patients' perceptions of treatment outcomes and the factors that influence them. Arch Intern Med 2001; 161:2133–2139.
58. Kottke TE, Wu LA, Hoffman RS. Economic and psychological implications of the obesity epidemic. Mayo Clin Proc 2003; 78:92–94.
59. Franklin PA. Impact of disability on the family structure. Soc Secur Bull 1977; 40:3–18.
60. Black DR. Weight changes in a couples program: negative association of marital adjustment. J Behav Ther Exp Psychiatr 1988; 19:103–111.

61. Wynick, M. Nutrition education in medical schools. Am J Clin Nut 1993; 58:825–827.
62. Davis CH. The report to Congress on the appropriate federal role in assuring access by medical students, residents and practicing physicians to adequate training in nutrition. Pub Health Reports 1994; 109:824–826.
63. Weinsier RL, Boker JR, Brooks CM, et al. Priorities for nutrition content in medical school curriculum; a national consensus of medical educators. Am J Clin Nutr 1989; 50:707–712.
64. Hill JO. Dealing with obesity as a chronic disease. Obes Res 1998; 6:34s–38s.
65. Galuska DA, Will JC, Serdula MK, Ford ES. Are health care professionals advising obese patients to lose weight? J A M A 1999; 282:1581–1582.
66. Kushner R. The treatment of obesity: a call for prudence and professionalism. Arch Int Med 1997; 157: 602–604.
67. Rossner S. Long-term intervention strategies in obesity treatment. Int J Obes 1995; 19:s29–s33.
68. Sayler ME, Goldstein DJ, Roback PJ, Atkinson RL. Int J Obes 1994; 18:742–751.
69. Atkinson RL. Proposed standards for judging the success of the treatment of obesity. Ann Int Med 1993; 119:677–680.
70. Frank A. Measuring maintenance: an index for measuring and comparing the maintenance of weight loss. Obes Res 1996; 4:54s.
71. Shekelle PG, Hardy ML, Morton SC, et al. Efficacy and safety of ephedra and ephedrine for weight loss and athletic performance: a meta-analysis. JAMA 2003; 289:1537–1545.
72. Fontanarosa PB, Rennie D, DeAngelis CD. The need for regulation of dietary supplements—lessons from ephedra. J A M A 2003; 289:1568–1570.
73. Bray GA. Drug treatment of obesity. Amer J Clin Nutr 1992; 550:538s–544s.
74. National Task Force on the Prevention and Treatment of Obesity. Towards prevention of obesity: research directions. Obes Res 1994; 2:571–584.
75. Klem ML, Viteri JE, Wing RR. Primary prevention of weight gain for women aged 25–34: the acceptability of treatment formats. Int J Obes 2000; 24:219–225.
76. Jeffery RW, Hellerstedt WL, Schmid TL. Correspondence programs for smoking cessation and weight control: a comparison of two strategies in the Minnesota Heart Health Program. Health Psychol 1990; 9:585–598.
77. Clothier N, Marvel MK, Cruickshank CS. Does presenting patients' BMI increase documentation of obesity? Med Educ Online 2002; 7:6. (Accessed Spetember 5, 2002.) Website: (http://www.med-ed-online.org).
78. Hash RB, Munna RK, Vogel RL, Bason JJ. Does physician weight affect perception of health advice? Prev Med 2003; 36:41–44.
79. Frank A. Conflicts in the care of overweight patients: inconsistent rules and insufficient money. Obes Res 1997; 5:268–270.
80. Hearn W. Healthy Eats. American Medical News, November 20, 1995, p. 25.
81. Tershakovec AM, Watson MH, Wenner MJ, Marx AL. Insurance reimbursement for the treatment of obesity in children. J Pediatr 1999; 134:573–578.
82. Campbell GR. A weighty problem: a new drug therapy stirs debate about how health plans ought to contain obesity's crushing costs. Managed Health Care 1996 (July);s11–s19.
83. Quesenberry CP, Caan B, Jacobson A. Obesity, health services use, and health care costs among members of a health maintenance organization. Arch Int Med 1998; 158:466–472.
84. Collins RW, Anderson JW. Medication cost savings associated with weight loss for obese non-insulin dependent diabetic men and women. Preventive Med 1995; 24:369–374.
85. Bray GA. Barriers to the treatment of obesity (editorial). Ann Int Med 1991; 115:152–3.
86. Krentzman B. State Laws on Obesity Medications. (Accessed March 17, 2003.) Website: (http://home.attbi.com/~bkrentzman/obesity/state.laws.html.)
87. American Obesity Association. AOA Fact Sheets: Obesity and Health Insurance. (Accessed March 12, 2003.) Website: (http://www.obesity.org/subs/fastfacts//Obesity)
88. American Obesity Association. AOA Fact Sheets: Obesity, Medicaid and Medicare. (Accessed March 12, 2003.) Website: (http://www.obesity.org/subs/fastfacts//Obesity).
89. American Obesity Association. AOA Fact Sheets: Obesity Research. (Accessed March 12, 2003.) Website: (http://www.obesity.org/subs/fastfacts//Obesity).

90. Ad Council to launch anti-obesity PSAs. AdAge.com.Crain Communications. (Accessed February 18, 2003.) Website: (http://www.adage.com/page>).

91. Wyden R. Deception and Fraud in the Diet Industry. Hearings before the Subcommittee on Regulation, Business Opportunity and Energy of the Committee on Small Business of the US House of Representatives. Serial Number 101-57, May 7, 1992.

25 Prevention of Obesity

Barbara C. Hansen

KEY POINTS

- The prevalence of obesity continues to increase worldwide.
- Obesity treatment is improving, but prevention should become the focus.
- Despite a genetic predisposition for weight gain, environmental conditions have resulted in the recent epidemic of obesity and overweight. Thus, appropriate altering of the environment should reverse this trend.
- Animal studies of caloric restriction suggest that increased longevity and other positive effects are likely to occur with prevention of weight gain.
- Establishing the efficacy of various approaches for long-term prevention of obesity will be difficult, but not impossible
- The search for the tools to support prevention efforts deserves to be enhanced.

1. INTRODUCTION

Faced with the extraordinary increases in prevalences of obesity and overweight in both developed and developing countries, and with the high rate of recidivism following weight-loss programs for the obese, we must turn our attention to primary prevention to stem this epidemic and its negative health consequences. The discussion that follows considers the questions shown in the Table 1.

2. WHY PREVENT OBESITY?

The 20-year increasing prevalence of obesity in the United States *(1,2)* as well as in many other countries including Brazil *(3)* and Japan *(4)*, as well as countries in Europe *(5)*, has been clearly demonstrated through epidemiological studies. In Japan, according to the criteria set by the Japan Association for the Study of Obesity (obesity defined as a body mass index [BMI] ≥ 25), the overall prevalence of obesity is 20% and the prevalence in men over 30 and women over 40 is 30%, a 34-fold increase over the past 40 yr *(4,6,7)*. The BMI threshold of 25 for obesity in the Japanese compares to the BMI of 30 for Americans on the basis of the sensitivity and specifically for detecting persons at risk for diabetes, cardiovascular disease (CVD), and other obesity-associated diseases *(8)*.

In 1990, the United States launched a national strategy to improve the health of America. Then-Secretary of Health and Human Services, Louis W. Sullivan, announced goals for the coming decade in an extensive report, *Healthy People 2000: National Health Promo-*

From: *The Management of Eating Disorders and Obesity, Second Edition*
Edited by: D. J. Goldstein © Humana Press Inc., Totowa, NJ

Table 1
Chapter Overview

tion and Disease Prevention Objectives (11), which included to "reduce the proportion of adults who are obese" and to "reduce the proportion of children and adolescents who are overweight or obese." The health risks of being overweight were cited, including increased risks of adult-onset diabetes mellitus, hypertension, coronary heart disease, gallbladder disease, and some forms of cancer. The epidemiological evidence for these risks is discussed in Chapter 10. In fact, 5 of the 10 leading causes of death are closely associated with overweight/obesity. Given the prominence of this national initiative for the year 2010, and the featured status of reducing excess weight and maintained (not increasing) body adiposity among the goals, it is disconcerting that still, the American population continues to grow fatter, not slimmer, and the prevalence of overweight is now 64.5% *(12).* Nevertheless, the extraordinary increase in the rate of obesity in the very short time interval of 20 to 30 yr precludes a genetic mutational explanation for this population change. Rather, we must infer that environmental factors have been changing in a direction that enhances or facilitates the expression of such obesity genes, and that those factors are potentially identifiable and, if found, may strengthen efforts directed toward the prevention or mitigation of obesity. Chapter 18 reviews the genetics of obesity. At this time, many contributing factors, collectively referred to as "lifestyle" factors, have been suggested to be participants in the growing problem of obesity. Some of these contributors have been surmised to be rooted in our sedentary or "Westernized" lifestyle, including declining levels of physical activity and increasing consumption of calorie-enriched diets, as summarized in Table 2.

3. IS IT POSSIBLE TO PREVENT OBESITY?

This apparently simple question has not been well addressed in free-living peoples; however, as noted here, studies of obesity-prone animals have already answered in the

Table 2
Factors Facilitating the Development and Sustaining of Obesity

• Increasing calorie consumption (diet/nutrition)	• Increasing longevity
• Reduced physical activity	• Parity
• Pregnancy	• Stress

affirmative. Yes, it is possible to prevent obesity, and yes, it is beneficial to health to do so. Toward this end *Healthy People 2010* recommends reducing dietary fat content to no more than 30% of calories, and increasing consumption of vegetables to at least three servings per day, fruits to at least two daily servings, and grain products to at least six daily servings, together with increasing moderate daily physical activity to at least 30 min a day. This report also notes several areas for more focused attention, including initiating the effort to maintain a healthful weight early in childhood and continuing into adulthood. Thus, *Healthy People 2010* avers that early efforts to prevent obesity are more likely to be successful than later efforts to lose substantial amounts of weight after obesity has developed *(11)*.

The Cholesterol Education Program has demonstrated that the behavior of the American public can be changed by intensive education and prevention efforts, as we have clearly altered our overall eating patterns in the direction of reduced cholesterol intake. It is, however, much less clear, when the goal is overall reduction in total daily calorie intake, that similar educational efforts will be as successful. Nevertheless, several initiatives are currently underway to educate the public on the risks of excess overweight and to coach the public on changes in behavior that may reduce these risks (*see* the following websites: www.cdc.gov; www.niddk.nih.gov; www.nih.gov). Only time will tell whether such initiatives can alter the prognosis for our population. Current government-sponsored research programs are seeking this answer (*see* websites: www.cdc.gov; www. niddk.nih.gov; www.nih.gov). In the mean time, it is extraordinarily clear that on an individual basis, the health of a patient will frequently be substantially enhanced by even modest weight loss *(6,7)*. It is therefore important to consider what is currently known about the consequences of prevention of obesity, the challenges to sustaining reduced weight, and the future for increasing the understanding of prevention methods.

4. CONSEQUENCES OF OBESITY PREVENTION

4.1. Lessons From Examination of Modest Weight Reduction in the Obese

The beneficial health effects of modest weight loss were thoroughly reviewed by Goldstein *(13)*, and studies to date provide unequivocal support for the positive effects of weight reduction of obese individuals. Under the sponsorship of the National Heart, Lung, and Blood Institute, methods used to achieve weight loss were reviewed and guidelines developed for the treatment of overweight and obese persons *(14)*. Most prominent among the positive benefits observed to date are improvement in glucose tolerance and reduction in the medical complications observed in obese persons with type 2 adult-onset diabetes mellitus (DM), reduction in blood pressure (BP) in those obese with hypertension, and improvement in lipid profiles in those obese with dyslipidemia and a high risk for CVD *(15)*. Benefits appear to be broadly related both to initial degree of obesity (the greater the degree of overweight, the greater the risk to health and the greater the benefit of losing weight) and to the proportion of excess weight lost. Nevertheless, losses as small as 5 to 10% also appear to convey important improvements in long-term health for the overweight person.

Clearly, targeting our efforts on weight reduction toward those individuals who already exhibit burdens of illnesses associated with obesity makes sense, as the near-term reduction in obvious risk parameters such as hyperglycemia, hypertension, and dyslipidemia provide direct indicators of improved health. Such patients may have heightened motivation to comply with a difficult and challenging dietary and activity regimen, and the likelihood of short-term weight reduction in such highly motivated persons may be enhanced. Nevertheless, these complications of obesity should be viewed as endpoints in a continuum of health impairments that undoubtedly begin to sow their seeds of ill health long before these specific features are fully manifest. Several studies have pointed to the long-time course of the development of obesity-associated disorders, often substantially proceeding the time at which a diagnosis is made of a pathological condition such as diabetes. In the case of diabetes associated with obesity, diagnosis itself may be substantially delayed because more than half of all diabetic persons in the United States are believed to be undiagnosed at this time (16), and similar statistics relate to CVD. Furthermore, increased cardiovascular risk has been demonstrated in obese pre-diabetics well before the diagnostic criteria for diabetes have been reached (17), and many diabetic persons have retinopathy at the time of diagnosis (11), again illustrating the importance of early identification of persons who are at risk so that preventive measures can be initiated.

4.2. Lessons for Prevention of Obesity From Modeling of Primary, Secondary, and Tertiary Prevention in Diabetes

Eighty to 90% of patients with adult-onset DM were obese before diagnosis, and, as is discussed here, prevention of obesity can prevent (or substantially delay) diabetes. The National Institute of Diabetes and Digestive and Kidney Diseases has examined the effects of modeling various interventions directed toward those at risk for diabetes and those with the disease. Primary prevention shifted the cumulative incidence of one complication of diabetes, retinopathy, to the right, representing postponement of the development of eye disease. Specifically, the model suggested that, with successful delay in the onset of type 2 DM by 6 yr, the cumulative incidence of proliferative retinopathy could be reduced by about 50% at age 65 yr. This example specifically focused on one complication of one obesity-associated disease, and such positive effects would be likely to be multiplied many fold by the effects of reduction of diabetes by broad reduction in the prevalence of overweight. Not only would the average age of onset of type 2 DM be postponed, but other associated risk factors would also be modified. Secondary prevention refers to early treatment once a diagnosis of disease is made. Such secondary prevention efforts also alter the course of disease, and have been modeled to shift the complication curve downward. Tertiary prevention, the area of current treatment focus, although important, is clearly operating at a time for each patient when much of the damage has already occurred and pathology is advanced. Often, this point of intervention is too late to restore health, although further deterioration may be slowed. The American Diabetes Association (ADA) has provided evidence-based nutrition principles that address obesity and diabetes *(18)*. The ADA recognized that long-term maintenance of weight loss is challenging and that often as few as 5 to 6% of those who lose weight can successfully maintain their loss. To accomplish long-term maintenance of reduced weight has required long-term involvement of a clinician. The ADA has affirmed what many in the field of appetite regulation have long recognized: the difficulty in maintaining reduced body weight is probably because both energy intake and energy expenditure are both controlled and regulated by the central nervous system. A variety of neural, endocrine, and gastrointestinal factors provide input to the brain on the status of energy balance, a control system that is likely to be genetically based *(see* Chapter 18).

4.3. Lessons From Rodent Models of Prevention of Obesity

The restriction of calories in rodent animal models has been carried out beginning just after weaning (and also, in separate studies, beginning at later ages) with the goal of extending longevity. That goal was clearly achieved in many rodent studies dating back as far as 1935 *(13)*. Interestingly, in the course of these and subsequent rodent studies to reduce or slow aging processes, the animals were kept in a very lean state. When obesity-prone rodent models were restricted, they, like the lean animals, had an extension in life (together with, of course, a reduction in fat mass). These anti-aging effects of long-term calorie restriction in rats and in mice are well accepted; specifically, in rodents, restriction of calories to 60 or 70% of the intake of control rats results in doubling of life span, increased life expectancy, reduced cancer incidence, decreased hypertension, reduction in hypertriglyceridemia, less atherosclerosis, and decreased nephropathy *(14–16)*. Such important health benefits have now been reported in non-human primates in continuing studies of the long-term effects of calorie restriction to improve health reduce various sources of morbidity, and postpone average age of death *(19)*.

4.4. Lessons From Non-Human Primate Models for Prevention of Obesity

Several groups currently have ongoing long-term calorie-restriction studies in non-human primates; and, although final answers to the question of effects on ultimate life span await longer study duration, the likelihood of increased longevity *(17)*, as well as many other positive effects, are already becoming apparent *(18–21)*. Bodkin et al. reported the significant reduction in morbidities in a group of monkeys that have been under a regimen of calorie restraint for more than 20 yr. In addition, the average age of death has been significantly postponed by maintenance of a normal healthy weight and prevention of obesity in non-human primates *(19)*.

4.4.1. BODY WEIGHT/BODY FAT

The effects of long-term calorie restraint are being evaluated in a group of adult non-human primates (rhesus monkeys) currently maintained in the University of Maryland Obesity and Diabetes Research Center. One group of monkeys has had its food intake restrained for more than 20 yr from the time they reached full-grown adulthood (~10 yr) to the present with the specific goal of preventing the development of obesity in monkeys. The other group has eaten *ad libitum*. For the calorie-restricted group, an individual calorie titration method was used, akin to a "bathroom scale model." Each monkey was weighed once a week and if the monkey gained weight its calorie allotment for the next

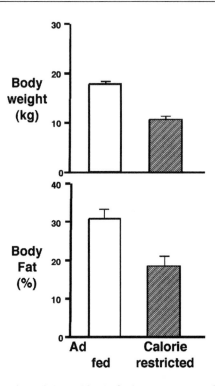

Fig. 1. Comparison of body weight and body fat in two groups of non-human primates, ad libitum fed and calorie-restrained. Both groups are older than 20 yr of age, similar to humans older than 60 yr. The calorie-restrained group has been prevented from gaining "middle-aged" obesity, whereas it is common in the ad libitum fed group. (Groups are the same for all figures.) (Redrawn with permission from ref. *21a.*)

week was reduced; and if the monkey lost weight, calorie intake was increased. The objective was to keep each monkey at its lean, young adult body weight (equivalent to body weight at about 25 yr of age in humans). Thus "middle-age" obesity was prevented, body weight stayed stable (whereas that of the *ad libitum*-fed animals increased), and body fat increased slightly, but remained much less than in the *ad libitum*-fed monkeys (*see* Fig. 1; *21a*), whereas the calorie intake per kilogram of body weight was significantly reduced *(20)*. Because of the physiological and genetic similarities of monkeys to humans, the lessons from this study have particular relevance to people at risk for obesity. This weekly calorie adjustment plan to prevent adult-onset obesity has already had profound positive effects on these animals and may be similar to possible positive health effects that may be achieved by people who are "restrained" eaters.

4.4.2. Glucose Metabolism

In these healthy, lean, calorie-restrained monkeys, diabetes and impaired glucose tolerance (IGT) have been completely prevented by the prevention of obesity, whereas about half of the *ad libitum*-fed monkeys have already shown defects in glucose regulation *(20–24)*. Figure 2 shows the fasting plasma glucose and the glucose disappearance rates in response to an intravenous glucose tolerance test in the two groups of monkeys.

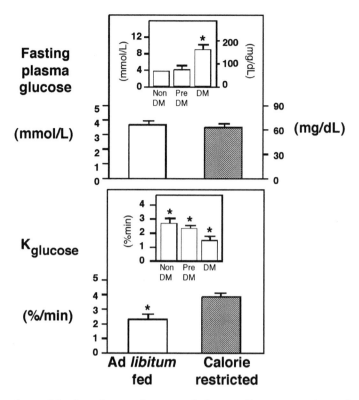

Fig. 2. Comparison of fasting plasma glucose and glucose disappearance rate during an intravenous glucose tolerance test (K glucose). The insert shows that within the *ad libitum* fed group some are normal non-diabetic (NON-DM), some are developing diabetes (pre-DM), and some are already overtly diabetic. (Redrawn with permission from ref. *21a*.)

Although it has long been appreciated that glucose intolerance is frequently associated with obesity, it is now clear that the simple prevention of obesity in non-human primates (and probably in humans as well), can prevent the deterioration of an obese individual to overt type 2 DM. The results of oral glucose tolerance testing (OGTT) in these monkeys (shown in Fig. 3) confirm that all of the calorie-restrained monkeys remained normal, whereas some of the *ad libitum* animals either became overtly diabetic or developed IGT.

As all professionals in the field of diabetes recognize, diet is the first line of treatment for the newly diagnosed patient with adult-onset diabetes *(18)*. We suggest that the non-human primate studies indicate the importance of earlier intervention and primary prevention of weight gain and obesity, even before the overt disease of diabetes is diagnosed, at least in high-risk potentially obese or already obese patients. As noted here, the positive effects of anti-obesity measures go well beyond the prevention of diabetes, and in fact, show positive effects in many other areas of health risk that are associated with obesity *(20–23,25–34)*.

4.4.3. INSULIN AND INSULIN RESISTANCE

Prevention of middle age-onset obesity in monkeys has also had a strong positive effect on insulin sensitivity, preventing the decline seen in many of the *ad libitum* animals

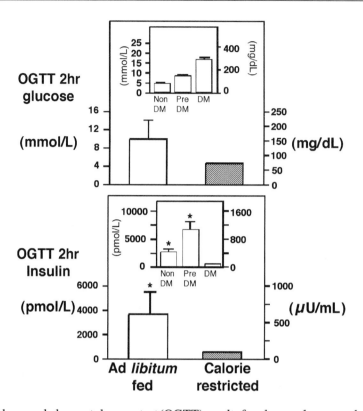

Fig. 3. Two-hour oral glucose tolerance test (OGTT) results for plasma glucose and plasma insulin. The insert shows that within the *ad libitum* fed group some are normal non-diabetic (NON-DM), some are developing diabetes (pre-DM), and some are already overtly diabetic. (Redrawn with permission from ref. *21a*.)

(35–38). Figure 4 shows that the insulin levels of the *ad libitum* animals were increased, whereas the fasting insulin levels of the animals in whom obesity had been prevented remained normal *(38–41)*. Two other studies by the University of Wisconsin Primate Center group and by the National Institute on Aging group have similarly found lower fasting plasma insulin levels in dietary-restricted primates. Furthermore, a measure of insulin action in the whole body showed normal glucose uptake in the obesity-prevented/ calorie-restrained monkeys, and reduced insulin action in the *ad libitum*-fed monkeys (Fig. 4, *41a*). In addition, direct measures of insulin action at the tissue level also confirm the enhanced basal activity of glycogen synthase, the rate-limiting enzyme for glycogen synthesis, in the monkeys with sustained prevention of obesity *(24,42,43)*. The actions of other enzymes of metabolism are also significantly changed by calorie restriction.

4.4.4. Energy Balance

Interestingly, the calorie-restrained monkeys show a greater efficiency in the utiliza- tion of energy compared to the *ad libitum*-fed monkeys *(20,38,44)*. There are other effects of calorie restriction with yet unknown benefits or consequences, for example, effects on hepatic enzymes *(45)* and other alterations in intermediary metabolism *(43)*. Dietary or calorie restriction in addition to altering energy balance has been found to alter the

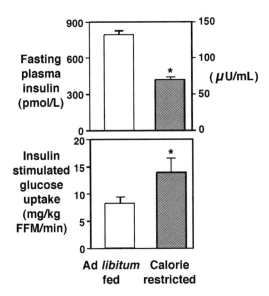

Fig. 4. Fasting plasma insulin and insulin-stimulated glucose uptake (measured during steady state with a euglycemic hyperinsulinemic clamp procedure). (Redrawn with permission from ref.*41a*.)

expression of many genes *(46,47)*. To date, it appears that such changes are likely to be beneficial, but further studies are needed to clarify the nature of the major metabolic shifts induced by chronic calorie restriction.

5. WHAT IS THE RELATIONSHIP OF OBESITY PREVENTION TO SYNDROME X?

5.1. Effects of Prevention of Obesity on Prevention of Hypertension

Loss of weight by obese hypertensive patients is clearly associated with an improvement in BP 9*see* Chapter 10 for more extensive discussion on the benefits of weight loss). It is likely that prevention of obesity will have even more profound effects in mitigating the untoward consequences of hypertension *(48–51)*. Evidence has been developed in the non-human primates *(53,54)*.

5.2. Effects of Prevention of Obesity on Prevention of Dyslipidemia

Obesity has been frequently found to be associated with dyslipidemia and with CVD *(55,56)*. Previous studies have shown reduced risk of CVD with reduction of dyslipidemia *(57)*. Reduction of weight in the obese can clearly lead to improvement in both triglyceride and cholesterol levels *(57,58)*. As with hypertension and other cardiovascular risk factors, dyslipidemia will clearly be improved by obesity prevention *(21)*.

6. IS PREVENTION MORE EFFECTIVE THAN TREATMENT?

This is a question that, *a priori,* appears to be answerable in the affirmative; however, prospective longitudinal prevention trials are still too few to clearly demonstrate that this is the case. The Diabetes Prevention Program trial has provided some evidence on this.

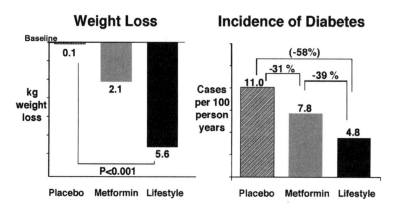

Fig. 5. Diabetes Prevention Program: Weight loss in human subjects at risk for diabetes in three groups of patients (placebo, Metformin, lifestyle intervention) showed related reductions in conversion from impaired glucose tolerance to overt type 2 diabetes. (Redrawn with permission from ref. *58a*.)

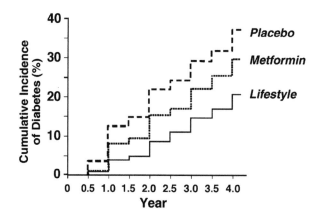

Fig. 6. Diabetes Prevention Program: The cumulative incidence of diabetes was most reduced by the intensive lifestyle intervention. (Redrawn with permission from ref. *58a*.)

This study successfully produced and maintained small amounts of weight loss, and showed a reduction in the conversion of at-risk patients from IGT to overt type 2 DM. The key findings of this study are shown in Figs. 5 and 6. There were three arms of this study, the control group (placebo), the Metformin-treated group, and the intensive lifestyle modification group. These groups showed overall weight loss after, on average 2.8 yr of study of 0.1, 2.1, and 5.6 kg, respectively and reduction in the conversion from IGT to overt diabetes. These results give promise that preventive efforts can have more long-term, sustained effects than seem to be currently possible when treating obesity after it has developed. Further evidence may emerge from the large multicenter obesity mitigation/prevention study underway with the support of National Institutes of Health (Look AHEAD [Action for HEAlth in Diabetes] trial; *see* Website: www.niddk.gov). The likelihood that prevention of obesity will have significant positive effects is further supported by epidemiological studies that show the possible increased risk for disease in those who gained weight compared to those whose weight remained stable in middle age. Furthermore, loss of excess weight followed by maintenance of that loss has been found to reduce the likelihood of diabetes and of hypertension (59). In the past, some have voiced concern about the consequences of repeated cycles of weight loss and regain (60), however, current consensus does not support an increased risk in those who lose weight purposefully and then regain it (61). Thus, even partially successful prevention efforts are likely to have positive benefits.

7. WHAT IS THE FUTURE FOR OBESITY PREVENTION?

Following up on the major Diabetes Prevention Program trial designed to prevent diabetes, the current Look AHEAD trial designed to prevent obesity, may result not only in lowering the number of obese persons developing obesity, but may positively affect all aspects of the metabolic syndrome with the expected consequence of reducing or slowing CVD as well. The non-human primate data indicate that prevention of obesity will carry the potential for far more widespread impact and improvement in health than any other preventive effort aimed at a single complication or associated risk.

8. CONCLUSION

There are many challenges ahead in the efforts to prevent or slow the obesity epidemic. Establishing the efficacy of various approaches for long-term prevention of obesity will be difficult but not impossible. Some of these challenges include the following:

1. We do not yet know all or even the majority of the factors contributing to the development of obesity.
2. It is neither easy to alter the rate of progression of a slow, long-term, progressive disorder nor to demonstrate that a change in rate has occurred.
3. We do not know the genetic basis for obesity, although much effort is being devoted to this area currently.
4. Aging processes and the timing of onset and progression of obesity vary across individuals, so long-term prospective studies will be necessary in cohorts representing various ages.
5. Intermediate responses or markers of success are not well established. For example, is the loss and sustained maintenance of a 10-lb reduction in body weight sufficient? In all individuals? For how long? Started when? As measured by what? (62). Despite these deterrents to initiating obesity prevention efforts, the potential benefits to health are unquestionable, and these efforts should be further developed and extended.

Obesity is common, costly, and potentially preventable. The search for the tools to support prevention efforts deserves to be enhanced, so that the epidemic of the 1980s and 1990s will be a memory in the 2000s.

REFERENCES

1. Flegal KM, Carroll MD, Ogden CL, Johnson CL. Prevalence and trends in obesity among US adults, 1999–2000. JAMA 2002; 288:1723–1727.
2. Chumlea WC, Guo SS, Kuczmarski RJ, et al. Body composition estimates from NHANES III bioelectrical impedance data. Int J Obes Relat Metab Disord 2002; 26:1596–1609.

3. Sichieri R, Coitinho DC, Leao MM, et al. High temporal, geographic, and income variation in body mass index among adults in Brazil. Am J Public Health 1994; 84:793–798.

4. Yoshiike N, Kaneda F, Takimoto H. Epidemiology of obesity and public health strategies for its control in Japan. Asia Pac J Clin Nutr 2002; 11:S727–731.

5. Schutz Y, Woringer V. Obesity in Switzerland: a critical assessment of prevalence in children and adults. Int J Obes Relat Metab Disord 2002; 26(Suppl 2):S3–S11.

6. Kanazawa M, Yoshiike N, Osaka T, et al. Criteria and classification of obesity in Japan and Asia-Oceania. Asia Pac J Clin Nutr 2002; 11:S732–S737.

7. Yoshiike N, Seino F, Tajima S, et al. Twenty-year changes in the prevalence of overweight in Japanese adults: the National Nutrition Survey 1976–95. Obes Rev 2002; 3:183–190.

8. Examination Committee of Criteria for "Obesity Disease" in Japan; Japan Society for the Study of Obesity. New criteria for "obesity disease" in Japan. Circ J 2002; 66:987–992.

9. National Institutes of Health Committee on Care and Use of Laboratory Animals. Guide to the care and use of laboratory animals. Washington DC, Government Printing Office, 1996

10. Schoenborn CA, Adams PF, Barnes PM. Body weight status of adults: United States, 1997–1998. Adv Data 2002;1–15.

11. U.S. Department of Health and Human Services. Healthly People 2010: Understanding and Improving Health, 2nd ed. Washington, DC: US Government Printing Office, 2000.

12. Allison DB, Kaprio J, Korkeila M, et al. The heritability of body mass index among an international sample of monozygotic twins reared apart. Int J Obesity 1996; 20:501–506.

13. Goldstein DJ. Beneficial health effects of modest weight loss. Int J Obesity 1992; 16:397–415.

14. NIH–NHLBI. Clinical guidelines on the identification, evaluation, and treatment of overweight and obesity in adults. Washington, DC: US Government Printing Office, 1998.

15. Capell WH, DeSouza CA, Poirier P, et al. Short-term triglyceride lowering with fenofibrate improves vasodilator function in subjects with hypertriglyceridemia. Arterioscler Thromb Vasc Biol 2003; 23: 307–313.

16. Harris MI, Eastman RC. Early detection of undiagnosed diabetes mellitus: a US perspective. Diabetes Metab Res Rev 2000; 16:230–236.

17. Haffner SM, Agostino RD, Jr., Saad MF, et al. Carotid artery atherosclerosis in type-2 diabetic and nondiabetic subjects with and without symptomatic coronary artery disease (The Insulin Resistance Atherosclerosis Study). Am J Cardiol 2000; 85:1395–1400.

18. Franz MJ, Bantle JP, Beebe CA, et al. Evidence-based nutrition principles and recommendations for the treatment and prevention of diabetes and related complications. Diab Care 2003; 26:S51–S61.

19. Bodkin NL, Alexander TM, Ortmeyer HK, et al. Mortality and morbidity in laboratory-maintained Rhesus monkeys and effects of long-term dietary restriction. J Gerontol A Biol Sci Med Sci 2003; 58: 212–219.

20. DeLany JP, Hansen BC, Bodkin NL, et al. Long-term calorie restriction reduces energy expenditure in aging monkeys. J Gerontol A Biol Sci Med Sci 1999; 54:B5–B11.

21. Hansen BC, Bodkin NL, Ortmeyer HK. Calorie restriction in non human primates: Mechanisms of reduced morbidity and mortality. Toxicol Sci 1999; 52S:56–60.

21a. Hansen BC, Bodkin NL. Primary prevention of diabetes mellitus by prevention of obesity in monkeys. Diabetes 1993; 42(12):1809–1814.

22. Hansen BC. The natural history of the early development of type 2 diabetes and the metabolic Syndrome X: Implications for cause and early intervention. J Endocrinol Metab Diab S Afr 1999; 89:460.

23. Hansen BC. Introduction. Symposium: Calorie restriction: effects on body composition, insulin signaling and aging. J Nutr Sci Vitaminol (Tokyo) 2001; 131: 900S–902S.

24. Ortmeyer HK. In vivo insulin regulation of skeletal muscle glycogen synthase in calorie-restricted and in ad libitum-fed rhesus monkeys. J Nutr 2001; 131:907S–912S.

25. Hansen BC. Prevention of obesity positively affects all features of the metabolic syndrome X, while producing unique shifts in metabolism. J Endocrinol Metab Diab S Afr 1999.

26. Pechacek AJ, Bodkin NL, Hansen BC, Ortmeyer HK. Calorie restriction results in significant changes in glycogen metabolism in the liver and skeletal muscle of monkeys. FASEB J 1999; A602:464.12.

27. Bodkin NL, Ortmeyer HK, Hansen BC. Reversal of obesity: differing effects on in vivo insulin resistance in prediabetic and diabetic rhesus monkeys. Int J Obes 1994; 18:119.

28. Hansen BC. Dietary considerations for obese diabetic subjects. Diabetes Care. 1988; 11:183–188.
29. Bodkin NL, Ortmeyer HK, Nicolson M, Hansen BC. Plasma leptin: Alterations associated with acute and chronic changes in insulin and glucose. Obes Res 1996; 4:15S.
30. Ortmeyer HK, Huang L, Larner J, Hansen BC. Insulin unexpectedly increases the glucose 6-phosphate K_a of skeletal muscle glycogen synthase in calorie-restricted monkeys. J Basic Clin Physiol Pharmacol 1998; 9:309–323.
31. Bodkin NL, Ortmeyer HK, Hansen BC. Variation in calorie requirement to maintain a reduced body weight is directly related to insulin sensitivity. Int J Obes 1998; 22:S60.
32. Hansen BC, Izuka M, Bjenning C, Knudsen LB. Obese rhesus monkeys show reduced food intake and weight loss during treatment with NN2211, a long-acting GLP-1 derivative. Am J Clin Nutr 2002; 75:393.
33. Standaert ML, Ortmeyer HK, Sajan MP, et al. Skeletal muscle insulin resistance in obesity-associated type 2 diabetes in monkeys is linked to a defect in insulin activation of protein kinase C-zeta/lambda/iota. Diabetes 2002; 51:2936–2943.
34. Erwin JM, Tigno XT, Gerzanich G, Hansen BC. Age-related changes in fasting plasma cortisol in rhesus monkeys: implications of individual differences for pathological consequences. J Gerontol A Biol Sci Med Sci. 2004; 59:424–432.
35. Bodkin NL, Ortmeyer HK, Hansen BC. Long-term dietary restriction in older-aged rhesus monkeys: effects on insulin resistance. J Gerontol: Biol Sci 1995; 50:B142–B147.
36. Ramsey JJ, Colman RJ, Binkley NC, et al. Dietary restriction and aging in rhesus monkeys: the University of Wisconsin study. Exp Gerontol 2000; 35:1131–1149.
37. Lane MA, Ingram DK, Roth GS. Calorie restriction in nonhuman primates: effects on diabetes and cardiovascular disease risk. Toxicol Sci 1999; 52:41–48.
38. Roth GS, Ingram DK, Black A, Lane MA. Effects of reduced energy intake on the biology of aging: the primate model. Eur J Clin Nutr 2000; 54(Suppl 3):S15–S20.
39. Anson RM, Guo Z, De Cabo R, et al. Intermittent fasting dissociates beneficial effects of dietary restriction on glucose metabolism and neuronal resistance to injury from calorie intake. Proc Natl Acad Sci USA 2003; 100:6216–6220.
40. Gresl TA, Colman RJ, Roecker EB, et al. Dietary restriction and glucose regulation in aging rhesus monkeys: a follow-up report at 8.5 yr. Am J Physiol Endocrinol Metab 2001; 281:E757–E765.
41. Roth GS, Ingram DK, Lane MA. Caloric restriction in primates and relevance to humans. Ann NY Acad Sci 2001; 928:305–315.
41a. Bodkin NL, Ortmeyer HK, Hansen BC. Long-term dietary restriction in older-aged rhesus monkeys: effects on insulin resistance. J Gerontol Biol Sci 1995; 50A:B142–B147.
42. Ortmeyer HK, Bodkin NL, Hansen BC. Chronic caloric restriction alters glycogen metabolism in rhesus monkeys. Obes Res 1994; 2:549–555.
43. Ortmeyer HK, Fried S, Rachuba M, et al. Impaired in vivo insulin regulation of skeletal muscle lipoprotein lipase in obese monkeys: normalization by calorie restriction. Diabetes 2003; 52:A319.
44. Kemnitz JW, Roecker EB, Weindruch R, et al. Dietary restriction increases insulin sensitivity and lowers blood glucose in rhesus monkeys. Amer J Physiol 1994; 266 (Endocrinol Metab 29):E540–E547.
45. Feuers RJ, Duffy PH, Leakey JA, et al. Effect of chronic caloric restriction on hepatic enzymes of intermediary metabolism in the male Fischer 344 rat. Mech Ageing Dev 1989; 48:179–189.
46. Han E, Hilsenbeck SG, Richardson A, Nelson JF. cDNA expression arrays reveal incomplete reversal of age-related changes in gene expression by calorie restriction. Mech Ageing Dev 2000; 115:157–174.
47. Weindruch R, Kayo T, Lee CK, Prolla TA. Microarray profiling of gene expression in aging and its alteration by caloric restriction in mice. J Nutr 2001; 131:918S–923S.
48. Stamler R, Stamler J, Gosch FC, et al. Primary prevention of hypertension by nutritional–hygienic means: Final report of a randomized, controlled trial. JAMA 1989; 262:1801–1807.
49. Langford HC, Blaufox MD, Oberman A, et al. Dietary therapy slows the return of hypertension after stopping prolonged medication. JAMA 1985; 253:657–664.
50. Van Itallie T B. Obesity: adverse effects on health and longevity. Am J Clin Nutr 1979; 32:2723–2733.
51. Pi-Sunyer FX. Medical hazards of obesity. Ann Intern Med 1993; 119:655–660.

52. Bodkin NL, Hansen BC. Prevention of Syndrome X by long-term dietary restriction (DR) in aged rhesus monkeys. The Gerontologist, 1995; 239.

53. Sasaki S, Higashi Y, Nakagawa K, et al. A low-calorie diet improves endothelium-dependent vasodilation in obese patients with essential hypertension. Am J Hypertens 2002; 15:302–309.

54. Suter PM, Sierro C, Vetter W. Nutritional factors in the control of blood pressure and hypertension. Nutr Clin Care 2002; 5:9–19.

55. Hubert HB, Feinleib M, McNamara PM, Castelli WP. Obesity as an independent risk factor for cardiovascular disease: a 26-year follow-up of participants in the Framingham heart study. Circulation 1983; 67:968–977.

56. Alpert MA, Hashimi MW. Obesity and the heart. Am J Med Sci 1993; 305:117–23.

57. Frick MM, Elo O, Hoopa K, et al. Helsinki heart study: primary-prevention trial with gemfibrozil in middle-aged men with dyslipidemia. N Engl J Med 1987; 317:1237–1245.

58. Pi-Sunyer FX. Short-term medical benefits and adverse effects of weight loss. Ann Intern Med 1993; 119:722–726.

58a. Knowler WC, Barrett-Conner E, Fowler SE, et al. Reduction in the incidence of type 2 diabetes with lifestyle intervention or metformin. N Engl J Med 2002; 346(6): 393–403.

59. French SA, Jeffery RW, Folsom AR, et al. Weight loss maintenance in young adulthood: prevalence and correlations with health behavior and disease in a population-based sample of women aged 55–69 years. Int J Obes 1996; 20:303–310.

60. Lissner L, Odell PM, D'Agostino RB, et al. Variability of body weight and health outcomes in the Framingham population. N Engl J Med 1991; 324:1839–1844.

61. National Task Force on the Prevention and Treatment of Obesity. Weight cycling. JAMA 1994; 272: 1196–1202.

62. Hansen B, Ortmeyer H, Bodkin N. Ageing, energy restriction, and the progressive development of pathophysiology in obese non-human primates. In: Angel A, ed. Progress in Obesity Research. London, UK: John Libbey, 1996; pp. 541–547.

63. Hansen BC, Bodkin NL. Primary prevention of diabetes mellitus by prevention of obesity in monkeys. Diabetes 1993; 42(12):1809-1814.

Index

About the Series Editor

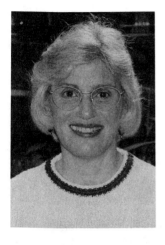

Dr. Adrianne Bendich is Clinical Director of Calcium Research at GlaxoSmithKline Consumer Healthcare, where she is responsible for leading the innovation and medical programs in support of TUMS and Os-Cal. Dr. Bendich has primary responsibility for the direction of GSK's support for the Women's Health Initiative intervention study. Prior to joining GlaxoSmithKline, Dr. Bendich was at Roche Vitamins Inc., and was involved with the groundbreaking clinical studies proving that folic acid-containing multivitamins significantly reduce major classes of birth defects. Dr. Bendich has co-authored more than 100 major clinical research studies in the area of preventive nutrition. Dr. Bendich is recognized as a leading authority on antioxidants, nutrition, immunity, and pregnancy outcomes, vitamin safety, and the cost-effectiveness of vitamin/mineral supplementation.

In addition to serving as Series Editor for Humana Press and initiating the development of the 15 currently published books in the *Nutrition and Health™* series, Dr. Bendich is the editor of nine books, including *Preventive Nutrition: The Comprehensive Guide for Health Professionals.* She also serves as Associate Editor for *Nutrition: The International Journal of Applied and Basic Nutritional Sciences,* and Dr. Bendich is on the Editorial Board of the *Journal of Women's Health and Gender-Based Medicine,* as well as a past member of the Board of Directors of the American College of Nutrition.

Dr. Bendich was the recipient of the Roche Research Award, a *Tribute to Women and Industry* Awardee, and a recipient of the Burroughs Wellcome Visiting Professorship in Basic Medical Sciences, 2000–2001. Dr. Bendich holds academic appointments as Adjunct Professor in the Department of Preventive Medicine and Community Health at UMDNJ, Institute of Nutrition, Columbia University P&S, and Adjunct Research Professor, Rutgers University, Newark Campus. She is listed in *Who's Who in American Women.*

About the Editor

David J. Goldstein, MD, PhD is a consultant to the pharmaceutical industry and adjunct Associate Professor of Pharmacology and Toxicology at the Indiana University School of Medicine in Indianapolis.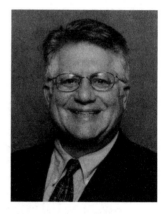

Dr. Goldstein was a Senior Clinical Research Physician in the Neuroscience and Endocrinology Research Divisions at Lilly Research Laboratories for 15 years before forming PRN Consulting, a pharmaceutical research and neurosciences consulting and writing services company in 2002.

Dr. Goldstein is a graduate of Franklin and Marshall College in Lancaster, Pennsylvania and of the University of Tennessee School of Medicine at Memphis where he earned MD and PhD degrees in biochemistry. He completed a residency in pediatrics at the Mayo Graduate School of Medicine in Rochester, Minnesota and a National Institutes of Health fellowship in human genetics under the supervision of Dr. Harry Harris at the University of Pennsylvania School of Medicine in Philadelphia. Subsequently, Dr. Goldstein was an Assistant Professor of medical genetics at the Indiana University School of Medicine.

Dr. Goldstein has investigated and published extensively on obesity, eating disorders, analgesia, migraine, depression and anxiety, effects of drug exposure in pregnancy and lactation, biochemical and clinical genetics, clinical trial methodology, and ethics.